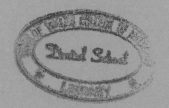

TEXTBOOK OF ENDODONTOLOGY

Edited by

Gunnar Bergenholtz
Preben Hørsted-Bindslev
Claes Reit

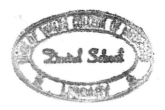

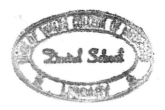

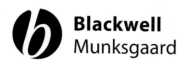
Blackwell
Munksgaard

© 2003 by Blackwell Munksgaard
a Blackwell Publishing company

Editorial Offices:
Blackwell Publishing Ltd, 9600 Garsington Road, Oxford OX4
2DQ, UK
   Tel: +44 (0)1865 776868
Iowa State Press, a Blackwell Publishing Company, 2121 State
Avenue, Ames, Iowa 50014-8300, USA
   Tel: +1 515 292 0140
Blackwell Publishing Asia Ltd, 550 Swanston Street, Carlton,
Victoria 3053, Australia
   Tel: +61 (0)3 8359 1011

First published 2003 by Blackwell Publishing Ltd

Library of Congress Cataloging-in-Publication Data
Textbook of endodontology/edited by Gunnar Bergenholtz,
Preben Hørsted-Bindslev, Claes Reit. – 1st ed.
   p. ; cm.
Includes bibliographical references and index.
ISBN 8-7161-2185-6 (hardback: alk. paper)1.   Endodontics.
[DNLM: 1. Dental Pulp Diseases–therapy.   2. Periapical
Diseases–therapy. WU 230 T355 2003] I. Bergenholtz, Gunnar.
II. Hørsted-Bindslev, Preben.   III. Reit, Claes.

RK351.T49 2003
617.6'342–dc21
2003004217

ISBN 8-7161-2185-6

A catalogue record for this title is available from the British Library

Set in 9.5/12.5 pt Palatino
by SNP Best-set Typesetter Ltd., Hong Kong
Printed and bound in Denmark using acid-free paper
by Narayana Press, Odder

For further information on Blackwell Publishing, visit our website:
www.blackwellpublishing.com

Contents

Preface

Textbook of Endodontology is intended to serve the educational needs of dental students, as well as of dental practitioners seeking updates on endodontic theories and techniques. The primary aim has been to provide an understanding of the biological processes involved in pulpal and periapical pathologies and how that knowledge impinges on clinical management, and to present that information in an easily accessible form. Therefore, we have supplemented the core text with numerous figures and photographs, as well as with boxes highlighting key facts, important clinical procedures and key research. Case studies are given at the end of some chapters in order to further illustrate topics described in the text. In these various ways, the book provides information both at a foundation level, and at a more detailed level for the graduating student and practitioner.

The key information boxes are colour coded as an easy-to-use navigational aid for readers. Core concepts are coloured pink, while advanced concepts are purple.

Clinical procedures are coded green and key literature boxes are blue.

This book is also intended to stimulate the reader to delve into the endodontic literature and the research methodology that forms our current knowledge base. To aid the reader, a selective reference list is provided and comments have been added to especially weighty or useful references. Important and interesting investigations are presented in the core and advanced concept boxes, and we hope that these features will encourage the reader to do his or her own research.

This book would not have been possible without the dedicated support of our co-authors – 18 highly respected clinicians and scientists, who, in addition to the editors, have contributed to this book. We thank them all sincerely for their time, effort and endurance during the editing process.

Gunnar Bergenholtz, Preben Hørsted-Bindslev
and Claes Reit

Contributors

Gunnar Bergenholtz	Department of Endodontology and Oral Diagnosis, Faculty of Odontology, Sahlgrenska Academy, Göteborg University, Sweden
Preben Hørsted-Bindslev	Department of Dental Pathology, Operative Dentistry and Endodontics, Royal Dental College, University of Aarhus, Denmark
Claes Reit	Department of Endodontology and Oral Diagnosis, Faculty of Odontology, Sahlgrenska Academy, Göteborg University, Sweden
Ilana Eli	Department of Occlusion and Behavioral Sciences, The Maurice and Gabriela Goldschleger School of Dental Medicine, Tel Aviv University, Israel
Risto-Pekka Happonen	Department of Oral and Maxillofacial Surgery, Institute of Dentistry, University of Turku, Finland
Eckehard Kostka	Department of Operative and Preventive Dentistry and Endodontics, School of Dental Medicine, Charité, Medical Faculty of the Berlin Humboldt University, Germany
Pierre Machtou	Department of Endodontics, Paris 7 University, France
Ingegerd Mejàre	Eastman Dental Institute and Faculty of Odontology, Center for Oral Sciences, Malmö University, Sweden
Olav Molven	Department of Odontology – Endodontics, University of Bergen, Norway
Matti Närhi	Department of Physiology, University of Kuopio, Finland
Leif Olgart	Division of Pharmacology, Karolinska Institute, Stockholm, Sweden
Kerstin Petersson	Department of Endodontics, Malmö University, Sweden
Jean-François Roulet	Department of Operative and Preventive Dentistry and Endodontics, Charité, School of Dental Medicine, Medical Faculty of the Berlin Humboldt University, Germany
Elisabeth Saunders	The Dental School, University of Dundee, Scotland
William P. Saunders	The Dental School, University of Dundee, Scotland
Gottfried Schmalz	Department of Operative Dentistry and Periodontology, University of Regensburg, Germany
Ib Paul Sewerin	Department of Oral Radiology, School of Dentistry, Faculty of Health Sciences, University of Copenhagen, Denmark
Nils Skaug	Department of Odontology – Oral Microbiology, Faculty of Dentistry, University of Bergen, Norway
Else Theilade	Department of Oral Biology, Royal Dental College, University of Aarhus, Denmark

Peter Velvart   Clinic for Periodontology, Endodontology and Cariology, Center of Dentistry, University of Basel, Switzerland

Paul Wesselink   Department of Cariology, Endodontology and Pedodontology, Academic Center for Dentistry Amsterdam (ACTA), The Netherlands

Part 1
FOUNDATIONS OF ENDODONTOLOGY

Chapter 1
Introduction to endodontology

Claes Reit, Gunnar Bergenholtz and Preben Hørsted-Bindslev

Endodontology

The word 'endodontology' is derived from the Greek language and is normally translated as 'the knowledge of what is inside the tooth'. Thus, endodontology concerns processes that take place primarily within the pulpal chamber. But what about 'knowledge'? What does it actually mean to 'know' things? Most people would probably say that knowledge has something to do with truth and providing reasons for things. It is often believed that dental and medical knowledge is simply scientific knowledge – science is concerned with how things are constructed and how they function. But as practising dentists we also need to have other types of knowledge. Although we need to know about tooth anatomy and how to produce good root canal preparations we also have to develop good judgment and make the 'right' clinical decisions.

There are at least three different forms of knowledge that the dental practitioner needs and, in a tradition that goes all the way back to Aristotle, we will refer to the Greek terms for these forms: *episteme*, *techne* and *phronesis* (1).

Episteme

Episteme is the word for theoretical–scientific knowledge. The opposite is *doxa*, which refers to 'belief' or 'opinion'. There is a major body of epistemic knowledge within endodontology, namely on pulp biology, root canal microbiota, root filling materials and clinical outcomes of endodontic therapy.

Science produces 'facts'. It must be understood that modern science is an industry and is affected by many factors, both internal and external. Although this is not the place to discuss the philosophy of science, the concept of 'truth' and the growth of knowledge in natural science is not unproblematic. There has been substantial contemporary philosophical discussion reflecting on epistemic knowledge, and the interested reader is referred to one of the many good introductory texts that are available (3).

The results of science are presented in lectures, articles and textbooks so from a student's point of view the learning situation is rather straightforward, provided that the subject is structured and ample time for reading and reflection is given. This book, in large part, is composed of epistemic knowledge.

Techne

The first person to challenge the deeply intrenched theoretical concept of knowledge was the British philosopher Gilbert Ryle. In his book *The Concept of Mind* (9) he introduces 'knowing-how' and distinguishes it from 'knowing-that'. 'Knowing-how' is practical in nature and concerns skills and the performance of certain actions. This concept of knowledge implies not only the ability to do things, but also to understand what you are doing. To say that you have practical knowledge, it is not enough to produce things out of mere routine or habit. You have to 'know' what you are doing and be able to argue about it. Practice must be combined with reflection.

The idea that there is a tacit or silent dimension of knowledge has had a great impact on the contemporary discussion. Michael Polanyi, for example, said that 'We know more than we can tell' (8). When trying to explain how we master practical things such as riding a bicycle or recognizing a face, it is not possible to articulate verbally all the knowledge that we have. Certain important aspects are 'tacit'. Likewise, it is not enough to teach students about root canal instrumentation simply by asking them to read a book or presenting a lecture. It has to be *demonstrated*. Knowledge is very often transmitted by the act of doing.

A substantial portion of endodontic knowledge must be characterized as *techne*. It is not possible to learn all about endodontology by studying a textbook, and a good clinical instructor, seeing other dentists at work, performing procedures oneself, and reflecting on what has been learned are all important.

Phronesis

According to Aristotle, *phronesis* is the ability to think about practical matters. This can be translated as 'practical wisdom' (5) and is concerned with why we might decide to act in one way rather than another. When thinking about the 'right' action or making the 'right' decision we enter the territory of moral philosophy. The person who has practical wisdom has good moral judgment. Modern ethical thinking has been influenced significantly by ideas that originated during the enlightenment. Morality is concerned with human actions and there are certain principles that can separate 'right' from 'wrong' decisions. Jeremy Bentham (2) and the utilitarians launched the utility principle and Immanuel Kant (6) invented the categorical imperative, each creating a tradition with great impact on today's medical ethics and decision-making.

Aristotle, on the other hand, believed that there are no explicit principles to guide us. He understood practical wisdom as a combination of understanding and experience and the ability to read individual situations correctly. He thought that *phronesis* could be learnt from one's own experience and by imitating others who had already mastered the task. He stressed the cultivation of certain character traits and the habit to act wisely.

The clinical situation demands that the dentist exercises practical wisdom, '*to do the right thing at the right moment*'. In order to develop *phronesis*, theoretical studies of moral theory and decision-making principles might be helpful. Neoaristotelians such as Martha Nussbaum (7) have suggested that reading literature should be part of any academic curriculum, the idea being that it increases our knowledge and understanding of other people. However, the essence of *phronesis* has to be learnt from practice.

Concepts of endodontology

From the above it can be concluded that endodontology encompasses not only theoretical thinking but also the practical skills of a craftsman and the practical thinking needed for clinical and moral judgment. Unfortunately, through the years, undue prestige has been given to theoretical–scientific thinking and this has hindered the development of a rational discussion of the other types of knowledge. The serious student of endodontology has to investigate all three aspects, but, as argued above, there are limits to what can be communicated within the covers of a textbook.

The dawn of modern endodontology

It all started with a speech at the McGill University in Montreal. In the morning of October 3, 1910, Dr William Hunter gave a talk entitled 'The role of sepsis and antisepsis in medicine'. Hunter said that:

'In my clinical experience septic infection is without exception the most prevalent infection operating in medicine, and a most important and prevalent cause and complication of many medical diseases. Its ill-effects are widespread and extend to all systems of the body. The relation between these effects and the sepsis that causes them is constantly overlooked, because the existence of the sepsis is itself overlooked. For the chief seat of that sepsis is the mouth; and the sepsis itself, when noted, is erroneously regarded as the result of various conditions of ill-health with which it is associated – not, as it really is, an important cause or complication.

Gold fillings, gold caps, gold bridges, gold crowns, fixed dentures, built in, on, and around diseased teeth, form a veritable mausoleum of gold over a mass of sepsis to which there is no parallel in the whole realm of medicine or surgery. The whole constitutes a perfect gold trap of sepsis.'

The cited text was published in the *Lancet* in 1911 but Hunter's words were also rapidly spread and intensively discussed among laymen and were given banner headlines in the newspapers. Essentially, Hunter proposed that micro-organisms from a focus of infection can spread to other body compartments and cause serious systemic disease. The waiting rooms of the dentists became filled with individuals who thought that their illnesses were caused by oral infections. These illnesses were often chronic or of unknown origin and teeth were removed in enormous numbers.

Although not directly stated by Hunter, teeth with necrotic pulp were seen as one of the main causes of 'focal infection'. Laboratory studies had disclosed the growth of bacteria in the dead pulp tissue. In the 1920s, dental radiography came into general use and radiolucent patches around the apices of necrotic teeth were detected. If such teeth were extracted and cultured, micro-organisms were often recovered from the detached periapical soft tissue. It was generally held that pulpally diseased teeth should be removed.

Reflecting on this period in the history of dentistry, Grossman (4) wrote: 'The focal infection theory promulgated by William Hunter in 1910 gave dentistry in general, and root canal treatment in particular, a black eye from which it didn't recover for about 30 years.' However, in hindsight this period can also be regarded as the dawn of modern endodontology. Researchers started to question and oppose the clinical consequences of the focal infection theory. Microbiologists began mapping out the intracanal microflora and pathologists investigated the reaction patterns of the pulp and periapical tissues. Clinicians invented aseptic methods to treat the root canal, and radiography made it possible to confine the procedures to within the root canal space. It was demonstrated that the intracanal microflora could be combated successfully and that periapical tissues subsequently would heal. Pulpally compromised teeth could be spared and endodontic treatment became a necessary skill of the modern dentist.

The objective of endodontic treatment

The consequences of inflammatory reactions in the pulp and periapical tissue (Fig. 1.1) have tormented mankind for thousands of years. Historically, therefore, the main task of endodontic treatment has been to cure toothache.

For a long period of time a commonly used method to remedy pain was to cauterize the pulp by a red-hot wire or by chemicals such as acid. In 1836, arsenic was introduced to devitalize the pulp, a methodology that would be used for well over 100 years. Procedures to remove the pulp were introduced in the early part of the 19th century and small, hooked instruments were used. The advent of local anesthesia at the beginning of the last century made vital pulpectomy a painless procedure.

Signs of chronic infection, such as abscesses with fistulae, also have been dealt with historically using highly toxic chemicals that were forced through the root canal and into the fistula. Often the treatment was more damaging than the disease, and the tooth and parts of the surrounding bone were lost.

Pain relief is still a primary goal of endodontic treatment, but patients also may want to exclude the compromised tooth, both as a general and local health hazard. This means that intra- as well as extraradicular infections should be eradicated and that materials implanted in the root canal should not cause adverse tissue reactions. Using modern endodontic treatment procedures, these goals can be accomplished to a great extent.

Clinical problems and solutions

The vital pulp

Under normal, physiological conditions the pulp is well protected by the hard tissue structures of the tooth and an intact periodontium (Fig. 1.2). However, the integrity of these tissue barriers might be breached. Microorganisms and the substances they release may gain access to the pulp and adversely affect its condition. The most common cause of bacterial challenge arises from caries. Substances from caries-causing bacteria may enter the pulp along exposed dentinal tubules. Like any connective tissue, the pulp responds to this with inflammation. An important aim of the inflammatory process is to neutralize and eliminate the noxious agents, but also to repair damaged tissue. Often the pulp may react in a manner that allows it to sustain the irritation and maintain a functional state. However, if the injury is severe or persists for an extended period of time, the

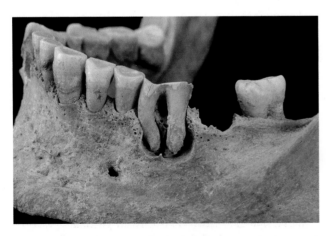

Fig. 1.1 A medieval skull found in Denmark showing seriously attritioned teeth. In the first left lower molar the pulpal cavity is exposed and the bone is resorbed round the root apices, indicating a once-present periapical inflammation.

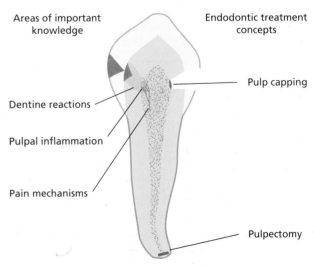

Fig. 1.2 The scope of endodontology: the vital pulp.

response may be destructive and result in total breakdown of the tissue.

An irreversibly inflamed or injured pulp ideally should be removed and replaced with a root filling because otherwise an infection may develop in the root canal system. This removal procedure is called *pulpectomy*. A pulpectomy is carried out under local anesthesia by the use of specially designed root canal instruments. These instruments remove the diseased pulp in its entirety and prepare the canal system so that it can be filled properly. The filling prevents microbial growth and multiplication in the pulpal chamber.

Exposure of the pulp may occur after clinical excavation of caries or after a traumatic insult or iatrogenic injury. If the pulp is judged to be injured reversibly it may not have to be removed. Simply by treating the open wound with a proper dressing and protecting it from the oral environment (so-called *pulp capping*), healing and repair are often possible.

The necrotic pulp

As mentioned above, injury to the pulp may lead to complete breakdown of the tissue (Fig. 1.3). The nonvital, or necrotic, pulp is defenceless against microbial invasion and will allow indigenous micro-organisms to reach the pulp chamber, either along a direct exposure or uncovered dentinal tubules or cracks in the enamel and dentine. Lateral canals exposed as a result of progressive marginal periodontitis may also serve as pathways for bacteria to reach the pulp.

The specific environment in the root canal, characterized by the degrading pulp tissue and lack of oxygen, will result in a microbiota dominated by proteolytic, anaerobic bacteria. Via the apical foramen, microbes and their by-products may reach the periapical tissue and elicit an inflammatory response. This response induces resorption of the surrounding bone, which often is visible in a radiograph as a localized periapical radiolucency. The inflammatory reaction may also stimulate epithelial cells in the periodontal membrane to proliferate and form a periapical cyst.

Treatment of the necrotic pulp is by *root canal treatment* (RCT) and is focused on combating the intracanal infection. The canal is cleaned with files in order to remove microbes as well as their growth substrate. However, owing to the complex anatomy of the root, instruments cannot reach all parts of the canal system and additional antimicrobial substances are usually needed to disinfect the canal. In order to avoid reinfection and to prevent surviving microbes from growing, the canal is then sealed with a root filling.

The root filled tooth

Pulpectomy and RCT do not always lead to a successful clinical outcome. For example, a tooth may continue to be tender or periapical inflammation may persist. Such treatment 'failures' are often associated with defective root fillings which allow organisms from the initial microbiota to survive in the root canal or new bacteria to enter the pulpal chamber via coronal leakage (Fig. 1.4).

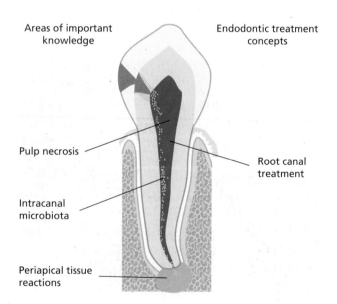

Areas of important knowledge

Endodontic treatment concepts

Pulp necrosis

Root canal treatment

Intracanal microbiota

Periapical tissue reactions

Fig. 1.3   The scope of endodontology: the necrotic pulp.

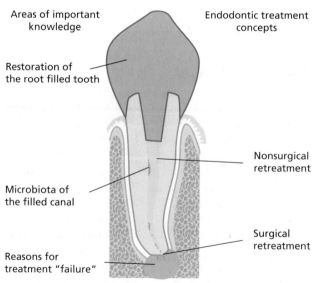

Areas of important knowledge

Endodontic treatment concepts

Restoration of the root filled tooth

Nonsurgical retreatment

Microbiota of the filled canal

Surgical retreatment

Reasons for treatment "failure"

Fig. 1.4   The scope of endodontology: the root filled tooth.

The root canal may be retreated using either a non-surgical or a surgical approach. In *non-surgical retreatment* the root filling is removed and the canal is reinstrumented. Antimicrobial substances are applied to kill the surviving microbes and the space is reobturated. Crowns, bridges and posts may mean that it is sometimes not feasible to reach the root canal in a conventional way. In such cases, a *surgical retreatment* is appropriate. A muco-periosteal flap is raised and entrance to the apical part of the root is made through the bone. Surgical retreatment may also involve cutting of the root tip and retrograde preparation and filling of the root canal.

The diagnostic dilemma

The disease processes in the pulp and periapical tissues take place in concealed body compartments that normally are not available for direct inspection. Instead, the clinician has to rely on indirect information to assess the condition of the tissues and reach a diagnosis. The interpretation of this information entails the risk of making false-positive and false-negative diagnoses. For example, the patient's report of pain has been shown to be an unreliable sign of pathology because most inflammatory episodes within the pulp or periapical bone pass by without symptoms. Furthermore, the discriminatory ability of the intrapulpal nerves is not perfect, which means that if a patient has toothache due to pulpitis there is a high risk that he or she may 'point out the wrong tooth'. Besides anamnestic information, vitality testing of the pulp and interpretation of periapical radiographs are the prime diagnostic sources of data. Such data have to be handled with utmost care and with in-depth knowledge of possible errors and the factors that influence diagnostic accuracy.

The tools of treatment

To many dentists, RCT can best be described by using Winston Churchill's words on golf: 'An impossible game with impossible tools'. The complexity of root canal anatomy, the relative stiffness of root canal instruments, being unable, often, to visualize the area properly, and the lack of space in the mouth provide substantial challenges to the skill and patience of the dentist. Intracanal work is exceptionally difficult; this is clearly demonstrated by radiographically based epidemiological surveys, which repeatedly report that many root fillings do not meet acceptable technical standards. Because clinical outcome is strongly related to the quality of treatment, the high frequency of substan-

dard performance is a subject of great concern to the profession.

The last decade has seen a tremendous technological development that hopefully will increase the overall standard of endodontic treatment. For example, the advent of superflexible nickel–titanium alloy has made it possible to fabricate instruments that follow much more easily the anatomy of the root canal and therefore produce good quality canal preparations. Furthermore, systems have been developed that allow the instruments to be maneuvered by machine rather than by hand, improving fine-scale manipulation and decreasing operator fatigue.

The microscope has brought light and vision into the pulp chamber and root canal (Fig. 1.5). Working under high magnification, it is now far easier to remove mineralizations, locate small root canal orifices and control intracanal procedures. However, high quality microscopes are expensive and, thus far, the technology has been adopted mostly by dentists specialized in endodontics.

In the midst of this technological boom it must not be forgotten that endodontics is basically about controlling infection. Luckily, there are few medical therapeutic procedures that can be carried out as aseptically as RCT. Shielding the operation field with a rubber dam is one of the oldest and still most effective ways to ensure that the area remains sterile, thus improving clinical success (Fig. 1.6).

Conclusions

Pulpal pain can be beyond endurance and pulpal infections can destroy supporting bone. To manage these

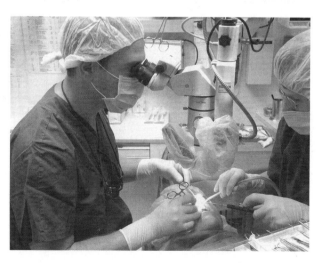

Fig. 1.5

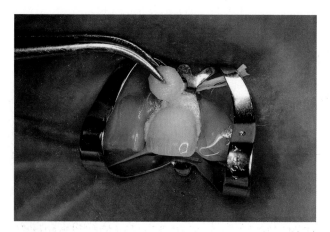

Fig. 1.6

clinical problems the dental profession has been forced to develop diagnostic skills, explore the microbial flora, investigate pharmacology and biocompatability of medicaments and materials, in addition to developing a broad range of specially designed tools. This combined knowledge concentrates on rendering the tooth asymp-tomatic and healthy, and capable of maintaining its functional place in the oral cavity.

References

1. Aristotle (Iruin, T. ed.). *Nicomachean Ethics.* London: Hackett Publishing, 1988.
2. Bentham J. *Introduction to the Principles of Morals and Legislation (1789)* (Burns JH, Hart DLA, eds). London: Methuen, 1982.
3. Chalmers AF. *What is this Thing called Science?* Buckingham: Open University, 1999.
4. Grossman LI. Endodontics 1776–1996: a bicentennial history against the background of general dentistry. *JADA* 1976; 93: 78–87.
5. Hughes GJ. *Aristotle on Ethics.* London: Routledge, 2001.
6. Kant I. *Foundations of the Metaphysics of Morals (1785).* Indianapolis: Bobbs–Merrill, 1959.
7. Nussbaum M. *Poetic Justice. The literary imagination and public life.* Boston: Beacon Press, 1995.
8. Polanyi M. *Personal Knowledge: Towards a Postcritical Philosophy.* London: Routledge, 1958.
9. Ryle G. *The Concept of Mind.* London: Penguin, 1949.

Chapter 2
Diagnosis of pulpal and periapical disease

Claes Reit, Kerstin Petersson and Olav Molven

Introduction

To diagnose diseases of the pulp and periapical tisssues is often a very demanding and sometimes frustrating procedure, e.g. when patients are in severe pain. Because the reactions mostly take place in concealed parts of the body, the disease picture frequently must be made 'visible' by indirect methods and tests. The clinician also must learn to navigate with a very limited diagnostic armamentarium at his or her disposal. In this situation, besides personal experience and intuition (which cannot be learnt from a textbook), the accuracy and correct interpretation of diagnostic information are all important. Evaluation and re-evaluation of data have to be carried out in a continuous process.

From textbooks, students normally learn about diagnosis through studying the various diseases. Expected symptoms, signs and test results of, for example, pulpal inflammation, are presented, the diseases are given and their clinical, radiographical and laboratory expressions are discussed. However, such a learning procedure is the reverse of what happens in the clinical situation. People rarely know what they suffer from and instead they present with certain symptoms, signs and test results. Suspicions often can be raised in several directions and the task of the clinician is to look through a wealth of information to find the right 'signal' or diagnosis. This chapter thus will start with a discussion on how diagnostic information may be evaluated.

Evaluation of diagnostic information

Making the right diagnosis is very often a complex task and clinicians easily may draw different conclusions. Many studies have demonstrated how physicians and dentists vary in the way they practice their profession, regardless of whether they are defining a disease, making a diagnosis or selecting therapeutic procedures. For example, in a study on microscopic investigation of biopsies from the uterine cervix, 13 pathologists were asked to read 1001 specimens and to repeat the readings at a later time. On average, each pathologist agreed with him or herself only 89% of the time (intraobserver agreement) and with a panel of 'senior' pathologists only 87% of the time (interobserver agreement). Looking only at patients who actually had cervical pathology, the intraobserver agreement was only 68% and the interobserver agreement was 51% (29).

Many similar studies on various signs and symptoms have been carried out and the literature on 'observer variation' has been growing for a long time (7, Key literature 2.1). From a diagnostic point of view it has been found that, in general, observers looking at the same thing will disagree with each other or even with themselves 10–50% of the time (8).

Many authors have regarded the diagnostic process more as an act of art than of science: 'Traditionally, the process of diagnosis was left undefined, a natural art, or explained as a process of intuition. Despite recent advances, this is still too often the case' (10). In Dorland's medical dictionary (6) 'diagnosis' is defined as 'The *art* of distinguishing one disease from another'. However, during recent years clinical reasoning has been the subject of substantial research, and both descriptive and normative models have been proposed (15).

Diagnostic accuracy

Let us assume that the question of whether or not a person has a certain disease D in a clinical situation can be determined only by a test T. It is possible to obtain two test results: one indicating that the patient has D (a positive test, T+) and one suggesting that the patient does not have D (a negative test, T–) (see Core concept 2.1). Unfortunately, T has the drawback (which it shares with almost all tests and procedures) that it cannot completely separate persons who have D and those who have not. Two types of error are possible. A person who has D can be informed that he or she has not (a false-negative diagnosis) and another person can receive a

---

Key literature 2.1   Observer variation in periapical radiographic diagnosis

In a study by Reit & Hollender (27) the radiographs of 119 endodontically treated roots were examined by six observers. Each root was visible on two separate radiographs. Three of the examiners were specialists in endodontics and three in oral radiology. The observers were asked to distinguish between 'normal periapical conditions', 'increased width of the periodontal membrane space' and 'periapical radiolucency'. In the opinion of one or more observers, 82 of the 119 roots presented normal periapical conditions. However, only at 33 (37%) of these roots was the decision shared by all six. The diagnosis of 'increased width of the periodontal membrane space' was made in agreement in only 9% of 65 recorded cases. Periapical radiolucency was reported at 37 of the roots, and at 10 of these (27%) all observers agreed. This study serves as an illustration of the difficulties in defining and maintaining criteria in radiographic evaluation of the periapical tissues.

Core concept 2.1   Measures of diagnostic accuracy

		Test results	
		T+	T−
Actual state	D+	TP (True positive)	FN (False negative)
	D−	FP (False positive)	TN (True negative)

T+ = positive test result
T− = negative test result
D+ = disease present
D− = disease absent

Sensitivity = the proportion of diseased patients (D+) correctly identified as positive (TP/TP + FN).

Specificity = the proportion of non-diseased patients (D−) correctly identified as negative (TN/TN + FP).

Positive predictive value = the proportion of positive tests (T+) that are true positive (TP/TP + FP).

Negative predictive value = the proportion of negative tests (T−) that are true negative (TN/TN + FN).

---

positive test although he or she does not have D (a false-positive diagnosis). Of course there are also two types of correct outcomes of the test: true-positive and true-negative diagnoses, respectively. The proportions of these four possible outcomes can be used to express the diagnostic value attached to the test. Sensitivity – or the true positive ratio – is a measure of the proportion of patients with D correctly identified as positive. Specificity – the true negative ratio – is a measure of the

proportion of persons without D correctly identified as negative.

In order to determine the sensitivity and specificity of a diagnostic test a comparison with some sort of ideal 'gold standard' has to be made. There must be some test-independent way of making a definitive diagnosis of whether the patient is diseased or not. Preferably, such a gold standard is created by means of a biopsy, but often another test normally not clinically available because of high costs or severe adverse effects may serve this purpose. In most cases investigators have to use gold standards that are below '24 carats'.

In the clinical situation the most interesting questions are formulated in a slightly different way. When the test indicates that the patient is diseased (T+), what is the probability that he or she really has D? And if the patient gets a negative test (T−), what is the probability that D is not present? These probabilities are given in the so-called *positive predictive value* (PPV) and the *negative predictive value* (NPV).

In contrast to sensitivity and specificity, PPV and NPV are dependent on the prevalence of the disease. Let us assume that a test has 90% sensitivity and 95% specificity for a certain disease. If the prevalence of the disease is 50%, then the PPV will reach 95%. This means that if a patient receives a positive test there is 95% probability that he or she is diseased. If the prevalence is 10%, the PPV will decrease to 67%; if the prevalence is 1%, the PPV is only 15%. This mathematical exercise tells us that tests do not work well when prevalences are low. Accordingly, in a clinical situation, tests should not be used on a routine basis. By history taking and oral examination the clinician selects patients in which a specific test may be used. What he or she actually does is to increase the prevalence of the suspected disease!

Receiver operating characteristic (ROC) analysis

If rates of true-positive response (TPR) and false-positive response (FPR) are calculated for different decision criteria (cut-offs), the obtained pairs of values may be plotted in a simple graph with the TPR placed vertically and the FPR horizontally. Various cut-off points may be obtained in many ways. For example, in radiographic diagnosis of periapical lesions the level of confidence of the observer often is used. Both the TPR and the FPR are calculated for five decision critera: definitely a lesion; probably a lesion; uncertain; probably no lesion; definitely no lesion. The plotted points form what is called the ROC curve.

The position of the ROC curve will tell us how good a test is at discriminating between people (or teeth) who have the disease from those who do not. The ROC curve of the perfect test coincides with the axes, whereas the curve of the worthless test lies along the 45° diagonal.

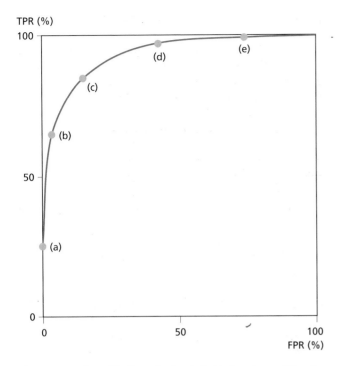

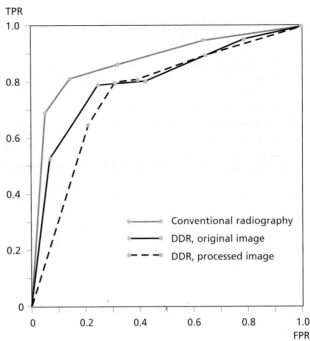

Fig. 2.1 In radiographic diagnosis of periapical lesions, true positive rates (TPR) and false positive rates (FPR) can be calculated for five decision criteria: (a) definitely a lesion, (b) lesion probable, (c) lesion uncertain, (d) probably no lesion, (e) definitely no lesion.

Fig. 2.2 ROC analysis of periapical radiography showing observer decisions for 59 radiographs (16).

We can measure the discriminatory power of a test by how close its ROC curve is to the axes and how far it is from the diagonal. More precisely, the discriminatory power is measured by the *area* under the curve, which is 100% for the perfect test and 50% for the worthless test. An ROC analysis demonstrates that changing the cut-off point will *not* influence the discriminatory power of a test, it just moves its position *along* the curve. However, different cut-off points can have momentous clinical consequences for those affected by the judgment, and a strategy for deciding the position to be taken on the curve must be developed (see next section).

Receiver operating characteristic (ROC) analysis of periapical radiography

In a study by Kullendorff *et al.* (16) the aim was to compare the observer performance of direct digital radiography, with and without image processing, with that of conventional radiography, for the detection of periapical bone lesions. For 50 patients a conventional periapical radiograph using E-speed film was taken and then a direct digital image of the same area was made. The images of 59 roots were assessed by seven observers using a five-point confidence scale: definitely no lesion; probably no lesion; uncertain; probably a lesion; definitely a lesion. A gold standard was created by

independent readings of 73 films by two experienced radiologists. Only images where they agreed (totalling 59) were included in the study. The ROC curves were established and mean values of the observers' decisions are shown in Fig. 2.2.

Conventional film radiography came out slightly better from the study than direct digital radiography. Image processing did not improve the observer performance.

Diagnostic strategy

The diagnosis is not a goal in itself but only, in the words of a Scottish clinician, 'a mental resting-place' for prognostic deliberation and therapeutic decisions (33). One of the main concerns for this deliberation is of course the fact that no diagnostic method has perfect sensitivity and specificity, which means that false diagnoses cannot be avoided completely. Also, from ROC analysis we learn that diagnostic decisions always have 'costs'. If we want to be sure that all cases treated are really diseased, we have to take a low position on the ROC curve. The cost for this will be a number of missed cases. In contrast, if we want to treat all diseased patients (or teeth), a high position on the ROC curve is needed and the cost will be a number of healthy cases being treated. If an analysis of an actual clinical situation results in a strategic decision to avoid overtreatment (low ROC position), then the clinician should signal for disease only when he or she is absolutely certain that it is present. If the problem is to avoid false-negative diagnoses, the best consequences will be obtained if disease is reported at the slightest suspicion of it (high ROC position). It is important to notice that a decrease of one type of error will lead to an increase in the other.

On which grounds should a certain strategy be chosen? This is a complex problem and an in-depth analysis is beyond the scope of this chapter. However, certain important factors may be identified: the consequences of untreated disease; risk of complications or adverse effects of instituted therapy; economic costs; and personal values.

In a situation where untreated disease will not lead to any serious complications of the general health or well-being, one normally wants to avoid overtreatment. The diagnostic process will be directed towards the avoidance of false-positive diagnoses and a low position on the ROC curve is taken. If untreated disease will lead to serious complications it is important to identify and find all or most of the diseased individuals. From a strategic point of view, false-positive diagnoses must be accepted and we have to move higher up the ROC curve.

It is obvious that if the available cure also implies great risk of severe complications or serious adverse effects you do not want to perform any unnecessary treatments. The price to pay for accepting false-positive diagnoses will be too high. In contrast, the diagnostic position should be moved higher up the ROC curve if treatment is simple and without any considerable risk.

All medical and dental care is associated with economic costs and thus resources must be regarded as limited. Diagnosis and treatment have to be cost-effective and if the available therapy is very expensive you want to be certain that you do not start treatment on a false-positive diagnosis. For example, you may start a non-surgical retreatment of a root filled tooth on a slight suspicion of apical periodontitis if the procedure is easily carried out in a tooth without complex prosthodontic restorations. But if you have to remove crown and post in order to reach the root canal, you probably want to be absolutely certain that this is the right thing to do and, accordingly, you will move to a lower position on the ROC curve.

Personal values have to be included in a decision strategy. Faced with the same clinical situation, people will not evaluate the benefits and risks of a treatment procedure in identical ways. This means that the position of the diagnostic criterion has to be discussed with the individual patient. Will the patient take a false-positive diagnosis before a false-negative diagnosis, or the other way around? Attempts have been made to measure patients' values in order to incorporate them in various decision

models (28). These possibilities are discussed in more detail in Chapter 14.

Clinical manifestations of pulpal and periapical inflammation

The clinical manifestations of inflammatory processes in the pulp and periapical tissues cover a broad range of expressions. Patients' experience of dental pain may vary from a barely noticeable discomfort to an unbearable torment, from the odd attack of short duration to a lingering continuous suffering. Patients may also display discolored teeth, fistulas, swellings and raised body temperature. In Core concept 2.2 the most commom symptoms and signs associated with pulp inflammation, pulp necrosis and periapical pathosis are collected and displayed. Strangely, however, patients most often are free of symptoms and the majority of pulpal inflammations in need of endodontic treatment are unveiled during operative procedures (26). Periapical inflammations are detected in most cases only by radiographic means.

Collecting diagnostic information

Inferences regarding disease processes in the pulp and periapical tissues have to be made with the help of a rather limited diagnostic armamentarium. The main sources of information are the patient's report on pain and other symptoms, the clinical examination of the tooth and surrounding structures, and the radiographic examination (Core concept 2.3).

The problem for which the patient seeks dental care (chief complaint) is the natural point of departure for the diagnostic process. If the patient is in acute distress, the examination and diagnosis must be focused on solving that problem as fast as possible and a complete examination and establishment of a definitive treatment plan will be postponed until later. A quieter situation will allow the examiner to expand on the present dental illness. The patient's report on character, intensity, frequency, localization and external influence of the symptoms will often give clues to a tentative diagnosis. This initial notion may be strengthened or refuted by penetrating the dental history, including information on such things as recently placed restorations, pulp cappings and potential bruxism.

When reviewing the medical history the endodontist will focus on illnesses, medication and allergic reactions. Consultation with the patient's physician is recommended when physical or mental illness is expected to interfere with diagnosis and treatment. There are no systemic disease conditions for which endodontic treat-

Core concept 2.2   Clinical manifestation of pulpal and periapical disease

Symptoms and signs of pulpal inflammation

- History of sharp pain, spontaneous or to thermal stimuli
- Pain attack may be provoked clinically by thermal stimuli (a)

Symptoms and signs of pulp necrosis (b)

- The pulp is insensitive to vitality testing
- The crown is discolored (grayish)

Symptoms and signs of periapical inflammation (c–e)

- Tooth is insensitive to vitality testing
- Dull, continuous pain
- Intra- or extraoral swelling
- Draining fistula
- Periapical radiolucency

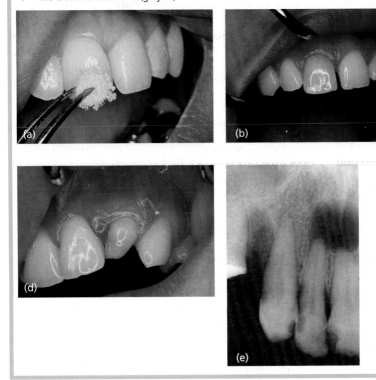

Core concept 2.3   Sources of diagnostic information

- **Anamnesis**
  — Chief complaint
  — Present dental illness
  — Dental history
  — Medical history
- **Clinical examination**
  — Evaluation of the crown
  — Evaluation of the pulp
  — Evaluation of the periapical tissues
- **Radiographic examination**

teeth are evaluated with regard to caries, defective fillings and discolorations. A fiber-optic light source may be used to try to disclose the presence of cracks in the enamel or dentine, and the patient may be asked to bite on a cotton roll or a firm object. The true condition of the pulp is very difficult to assess but pain provocation and vitality testing are helpful. Tenderness to percussion and palpation confirms a suspicion of periapical inflammation, as of course does the presence of a fistula and swelling or a periapical radiolucency in the radiograph.

Some informative sources are more important than others. In the following information gathered from pain reports, both pulp vitality testing and periapical radiographs will be discussed.

ments are contraindicated, other than those affecting any dental procedure.

The status of the tentative diagnosis is explored further at the clinical examination. Crowns of suspected

Evaluation of reported pain

From a subjective point of view the main sign of pulpal and periapical disease is the experience of pain. Patients usually associate pathology with pain, and a pain-free situation with non-disease. However, studies have pointed at a low correlation between pulp pathology and patients' symptoms (1, 30). In most cases inflammatory reactions in the pulp and periapical tissues will not give rise to pain. Thus, the sensitivity of pain as a diagnostic criterion of endodontic disease is very low.

The clinical picture is even more complicated. Studies have shown that when a patient reports spontaneous dental pain and locates the origin of symptoms to a certain tooth, the clinician cannot act on only this information. The discriminatory power of the pulpal nerves is not perfect. When healthy teeth were stimulated electrically, Mumford & Newton (23) found that only 46% of subjects correctly identified the right tooth. Friend & Glenwright (9) reported that 73% of subjects made a correct area localization (one neighboring tooth on each side included). In these studies electric pulp testers were used, which stimulate mostly A-delta fibers. When pain is elicited by pulp inflammation, nerve impulses will originate mostly from C-fibers. Those fibers have a lesser discriminatory ability, which means that the chance of correct patient identification in a clinical situation will decrease further. Thus, patients may experience pain in one tooth while the pathosis is to be found in another. This phenomenon is called referred pain (11, 31). Pain may be referred to teeth also from pathological processes in the ear, salivary glands, maxillary sinus and masticatory muscles (13). Even organs outside the head may generate an experience of 'toothache'. Bonica (4) reported that patients with angina pectoris rather frequently referred the pain to their teeth.

In order to find the right source of the pain, the most informative diagnostic move is to try to provoke or extinguish the symptoms. Pulpal pain may be triggered or aggravated by applying cold or hot stimuli to the tooth. In cases with continuous pain that is hard to localize, it may be very helpful to inject anesthetics systematically and find the site where the symptom can be relieved.

A lot of important diagnostic information can be found in the patient's description of the pain. Pulpal pain has a wide experience range: from a slightly increased sensitiveness, to intraoral temperature changes, to very intense, almost unbearable pain. In a typical case the pain comes in attacks often elicited by hot or cold food (Advanced concept 2.1). Initially, with such a provoked attack a sharp pain is felt (A-delta fibers). After the stimulus is removed, the pain lingers on for varying amounts of time (seconds to hours), often described as deep, dull and throbbing (C-fibres). Paradoxically, in some cases, taking a solid dose of ice water into the mouth may relieve the symptoms. This observation is mostly made when pain is continuous and very

---

> **Advanced concept 2.1   Temperature changes and pulpal pain**
>
> The hypothetical explanation to the phenomenon that temperature changes influence pulpal pain is that such changes influence the tissue pressure inside the pulpal chamber with its rigid dentine walls. Because of low compliance in the pulpal chamber, even modest changes in pulpal fluid volume will be reflected in the tissue pressure (20). An increased pressure in the pulpal tissue due to increased temperature, for example, would start a pain attack because the biochemical inflammatory mediators already maintain subclinical pain signals and a decreased pain threshold. Congruent to this reasoning, a significant decrease in temperature would decrease the tissue pressure and thus also the pain sensation. Tooth-related pain in patients subjected to pressure changes, called barodontalgia, is sometimes experienced by airborne or diving people and is important as an indicator of pulpal inflammation.

intense and is held to be a sign of excessive and irreversible pulpal inflammation.

As soon as the inflammatory reaction spreads out of the pulp chamber or root canal to involve the periodontal membrane, the tooth may be tender to percussion, palpation and chewing. Pain associated with periapical inflammation is mostly continuous and described as dull in character. The symptoms will not be influenced by changes in the temperature and thus may not be provoked.

Assessment of pulp vitality

Traditionally, pulp vitality has been determined by investigating its sensitivity. Because this is an indirect methodology the clinician has to work with hypotheses of the relation between the test result and the reality. Two main assumptions about this relation usually are made:

(1) If the pulp is sensitive, it is vital.
(2) If the pulp is sensitive and the patient has no symptoms, the pulp is healthy.

There are three types of pulp vitality test:

- Mechanical
- Thermal
- Electrical.

The rules for the use of vitality tests are given in Core concept 2.4.

Mechanical tests

Probing exposed dentine in a cavity or cervically at the neck of the tooth often results in a sensitive reaction in a vital tooth. Pulp sensitivity also may be disclosed during

---

Core concept 2.4   Guiding rules for the clinical use of vitality tests

- Explain the procedures to the patient.
- Do not rely on only one test; use combinations.
- Make comparisons with other teeth, preferably contralaterals but also with neighboring teeth.
- In cases with doubtful reactions, repeat the tests in a different order, 'hiding' the suspicious tooth.

Key literature 2.2   Diagnostic accuracy of thermal and electrical pulp tests

In a study by Petersson *et al.* (25), the pulpal status of 75 teeth was investigated by cold (ethyl chloride), heat (hot gutta-percha) and electricity (Analytic Technology Pulp Tester). True-positive, false-positive, true-negative and false-negative test results were calculated for each method compared with a gold standard. The gold standard was established by direct pulp inspection (59 teeth in need of endodontic treatment) and by judging radiographs (16 intact teeth). Twenty-nine teeth (39%) were judged to be necrotic. The authors found that an insensitive reaction represented a necrotic pulp in 89% with the cold test, in 48% with the heat test and in 88% with the electrical test. A sensitive reaction was found to correspond to a vital pulp in 90% with the cold test, in 83% with the heat test and in 84% with the electrical test.

---

removal of caries or defective fillings. It is sometimes recommended to drill a small test cavity, especially in teeth with full crown restorations. Such test cavities can be used also for thermal and electrical tests. Mechanical stimulation is generally considered to have a high sensitivity and specificity. However, scientifically obtained data on the diagnostic accuracy seem to be lacking.

Thermal tests
Cold air, water or a cold object may elicit a sensible response when placed at a tooth surface covering dentinal tubules. The temperature changes will influence the flow of dentine liquor, which leads to movement of the odontoblast process and subsequent mechanical stimulation of the pulpal nerves. A common method is to apply a cotton pellet soaked in a fast evaporating fluid, such as ethyl chloride or dichlorodifluoromethane. Dry ice sticks – made by filling empty cylindrettes with water and placing them in the freezer – also can be used.

Application of heat to the tooth surface also has been recommended for vitality testing, conveniently carried out by using temporary stopping. A gutta-percha bar is heated in an open flame for a few seconds until it softens. It is then placed on the buccal surface of the tooth, away from the gingiva. The bar is removed as soon as the patient signals a reaction. Because studies indicate that the diagnostic accuracy is very low (25, Advanced concept 2.1, Key literature 2.2), heat should not be used as a single test of pulp vitality.

Electrical test
An electric pulp tester sends a weak electric current through the tooth, which stimulates the pulpal nerves. An electrode coated with a conducting medium is placed on a tooth surface away from the gingiva. In order to avoid transduction of the current to its neighbors, the tooth to be tested should be isolated with rubber dam or plastic strips. The current is slowly increased. Electric pulp testers should not be used in individuals with cardiac pacemakers.

Vitality testing by electrical stimulation has good diagnostic accuracy (21, 25, Advanced concept 2.1) but its use is often prohibited if metallic restorations cover most of the tooth structure. To overcome this problem, Pantera *et al.* (24) suggested the use of a bridging technique. The tip of an explorer coated with toothpaste was placed against an exposed part of the tooth surface and the pulp tester then was placed against the explorer.

Studies have shown that the pain threshold is influenced by the placement of the electrode. Several authors registered the lowest threshold values when the pulp tester was placed on the incisal tip (3). At this part of the tooth the enamel layer usually is very thin (the enamel has greater electrical resistance than the dentine) and the concentration of sensory nerves is highest in the pulpal horns (17).

Interpretation of the test results
The outcome of a sensitivity test is the result of an interaction between the given stimulus and the patient's reaction to it. Accordingly, a failing correlation between sensibility and vitality may be either *stimulus* or *reaction dependent*. The former situation may be illustrated by an electric impulse that does not reach a vital pulp tissue owing to, for example, excessive amounts of reparative dentine. False recordings also may be obtained if the pulp is necrotic and the impulse reaches nerve fibers in the periodontal membrane or in a neighboring tooth. Such possibilities have been discussed in detail by several authors (12, 22). Sometimes a vital pulp cannot respond to stimulation owing to a traumatic injury of the intradental nerves. The accuracy of the test also may be impaired by the patient's behavior. He or she may be anxious or feeling uneasy and thus have difficulty in giving a correct report. Therefore, when test results are

doubtful and difficult to interpret, a combination of methods must be used (Core concept 2.4).

Interpretation of periapical radiographs

Because inflammatory reactions of the periapical tissues often proceed without any clinical symptoms, cases are frequently diagnosed by radiographic means only. The sensitivity of periapical radiography has been studied by numerous investigators and a common approach has been to create artificial bone lesions in cadavers and determine the minimum amount of bone loss that will result in a visible radiolucency. A now classic study was set up by Bender & Seltzer (2), who reported that a bone lesion was not visible until the cortex or the interface between cortical and cancellous bone was involved. They also stated that bone destructions were always larger than that suspected from studying the radiographs. In a study of human autopsy material, Brynolf (5) compared the radiology and histology of periapical areas of upper incisors. She reported a high frequency of radiographically undetected inflammatory lesions. Several later investigators have confirmed the findings of Bender & Seltzer (2) and Brynolf (5), and pointed out the high risk of false-negative recordings, which in turn will influence the sensitivity of the test.

Clinicians arrive at false-positive diagnoses mainly by erroneous interpretation of normal anatomical structures. Major blood vessels and spaces in the bone marrow, for example, might simulate the image of an inflammatory periapical lesion. The specificity of the radiographic diagnosis is also influenced by other disease processes that might cause periapical bone lesions, such as marginal periodontitis and cementoma. In such cases, sensitivity testing of the tooth is decisive. When testing of the pulp vitality is not possible, as in root filled teeth, the risk of making false-positive diagnoses increases. For example, cases in which healing has not resulted in periapical bone-fill but in scar tissue formation might be classified as 'failures'.

Diagnostic classification

The end of the diagnostic process is the formulation of a diagnosis. The collected information has to be related to a disease entity. In the literature, several classification systems have been suggested and various terms used to denote disease processes in the pulp and periapical tissues. At first glance this situation may appear confusing to the reader but a closer look will disclose that the systems express rather small variations on a common theme and 'translations' between them are not as difficult to carry out. It is important to recognize that a useful

---

> ### Core concept 2.5   Clinical diagnoses of the pulp and periapical tissues
>
> **Pulpa sana**: the tooth reacts positively to vitality testing and the pulp is covered by healthy, hard dentine. No clinical or radiographic signs of inflammation are present.
>
> **Pulpitis**: the pulp reacts positively to vitality testing and subjective or objective signs of inflammation are present.
>
> **Necrosis pulpae**: the pulp is insensitive and does not bleed.
>
> **Periodontitis apicalis chronica**: the pulp is non-vital and there are radiographic and/or clinical signs of chronic periapical inflammation (e.g. fistula). The patient has no symptoms.
>
> **Periodontitis apicalis acuta**: the pulp is non-vital and there are clinical signs of acute periapical inflammation (pain, swelling, raised body temperature).

diagnostic system must be based on *clinically available* information only. Therefore, in an attempt to distinguish clearly between clinical and histopathological diagnosis, the present book always refers to the former in their Latin form (Core concept 2.5).

Pulpa sana

There are situations when teeth with healthy pulps are treated endodontically. These cases are not unveiled through a pulp diagnostic procedure. The barrier function in the tooth may be violated through operative procedures by penetrating the dentine and exposing the pulp tissue. Occasionally root canal retention is needed when the possibilities for coronal retention are insufficient. Hemisection of multi-rooted teeth also initiates the need for endodontic treatment of the healthy pulp.

Pulpitis

As mentioned above, findings from numerous studies indicate that the presence or absence of clinical symptoms provides little information about the true condition of the pulp (1, 18, 19, 30, 32). However, because the cardinal symptom of pulp inflammation is pain, the magnitude of the experience is used to try to distinguish between cases in need of pulpectomy (irreversible inflammation) and those that are not (reversible inflammation). To make this important distinction, the presence or absence of pulp exposure is an informative finding. The severe inflammatory reactions often observed, even in symptom-free teeth with carious pulp exposures (14), in combination with the broken dentine barrier make the prognosis of pulpal healing doubtful.

From a practical point of view it is helpful to regard excavation of caries and removal of fillings as part of the diagnostic process, and painful pulps found to be covered by dentine are provisionally regarded to be reversibly inflamed. Such cases should be treated temporarily by filling the cavity with ZOE cement, for example, and only when pain persists should a pulpectomy be performed. Thus, the diagnosis of 'pulpitis' covers a broad range of pathological situations and cases will receive different clinical monitoring. As in most endodontic diagnostic and treatment decision situations, underdiagnosis and undertreatment are preferred to overdiagnosis and overtreatment.

Necrosis pulpae

A failing reaction to a vitality test is not sufficient information to act on this diagnosis. However, in combination with a discolored crown or periapical radiolucency, an access preparation to the pulp chamber is justified and the diagnosis is confirmed with the finding of a non-bleeding pulp.

Periodontitis apicalis chronica/acuta

Pathological processes of the periapical tissues are most often asymptomatic and the diagnosis is verified only by radiographic examination. Sometimes, in clinically acute situations, bone resorption may not have reached the level at which radiolucency is detectable in the radiograph. The clinical diagnosis of 'periodontitis apicalis' makes no attempt to differentiate between various histopathological situations such as granulomas and cysts.

References

1. Baume LJ. Diagnoses of diseases of the pulp. *Oral Surg.* 1970; 29: 102–16.
2. Bender IB, Seltzer S. Roentgenographic and direct observation of experimental lesions in bone. *JADA* 1961; 62: 150–60, 708–16.
3. Bender IB, Landau MA, Fonsecca S, Trowbridge HO. The optimum placement-site of the electrode in electric pulp testing of the 12 anterior teeth. *JADA* 1989; 118: 305–10.
4. Bonica JJ. *The Management of Pain.* Philadelphia: Lea & Febiger, 1953.
5. Brynolf I. Histological and roentgenological study of periapical region of human upper incisors. *Odontol. Revy* 1967; 18: suppl. 11.
6. *Dorland's Illustrated Medical Dictionary.* Philadelphia: Saunders, 1965.
7. Eddy DM. Variations in physician practice: the role of uncertainty. *Health Affairs* 1984; 3: 74–89.
8. Feinstein AR. A bibliography of publications on observer variability. *J. Chron. Dis.* 1985; 38: 619–32.
9. Friend LA, Glenwright HD. An experimental investigation into the localization of pain from the dental pulp. *Oral Surg.* 1968; 25: 765–74.
10. Gale J, Marsden P. *Medical Diagnosis: from Student to Clinician.* Oxford: Oxford University Press, 1983.
11. Glick DH. Locating referred pulpal pain. *Oral Surg.* 1962; 15: 613–23.
12. Himmel VT. Diagnostic procedures for evaluating pulpally involved teeth. *Curr. Opini. Dent.* 1992; 2: 72–7.
13. Ingle JI, Glick DH. Differential diagnosis and treatment of dental pain. In *Endodontics* (Ingle JI, Bakland LK, eds). Philadelphia: Williams & Wilkins, 1994; 524–49.
14. Izumi T, Kobayashi I, Okamura K, Sakai H. Immunohistochemical study on the immunocompetent cells of the pulp in human non-carious and carious teeth. *Archs. Oral Biol.* 1995; 40: 609–14.
15. Kassirer JP, Kopelman RI. *Learning Clinical Reasoning.* Baltimore: Williams & Wilkins, 1991.
16. Kullendorff B, Peterson K, Rohlin M. Direct digital radiography for the detection of periapical bone lesions: a clinical study. *Endodont. Dent. Traumatol.* 1997; 13: 183–9.
17. Lilja J. Sensory differences between crown and root dentine in human teeth. *Acta Odontol. Scand.* 1980; 38: 285–94.
18. Lundy T, Stanley HR. Correlation of pulpal histopathology and clinical symptoms in human teeth subjected to experimental irritation. *Oral Pathol.* 1969; 27: 187–201.
19. Mitchel DF, Tarplee RE. Painful pulpitis. A clinical and microscopic study. *Oral Surg.* 1960; 38: 1360–81.
20. Mjör I, Heyeraas K. Pulp-dentine and periodontal anatomy and physiology. In *Essential Endodontology* (Örstavik D, Pitt Ford TR, eds). Oxford: Blackwell Science, 1998; 9–41.
21. Mumford JM. Evaluation of gutta percha and ethyl chloride in pulp testing. *Br. Dent. J.* 1964; 116: 338–42.
22. Mumford JM. *Toothache and Orofacial Pain.* London: Churchill Livingstone, 1976.
23. Mumford JM, Newton AV. Convergence in the trigeminal system following stimulation of human teeth. *Arch. Oral Biol.* 1971; 16: 1089–97.
24. Pantera EA, Anderson RW, Pantera CT. Use of dental instruments for bridging during electric pulp testing. *J. Endodont.* 1992; 18: 37–8.
25. Petersson K, Söderström C, Kiani-Anaraki M, Lévy G. Evaluation of the ability of thermal and electrical tests to register pulp vitality. *Endodont. Dent. Traumatol.* 1999; 15: 127–31.
26. Petersson K, Wennberg A, Olsson B. Radiographic and clinical estimation of endodontic treatment need. *Endodont. Dent. Traumatol.* 1986; 2: 62–4.
27. Reit C, Hollender L. Radiographic evaluation of endodontic therapy and the influence of observer variation. *Scand. J. Dent. Res.* 1983; 91: 205–12.
28. Reit C, Kvist T. Endodontic retreatment behaviour: the influence of disease concepts and personal values. *Int. Endodont. J.* 1998; 31: 358–63.

29. Ringsted J, Amtrup C, Asklund P, Baunsgaard HE, Christensen L, *et al.* Reliability of histopathological diagnosis of squamous epithelial changes of the uterine cervix. *Acta Pathol. Microbiol. Immunol. Scandi.* 1978; 86: 273–8.

30. Seltzer S, Bender IB, Zionz M. The dynamics of pulp inflammation: correlation between diagnostic data and actual histologic findings in the pulp. *Oral Surg.* 1963; 16: 846–77.

31. Sharav Y, Leviner E, Tzukert A, McGrath PA. The spatial distribution, intensity and unpleasantness of acute dental pain. *Pain* 1984; 20: 363–70.

32. Warfvinge J, Bergenholtz G. Healing capacity of human and monkey dental pulps following experimentally induced pulpitis. *Endodont. Dent. Traumatol.* 1986; 2: 256–62.

33. Wulff HR & Gotzsche PC. *Rational Diagnosis and Treatment.* Oxford: Blackwell Science, 2000.

Part 2
THE VITAL PULP

Chapter 3
The dentine–pulp complex: responses to adverse influences

Leif Olgart and Gunnar Bergenholtz

Introduction

The extent to which the dental pulp will sustain impairment in the clinical environment depends on its potential to oppose bacterial challenges and withstand injury by various forms of trauma. To understand the biological events that operate and most often prevent the pulp from suffering a permanent breakdown, the specific biological functions of both dentine and pulp under pathophysiological conditions will be addressed in this chapter. These two tissue components of the tooth form a functional unit that often is referred to as the *dentine – pulp complex* (Fig. 3.1).

Basal functions of the dentine–pulp complex

Dentine and dentinal tubules

Under normal conditions, when dentine is covered by enamel and cementum, fluid in the dentinal tubules can contract or expand to impinge on the cells in the pulp in response to thermal stimuli applied on the tooth surface. Hence, dentine of the intact tooth can transform external stimuli into an appropriate message to cells and nerves in the pulp – a feature that is useful clinically to test its vital functions (see Chapter 2).

When enamel and cementum are lost for any reason, the exposed dentinal tubules provide diffusion channels from the surface to the pulp (Fig. 3.2). In the periphery there are about 20 000 tubules per square millimeter, each having a diameter of 0.5 μm. At the pulpal ends the tubular apertures occupy a greater surface area because the tubules converge centrally and become wider (2.5–3 μm) (25). Thus, at the inner surface of dentine there are more than 50 000 tubules per square millimeter. In root dentine, especially towards the apex, the tubules become more widely spaced. Also, in the pulpal portion of root dentine they are thinner and assume a lesser diameter of ca. 1.5 μm. There are extensive branches between the tubules that allow intercommunication.

The dentinal fluid serves as a vehicle for the transport of particulate matter and macromolecules in either direction. From the pulp, plasma proteins may enter the tubules, especially following an injury (42), which results in disruption of the tight junctions between the odontoblasts (80). Similarly, following exposure to the oral environment, bacterial macromolecules may penetrate the tubules and provoke an inflammatory response in the pulp (7; see further below).

The permeability of the dentinal tubules is normally greatly restricted by a variety of tissue structures, including collagen fibers and cellular processes. The odontoblasts normally extend cytoplasmic processes into the tubules of the innermost part (0.5–1 mm) of the dentine (23, 18). Some believe that these processes extend all the way to the dentine–enamel or dentine–cementum junction. A large number of the tubules also contain nerve terminals (Fig. 3.3). Furthermore, cells belonging to the immunosurveillance system of the pulp extend dendrites into the tubules of the predentine layer (59). Consequently, the space available in the tubules for the transport of particulate matter and macromolecules

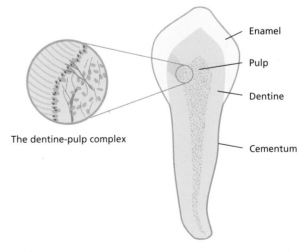

The dentine-pulp complex

Fig. 3.1 Soft tissue of the pulp surrounded by dentine and enamel and cementum. Inset depicts the interface between dentine and pulp.

is normally much smaller than the tubular space *per se* (67). This is especially true at their pulpal ends.

Primary odontoblasts

The primary odontoblasts that line the periphery of the pulp (Fig. 3.4) are highly differentiated cells. They produce primary dentine both during tooth development and after completion of root formation (Core concept 3.1). Intratubular cellular processes make the primary dentine tubular in nature. Owing to the continued function of the odontoblasts, the pulpal space gradually narrows over time and in old individuals become so small that endodontic treatment becomes difficult (see Chapter 16).

The rate at which tubular dentine forms in the adult tooth is low and seems to be influenced by sensory nerves in the pulp, because it has been shown that the absence of nerve supply to animal teeth slows down dentine formation (33). Hormonal factors also influence the secretory activity of the odontoblasts. Thus, high systemic dosages of corticosteroids, given for immunosuppression in organ-transplanted patients, strongly stimulate dentine production (57).

The primary odontoblasts may also produce new dentine at an increased rate in response to mild stimuli:

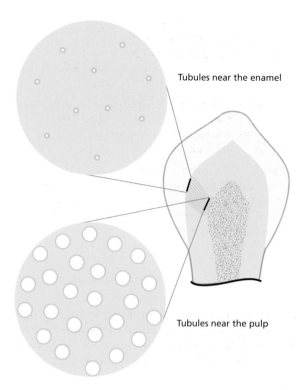

Fig. 3.2 Density of dentinal tubules in various portions of the crown region in teeth. It has been estimated that the surface area taken by cross-cut tubules is ca. 2–3% in the periphery but near the pulp the dentinal tubules assume ca. 25% of the surface area (67).

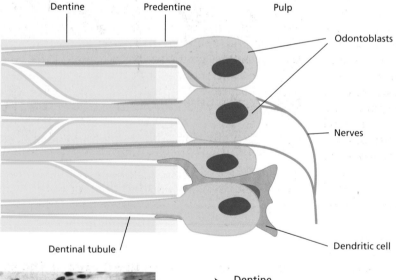

Fig. 3.3 Cellular extensions of odontoblasts, nerves and cells of the immune system (dendritic cells) that occupy the pulpal ends of the dentinal tubules.

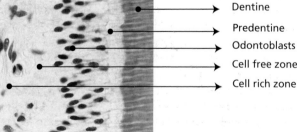

Fig. 3.4 Tissue section stained with hematoxylin and eosin showing dentine, predentine and pulp tissue proper with odontoblasts lining the periphery.

Core concept 3.1   Various terms used for different types of dentinogenesis

Primary dentine: dentine formed by primary odontoblasts.

Reparative dentine: dentine formed in response to injury by either primary or secondary odontoblasts (repairing odontoblasts). Equivalent terms commonly used are *irregular secondary dentine*, *irritation dentine* and *tertiary dentine*.

Note that primary dentine and secondary dentine are terms sometimes used to designate dentine formed by primary odontoblasts before and after termination of root development, respectively. Consequently, the term tertiary dentine has emerged to denote dentine formed in response to irritation or injury. The current text makes no such distinction.

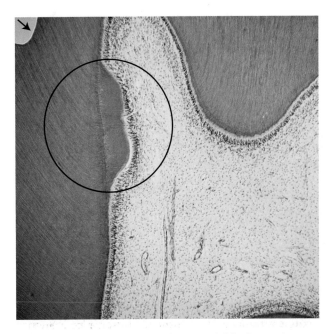

Fig. 3.5 Microphotograph shows hard tissue repair following a cavity preparation (arrow). The circle indicates the bulk of new dentine being formed.

e.g. during initial precavitated stages of enamel caries (14); by slowly progressing caries in general (13); or during a shallow preparation for restorative purposes. This is sometimes termed reactionary dentine (73).

Secondary odontoblasts

Following injury or irritation (e.g. induced by a restorative procedure or rapidly progressing caries), primary odontoblasts may die. Because these cells are postmitotic cells, they are unable to regenerate by cell division. Although the origin of the repairing cells has been the subject of much debate, mesenchymal cells in the pulp tissue *per se* have been implicated as their likely source (24). It is plausible that these repairing odontoblasts represent a population of pulpal stem cells that are recruited to the site of injury. Following their upregulation, a mineralizing matrix is laid down on the dentinal wall. Repair by secondary odontoblasts is also possible against an appropriate wound-healing agent applied to treat direct exposure of the tissue (see Chapter 6). Hence, a new generation of odontoblast-like cells, capable of making new dentine locally, can evolve in the pulp upon injury.

Secondary odontoblasts produce dentine at a rate that is dependent on the extent and duration of the injury. The development of this hard tissue leads to a compensatory increase in dentine thickness (Figs 3.5 and 3.6).

It should be noted that dentine formed by secondary odontoblasts becomes more irregular and amorphous and contains less dentinal tubules (15). These tubules will not necessarily be in direct line with the tubules of the primary dentine (Fig. 3.7). Consequently, a complex of primary and reparative dentine becomes less permeable to externally derived matter. It also follows that such dentine is less sensitive to thermal, osmotic and

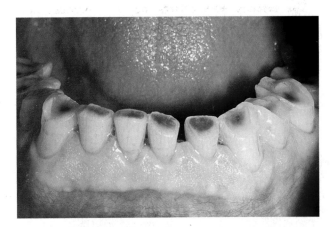

Fig. 3.6 Clinical photograph of anterior lower teeth showing extensive loss of tooth structure due to tooth wear. Reparative dentine formed in the pulp has prevented direct exposure of the tissue to the oral environment.

evaporative stimuli (15; see also Chapter 4). Yet, the quality of the new hard tissue is not always as good as that of primary dentine. When formed at a rapid pace, tissue inclusions are formed, rendering it a highly porous configuration. Similarly, hard tissue repair of pulpal wounds may occasionally show substantial defects, which makes it highly permeable to bacteria and bacterial elements. Therefore, hard tissue repair in the pulp, although adding to the defence potential of the tissue in certain aspects, should be viewed as a scar.

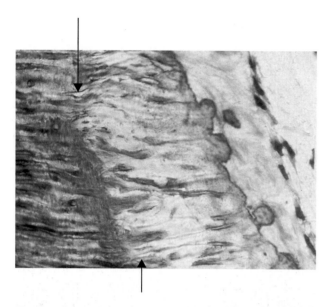

Fig. 3.7   Tissue section of an interface zone between primary dentine and reparative dentine as indicated by arrows. Note that the dentinal tubules are less numerous in the secondary dentine than in the primary dentine to the left. Also, few of the tubules are in direct line with those of the primary dentine, thus making the entire complex less permeable. Pulpal tissue and nuclei of odontoblasts are to the right. (Courtesy of Dr Lars Bjørndal and with permission of Caries Research, Karger.)

Nerves

Pulpal nerves monitor painful sensations. By virtue of their peptide content they also mediate a variety of biological functions, including the control of dentine formation, inflammatory events and tissue repair (Fig. 3.8).

There are two types of nerve fiber that mediate the sensation of pain: A-fibres conduct rapid and sharp pain sensations and belong to the myelinated group, whereas C-fibres are involved in dull aching pain and are thinner and unmyelinated. The A-fibres, mainly of the A-delta type, are preferentially located in the periphery of the pulp, where they are in close association with the odontoblasts and extend fibers to many but not all dentinal tubules. The C-fibres typically terminate in the pulp tissue *per se*, either as free nerve endings or as branches around blood vessels (61). The nature of A- and C-fibres and their respective roles in pain transmission are reviewed in Chapter 4.

Nerves belonging to the autonomic nervous system, such as sympathetic vasoconstrictor fibers, are also present (52). They enter the pulp together with blood vessels and sensory axons. Histochemically, they can be traced in the pulp via their content of noradrenaline and

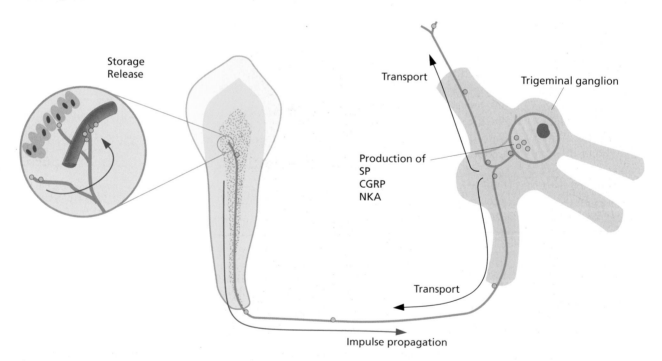

Fig. 3.8   A large portion of the sensory fibers, including C-fibers and some A-delta fibers, contain vasoactive neuropeptides such as calcitonin gene-related peptide (CGRP), substance P (SP) and neurokinin A (NKA) (83). The neuropeptides are produced in the trigeminal cell bodies and are transported via axonal flow to the nerve terminals in the pulp, where they are stored. In addition to their effect on pulpal blood flow and vessel permeability, SP and CGRP exert stimulatory effects on the growth of pulpal cells, such as fibroblasts (79), and repair odontoblasts. They are also active in the recruitment of immunocompetent cells in responses to bacterial infection.

neuropeptide Y. Upon release these substances exert contraction of the smooth-muscle sphincters in arteries and small arterioles apical to and within the pulp (63).

A parasympathetic vasodilator control implies that autonomic nerves, upon reflexogenic activation, release the classical transmitter acetylcholine and the co-stored vasoactive intestinal polypeptide (VIP). Both transmitters have been found in the pulp of many species and they have vasodilator actions (62). As yet, there is little evidence that this remote blood flow control plays an important role in the local defense of the pulp.

Vascular supply

Current knowledge of the vascular architecture of the pulp has been influenced greatly by the use of the microvascular resin cast method (Fig. 3.9) (76). This technique allows resin to fill up even the smallest capillaries of the pulp. A vascular cast is then obtained, which, following corrosion of surrounding tissue structures, can be examined in the scanning electron microscope.

In all developmental stages the crown pulp shows a larger vascular network than the root pulp, where the

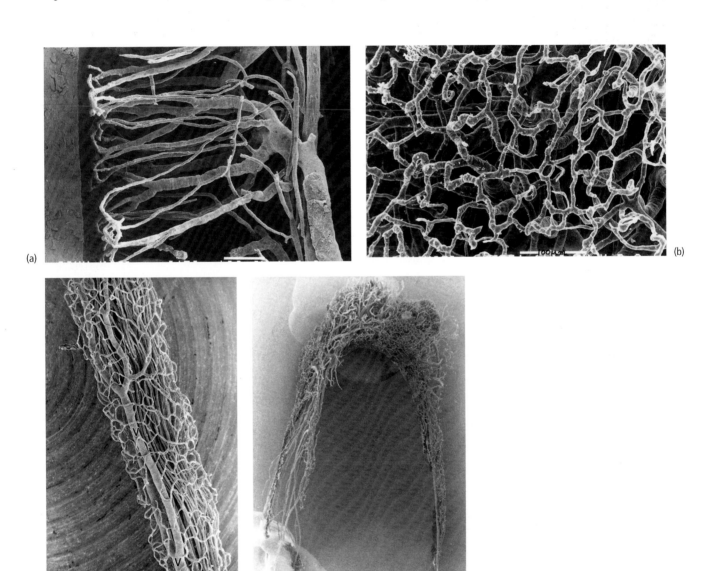

(a)

(b)

(c)

(d)

Fig. 3.9 Series of microphotographs of the vascular network in the pulp of teeth. (a) In the young tooth of dogs there is a dense terminal capillary network in the pulp–dentine border zone. (b) The superficial capillary network in the odontoblast region in a view perpendicular to the pulpal surface. (c) Blood vessels in the distal root canal of a mature dog premolar. The superficial capillaries drain directly into large venules (V). In the mature tooth, continuous dentine formation and narrowing of the pulp cavity lead to remodeling of the vascular tree. (d) The vascular network of an adult human tooth. With a narrow apical foramen, the number of arterioles is reduced to 5–8 and venules to 2–3 (41). The number of main vessels, arterioles and venules in the central pulp are also reduced and the typical hairpin loops of the terminal capillary network become less pronounced. (Courtesy of Dr K. Takahashi.)

capillary network is much denser than in more central portions of the pulp. Anastomosis between incoming and outgoing blood vessels has been observed in the central pulp of adult animal teeth (43) and seems to be more numerous in the apical pulp than in the crown pulp (39). Shunt connections between supplying and draining pulpal vessels have also been found just outside the apical foramen in the periodontal ligament (77). It is reasonable to assume that these shunts provide control of blood perfusion through the pulpal tissue. Hence, in the case of a local inflammatory event causing increased resistance to pulpal blood, arteriovenous shunts may come into play and redirect incoming blood.

Lymphatics

Both morphological and functional studies in animals show the existence of lymphatic vessels in the pulp (12, 27). These vessels are important to adjust for increased colloid osmotic pressures exerted by proteins and macromolecules accumulating extracellularly in inflamed areas. Another important function is to serve as pathways to the regional lymph nodes for antigen-presenting cells.

Cells of the immune system

The dental pulp is equipped with the necessary cells to initiate and maintain immune responses. Hence, T-lymphocytes and antigen-presenting cells (APCs) of various kinds have all been identified as residents of the normal dental pulp (36). B-cells, on the other hand, will not appear in the pulp tissue *per se* unless there is an inflammatory event.

The APC is a cell that carries stimulatory molecules of importance for T-cell activation on its surface. The Class II molecule is one such molecule and is a gene product of the major histocompatibility complex (MHC). It is able to display fragments of foreign protein for recognition by T-cells. Together with other co-stimulatory molecules, Class II molecules are found on all so-called professional APCs.

There are two types of professional APCs in the normal pulp. One type has a pronounced dendritic configuration and most likely represents the dendritic cells, which constitutively carry Class II MHC molecules on their cell surface. These dendritic cells are strategically positioned in the periphery of the pulp, where foreign antigens are most likely to enter the tissue (Figs 3.10 and 3.11). Here, they compete for available space with the odontoblasts and thus make contact with these cells via their cytoplasmatic processes (59).

As with all white blood cells, dendritic cells derive from the hematopoietic stem cell in the bone marrow.

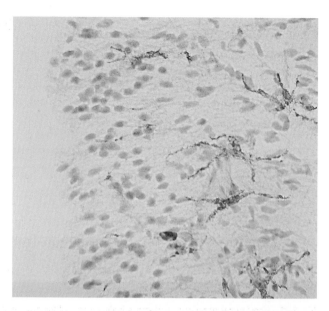

Fig. 3.10 Tissue section showing dendritic cells (stained brown) within the odontoblastic and subodontoblastic layer. Immunohistochemical staining was carried out with OX6-antibody, which is a marker for Class II MHC molecules.

They occur in most body compartments and are characterized by:

- Highly dendritic morphology
- High amounts of Class II molecules on their cell surface
- High motility
- Limited phagocytic capacity
- Efficient activation of naïve T-cells.

The Class II molecule-expressing macrophage is the other professional APC of the normal, non-inflamed pulp. These macrophages are distributed in a remarkably high number in the pulp and seem to form a dense network together with pulpal dendritic cells (35). As in other connective tissues, macrophages in the pulp are heterogeneous in terms of phenotype and function. Hence, there are resident macrophages (histiocytes) that do not carry Class II molecules. These cells are primarily located perivascularly. Other macrophages express various combinations of cell surface markers, including Class II molecules.

The normal pulp also harbors a limited number of T-helper and T-cytotoxic cells. These cells may represent circulating memory cells (Fig. 3.12).

Basal maintenance

Blood flow

The blood flow through the young adult pulp during resting conditions is relatively high compared with

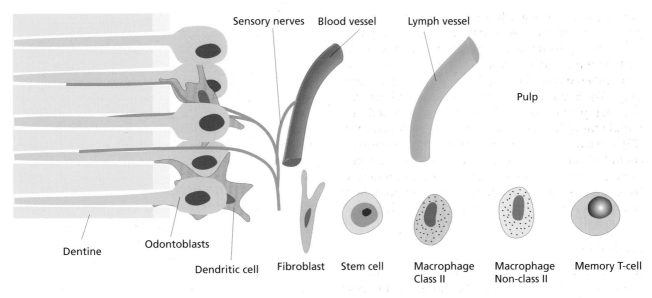

Fig. 3.11 Constituents of primary significance in the defense of the pulp against foreign substances, including bacterial elements, make up the innate 'first line of defense'.

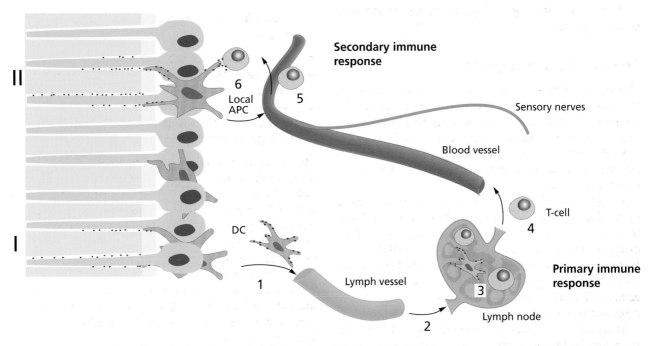

Fig. 3.12 Antigen-specific T-cells are developed in the pulp following primary (I) and secondary (II) antigen exposures along dentinal tubules. Dendritic cells (1 in figure) capture protein antigen for processing to peptide fragments and carry (2) and present peptide fragments in the context of the Class II molecules on their cell surface to naïve T-cells in the regional lymph nodes (3: primary immune response). Following clonal expansion, these cells enter the circulation (4 in figure). Following their patrolling of tissues as memory T-cells, they may participate in secondary immune responses at local sites, e.g. in the pulp (5 in figure), if exposed to the appropriate antigen by local APC (6 in figure). This route constitutes adaptive pathogen-specific immunity.

that of other oral tissues (54). In the adult dog, blood flow per 100 g of tissue is ca. 40 ml/min in teeth with a fully formed apex. By comparison, in the gingiva it is ca. 30 ml/min.

Local control

The level of the resting blood flow in the pulp is to a great extent controlled by the neuropeptides, substance P (SP) and calcitonin gene-related peptide (CGRP). Both CGRP and SP maintain a continuous relaxation of feeding arterioles (11). This continuous influence on the blood supply to the pulp depends on a basal release of the peptides without apparent nerve activation.

Nitric oxide (NO) – a short-lived gas molecule that is produced enzymatically in the endothelial cell lining of the vessels – also serves to maintain a physiological blood perfusion of the pulp (38). It has a powerful vasodilator action and, unlike neuropetides, exerts relaxation of the draining venules in the pulp under physiological conditions (11). (See Advanced concept 3.1.)

Remote control

The regulatory control of pulpal blood flow also involves autonomic nerves. This remote system influences blood circulation in the pulp as well as in adjacent tissues within the same innervation territory.

Although parasympathetic vasodilator nerves do not seem to play a significant role, there is firm evidence for sympathetic vasoconstrictor control in the dental pulp. The system does not seem to be active tonically and may not support local moment-to-moment demands of the tissue. However, physical and mental stress trigger sympathetic vasoconstriction in the oral region, including the pulp, as part of the general fight-and-flight reaction (63).

Advanced concept 3.1   Mechanisms regulating pulpal blood flow

The physiological regulation of blood flow and tissue pressures in the pulp has been studied in some detail in animal teeth. For example, treatment with antagonists to neuropeptides, or axotomy leading to degeneration of the sensory innervation, almost halves the pulpal blood flow and reduces the interstitial fluid pressure in the pulp. Pharmacological blocking of NO production also reduces blood flow but, at the same time, increases tissue pressure. Thus, when the physiological action of NO is intact, flow resistance in draining vessels is low (dilated vessels), allowing appropriate blood flow, volume and tissue pressure in the pulp (11).

In general terms, both the sympathetic and the parasympathetic systems operate at the general or segmental levels and tend to ignore the needs of an individual tissue such as the pulp. Therefore, the locally active mechanisms most favorably meet the nutritional demands of the healthy pulp. Suitable adjustment of the resting blood flow in the pulp is mainly the result of a balance between the locally governed relaxing factors and a certain myogenic constrictive tone of the vessels.

Appropriate responses of the healthy pulp to non-destructive stimuli

Functionally, the unique dentine–odontoblast unit acts as a transducer of various external stimuli of moderate intensity. This enables the tissue constituents of the peripheral pulp to be alerted appropriately. Thus, in the intact healthy tooth, a limited cold stimulus or elastic deformation of dentine due to a sudden heavy load on the tooth is transformed to minute and rapid movements of the dentinal fluid (17, 82). Such movements excite adjacent nerves, resulting in a rapid reflex withdrawal reaction; this is immediately followed by a brief, sharp pain, alerting the individual to further withdrawal. This is an important alarm system protecting the tooth from overload by mastication forces for example.

In parallel there is a transient increase in blood perfusion in the pulp (53). This is part of an instant local defense reaction and is brought about by the fine terminal branches of sensory nerves supplying both cells in the odontoblast region as well as small feeding arterioles deeper in the pulp. Excitation of the most terminal branches in the peripheral area of the pulp results in a reflex propagation of impulses in adjacent nerve terminals belonging to the same nerves (axon reflex) (64, 82). Because these nerves contain vasodilating neuropeptides (66, 52), it takes only a few seconds for a short-lasting (< 10 min) increase in blood perfusion of the pulp. The CGRP is the dominating mediator of this response. As a result of the transient increase in local blood volume, pulpal tissue pressure increases. (See Advanced concept 3.2.)

Collectively, the reflex withdrawal, the pain and the local blood flow increase are judged as being appropriate and essential responses for the protection and maintenance of normal function of the pulp.

Effects of intermittent and longstanding irritation

Episodes of sustained and iterated irritation of the intact tooth or an exposed dentine surface cause extended

Advanced concept 3.2 Spreading of vascular reactions

A transient increase in pulpal blood flow is produced by electrical or noxious stimulation of adjacent tissues and teeth, as demonstrated in anesthetized animals (71, 62). Thus pinching or insertion of an injection needle in the vestibular oral mucosa and delivery of a short train of electrical impulses to the lip or adjacent teeth give rise to a blood flow increase several minutes long. This phenomenon demonstrates the extensive branching of sensory nerves in and around teeth and their wide receptive fields, implying that spreading of neurogenic vascular reactions may take place between different oral tissues within the same nerve territory.

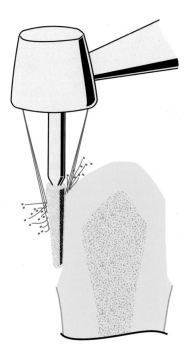

Fig. 3.13 Preparing teeth for restorations generates frictional heat, which causes dehydration and tissue damage to the pulp. Such injury is lessened by proper water irrigation during the cutting procedure.

pulpal reaction and mobilize elements in a proinflammatory response. The predisposition of the pulp to react with more complex but transient cascades of events is shared by most peripheral tissues and is an important function to maintain and regain health. As far as the pulp is concerned, there are some unique features that affect its ability to sustain injury:

- The encasement within rigid hard tissue walls restricts edema formation and expansion. In other words, the pulpal tissue is confined to a *low-compliance system*.
- The lack of collateral blood supply in one-rooted teeth limits the supply and drainage of blood.

Both of these factors have implications for the way in which inflammatory responses develop in the pulp and may, on severe challenge, be contributory to pulpal tissue breakdown.

Restorative procedures

Restorative procedures undertaken in dentistry to manage caries, fractures and tooth losses cannot normally be undertaken without generating damage to the pulp. It is primarily the cutting procedure that causes pulpal irritation, related primarily to the release of frictional heat from the use of rotary instruments. Because the thermal conductivity of dentine is low, it is primarily dehydrating effects that are damaging; this will be the case with insufficient water irrigation (Fig. 3.13). Direct heat injury does not normally occur unless the procedure is carried out close to the pulp. Also, the frequent touching of the tooth structure by improperly centered instruments may cause traumatic effects. All these injuries cause neurovascular responses of a nature similar to those described above.

A preparation trauma with rotary instruments is likely to injure the odontoblast layer (80). Owing to dehydra-

tion of the tubular content, odontoblasts may even be sucked into the dentinal tubules. This particular feature is termed *odontoblast aspiration* and can be observed in tissue sections by the presence of their nuclear profiles within the dentinal tubules.

Injury by preparation trauma to the odontoblast layer opens up pathways for a peripherally directed flow of tissue fluid along the tubules. The fluid flow is possible due to the higher tissue pressure in the pulp than externally. Under normal conditions it is 5–10 mmHg higher in the pulp (27). This corresponds fairly well with the local blood pressure. Under inflammation, the pulp tissue pressure increases. By contrast, it may be reduced during flight-and-fight reactions, apprehension (9) and in the use of anesthetic solution containing vasoconstrictor (82).

Potential protective roles of the dentinal fluid

Provided that anesthesia with a vasoconstrictor is not used and as long as a dentine exposure remains open, there will be a slow continuous outward flow of fluid along the dentinal tubules ($0.4\,\mu l/min/cm^2$) (Fig. 3.14). It has been estimated that the individual tubule can be emptied and refilled ten times a day (15).

Both the continuous and the stimulus-induced dentinal fluid flow may serve to limit invasive threats. Following exposure of dentine to the oral environment,

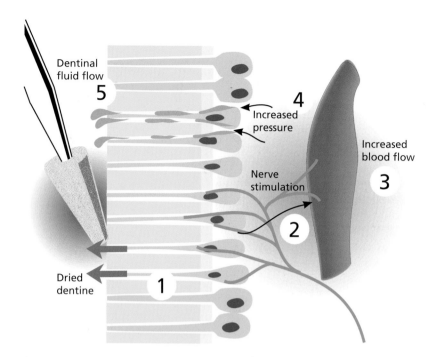

Dentinal fluid flow

5

4

Increased pressure

Nerve stimulation

Increased blood flow

3

2

Dried dentine

1

Fig. 3.14 When exposed dentine is dried (1 in figure) or subjected to a painful stimulus such as a blast of compressed air or scraping with an explorer, the outward movement of the dentinal fluid is rapidly accelerated. This results in nerve stimulation (2 in figure) and a nerve-mediated increase of pulpal blood flow (3 in figure). Consequently, many vessels, which during resting conditions were only partly blood-filled, now fill up and increase the volume of filled blood vessels in the pulp. This in turn requires room for expansion (4 in figure). Because the space for the encapsulated pulp is restricted, the instant fill-up of vessels prompts an increase in the interstitial tissue pressure (28). The resultant force enhances the outward filtration of dentinal fluid (5 in figure) (9, 53).

bacterial elements may enter the pulp along the tubules by diffusion. However, a peripheral flow of dentinal fluid both dilutes and opposes such an inward transport of elements. Thus, freshly exposed dentine subjected to a painful stimulus has some capacity to flush the tubules, whereby diffusion of harmful agents is counteracted (81, 1). It needs to be recognized, however, that the peripheral flow of fluid cannot completely prevent the inward diffusion of bacterial elements (8). Also, under periods of negative tissue pressure noxious agents on the surface of dentine, by virtue of the fluid, may be drawn into the pulp and aggravate a pulpal lesion (82, 9).

Nevertheless, the protective effect of the fluid is likely to be enhanced during pulpal inflammation and may contribute to the process of pulpal healing and repair seen following bacterial challenge of dentine (51, 84, 8). Along with the increase of plasma proteins in the extravascular tissue compartment, the content of plasma proteins will increase in the dentinal fluid as well. This means that a variety of antimicrobial elements, such as immunoglobulin and complement factors, are carried to the periphery of dentine and may bind to bacteria and bacterial macromolecules. Such a binding is likely to impede their further penetration to the pulp. The increased concentration of plasma proteins further affects the viscosity of the fluid and makes it less pervious. Thus, several factors associated with the dentinal fluid may aid in limiting threats that may follow exposure of dentine to the oral environment.

Core concept 3.2

- Neurovascular reactions, including vasodilation and increased vessel permeability in response to external, relatively innocuous stimuli, are proinflammatory events.
- They are reversible in the normal pulp and serve to support the tissue in overcoming potential threats.
- The responses are significant because:
  — challenged cells are dependent on optimal nutrition;
  — clearance of harmful products from the affected tissue compartment is augmented; and
  — a moderate increase in tissue pressure tends to limit invasion of noxious elements along patent dentinal tubules by increasing the peripheral flow of dentinal fluid.

Blood flow changes

Preparation of dentine by rotary instruments results instantaneously in increased pulpal blood flow (Fig. 3.15). Activation of the peptide-containing sensory nerve arrangement, described above, mediates this response (see Core concept 3.2).

In deep-cavity or crown preparations, a direct effect of moderate heat on pulpal cells and vessels also augments pulpal blood flow. Excessive generation of heat represents an inappropriate operative procedure and cannot be abated by the local protective mechanisms, thus potentially causing serious damage to the tissue. For this

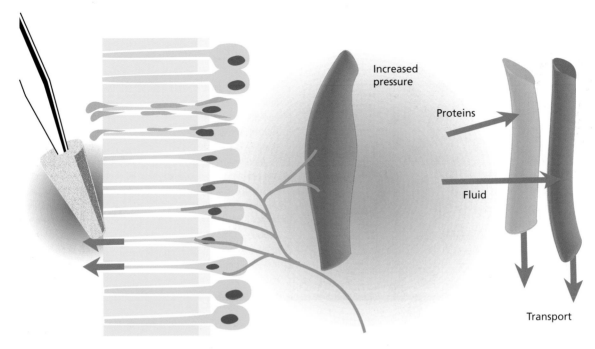

Fig. 3.15 Preparation of dentine for restoration causes an increased pulpal blood flow that results in accumulation of fluid and macromolecules outside the leaking vessels. In turn, this will cause a sustained increase in intrapulpal pressure, which may be double that in the normal pulp (33). The fluid pressure promptly causes an enhanced outward dentinal fluid flow in exposed dentine. The interstitial fluid accumulation is, however, limited by the counteracting pressure increase and by removal of the proteins via lymph vessels. The surplus fluid is slowly transported away by absorption via intact venules in adjacent tissue compartments (28). Adjacent lymph and blood vessels also contribute to the clearance of noxious substances.

reason, it is essential that a proper water-cooling system is in effect when cutting teeth with rotary instruments.

Preparation in vital dentine usually makes the use of local anesthetics necessary. As a result, the appropriate nerve-mediated vascular responses to the preparation trauma will be attenuated for a while. This is not regarded as a serious problem because pulpal nerves are only blocked for a few minutes after injection. However, when a vasoconstrictor (adrenaline/epinephrine) is used, there will be a long-lasting period of reduction of basal blood flow: infiltration anesthesia in the upper front tooth region may lower blood perfusion of the pulp in adjacent teeth by 70–80% for > 1h (65, 26, 58). These changes are not as prominent with a mandibular block but the pulp is likely to be vulnerable to the clinical procedures directed to the tooth structure. It is therefore advisable to avoid catecholamine vasoconstrictors when preparing for restorations in teeth with vital pulp.

Migration of inflammatory cells

A local injury to the pulp activates the migration of inflammatory cells. Following the injury, a variety of soluble chemotactic factors are formed that prompt neutrophils, monocytes and T- and B-cells to leave the vasculature. The neutrophils arrive in large numbers

and their primary function is to kill bacteria. If there is no or little bacterial exposure in conjunction with the injury, e.g. after a preparation trauma, the infiltration of neutrophils will be limited and they will disappear within a few days. On bacterial challenge in conjunction with leaky restorations, neutrophils may accumulate in large numbers and enter the pulpal ends of the dentinal tubules (Fig. 3.16). In such a position they contribute to pulpal protection by blocking both the diffusion of bacterial macromolecules as well as the invasion of bacterial organisms (8). (See Advanced concept 3.3.)

Peripheral blood monocytes also infiltrate the site of injury. Once in the tissue, monocytes become activated and turn into macrophages with a multitude of important functions, such as:

- Bacterial killing
- Cleansing the tissue of cellular debris
- Antigen presentation
- Tissue repair by stimulating angiogenesis and fibroblast proliferation.

Effects of potentially destructive stimuli

In the clinical environment a variety of potentially destructive elements, primarily of a bacterial nature,

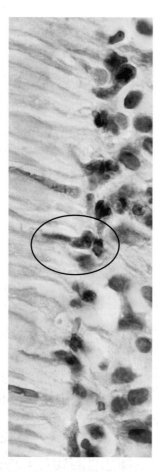

Fig. 3.16   Following a bacterial challenge of exposed dentine, neutrophils may enter the tubules of the affected dentine at the pulpal end (encircled) and prevent the dissemination of bacterial elements to the pulp. (From Bergenholtz and Lindhe (10).)

can endanger the continued vital function of the pulp. Also, dental procedures and various forms of accidental trauma may cause injury leading to pulpal breakdown.

Caries

Caries is a most common cause of bacterial provocation of the pulp. In the process of destroying the tooth structure, a variety of substances are produced that evoke inflammatory lesions. Most often the pulp is able to sustain the irritation, especially when caries is confined to primary dentine only. By contrast, once into reparative dentine or the pulp tissue proper, severe inflammatory involvement usually emerges (69, 45) that may jeopardize the continued vital function of the tissue.

Caries is defined as *initial caries* as long as the process has not resulted in macroscopic destruction of the enamel (cavitation). In reality, dentine is often involved early on, in spite of the fact that the lesion may be detected only following plaque removal and air-drying. Consequently, the pulp becomes alerted and prompted to respond to caries at a very early phase (14, 16, 45).

The progression of caries tends to be intermittent, with periods of rapid destruction interchanged with periods where caries advances at a slow pace. Sometimes it may be stopped temporarily or permanently (arrested caries; Fig. 3.17). The character of the caries lesion in these respects influences the degree of pulpal inflammatory involvement.

Pulpal responses to caries confined to primary dentine

Given the nature of the carious process, inflammatory tissue changes as well as repair phenomena can be seen in the pulp at all stages of an active lesion. The extent of the response depends on the quantity of bacterial irritants that reach the pulp at a given point. It is also a function of distance. Consequently, while still in the periphery, bacteria will release substances that will have to travel much further than in a lesion close to the pulp. However, the distance factor is generally of lesser significance when reactive processes in terms of intratubular mineralization (*dentinal sclerosis*) have emerged.

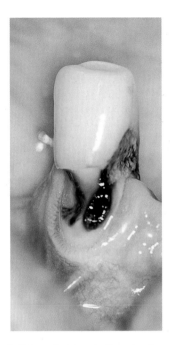

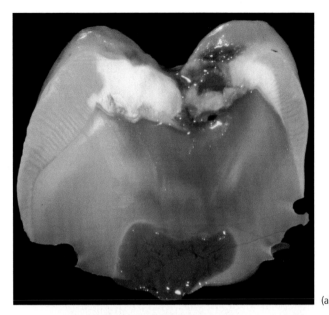

(a)

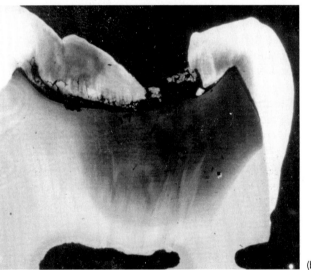

(b)

Fig. 3.17 Clinical photograph demonstrating extensive caries in the cervical region of a lower canine. Part of the lesion seems to be arrested, as indicated by the pigmented, leather-like appearance at the buccal aspect. At the mesial surface there is plaque accumulation and the lesion is soft to probing, indicating progression.

Fig. 3.18 (a) Central part of an active caries lesion in a molar. (b) Microradiograph shows radiopacities within the demineralized dentine, which, towards the pulpal aspect, is bordered by a rim of hypermineralized dentine. (Courtesy of Dr L. Bjørndal with permission of Caries Research, Karger.)

Dentinal sclerosis

In relatively deep carious lesions the dentine may become hypermineralized within a limited area pulpally to the advancing demineralization front, including areas within the zone of demineralization (Fig. 3.18). Depending on the size and rate of penetration of the caries lesion, the formation of dentinal sclerosis can be explained in the following manner: the transmission of bacterial irritants takes place (in initial caries) through the demineralized precavitated enamel and may cause a pulpal response that leads to dentinal sclerosis even before evidence of mineral loss in dentine. Consequently, hypermineralization may be an effect of enhanced growth of peritubular dentine (14), which may continue in particular on slowly progressing caries. Such dentine receives a transparent and glass-like appearance. At least temporarily, dentinal sclerosis may block or reduce the permeability of the involved dentine to bacterial elements.

At a certain point during initial caries, the enamel will be demineralized through the entire enamel layer thickness and the initial dentinal sclerosis will be dissolved. The pattern of sclerosis from this point will include reprecipitation of crystals of various forms and composition of hydroxyapatite in the caries process. Upon further advancement of the caries process, these miner-

alizations continue to be dissolved and new precipitates may appear in tubules even closer to the pulp. Hence, a caries lesion in dentine is a dynamic process that includes events of breakdown and remineralization in different parts of the tooth structure where caries is active (72) (Fig. 3.18).

Dentinal sclerosis can also occur in the absence of caries. It is a common change associated with ageing and develops successively in a coronal direction from the apical region of the tooth, as individuals grow older (56). It may also develop at the peripheral ends of the tubules subsequent to their oral exposure by abrasion and cervical erosion. After a period of time, mineral salts are deposited, which will reduce the sensitivity of the involved dentine.

Mechanisms and nature of the pulpal response

It is important to understand that, already during its initial penetration of dentine, caries evokes inflammatory responses in the pulp long before bacteria in the caries process have reached the pulp. Support for this view has been gained from experimental studies in humans and animals where known components of bacteria in dental plaque were topically applied to freshly cut dentine (10, 7). Within hours, and in association with the pulpal ends of the challenged dentine, an acute inflammatory response developed in the pulp. These experiments suggest that dentinal tubules indeed are permeable to bacterial elements and support the view that even a small caries lesion when just penetrating the enamel is able to provoke an inflammatory pulpal lesion (16). In this aspect, however, it should be mentioned that the pulpal response, including changes in the odontoblast–predentine region, has shown a more pronounced pattern in active initial caries lesions compared with similarly sized slowly progressing lesions, hereby indicating the reversible nature of the early pulpal response (14).

During growth and cell death of micro-organisms in the caries process, elements are liberated that may initiate pulpal responses by different mechanisms. These include:

(1) Release of inflammatory mediators from pulpal cells, including odontoblasts (prostaglandins, leukotrienes and proinflammatory cytokines).
(2) Penetration of bacterial components, which act as antigens and evoke an immune response.

The first cells to encounter the bacterial challenge are the peripherally located odontoblasts and dendritic cells. Both are capable of activating a variety of effector cells of innate and specific immunity. The highly motile dendritic cells, after obtaining protein fragments, will move to regional lymph nodes and initiate a primary immune response upon which there will be recruitment of antigen-specific T-cells (see Fig. 3.12).

Neutrophils will not normally infiltrate the pulp during early dentinal caries. Instead, the infiltrate is most often composed of macrophages, T-cells and plasma cells. These mononuclear cell infiltrates can be seen either in clusters or dispersed in the pulp tissue proper underneath the caries lesion.

Also, the number of Class II molecule-expressing cells is increased (37), represented by an accumulation of dendritic cells and Class II molecule-expressing

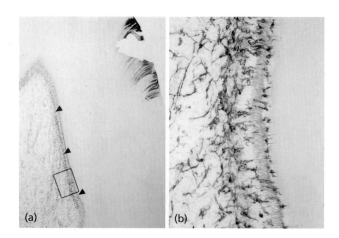

Fig. 3.19 (a) Numerous Class II molecule-expressing cells (stained brown) accumulated underneath a superficial caries lesion, extending into the dentine of a human tooth (dark stain, upper right). (b) Extension of dendrites into the tubules. (Courtesy of Dr T. Okiji.)

macrophages (Fig. 3.19). These cells participate in the secondary immune response taking place in the pulp and are likely to enhance the defense capacity of the tissue.

Although the inflammatory reaction may be pronounced on rapidly progressing caries in a young tooth where the distance to the pulp is short, it is less distinct in a mature tooth where caries is progressing slowly (Fig. 3.20). In fact, in the latter the inflammatory activity is limited and sometimes the only evidence of bacterial irritation is the emergence of a small rim of reparative dentine (13). The number of Class II molecule-expressing cells is also decreased, suggesting that the influx of inflammatogenic substances in these lesions is reduced or inhibited (37). The fact that the tissue change becomes so limited is likely to be explained by the previously described reactive processes taking place in dentine. The formation of reparative dentine also contributes to a reduction of dentine permeability. Yet, in the periphery of the caries lesion where new dentinal tubules become involved, inflammatory/immunological responses and subsequent repair phenomena continue to emerge.

In teeth where caries has progressed at a slow pace, pulps display increased fibrosis at the expense of the nervous and vascular supply. Intrapulpal mineralizations also may develop. Thus, tissue changes of this nature render the pulp tissue less cellular and less resistant to iterated injury.

Response to deep caries

Once the caries lesion with its bacterial front has penetrated the primary dentine and advanced to reparative dentine and/or to the pulp tissue proper, a massive mobilization of the inflammatory response will take

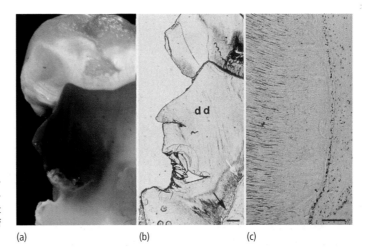

Fig. 3.20 (a) Microphotograph giving overview of a slowly progressing carious lesion with a total surface breakdown. (b) Microradiographic view shows tubular reparative dentine in the adjacent pulp. (c) Pulpal tissue is free of inflammatory infiltrates. (Courtesy of Dr Lars Bjørndal.)

(a)   (b)   (c)

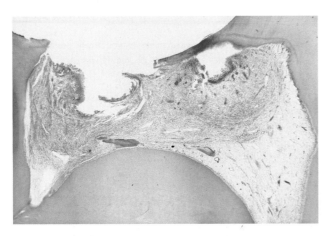

Fig. 3.21 Histological section of a pulp specimen demonstrating a microabscess associated with a caries exposure. Note that the remainder of the pulp shows a fairly normal appearance. (Courtesy of Dr Nicola Perrrini.)

place (69, 45) (Fig. 3.21). A most conspicuous feature is the aggregation of neutrophils. Often a local abscess has developed (Fig. 3.22). Clinically, upon excavation of caries, a droplet of pus may sometimes appear from the exposure site.

Although short-lived in an acute inflammatory lesion, neutrophils release tissue-destructive elements, including oxygen radicals, lysosomal enzymes and excessive amounts of nitric oxide. Collectively these agents contribute to degradation of the pulpal tissue (see Advanced concept 3.4). There will also be renewed and intense immunological activity, as expressed by an accumulation of Class II molecule-expressing cells (dendritic cells and macrophages) (37). Collectively, this means that the microbial load on the pulp has increased dramatically and the vital functions of the pulp at this stage are clearly threatened (Fig. 3.22). Nevertheless, in spite of the massive bacterial attack and the intense

---

Advanced concept 3.4   Nitric oxide in the pulpal response to a carious exposure

In acute pulpal inflammatory lesions the formation of nitric oxide (NO) is dramatically increased (46). Endotoxins from Gram-negative bacteria and cytokines, such as interleukin-1, tumor necrosis factor and interferon-gamma, are typical activators triggering a rapid production of NO-producing enzymes (74). This occurs both in immune cells and in vascular endothelium in areas close to and around an inflammatory site (55). Although the functional importance of this massive and long-lasting NO formation has not been specifically addressed for the pulp, NO is regarded as a central component in natural (innate) immunity aimed at eliminating invading microorganisms. Hence, NO can increase the blood flow and relax the draining vessels, thereby supporting appropriate outflow and pressure adjustment (11). In addition, NO may exert antibacterial activity and has an inhibitory effect on neutrophil infiltration in the acute phase of inflammation (44). In fact, the final destruction of microorganisms phagocytized by macrophages is due to NO (29). These immune cells produce large amounts of NO. Thus, NO may assist in modifying the acute inflammatory response.

Excess of NO, although beneficial, may also provide destructive effects. It can react with free oxygen radicals produced during the inflammatory process to form the stable peroxynitrite. Peroxynitrite is a strong oxidant that causes tissue injury (5). Thus, although NO supports the defense response in moderate tissue inflammation, in severe reactions such as that upon caries exposure of the pulp it may become severely toxic and contribute to the breakdown of the tissue.

---

inflammatory response, the pulp may retain vital functions for a period of time, although survival is unpredictable.

Neurovascular events
Besides the accumulation of neutrophils and immunocompetent cells near the caries lesion, the inflammatory

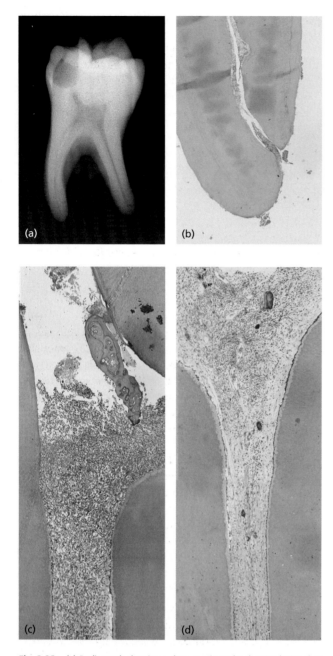

Fig. 3.22 (a) Radiograph showing a deep, mesio-occlusal caries lesion that has advanced to the pulp in a lower molar. Histological examination of the pulp in the extracted tooth reveals partial pulpal breakdown at the breakthrough of the caries lesion. (b) The apical pulp displays a normal appearance. (c) An intense inflammatory infiltrate extends into the orifice of the mesial root canal. (d) The pulp tissue of the distal root canal shows less leukocyte infiltration with an intact odontoblast cell layer. (Courtesy of Dr Domenico Ricucci.)

response also involves extensive neurovascular reactions. These responses consist of branching and sprouting of neuropeptide-containing nerve terminals, increased pulpal blood flow, increased vascular permeability and extravasation of fluid and plasma proteins.

Core concept 3.3   Tissue changes in the pulp to caries

Caries confined to dentine

- During its course towards the pulp, caries completely destroys dentine and transforms it into a mushy mass of decomposed tissue containing an abundance of bacterial elements that can provoke inflammatory changes in the pulp. Yet, owing to reactive processes in dentine (dentinal sclerosis) and defense responses of the pulp, the vital functions of the tissue are seldom endangered as long as caries is confined to primary dentine.
- The inflammatory involvement with superficial and medium-deep caries in dentine is normally limited to the superficial portions of the pulp. Inflammatory cells, primarily mononuclear leukocytes (macrophages, plasma cells and T-cells), infiltrate the tissue but to a limited degree. Signs of repair (e.g. the formation of reparative dentine) are often, but not always, a prominent feature.
- Pulp in teeth with longstanding and/or slowly progressing caries may display increased fibrosis, reduced nervous and vascular supply and intrapulpal mineralizations.

Direct exposure

- Next to the bacterial front there is accumulation of neutrophils and tissue destruction.
- In adjoining areas there is:
  — immune cell activation and accumulation of macrophages
  — branching and sprouting of neuropeptide-containing nerve terminals
  — intense vascular activity and localized increased tissue pressure.

Total necrosis of the pulp may develop after a period of time.

In the process, severe painful symptoms may or may not appear (see Chapter 4). The locally increased tissue pressure as a result of vascular leakage may lead to stasis and local ischemia, thus contributing to the risk of pulpal necrosis.

The previous assumption that increased pulpal tissue pressure as a dominant factor would compress thin-walled veins in a vicious circle resulting in a dramatic reduction of pulpal blood flow and possibly pulpal necrosis (strangulation theory) is misleading and has found no support in recent literature (67). Thus, the clearance of excess fluid and proteins via blood and lymph vessels (28) in the vicinity of the reaction zone, as described above, gives the pulp relief and may allow it to survive for a period of time.

A summary of the tissue changes in the pulp as a response to caries can be found in Core concept 3.3.

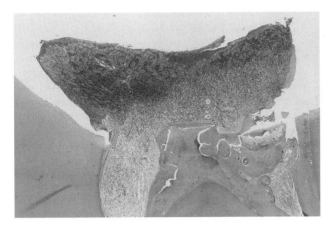

Fig. 3.23 Microphotograph of a pulp polyp extending from the pulp of a young tooth broken down by caries. Note the dense inflammatory infiltrate in the proliferating tissue. (Courtesy of Dr Domenico Ricucci.)

Response of the periapical tissue

The inflammatory response of the pulp to an open exposure by caries is often confined to the site of breakthrough, with the apical portion of the pulp remaining non-inflamed. The lesion in certain cases may be extensive and involve the periapical tissue adjacent to apical foramina. These changes include mobilization of APCs (60), edema formation and some bone resorption, which may be visible radiographically (Chapters 9 and 15).

Pulp polyp

When the pulp chamber is wide, as in young individuals, caries may initiate a proliferative response and cause what is termed a *pulp polyp* (Fig. 3.23). A prerequisite is that the roof of the pulpal chamber has been totally destroyed. The tissue proliferation is an expression of the reparative phase of the pulpal response and is made possible by the fact that the process no longer occurs within a closed system. Subsequently, pulpal polyps may become epithelialized upon making contact with the gingival tissue.

Dental treatment procedures

The primary objective of dental treatment procedures is to eliminate infectious agents in the treatment of caries and periodontal disease and to restore tooth function and aesthetics, but these procedures can seldom be carried out without causing pulpal injury. In the short term, most irritation occurring in this context is sustainable by the pulp. It is only following advanced disease and the use of too damaging or inappropriate procedures that the risk of severe injury is imminent.

Common threats to the pulp relate to:

- The damage inflicted in conjunction with the use of rotary instruments.
- Leakage of bacterial elements from the oral environment along margins of restorations that show poor adaptation to the remaining tooth structure.
- Toxic effects of medicaments and components of materials used to restore cavities and cement crowns and inlays.

It is reasonable to assume that preparation traumas, bacterial influences and material toxicities in combination cause a cumulative effect and are thus more detrimental to the pulp than each of these factors alone (8).

Preparation trauma

A cutting procedure by rotary instruments will not normally cause damage to the extent that the vital function of the pulp is jeopardized. Preparation for restoration close to the pulp may, however, generate substantial frictional heat to cause a significant and detrimental temperature increase in the pulp. Repair will usually ensue, but the formation of reparative dentine can be extensive and render the pulp vulnerable to repeated injury. In fact, clinical follow-ups of teeth restored with cast restorations (full crowns and teeth included as abutments in bridgeworks) have shown that pulpal necrosis may occur with a frequency of 10–15% over a period of 5–10 years (8). Often one will find that the coronal portion of the pulp in such teeth is obliterated by reparative dentine, making endodontic therapy precarious.

Another complication to cavity and crown preparation is internal bleeding. In rare cases it may be so extensive that pulpal necrosis occurs almost instantaneously. The tooth structure of such teeth may turn red and later a gray color.

Bacterial leakage

In spite of substantial efforts over the years to improve restorative materials, including resin composites, and the techniques for their use, the shrinkage of these materials after setting is critical (75, 21). Shrinkage builds up strains in the filling that later may result in gaps at the tooth/restoration interface. This may allow bacteria and bacterial elements in the oral environment to affect the pulp. The term *bacterial leakage* is used to imply this form of pulpal irritation.

Research in recent years has indeed demonstrated that bacterial leakage in restoration margins is a major threat to the vital functions of the pulp subsequent to restorative therapies (8, 67). In particular on deep and extensive exposures of dentine, the infectious load on the pulp can be substantial (Fig. 3.24).

In principle, the inflammatory events of the pulp in response to these bacterial exposures are similar to those

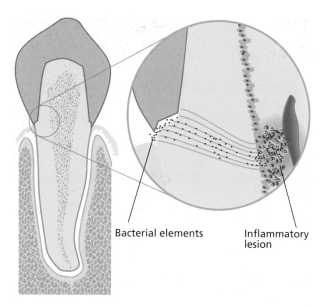

Bacterial elements   Inflammatory
                            lesion

Fig. 3.24 In contraction gaps or after incomplete coverage of dentine following restorative procedures, bacterial elements in the oral cavity may gain access to pulp along the exposed dentinal tubules. This is regarded as a serious threat to the pulp because it may induce painful symptoms and inflammatory lesions in the pulp.

Key literature 3.1

Lundy and Stanley (51), in an experimental study in humans, prepared small but deep dentine cavities in teeth scheduled for extraction. The cavities were left unrestored to the oral environment for various periods of time to observe and correlate pulp tissue responses to the degree of occurring painful symptoms. The initial response of the pulp after 1–2 days consisted of severe infiltrates of neutrophils. However, at subsequent observations there was no breakdown of the pulps even if the remaining dentine wall to the pulp was thin. Instead, reduced inflammation and evidence of repair were seen as early as 9 days after dentine exposure. Weeks and months after the initiation of oral exposure, normal pulpal tissue and the formation of reparative dentine were seen in the large majority of specimens. On testing for sensitivity, teeth became increasingly painful over the first few days. These symptoms subsequently subsided, along with recovery of the pulp. Findings confirm the potential of the pulp to withstand bacterial challenges when there is still a wall of dentine separating the pulp from the oral environment. Both reduced or blocked dentine permeability and inflammatory and immunological responses in the pulp are mechanisms that are likely to impede further bacterial irritation. Experiments in both humans and primates employing challenges of carious dentine or a mixture of bacterial products corroborate these findings (48, 84).

detailed for caries, but there are some distinct differences. Neutrophils play an important role in the initial responses owing to the more sudden and extensive bacterial exposure than that in the relatively slowly progressing caries lesion. These cells accumulate in areas of the pulp that correspond to the involved dentinal tubules. Chemotactic stimuli also prompt neutrophils to migrate into the tubules. This is probably the most significant defense factor that, in addition to the protective effects of the dentinal fluid (described above), helps to block further penetration of bacteria and bacterial elements into the pulp. Collectively, these mechanisms are likely to explain why pulpal repair and healing are still possible even when a restoration does not completely seal its margin (8, Key literature 3.1).

Contrary to caries, occlusion of dentinal tubules by mineral deposits seldom occurs underneath fillings. Thus, dentine in areas unaffected by caries may remain permeable and sensitive unless reparative dentine has been formed in the pulp.

Toxic effects of restorative materials

In addition to the trauma from preparing teeth for restoration and the subsequent leakage of bacterial elements, constituents of restorative materials may have an adverse influence on the pulp. For many years the toxicity of restorative materials was regarded as the major cause of adverse pulpal responses in restorative proce-

dures. However, research in recent years has shown that, contrary to previous beliefs, toxic components in restorative materials are a lesser threat to the pulp than previously anticipated (8). This has been best demonstrated in experimental studies where dental materials in common use (amalgam, zinc phosphate cement, resin composites) were applied directly on pulpal tissue and where the surface of the restoration was sealed bacterial-tight (19, 20). These experiments demonstrated that the pulp around sealed restorations often resumed a healthy state, but without a bacterial-tight surface seal the bacteria were present at the pulp/restoration interface and severe inflammation developed in the pulp.

The risk of severe pulpal complication is even less when a dentine barrier remains. Dentine seems to serve as a detoxifying tissue, in that highly toxic materials may be absorbed to the inner walls of the dentinal tubules (30). It has been shown also that dentine buffers the effects of acids and bases (31). It needs to be recognized that experiments *in vitro* (32) and *in vivo* have demonstrated that cytotoxic components of resin monomers – triethylene glycol dimethacrylate (TEGDMA) and 2-hydroxyethyl methacrylate (HEMA) – readily penetrate thin dentine walls upon topical application. The effect of such leakage is not well understood. However, observations in animals suggest that the toxic effect on the pulp

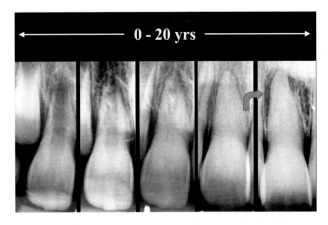

Fig. 3.25 Series of radiographs of a tooth that suffered a luxation injury at a young age. Hard tissue is successively deposited in the pulp. Arrow indicates change in status between the 15-year and 20-year follow-up radiographs. In the radiograph to the right, a periapical radiolucency is seen, suggesting pulpal infection. (From Robertson *et al.* (70) with permission of the *Journal of Endodontics*.)

of these agents is short lasting. It has been shown, furthermore, that most leachable substances from resin composites are released within the first few days after placement and then little will be discharged (22). Therefore, the threat to the pulp in conjunction with restorative procedures does not seem to be as much related to the materials *per se* as it is to the improper seal that often results (Core concept 3.4).

Dental trauma

Traumatic injuries to teeth include fractures and luxations or combinations of fractures and luxations (2). Luxation is an injury where the tooth has been loosened from its alveolus. Luxation may or may not be associated with various degrees of dislocation. A traumatic injury, regardless of whether there is loss of tooth structure, may have serious implications for the vital functions of the pulp both in the short and the long term. Most significant is whether or not the neurovascular supply of the tissue has become severed. There are two mechanisms for such an injury:

(1) The trauma may have resulted in severe internal bleeding due to rupture of the larger blood vessels supplying the pulp. The bleeding reaction, if extensive, may cause the breakdown of the entire tissue within a very short period of time.

(2) Separation of the tooth from the alveolus following dislocation may have severed the blood vessels and the nerves at the apical foramen to a complete cessation of the nutritional supply of the pulp. Nutrition also may be terminated from the compression in conjunction with an intrusion injury. If the blood supply is not restored, these complications may

result in successive degradation of the pulpal tissue by autolysis.

Along cracks in the enamel (infractions) or along direct exposures of dentine, bacteria may sooner or later access the necrotic tissue and infect it (6). Phagocytosis and replacement of the necrotic tissue in the pulpal chamber with connective tissue from the periodontal tissue is possible only if there is a wide apical foramen in a young tooth (85, 4). Otherwise, necrotic tissue will remain aseptic until becoming infected.

In teeth suffering a fracture, whether limited to the crown or extensive and involving the pulpal tissue, pulpal necrosis is a much less common outcome than in a luxated tooth (2, 3). Pulp most often survives and remains vital even though the loss of tooth structure may allow the oral microbiota to affect the pulpal tissue secondarily. The response pattern to the microbial challenge is similar to that associated with caries and dental procedures and shall not be detailed further.

Luxations may cause a temporary ischemic injury to the pulp that does not necessarily lead to necrosis. However, such an injury may trigger pulpal cells to respond with an accelerated hard tissue deposition, leading to more or less complete obliteration of the pulpal chamber (34). This type of pulpal reaction is particularly common in traumatized teeth of young individuals (Fig. 3.25). Over a period of 15–20 years about 20% of these teeth may develop pulpal necrosis and root canal infection, as indicated by the appearance of a periapical lesion (34, 70).

Core concept 3.5   Pulpal response to trauma

- Traumatic injuries to teeth may result in both immediate and late effects on the pulp.
- If pulp survives the trauma, inflammatory responses develop due to the tissue damage induced and due to any microbial irritants that accessed the pulp subsequently.
- Ischemic injury may develop in the pulp due to more or less extensive internal bleeding or rupture of the neurovascular supply at the apex. This complication may lead to pulpal necrosis.
- Repair is possible in young teeth with open apices. Such repair frequently is accompanied by hard tissue repair, resulting in more or less complete obliteration of the pulpal chamber.

For a summary of the pulpal response to trauma, see Core concept 3.5.

References

1. Abou Hashieh I, Franquin JC, Cosset A, Dejou J, Camps J. Relationship between dentine hydraulic conductance and the cytotoxicity of four dentine bonding resins in vitro. *J. Dent.* 1998; 26: 473–7.
2. Andreasen J-O, Andreasen FM. *Textbook and Color Atlas of Traumatic Injuries to the Teeth.* Munksgaard: Copenhagen, 1994.
3. Andreasen FM, Pedersen BV. Prognosis of luxated permanent teeth – the development of pulp necrosis. *Endodont. Dent. Traumatol.* 1985; 1: 207–20.
4. Andreasen FM, Zhijie Y, Thomsen BL. Relationship between pulp dimensions and development of pulp necrosis after luxation injuries in the permanent dentition. *Endodont. Dent. Traumatol.* 1986; 2: 90–98.
5. Beckman JS, Koppenol WH. Nitric oxide, superoxide, and peroxynitrite: the good, the bad, and ugly. *Am. J. Physiol.* 1996; 271: C1424–37.
6. Bergenholtz G. Micro-organisms from necrotic pulp of traumatized teeth. *Odontol. Rev.* 1974; 25: 347–58.
7. Bergenholtz G. Effect of bacterial products on inflammatory reactions in the dental pulp. *Scand. J. Dent. Res.* 1977; 85: 122–9.
8. Bergenholtz G. Evidence for bacterial causation of adverse pulpal responses in resin-based dental restorations. *Crit. Rev. Oral Biol. Med.* 2000; 11: 467–80.
   Review paper for further reading on pulpal responses to iatrogenic injuries, including resin composites.
9. Bergenholtz G, Knutsson G, Jontell M, Okiji T. Albumin flux across dentin of young human premolars following temporary exposure to the oral environment. In *Proceedings of the International Conference on Dentine/Pulp Complex 1995*, Chiba, Japan (Shimono M, Maeda T, Suda H, Takahashi K, eds). Tokyo, Japan: Quintessence Publishing, 1996; 51–7.
10. Bergenholtz G, Lindhe J. Effect of soluble plaque factors on inflammatory reactions in the dental pulp. *Scand. J. Dent. Res.* 1975; 83: 153–8.
11. Berggren E, Heyeraas K. The role of sensory neuropeptides and nitric oxide on pulpal blood flow and tissue pressure in the ferret. *J. Dent. Res.* 1999; 78: 1535–43.
12. Bishop M, Malhotra M. An investigation of lymphatic vessels in the feline dental pulp. *Am. J. Anat.* 1990; 187: 247–53.
13. Bjørndal L, Darvann T. A light microscopic study of odontoblastic and non-odontoblastic cells involved in tertiary dentinogenesis on well-defined cavitated carious lesions. *Caries Res.* 1999; 33: 50–60.
    Histology and microradiographic techniques were used to study the events taking place in dentine and pulp on both advanced and slowly progressing caries lesions.
14. Bjørndal L, Darvann T, Thylstrup A. A quantitative light microscopic study of the odontoblast and subodontoblastic reactions to active and arrested enamel caries without cavitation. *Caries Res.* 1998; 32: 59–69.
15. Brännström M. *Dentine and Pulp in Restorative Dentistry.* London: Wolfe Medical, 1982.
16. Brännström M, Lind P-O. Pulpal response to early dental caries. *J. Dent. Res.* 1965; 44: 1045–50.
    In this study, clusters of mononuclear leukocytes and small areas of reparative were observed in the pulp of young premolars underneath initial caries lesions.
17. Brännström M, Lindén L-Å, Åström A. The hydrodynamics of the dental tubule and of pulp fluid. A discussion of its significance in relation to dentinal sensitivity. *Caries Res.* 1967; 1: 310–17.
18. Byers MR, Sugaya A. Odontoblast processes in dentin revealed by fluorescent Di-I. *J. Histochem. Cytochem.* 1995; 43: 159–68.
19. Cox CF, Keall CL, Keall HJ, Ostro E, Bergenholtz G. Biocompatibility of surfaced sealed dental materials against exposed pulps. *J. Prosthet. Dent.* 1987; 57: 1–8.
20. Cox CF, Sübay RK, Suzuki S, Suzuki SH, Ostro E. Biocompatibility of various dental materials: pulp healing with a surface seal. *Int. J. Periodont. Restorat. Dent.* 1996; 16: 241–51.
21. Davidson CL, Feilzer AJ. Polymerization shrinkage and polymerization shrinkage stress in polymer-based restoratives. *J. Dent.* 1997; 25: 435–40.
22. Ferracane JL, Condon JR. Rate of elution of leachable components from composite. *Dent. Mater.* 1990; 6: 282–7.
23. Frank RM. Ultrastructural relationship between the odontoblast, its process and nerve fibre. In *Dentine and Pulp: their Structure and Reactions* (Symons BN, ed.). London: Livingstone, 1968; 113–43.
24. Fitzgerald M, Chiego D, Heys DR. Autoradiographic analysis of odontoblast replacement following pulp exposure in primate teeth. *Arch. Oral Biol.* 1990; 35: 707–15.
25. Garberoglio R, Brännstrom M. Scanning electron microscopic investigation of human dentinal tubules. *Arch. Oral Biol.* 1976; 21: 355–62.
26. Gazelius B, Olgart L, Edwall B, Edwall L. Non-invasive recording of blood flow in human dental pulp. *Endodont. Dent. Traumatol.* 1986; 2: 219–21.

27. Heyeraas KJ. Pulpal hemodynamics and interstitial fluid pressure: balance of transmicrovascular fluid transport. *J. Endodont.* 1989; 15: 468–72.

28. Heyeraas KJ, Kvinnsland I. Tissue pressure and blood flow in pulpal inflammation. *Proc. Finn. Dent. Soc.* 1992; 88 (Suppl. 1): 393–401.

29. Hibbs Jr JB, Taintor RR, Vavrin Z, Rachlin EM. Nitric oxide: a cytotoxic activated macrophage effector molecule [published erratum appears in *Biochem. Biophys. Res. Commun.* 1989; 158: 624]. *Biochem. Biophys. Res. Commun.* 1988; 157: 87–94.

30. Hume WR. An analysis of the release and the diffusion through dentin of eugenol from zinc oxide-eugenol mixtures. *J. Dent. Res.* 1984; 63: 881–4.

31. Hume WR. Influence of dentine on the pulpward release of eugenol or acids from restorative materials. *J. Oral Rehabil.* 1994; 21: 469–73.

32. Hume WR, Gerzina TM. Bioavailability of components of resin based materials which are applied to teeth. *Crit. Rev. Oral Biol. Med.* 1996; 7: 172–9.
    The potential hazards for the pulp when using composite resin materials as dental restorative materials are detailed in this review paper.

33. Jacobsen EB, Heyeraas KJ. Effect of capsaicin treatment or inferior alveolar nerve resection on dentine formation and calcitonin gene-related peptide- and substance P-immunoreactive nerve fibres in rat molar pulp. *Arch. Oral Biol.* 1996; 41: 1121–31.

34. Jacobsen I, Kerekes K. Long-term prognosis of traumatized permanent anterior teeth showing calcifying processes in the pulp cavity. *Scand. J. Dent. Res.* 1977; 85: 588–98.

35. Jontell M, Bergenholtz G. Accessory cells in the immune defense of the dental pulp. *Proc. Finn. Dent. Soc.* 1992; 88: 345–55.

36. Jontell M, Okiji T, Dahlgren U, Bergenholtz G. Immune defense mechanisms of the dental pulp. *Crit. Rev. Oral Biol. Med.* 1998; 9: 179–200.

37. Kamal AM, Okiji T, Kawashima N, Suda H. Defense responses of dentine/pulp complex to experimentally induced caries in rat molars: an immunohistochemical study on kinetics of pulpal Ia antigen-expressing cells and macrophages. *J. Endodont.* 1997; 23: 115–20.
    Studies on pulpal responses to dental caries mostly rely on observations in extracted human teeth. Therefore, little is known on the dynamic events that may take place in the pulp. This report is one of the few experimental studies available. It shows findings in rats where the cellular responses of the pulp to experimentally induced caries were explored.

38. Kerezoudis NP, Olgart L, Fried K. Localization of NADPH-diaphorase activity in the dental pulp, periodontium and alveolar bone of the rat. *Histochemistry* 1993; 100: 319–22.

39. Kim S, Dorscher-Kim JE, Liu M, Grayson A. Functional alterations in pulpal microcirculation in response to various dental procedures and materials. *Proc. Finn. Dent. Soc.* 1992; 88 (Suppl. 1): 65–71.

40. Kimberly CL, Byers MR. Inflammation of rat molar pulp and periodontium causes increased calcitonin gene-related peptide and axonal sprouting. *Anat. Rec.* 1988; 222: 289–300.

41. Kishi Y, Takahashi K. Change of vascular architecture of dental pulp with growth. In *Dynamic Aspects of Dental Pulp* (Inoki R, Kudo T, Olgart L, eds). New York: Chapman and Hall, 1990; 97–129.

42. Knutsson G, Jontell M, Bergenholtz G. Determination of plasma proteins in dentinal fluid from cavities prepared in healthy young human teeth. *Arch. Oral Biol.* 1994; 39: 185–90.

43. Kramer IR. The vascular architecture of the human dental pulp. *Arch. Oral Biol.* 1960; 2: 177–89.

44. Kubes P, Suzuki M, Granger DN. Nitric oxide: an endogenous modulator of leukocyte adhesion. *Proc. Natl. Acad. Sci. USA* 1991; 88: 4651–5.

45. Langeland K. Tissue response to dental caries. *Endodont. Dent. Traumatol.* 1987; 3: 149–71.

46. Law A, Baumgardner K, Meller S, Gebhart G. Localization and changes in NADPH-diaphorase reactivity and nitric oxide synthase immunoreactivity in rat pulp following tooth preparation. *J. Dent. Res.* 1999; 78: 1585–95.

47. Lawman MJ, Boyle MD, Gee AP, Young M. Nerve growth factor accelerates the early cellular events associated with wound healing. *Exp. Mol. Pathol.* 1985; 43: 274–81.

48. Lervik T, Mjör IA. Evaluation of techniques for the induction of pulpitis. *J. Biol. Bucc.* 1977; 5: 137–48.

49. Lewin GR, Mendell LM. Nerve growth factor and nociception. *Trends Neurosci.* 1993; 16: 353–9.

50. Lindsay RM, Lockett C, Sternberg J, Winter J. Neuropeptide expression in cultures of adult sensory neurons: modulation of substance P and calcitonin gene-related peptide levels by nerve growth factor. *Neuroscience* 1989; 33: 53–65.

51. Lundy T, Stanley H. Correlation of pulpal histopathology and clinical symptoms in human teeth subjected to experimental irritation. *Oral Surg.* 1969; 27: 187–201.

52. Luthman J, Luthman D, Hökfelt T. Occurrence and distribution of different neurochemical markers in the human dental pulp. *Arch. Oral Biol.* 1992; 37: 193–208.

53. Matthews B, Vongsavan N. Interactions between neural and hydrodynamic mechanisms in dentine and pulp. *Arch. Oral Biol.* 1994; 39 (Suppl.): 87S–95S.

54. Meyer MW. Pulpal blood flow: use of radio-labelled microspheres. *Int. Endodont. J.* 1993; 26: 6–7.

55. Moncada S, Palmer RM, Higgs EA. Nitric oxide: physiology, pathophysiology, and pharmacology. *Pharmacol. Rev.* 1991; 43: 109–42.

56. Nalbandian J, Gonzales F, Sognaes RF. Sclerotic age changes in root dentine of human teeth observed by optical and x-ray microscopy. *J. Dent. Res.* 1960; 39: 588–607.

57. Näsström K, Forsberg B, Petersson A, Westesson PL. Narrowing of the dental pulp chamber in patients with renal diseases. *Oral Surg.* 1985; 59: 242–6.

58. Odor TM, Pitt Ford TR, McDonald F. Adrenaline in local anaesthesia: the effect of concentration on dental pulpal circulation and anaesthesia. *Endodont. Dent. Traumatol.* 1994; 10: 167–73.

59. Ohshima H, Maeda T, Takano Y. The distribution and ultrastructure of class II MHC-positive cells in human dental pulp. *Cell Tissue Res.* 1999; 295: 151–8.

60. Okiji T, Kawashima N, Kosaka T, Kobayashi C, Suda H. Distribution of Ia antigen-expressing nonlymphoid cells in various stages of induced periapical lesions in rat molars. *J. Endodont.* 1994; 20: 27–31.

61. Olgart L. Local mechanisms in dental pain. In *Mechanisms of Pain and analgesic compounds* (Beers Jr RF, Borrett EG, eds). New York: Raven Press, 1979; 285–94.

62. Olgart L. Neurogenic components of pulpal inflammation. In *Proceedings of the International Conference on Dentine/Pulp Complex 1995*, Chiba, Japan (Shimono M, Maeda T, Suda H, Takahashi K, eds). Tokyo, Japan: Quintessence Publishing, 1979; 169–75.

63. Olgart L. Neural control of pulpal blood flow. *Crit. Rev. Oral Biol. Med.* 1996; 7: 159–71.
    Review paper describing mechanisms governing pulpal hemodynamics.

64. Olgart L, Edwall L, Gazelius B. Involvement of afferent nerves in pulpal blood-flow reactions in response to clinical and experimental procedures in the cat. *Arch. Oral Biol.* 1991; 36: 575–81.

65. Olgart L, Gazelius B. Effects of adrenaline and felypressin (octapressin) on blood flow and sensory nerve activity in the tooth. *Acta Odontol. Scand.* 1977; 35: 69–75.

66. Olgart L, Hökfelt T, Nilsson G, Pernow B. Localization of substance P-like immunoreactivity in nerves in the tooth pulp. *Pain* 1977; 4: 153–9.

67. Pashley DH. Dynamics of the pulpo-dentine complex. *Crit. Rev. Oral Biol. Med.* 1996; 7: 104–33.
    Comprehensive review on functions and responses of the dentine–pulp complex to injurious elements.

68. Payan BG, Brewster DR, Goetzl EJ. Specific stimulation of human T lymphocytes by substance P. *J. Immunol.* 1983; 133: 3260–65.

69. Reeves R, Stanley HR. The relationship of bacterial penetration and pulpal pathosis in carious teeth. *Oral Surg.* 1966; 22: 59–65.

70. Robertson A, Andreasen FM, Bergenholtz G, Andreasen JO, Norén JG. Incidence of pulp necrosis subsequent to pulp canal obliteration from trauma of permanent incisors. *J. Endodont.* 1996; 22: 557–60.

71. Sasano T, Kuriwada S, Shoji N, Sanjo D, Izumi H, Karita K. Axon reflex vasodilatation in cat dental pulp elicited by noxious stimulation of the gingiva. *J. Dent. Res.* 1994; 73: 1797–802.

72. Schüpbach P, Guggenheim B, Lutz F. Histopathology of root surface caries. *J. Dent. Res.* 1990; 69: 1195–204.

73. Smith AJ, Cassidy N, Perry H, Begue-Kirn C, Ruch JV, Lesot H. Reactionary dentinogenesis. *Int. J. Dev. Biol.* 1995; 39: 273–80.

74. Stuehr DJ, Cho HJ, Kwon NS, Weise MF, Nathan CF. Purification and characterization of the cytokine-induced macrophage nitric oxide synthase: an FAD- and FMN-containing flavoprotein. *Proc. Natl. Acad. Sci.* USA 1991; 88: 7773–7.

75. Swift EJ Jr, Perdigao J, Heymann HO. Bonding to enamel and dentine: a brief history and state of the art. *Quintess. Int.* 1995; 26: 95–110.

76. Takahashi K, Kishi Y, Kim S. A scanning electron microscope study of the blood vessels of dog pulp using corrosion resin casts. *J. Endodont.* 1982; 8: 131–5.

77. Takahashi K, Sakai S. Regulation mechanisms of pulpal blood flow outside the dental pulp. In *Dentine/Pulp Complex* (Shimono M, Takahashi K, eds). Tokyo, Japan: Quintessence Publishing, 1996; 158–61.

78. Taylor PE, Byers MR, Redd PE. Sprouting of CGRP nerve fibers in response to dentine injury in rat molars. *Brain Res.* 1988; 461: 371–6.

79. Trantor IR, Messer HH, Birner R. The effects of neuropeptides (calcitonin gene-related peptide and substance P) on cultured human pulp cells. *J. Dent. Res.* 1995; 74: 1066–71.

80. Turner DF, Marfurt CF, Sattelberg C. Demonstration of physiological barrier between pulpal odontoblasts and its perturbation following routine restorative procedures: A horseradish peroxidase tracing study in the rat. *J. Dent. Res.* 1989; 68: 12162–8.

81. Vongsavan N, Matthews B. The permeability of cat dentine in vivo and in vitro. *Arch. Oral Biol.* 1991; 36: 641–6.

82. Vongsavan N, Matthews B. Changes in pulpal blood flow and in fluid flow through dentine produced by autonomic and sensory nerve stimulation in the cat. *Proc. Finn. Dent. Soc.* 1992; 88 (Suppl. 1): 491–7.

83. Wakisaka S, Akai M. Immunohistochemical observation on neuropeptides around the blood vessel in feline dental pulp. *J. Endodont.* 1989; 15: 413–16.

84. Warfvinge J, Bergenholtz G. Healing capacity of human and monkey dental pulps following experimentally induced pulpitis. *Endodont. Dent. Traumatol.* 1986; 2: 256–62.

85. Öhman A. Healing and sensitivity to pain in young replanted teeth. An experimental, clinical and histological study. *Odontol. Tidskr.* 1965; 73: 165–228.

Chapter 4
Dentinal and pulpal pain

Matti Närhi

Introduction

The dental pulp is exceptionally richly innervated by trigeminal afferent axons (7, 10) that seem to subserve mostly, if not exclusively, nociceptive function (23, 31, 35). Accordingly, they respond to stimuli that induce or threaten to induce injury to the pulp tissue, and their activation may induce defensive, withdrawal-type reflexes in the masticatory muscles (30, 35, 41). The pain responses induced by external stimuli can be extremely intense. The dense innervation of the pulp and dentine gives a morphological basis for the sensitivity of these tissues. In addition to the afferent sensory nerves, the dental pulp is innervated by autonomic sympathetic efferents that play a role in the regulation of the blood flow in the pulp (39). The existence and functional significance of parasympathetic innervation are still controversial (39).

Classification of nerve fibers

Nerves can be divided into different groups according to axon size and structure, which determine the conduction velocities of the individual fibers (17) (Table 4.1). In the nervous system the different-sized fibers are distributed in a functionally meaningful manner, namely thick myelinated fibers in those nerve tracts where fast conduction is demanded and fine-caliber fibers in those tracts where the speed of conduction is not as critical. For example, the efferent $A\alpha$-motoneurons, which transmit nerve impulses to the skeletal muscles, have thick myelinated axons and conduction velocities of up to 120 m/s (17). The afferent $A\beta$-type sensory axons (with conduction velocities of 30–70 m/s) transmit touch and pressure sensations and, usually, their receptors respond to light mechanical forces, i.e. they have low stimulation thresholds (17).

Pain is conducted by two different sets of neurons: thin myelinated $A\delta$-fibers with conduction velocities of 12–30 m/s and neurons with unmyelinated axons with con-

duction velocities of 0.5–2.5 m/s. Because of this organization, the sensation perceived in response to noxious stimulation consists of two discrete and different components: first sharp and well-localized pain mediated by $A\delta$-fibers and then delayed, dull pain that is mediated by C-fibers and can radiate to a wide area surrounding the affected tissue (31). Under experimental conditions, the temporal discrimination and the quality differences of the two pain components can be demonstrated clearly in response to stimulation of extremities (31). The same dichotomy in the quality of pain can be shown when stimulating teeth (23), although temporal discrimination is not as obvious because of the short distance between the brain and the site of stimulation.

Morphology of intradental sensory innervation

The sensory neurons of the dental pulp have their cell bodies in the trigeminal ganglion (7, 10). The teeth of the upper jaw are innervated by neurons of the maxillary and those of the lower jaw by neurons of the mandibular division of the trigeminal nerve. The pulpal axons are located in the alveolar branches of the nerve and finally enter the pulp through the apical foramen or multiple foramina of the root apex in close proximity to the intradental blood vessels (Fig. 4.1).

Several hundred axons per tooth enter the pulp at the root apex; for premolars, this number is close to a thousand (7, 19, 22). The nerve fibers enter the tooth pulp in multiple bundles that contain both myelinated and unmyelinated axons (Fig. 4.2) (7, 19, 22). The majority of the axons (70–80%) are unmyelinated (7, 19, 22).

In species as varied as human, cat, dog, monkey and ferret, it appears that there are no gross differences in intradental innervation (7, 10). Rat molars also have similar innervation but in the incisors, which are continuously erupting, the innervation is sparse and of a different structure. For example, these teeth lack dentinal nerve fibers (7, 10).

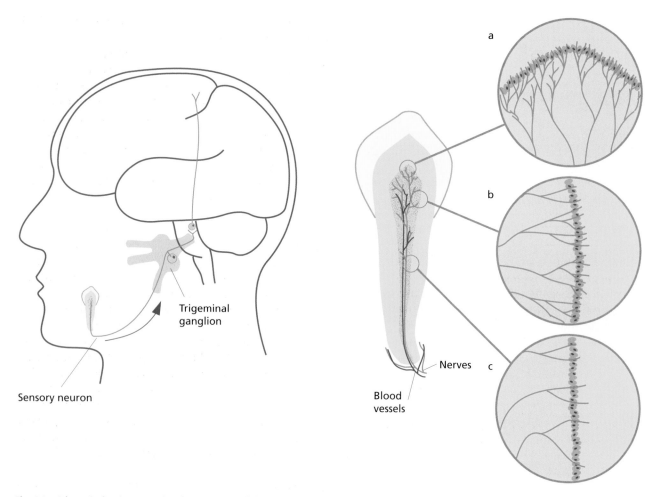

Fig. 4.1 Schematic drawing presenting the innervation of the dental pulp. Several branches from the alveolar nerve enter the apical area of the tooth. A part of the nerve bundles innervate the periodontal tissues. Multiple bundles enter the pulp in close proximity to the blood vessels through the apical foramen; they branch further on their way to the tooth crown. Most of the intradental axons have their terminals in the pulp/dentine border of the coronal pulp, which is the most densely innervated area in the tissue (a). There are fewer nerve endings in the cervical area (b) and the pulp/dentine border in the root pulp is sparsely innervated (c).

Table 4.1 Examples of different nerve fiber types, their functions, diameters and conduction velocities.

Fiber type	Function	Diameter (µmm)	Conduction velocity (m/s)
Aα	Motoneurons Muscle affererents	12–20	70–120
Aβ	Mediation of touch and pressure sensations	5–12	30–70
Aδ	Mediation of pain, temperature and touch	2–5	12–30
C	Mostly mediation of pain	0.4–1.2	0.5–2.5

Only a small proportion of the pulpal afferents terminate in the root. Most of the nerve bundles extend to the coronal pulp, branching on their way (Fig. 4.1). The terminal branch endings are located mostly in the pulp/dentine border area of the coronal pulp (Fig. 4.3). A dense network of fine nerve filaments, known as the nerve plexus of Raschkow, is formed close to the odontoblasts. A number of nerve terminals also enter the odontoblast layer and many of them extend into the dentinal tubules (7, 10) (Fig. 4.3). Both morphological and functional studies indicate that the fine nerve filaments in the dentinal tubules are mostly terminals of the myelinated intradental axons (7, 10, 32, 35). A part of the axons also terminate in the deeper parts of the pulp, often in close proximity to the pulpal blood vessels, and they may have a significant role in the mediation of pulpal blood flow responses to external irritation, as

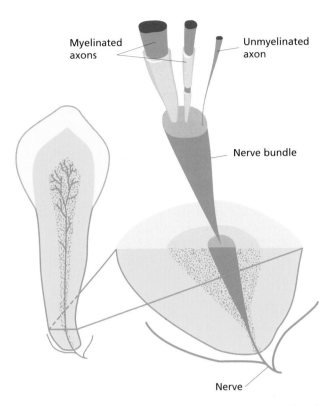

Fig. 4.2 A schematic drawing showing a nerve bundle entering the pulp chamber in the apical area of the tooth. The nerve bundle contains both unmyelinated and myelinated axons of variable sizes.

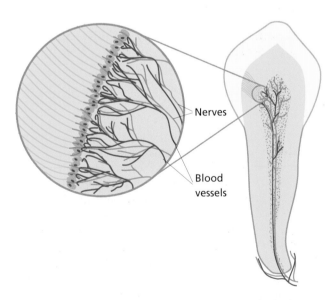

Fig. 4.3 Innervation of the pulp/dentine border in the coronal pulp. The nerve fibers entering the area form a dense network known as the plexus of Raschkow. The fibers form free nerve endings in the peripheral pulp and in the odontoblast layer. Many nerve terminals are also located in the dentinal tubules. Some fibers branch to innervate the adjacent blood vessels (see text for details).

well as in pulp tissue inflammation and repair (9, 10, 39, 40; see also Chapter 3).

The terminal branching of the pulpal nerve fibers is extensive (7). Individual myelinated axons may innervate more than a hundred dentinal tubules. Accordingly, innervation of the pulp/dentine border is extremely dense. Both myelinated and unmyelinated fibers terminate as free nerve endings. These are the receptors or nociceptors, which respond to various external stimuli in normal teeth and to the environmental changes and various inflammatory mediators that occur under pathological conditions.

As in other tissues, the sensory nerves of the dental pulp contain neuropeptides such as substance P and calcitonin gene-related peptide (CGRP) (8–11). A number of different neuropeptides have been identified in various parts of the nervous system (16, 27) that act as neuromediators or modulators and have significant regulatory effects on impulse transmission in the central nervous system. Many of them also have been shown to function in peripheral tissues as, for example, mediator substances in the effector organs of the autonomic sympathetic and parasympathetic nerves (27). The sensory neuropeptides in the afferent nerves play an important role in the initial stages of the inflammatory process (neurogenic inflammation) following injury in the peripheral tissues (39, 40) and also seem to regulate the later stages of inflammation and repair (8–11).

The location of the nerve terminals in dentine is limited to the inner 150–200 μm of the tubules (7, 10). The outer layers of dentine are not innervated. It should be noted also that innervation of the dentine is densest in the coronal part, especially in the pulp tips under the cusps, where about 50% of the tubules have been shown to contain nerve fibers (7). Many tubules contain several nerve endings (7, 21). Innervation of the pulp/dentine border becomes less dense towards the cervical areas and the number of innervated tubules becomes considerably lower (7, 10). In addition, the distance that the nerve fibers penetrate into the tubules is much shorter compared with the coronal areas. In the root, the innervation of the peripheral pulp and dentine is sparse (7). In this respect the structural organization of intradental innervation seems to be poorly correlated to the sensitivity of different dentine areas in the clinical situation, namely, that exposed cervical dentine seems to be especially sensitive. However, this obvious discrepancy can be due to differences in the time the dentine has been exposed and in the responses of the pulp–dentine complex to irritation in the coronal dentine compared with the cervical dentine (see section on dentine hypersensitivity below). The variation in dentinal innervation in different parts of the tooth may explain the different types of pain response induced in the coronal versus the root dentine in human teeth (25).

Some afferent nerve fibers may branch to innervate both the dental pulp and the adjacent tissues or multiple teeth. Such organization may, to some extent, contribute to the poor localization of dental pain and may also allow neurogenic vasodilation and inflammatory reactions to occur in an area of tissue wider than that affected by the original insult. Correspondingly, within the dental pulp the terminal branching of the nerve fibers may contribute to the spread of the inflammatory reactions (36).

Function of intradental sensory nerves under normal conditions

Knowledge of the function of intradental nerves is mostly based on electrophysiological recordings performed on experimental animals (32, 35, 36, 38). Comparison of the nerve responses to the sensations induced from human teeth with the same stimuli, as well as to the clinical cases of dental pain, has given insight to the contribution of the different intradental nerve fiber groups to different dental pain sensations. The apparently similar structure and function of the innervation in the different species examined (man, monkey, dog, cat and ferret) gives a reasonable basis for such comparisons (Advanced concept 4.1).

As already mentioned, the pulp and dentine are innervated by two different groups of afferents: A- and C-fibers (23, 32, 35). The functional classification is based on the conduction velocities of the axons and corresponds to the morphological findings showing the existence of both myelinated and unmyelinated nerve fibers in the pulp (7, 19, 22).

Intradental A- and C-fibres are functionally different (10, 23, 35, 36). The A-fibers respond to various 'hydrodynamic' stimuli applied to dentine, such as drilling, probing, air-drying and hypertonic chemical solutions (32, 34, 35). The mechanism of the nerve fiber activation in response to the different stimuli seems to be common. This hydrodynamic mechanism will be described and discussed in detail later in this chapter. The pulpal C-fibers are polymodal, which means that they respond to several different stimuli when they reach the pulp proper (23, 32, 35). The fibers have high thresholds and are activated by intense thermal (heat and cold) and mechanical stimulation (23, 32, 35). They also respond to such inflammatory mediators as bradykinin and histamine (32, 35), which are both formed and/or released in response to tissue injury and associated inflammatory reactions. Thus, the results from the electrophysiological studies indicate that intradental A-fibers are responsible

Advanced concept 4.1   Electrophysiological methods for the recording of pulp nerve activity

Two different methods have been applied in the electrophysiological recordings of pulp nerve function. Recording from dentine is performed by placing the electrodes in dentinal cavities (43). This method allows the discrimination of the action potentials of faster-conducting A-fibers. The activity of the C-fibers cannot be recorded and classification of the individual nerve fibers with respect to their conduction velocities and electrical thresholds is not possible. The recordings were performed initially on cat canine teeth (43) but it is important to note that the method has been applied to human teeth as well and those experiments have shown that intradental nerve activity is related to pain sensations perceived by the subjects in response to the external stimuli applied, showing that pulpal nerves are able to conduct nociceptive information (15). In the cat teeth the recordings from dentine have shown that pulpal A-fibers respond to mechanical and osmotic stimulation of dentine (38) and are activated or sensitized by certain inflammatory mediators and heat injury (1, 37, 40). It was also shown that the activity of the intradental A-fibers is greatly affected by changes in the pulpal blood flow.

In single-fiber recordings the individual fibers innervating the examined teeth are dissected from the alveolar nerve and are identified by electrical stimulation of the tooth crown (32). The method has been used in dog, cat and ferret teeth and it allows detailed functional classification of the examined nerve fibers with respect to their electrical thresholds, conduction velocities, receptive fields (the area in the dentine or pulp where an individual fiber can be activated) and sensitivity to a variety of stimuli applied to the dental hard tissues or to the pulp (32, 35).

for the sensitivity of dentine and may give the first warning signals whenever dentine is exposed, whereas the C-fibers may be activated mostly under pathological conditions.

Discrete receptive fields of the intradental nerve fibers can be located in either the pulp or dentine (23, 32, 36, 50). The receptive fields of C-fibers are found in the pulp proper and for their location the pulp tissue has to be exposed. Also, a part of the A-fibers, mostly slowly conducting, have their receptive fields in the pulp and thus cannot be activated by dentinal stimulation (36, 50). On the other hand, the receptive fields of those A-fibers that are activated by hydrodynamic stimulation of dentine can be located by probing the exposed dentine surface (36, 50). In normal teeth the receptive fields are usually small spots of a few mm diameter (Fig. 4.4). Some fibers may have two or even three separate receptive fields that can be located at a considerable distance from each other, in the coronal dentine and cervical area in some cases (50). Typically, the receptive fields of individual fibers overlap extensively, meaning that stimulation of a

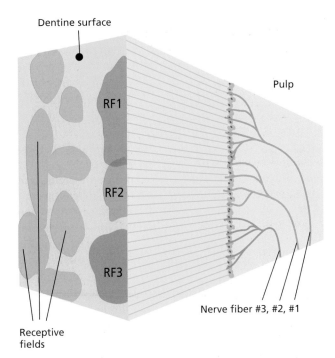

Dentine surface

RF1

RF2

RF3

Pulp

Nerve fiber #3, #2, #1

Receptive
fields

Fig. 4.4 Schematic drawing showing the receptive fields of ten individual pulp nerve fibers on the exposed dentine surface. The receptive fields are of variable shape and overlapping, and in a normal tooth are rather small. The terminal branching of three nerve fibers (fibers 1, 2 and 3) in the pulp/dentine border on the right side of the figure and the corresponding receptive fields (RFI, RF2 and RF3) on the dentine surface are shown as examples. The RF of each individual fiber corresponds to the area in the pulp/dentine border innervated by the particular axon and connected to the receptive field on the dentine surface by the dentinal tubules.

small area in dentine or pulp can activate multiple nerve fibers; this is an important factor, considering the intensity of the pain responses induced by external stimulation. These functional findings are in accordance with the structure of innervation of the pulp/dentine border area, with the extensive and overlapping terminal branching of the individual axons (see above) (Fig. 4.4).

The intradental C-fibers are activated by a direct effect of the applied stimuli on the nerve endings (23, 32, 35). For example, in thermal stimulation the response latencies are rather long and the nerve firing does not begin until the temperature within the pulp has changed by several degrees centigrade (23, 32). Similarly, activation of the most slowly conducting Aδ-fibers seems to result from a direct effect of the stimuli on the nerve endings (36, 50). It also seems that the pulpal C-fibers and slowly conducting Aδ-fibers are 'silent' in normal healthy teeth and may become active only in cases of pulp injury and inflammation. On the contrary, the A-fibers (mostly faster conducting) responsible for the sensitivity of dentine respond readily whenever dentine is exposed. The nerve activation is immediate or of a very short

latency compared with C-fibers, which is in accordance with their activation mechanism (see below).

Comparison of the above-described nerve responses to the pain sensations induced from human teeth under similar stimulation conditions has revealed how different intradental nerve fiber groups may contribute to the different dental pain conditions. For example, 'hydrodynamic' stimuli, which activate only pulpal A-fibers, induce sharp pain when applied to dentine in human subjects (34, 35). Intense thermal stimulation of human teeth has been shown to induce an initial sharp pain sensation followed by delayed dull and lingering pain if the stimulation is continued (23). Similar stimulation of the cat canine tooth induces a brief, short latency firing of intradental A-fibers followed by a long latency activation of C-fibers (23, 32, 35). Consequently algogenic (pain-producing) agents, which activate selectively either A- or C-fibers in experimental animals (32, 35), induce sharp or dull and lingering pain in human subjects (2). Altogether, the above results indicate that intradental A-fibers mediate the sharp dental pain sensations and are responsible for dentine sensitivity, whereas C-fibers mediate the dull pulpal pain or toothache connected with pulpitis.

In spite of the type of stimulus applied to a tooth, pain is the only sensation induced in response to activation of the pulpal sensory nerves, according to most studies. The only exception is low-intensity electrical stimulation (31, 35), which can induce so-called prepain sensations that probably result from low-level (liminal) activity in the pulpal nociceptive afferents. Considering any clinical situations when an electric pulp tester is used, it is important to note that the initial sensation at threshold level is usually not painful. When the stimulus intensity is increased, the sensation becomes painful and any other stimulus applied to the tooth induces pain, although its quality may vary in response to different stimuli. The variation is due to differences in the nerve response patterns and the activation of different types of nerve fibers (35).

Sensitivity of dentine: hydrodynamic mechanism in pulpal A-fiber activation

The 'hydrodynamic hypothesis' explaining the sensitivity of dentine was first presented by Gysi (18) in 1900. Today it is widely accepted that the sensitivity of dentine is based on hydrodynamic activation of the intradental A-fibers (Fig. 4.5). This concept is supported by a considerable amount of *in vitro* and *in vivo* data from both human and animal experiments (5, 6, 32, 34, 36). It was shown in the early 1960s and in a number of later studies that stimuli inducing pain when applied to human

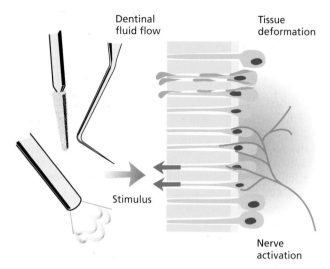

Dentinal fluid flow

Tissue deformation

Stimulus

Nerve activation

Fig. 4.5 The hydrodynamic mechanism of pulp nerve activation. Any stimulus capable of removing fluid from the outer ends of the dentinal tubules activates hydrodynamic fluid movement. The lost fluid is replaced by an immediate outward flow due to the high capillary forces in the dentinal tubules. The fluid flow causes mechanical distortion of the tissue with the nerve endings in the pulp/dentine border.

dentine are able to induce fluid flow in dentinal tubules *in vitro* (5, 6). The strong capillary forces in the fine tubules cause the hydrodynamic fluid flow. In general, desiccating or evaporative stimuli are the most effective because the capillary force contributes to the outward movements of the tubule contents. It is much more difficult to induce inward fluid flow (6, 42). The fluid flow causes mechanical distortion of the tissue in the pulp/dentine border area where most of the nerve endings are located (Figs 4.1 and 4.3–4.5). Accordingly, with all hydrodynamic stimuli the final factor inducing activation of the nerve endings or receptors is a mechanical effect. The results from single pulp nerve recordings showing that individual nerve fibers respond to several different hydrodynamic stimuli are in line with this concept (32, 35, 36).

The fluid flow in the dentinal tubules must be rapid enough to induce sufficient mechanical effect for activation of the nerve endings in the pulp/dentine border. Although there is continuous, slow outward flow in the tubules of exposed dentine due to the high capillary and tissue fluid pressure in the pulp, such a flow is not sufficient to cause nerve activation (42, 49). As already mentioned, stimuli that are able to remove fluid from the tubule apertures, e.g. evaporative or desiccating, are the most effective in activating the pulpal nociceptors because the capillary forces contribute to their effect, resulting in an immediate rapid outward flow (5, 6).

Thermal stimulation also is able to induce hydrodynamic nerve activation because temperature changes cause volume changes in the dentine and tubule contents. However, the temperature change must be rapid enough to cause sufficient fluid flow for the nerve activation. In general, cold is more effective than heat because it induces outward fluid movement (6). If intense enough, thermal stimulation (both heat and cold) is able to induce hydrodynamic nerve activation in an intact tooth without any dentine exposure (23). In cases of pulpal inflammation, the intradental nociceptors may become sensitized and activated by a direct effect of heat or cold (35, 36), resulting in a significant increase in the thermal sensitivity of the affected teeth.

Various hypertonic solutions can induce pain when applied to human dentine and activate intradental nerves in experimental animals (3, 5, 35). This action is based on their ability to extract fluid from the dentinal tubules, owing to their high osmotic pressure, resulting in activation of the capillary forces and fluid movement (5, 6). Several studies have shown that the capability of hypertonic solutions to induce pain in human teeth (3, 5, 6) and to activate intradental nerves in experimental animals (35) is related to their osmotic pressure rather than to the chemical composition of the applied solution. Such results give further support to the view that the intradental nerves are activated by the hydrodynamic mechanism.

The experimental induction of pain with hypertonic solutions corresponds to a clinical situation: when a patient complains of dental pain in connection with eating sweets (which form a saturated sucrose solution when mixed with the saliva on the tooth surface), this indicates that dentine with patent tubules is exposed in a tooth or teeth. The exposure can be found on visible occlusal or cervical surfaces but also in the margins of leaky fillings.

A major characteristic of sensitive human dentine is that the dentinal tubules are patent (5, 6, 33, 34). The hydraulic conductance of dentine and the amount and speed of the dentinal fluid flow are, to a great extent, dependent on the dentine having open or blocked tubules (6, 42). In practice, this means that all exposed dentine is not sensitive. For the induction of hydrodynamic fluid flow by capillary forces, removal of fluid from the tubule apertures is essential. Blocking of the tubule openings prevents or reduces the removal of dentinal fluid by the applied hydrodynamic stimuli and thus reduces dentine sensitivity.

The effect of the condition of dentine on its sensitivity has been shown in a number of human and animal experiments. For example, after drilling, the dentine surface is covered with a smear layer (drilling debris) and the tubule openings are blocked by the smear plugs. Etching of the exposed surface with acid is able to remove the smear and open the tubules, thus increasing the sensitivity of the dentine to a great extent (5, 6, 32, 34, 35). Blocking of the dentinal tubules, e.g. with oxalates or resins, reduces or abolishes the pulp nerve responses in experimental animals (32, 34, 35) and desensitizes dentine in human subjects (6, 34). It has been reported also that a significant positive correlation exists between the density of the open dentinal tubules and the intensity of the pain responses induced from exposed cervical dentine surfaces (33). In addition to the surface condition, changes occurring deeper in dentine, such as intratubular mineralization and secondary or irritation dentine formation in the pulp, may affect the hydraulic conductance of dentin and thus its sensitivity (6, 42).

The results of the studies listed above give strong but still only indirect evidence supporting the idea that the sensitivity of dentine and intradental A-fiber activation are based on the hydrodynamic mechanism. Recently, Vongsavan and Matthews (49) have shown a direct relationship between the measured dentinal fluid flow and intradental nerve activity in response to hydrostatic pressure changes in cat teeth.

Other suggested mechanisms of pulp nerve activation include the possibility of direct activation of the nociceptors when dentine is stimulated. However, such a mechanism does not fit with the findings regarding the response properties of intradental nerve fibers and sensory responses in human subjects, showing that algogenic agents are unable to induce nerve activity or pain when applied to peripheral dentine (32, 37). Moreover, as described earlier, neuroanatomical studies have shown that peripheral dentine is not innervated (7). The possible role of the odontoblasts in pain impulse transmission has been discussed and studied but the evidence supporting such a view is vague (see Advanced concept 4.2).

It can be concluded that the sensitivity of dentine is based on hydrodynamic activation of intradental A-fibers and, because patent dentinal tubules are the most important factor for nerve activation, blocking of the tubules would be the method of choice to abolish or prevent dentinal pain symptoms.

Responses of intradental nerves to tissue injury and inflammation

In normal intact teeth quite intense external stimuli are needed for the induction of any activity in the pulpal nociceptors. They stay mostly 'silent' because their thresholds to various stimuli are high and they are also well protected by the dental hard tissues. As a result, hot or cold foods and drinks do not cause any significant discomfort or pain in a healthy dentition. When dentine

---

Advanced concept 4.2   Odontoblasts as receptor cells?

The possible function of odontoblasts – with their cell processes in the dentinal tubules – as receptor cells has been discussed for a long time (4, 29, 32). It has been suggested that these cells have membrane properties like those of excitable cells and thus would be able to respond to external stimulation by creating a receptor or generator potential (29). This potential would then cause propagation of action potentials, which would be transmitted further in the nerve fibers. However, evidence supporting the idea of receptor cell function of the odontoblasts is controversial. Although the membrane properties with the characteristics of the ion channels and consequent electrical responses of the cells possess some properties similar to neuronal satellite cells (14), their electrophysiological responses do not resemble those of sensory receptors (14, 29). Moreover, morphological studies have been unable to identify any cell contacts between odontoblasts and the adjacent nerve fibers, which would be typical for synaptic connections or electric coupling of the two cells (7, 10, 29). According to morphological studies, the odontoblast process is limited to the inner third or half of the dentinal tubule (7, 21) and thus might not contribute to the sensitivity of the peripheral dentine. Also, studies on human teeth and electrophysiological recordings on experimental animals have indicated that dentine can remain sensitive and the intradental nerve fibers are activated even when the odontoblast layer has been destroyed (5, 6, 20). In conclusion, on the basis of the currently available evidence, the proposed receptor cell function of the odontoblasts seems improbable. However, odontoblasts may have important functions as supporting cells for the fine nerve terminals and in the regulation of the environmental conditions, including the composition of the dentinal and tissue fluid around the nerve endings (10). Such environmental changes may modify the sensitivity of the intradental nociceptors.

---

is exposed, activation of the hydrodynamic forces can intensify the effects of the external stimuli to a great extent. This allows activation of the intradental A-fibers, mediating sharp dentinal pain. The intensity of the pain is most often still mild or, at greatest, moderate and considerably well localized. Such initial pain responses after dentine exposure can be regarded as a warning signal indicating that dentine is exposed and there are patent dentinal tubules that form a connection between the pulp and the dentine surface. In addition, the protective or withdrawal reflexes induced by the pulpal A-fiber activation in the jaw muscles can modify the masticatory function and contribute to the prevention of excess tooth wear or, in some extreme cases, even cracking of the tooth crown (30, 35, 41).

In inflamed teeth, external stimuli that are not painful in healthy dentition can induce extremely intense pain responses. For example, patients with pulpitis often complain that temperature changes caused by hot or

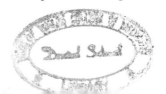

cold foods or drinks induce pain. Also, spontaneous pain without any obvious external irritation may be present. Such symptoms indicate that the pulpal nociceptors have been sensitized, which means that their thresholds to heat, cold and other stimuli are decreased. The sensitization can be induced by a number of inflammatory mediators that are released and/or formed in the pulp as a result of the insult (32, 35, 36, 38). Owing to the environmental changes and the activation of different mediators, intradental A- and C-fibers may be affected differentially during the progress of the inflammation (32, 35, 36), which may explain the changes in the type of pain symptoms found in clinical cases of pulpitis.

Peripheral neural changes affecting pain responses in inflamed teeth

As in other tissues, injury to the pulp results in an inflammatory reaction, which is an initial promoter of the healing and repair processes. Stimulation of exposed dentine is able to induce injury, which includes dislocation of the odontoblasts into the dentinal tubules as shown in histological studies (5, 6, 20). Also, nerve endings located in the tubules or adjacent to the odontoblasts become damaged (10, 26). Such morphological changes are prominent after dehydrating stimuli and clearly show the efficacy of the hydrodynamic link in the mediation of the stimulation effects from the dentine surface to the pulp. Thus, even a light stimulus such as an air blast can, in fact, be noxious to the pulp owing to the amplifying effect of the capillary and hydrodynamic forces. In spite of the morphological changes with destruction of the odontoblast layer and dentinal nerve endings, the exposed dentine surface remains sensitive in human subjects (5, 6, 26) and intradental nerve fibers in experimental animals maintain their responsiveness

to dentinal stimulation (20). Thus, dentine sensitivity is not dependent on the existence of intact odontoblasts or nerve endings in the dentinal tubules.

Neurogenic vasodilation and inflammation

Whenever an insult causes activation of the intradental nociceptors, the initial reaction in the pulp tissue is neurogenic vasodilation mediated by the terminals of the afferent nerve fibers (Fig. 4.6). The propagated action potentials are conducted over the entire cell membrane of the neuron. As a result of ortodromic conduction the impulses reach the trigeminal nuclei and then higher brain centres, including the cortex, to evoke a pain sensation. Antidromic transmission along the collateral terminal branches of the axons results in the release of CGRP and substance P, which induce vasodilation and an increase in the permeability of the blood vessel walls. Because the responses are evoked by the propagated nerve impulses, they are induced immediately by external irritation. Thus, this initial component of the inflammatory reaction is dependent on afferent nerve fibers and is called neurogenic inflammation.

The extensive branching of the pulpal afferents also allows a spread of the neurogenic effects in a wider area of the pulp than was originally stimulated. It is also possible that activation of axons innervating the pulp and the surrounding structures may result in a spread of the neurogenic inflammatory reactions between the adjacent tissues in rather early stages of inflammation (39, 40).

Inflammatory mediators

As outlined in Chapter 3, many different mediators are activated at different stages during the inflammatory reaction and tissue repair, originating from numerous

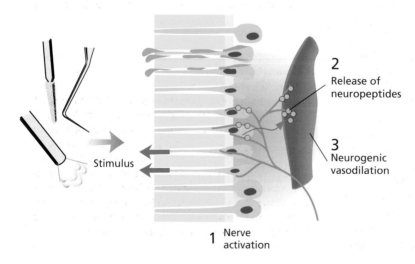

2
Release of neuropeptides

3
Neurogenic vasodilation

Stimulus

1 Nerve activation

Fig. 4.6 Schematic drawing presenting the induction of neurogenic vasodilation and inflammation in the pulp/dentine border. Activation of the nociceptors by external stimulation results in nerve impulse conduction along all collateral endings of the same axon. Some of the endings are located adjacent to the blood vessels. In response to their activation, the terminals release sensory neuropeptides, which induce vasodilation and increase the permeability of the vessel wall.

sources, e.g. various tissue components of the pulp, migrating inflammatory cells and the circulating blood. These mediators have important effects in the regulation of the inflammatory reaction and tissue repair. The neurogenic factors interact closely with other mediators (40), e.g. sensory neuropeptides can induce the release of histamine. Autonomic nerves also seem to be involved and it has been suggested that sympathetic nerve endings form contacts with the afferent nociceptive terminals to prevent the release of sensory neuropeptides by a preterminal inhibitory effect (40).

After heat injury, intradental nerves are sensitized and show ongoing firing and increased responses to thermal stimulation (1). The fact that the induced activation is inhibited by anti-inflammatory drugs indicates that the sensitization is mediated by prostaglandins (1). Serotonin has been shown to sensitize pulpal A-fibers (35, 37). After local application of serotonin into deep dentinal cavities, the responses of A-fibers to hydrodynamic stimulation of dentine are enhanced and they show ongoing activity (35). Bradykinin and histamine activate pulpal C-fibers (32, 35). The differential sensitivity of the intradental A- and C-fibers to various inflammatory mediators may give an explanation to the changes in the type and intensity of the pain symptoms during the progress of pulpal inflammation. The conditions in the pulp tissue, such as alterations in the blood flow and consequently the amount of available oxygen, may also play a role. In general, the unmyelinated C-fibers are more resistant than the myelinated A-fibers against reduced oxygen pressure (17), and single-fiber recordings in cats suggest a similar difference in the intradental nerves (35).

Morphological versus functional changes of pulpal nerves in inflammation

In addition to the nerve impulse transmission there is another, slower type of signalling between the nerve terminals in the peripheral tissues and the soma of the neuron via axonal transport. This process is bidirectional, including both antero- and retrograde transportation of various cytochemical signaling agents. It allows transmission of information regarding the conditions of the tissues around the nerve endings to the soma of the neuron (10). An injury to the nerve terminals and other tissue components in the pulp results in metabolic activation of the neurons in the trigeminal ganglion. As a result, various signaling molecules, receptors, mediators and modulators are synthesized and transported to the nerve endings in the injured tissue, where they take part in regulation of the inflammatory process and tissue repair (8, 10). Also, profound morphological changes take place in the peripheral nerve terminals (11). These

changes are regulated by growth factors and other signaling molecules activated during the process (8, 10). It should be noted also that the action of potential firing and the transport of signal molecules into the central nervous system result in discrete cytochemical changes in the second-order neurons of the trigeminal pain pathways (12).

The sensory neuropeptides, CGRP and substance P present in the afferent nerves of normal healthy tissues (8–11) seem to be confined to the fine-caliber pain-mediating afferents (10, 16). It is also indicated that the neuropeptides are predominantly located in the unmyelinated C-fibers and that some small Aδ-fibers are CGRP-immunoreactive (24, 28, 40).

Morphological changes shown to take place in response to injury and inflammation in the intradental nerve endings include an increase in their neuropeptide content and sprouting of the nerve terminals (8, 9). As already mentioned, the sensory neuropeptides are able to induce vasodilation and an increase in the permeability of the vessel walls (39, 40). Such vascular reactions are an essential part of the inflammatory reaction and are necessary to satisfy the nutritional needs related to the increased metabolic activity in connection with tissue repair and healing. The above-described structural neural responses are probably important for tissue repair because they allow more effective regulatory function of the nerve terminals in the healing process (11, Key literature 4.1). Also, the time course of the morphological changes in the nerve terminals indicates that they are an essential part of the tissue responses. They are obvious within a couple of days after the insult in the rat molars and they disappear concomitantly with tissue repair and resolution of the insult in reversible cases (8, 9).

The experimental findings regarding the functional correlates of the morphological changes in the pulpal nociceptors described above are limited. Considering the extent of the changes, they may have important

---

Key literature 4.1

Byers and Taylor (11) compared the responses after pulp exposure in denervated and normally innervated rat molars and found that the absence of the sensory nerves affected the tissue response significantly. Six days after occlusal pulp exposure, the denervated teeth showed more advanced pulp necrosis and less remaining vascular, vital pulp tissue compared with the control teeth with normal sensory innervation. The results indicate that the existence of intact sensory innervation with its responses to tissue injury may be important for regulation of the inflammatory response and consequently for the tissue defense and repair reactions in the pulp.

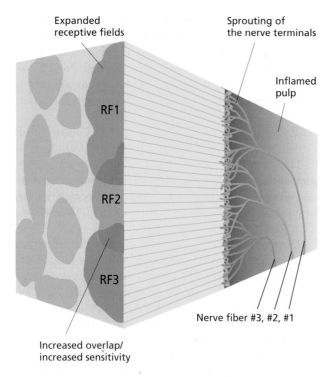

Expanded receptive fields

Sprouting of the nerve terminals

Inflamed pulp

RF1

RF2

RF3

Nerve fiber #3, #2, #1

Increased overlap/ increased sensitivity

Fig. 4.7 Schematic drawing showing receptive fields of the same intradental nerve fibers as presented in Fig. 4.4. Terminal sprouting of three fibers (fibers 1, 2 and 3) in the pulp/dentine border is shown on the right and consequently the receptive fields (RFI, RF2 and RF3) on the dentine surface have expanded and show increased overlap (cf. Fig. 4.4).

Local control of pulpal nociceptor activation

A puzzling clinical finding is that pulpitis may often result in total pulp necrosis without any symptoms. Recent studies have revealed a number of local mediators in the peripheral tissues that regulate the inflammatory process and consequently the sensitivity of the nociceptors (40, 47). In the dental pulp, for example, peripheral endogenous opioids, somatostatin and noradrenaline have been suggested to possess such effects (10, 36, 40). It is indicated that the release of the mediators is closely linked to specific steps in the inflammatory process and is regulated by a negative feedback loop (40). The inhibitory factors may be needed to attenuate the inflammatory reaction and at the same time they inhibit the activation of the pulpal nociceptors. In addition, environmental changes due to alterations in the local blood flow are able to modify the responsiveness of the intradental nerves (35, 38).

In addition to the described local factors in the pulp tissue itself, a large number of chemical agents released from carious lesions in decayed teeth and diffusing from the dentine surface through patent tubules may modulate the nerve activity (38). Thus, numerous local mechanisms may affect the activation of the intradental nerves and contribute to the wide variability of pulpitis symptoms.

Dentine hypersensitivity

Dentine hypersensitivity is a pain condition that develops following exposure of dentine surfaces. The condition is most often located in the cervical area of the tooth (6, 34, 42) and can be a considerable clinical problem. Typically, patients complain of a sharp or shooting pain that is induced by cold foods or drinks, tooth cleaning or even a light touch of the exposed dentine surface (34, 42). The pain symptoms can be extremely intense, continue for years and thus have great impact on the patient's everyday life. The condition and main features of sensitive dentine, as well as the hydrodynamic nerve activation mechanism as the basis for dentine sensitivity, have been described in detail in an earlier section on dentine sensitivity. The following text will focus on the factors that may prolong the condition, especially the role of inflammatory mechanisms and neural effects.

In favorable cases the repair reactions of the pulp–dentine complex in response to dentine exposure usually lead to a gradual tubule block by intratubular mineralization and/or irritation dentine formation to protect the pulp, leading to natural desensitization of dentine. However, sometimes the dentinal tubules may

effects on the tooth sensitivity. Electrophysiological studies indicate that the receptive fields of single intradental nerve fibers in inflamed dog teeth are wider compared with uninflamed controls (36) (Fig. 4.7). Such a change correlates with the morphological findings showing sprouting of the axon terminals (8, 9). Along with the expansion, overlap of the receptive fields of single afferents in dentine is increased, resulting in an increase in the number of fibers activated by stimulation of any particular area in dentine (Fig. 4.7). Accordingly, such changes may contribute to increased dentine sensitivity in inflamed teeth (34, 36).

Electrophysiological experiments have shown that in inflamed teeth the proportion of A-fibers that respond to dentinal stimulation is increased significantly (36), especially in slowly conducting A-δ fibers (36). Many of these fibers are 'silent' under normal conditions but seem to become active as a result of the inflammatory reaction (36). The change may be caused by sprouting and consequent formation of new nerve endings and also by sensitization of the original nerve terminals by the inflammatory mediators. Activation of the 'silent' nociceptors may significantly increase the sensitivity of the affected teeth.

stay open and the sensitivity of dentine is maintained (6, 34, 42). Such a variation in the local responses in dentine is poorly understood. It may be due to a compromised defense capability of the pulp tissue or too intense and continuous external irritation. Possible differences in the repair reactions in the coronal versus cervical pulp–dentine complex may explain why persistent symptoms of dentine hypersensitivity are often found in the cervical and root areas but rarely in the coronal dentine (34, 42). In this respect the structure of the intradental innervation is interesting, showing a dense network of nerve endings in the crown (7). Namely, the afferent nerves may play an important role in the repair and defense reactions of the pulp (11). Also, the time course of the dentine exposure may be significant. Gingival recession in the cervical area may cause much faster exposure compared with that caused by attrition on the occlusal or incisal tooth surfaces and thus not allow sufficient time for favorable repair reactions to take place in the pulp. If the dentinal tubules remain open, it may result in an inflammatory reaction in the pulp (6) and a more or less persistent pain condition.

The method of choice in the treatment of dentinal pain would be blocking of the patent tubules. The action mechanism of a number of products marketed for hypersensitive dentine is based on this principle but in some cases dentine sensitivity may remain even when the tubules have been blocked completely (34). This may be an indication of pulpal inflammation and consequent sensitization of the intradental nociceptors. Thus, the products used in the clinic for the treatment of dentine hypersensitivity may, in some cases, have diagnostic value in the discrimination of inflamed teeth.

Exposed dentine with patent tubules is sensitive if the underlying pulp is vital. The definition 'hypersensitive dentine' would implicate that dentine can be more sensitive than normal and it is tempting to state this, considering how extremely intense the dentinal pain responses sometimes can be (34). In fact, the electrophysiological and morphological studies presented before give support to this concept. Namely, local application of serotonin in healthy teeth can increase the sensitivity of intradental A-fibers to dentinal stimulation (34, 35). Moreover, morphological and functional changes showing sprouting of the pulp nerve terminals (8–11), expansion of the receptive fields of pulpal A-fibers (10, 36) and activation of 'silent' nociceptors (36) may contribute to an increase in dentine sensitivity in inflamed teeth. Accordingly, in teeth with hypersensitive dentine, pulpal inflammatory reactions may play a significant role in the development and maintenance of the pain symptoms. It should be noted, however, that the above neural changes are reversible. They can be resolved if the pulpal irritation can be abolished and

consequently the inflammatory reaction attenuated (8, 9). Thus, effective tubule block may contribute to the reduction of dentine sensitivity both directly, by reducing the hydraulic conductance, and indirectly, by allowing resolution of the pulpal neural changes induced by inflammation.

Central nervous system mechanisms

Both structural and functional changes in the central nervous system take place following peripheral nociceptor activation in response to tissue injury and inflammation. These changes become more prominent in long-lasting pain and may result in persistent alterations in those parts of the pain pathways that participate in the regulation of pain impulse transmission from the periphery to the higher centers of the brain. Results from psychophysiological studies and neurophysiological experiments indicate that central regulation is also important in various dental pain conditions.

The human experiments of Sigurdsson and Maixner (46) showed that radiation of the pain in pulpitis is via secondary hyperalgesia due to central sensitization. By conditioning painful stimulation of the arm, the secondary hyperalgesia could be abolished and the primary source of the pain more accurately localized.

Electrophysiological studies have shown that noxious stimulation of teeth results in discrete cytochemical responses in the second-order neurons of the trigeminal brainstem nuclei mediating orofacial pain (12, 13). These morphological changes are obvious within a few hours after stimulation of the peripheral nociceptors and may represent the first signs of initial sensitization of the central pain pathways. Injuries to the dental nerves caused by tooth extractions and pulpotomies have been shown to induce long-lasting functional changes in the trigeminal brainstem neurons (45). The neurons show increased spontaneous activity and expansion of their peripheral receptive fields, indicating that they have formed connections to peripheral neurons that do not normally activate them.

In summary, it is indicated that inflammation and injury in the peripheral tissues may result in changes in the impulse transmission in the central pain pathways. It is not known exactly to what extent the central mechanisms play a role in the dental pain conditions but they may be significant, especially in cases of long-lasting pain.

Pain symptoms and pulpal diagnosis

At its worst, pulpitis can cause extremely intense pain. On the other hand, it is a common clinical finding that a large number of teeth develop total pulp necrosis without being painful and with no symptoms (6). As described above, local mechanisms affecting nociceptor activation in the pulp (10, 36, 40) and regulation of the impulse transmission in the central nervous system (46) have significant modulatory effects on the development of pain in pulpitis. The poor correlation between the pain symptoms and the actual condition of the pulp in inflamed teeth has been established in histopathological studies (6, 44). From a diagnostic point of view, the great variation of symptomology in pulpal inflammation is important to note (see Chapters 2 and 6).

The nerve fibers in the pulp may maintain their structural identity even in advanced pulpitis showing a considerable destruction of the other components of the pulp tissue (48). It is not known if the remaining axons are capable of impulse transmission under such conditions but clinical experience shows that pain can be evoked in connection with the endodontic treatment of teeth where most of the pulp tissue is necrotic. Comparison of the electrical thresholds of single intradental nerve fibers and those of human teeth also indicates that activation of only a few intradental axons is sufficient to evoke prepain or pain sensations in human teeth (31, 35). With pulp diagnosis such results are significant because they indicate that a few surviving nerve fibers in a pulp with advanced tissue necrosis may give a positive sensory response to dental stimulation. Thus, evoked sensations in response to electrical stimulation with a pulp tester do not necessarily mean that the pulp is healthy. In fact, dentine can be sensitive in spite of considerable tissue damage in the underlying pulp tissue. All these findings indicate that the correlation between the dental sensory responses and the condition of the pulp tissue is poor. Accordingly, it should be noted that pain symptoms are not a reliable basis for pulp diagnostics.

In inflammatory lesions, mediators such as histamine and bradykinin activate C-fibers (32, 35). After reduction of the pulpal blood flow by periapical adrenaline injections they maintain their functional capacity better than A-fibers (35), where the impulse conduction is blocked, probably because of hypoxia in the pulp tissue. This means that during the progress of pulpitis, pulpal C-fibers may maintain their capability for nerve impulse conduction longer than A-fibers. In fact, they can become even more active in the advanced stages of pulpal inflammation owing to their susceptibility to inflammatory mediators.

The functional properties of the two pulp nerve fiber groups may explain the changes in the quality of the pain symptoms during pulpitis: from rather sharp or shooting and quite well localized, to dull and lingering. Thus, the type and duration of the symptoms in patients with pulpal inflammation are of diagnostic value and may give some indication of the pulp's condition. However, it must be underlined again that the correlation between the symptoms and histopathological changes in pulpitis is poor and determination of the type and extent of the inflammatory changes on the basis of the symptomology is inaccurate.

References

1. Ahlberg KF. Dose dependent inhibition of sensory nerve activity in the feline dental pulp by antiinflammatory drugs. *Acta Physiol. Scand.* 1978; 102: 434–40.
2. Ahlquist ML, Franzen OG, Edwall LGA, Fors UG, Haegerstam GAT. Quality of pain sensations following local application of algogenic agents on the exposed human tooth pulp: a psychophysiological and electrophysiological study. In *Advances in Pain Research and Therapy* (Fields HL, ed.), vol. 9. New York: Raven Press, 1985; 351–9.
3. Anderson DJ. Chemical and osmotic excitants of pain in human dentine. In *Sensory Mechanisms in Dentine* (Anderson DJ, ed.), Oxford: Pergamon Press, 1963; 88–93.
4. Avery JK, Rapp R. An investigation of the mechanism of neural impulse transmission in human teeth. *Oral Surg.* 1959; 12: 190–98.
5. Brännström M. A hydrodynamic mechanism in the transmission of pain-producing stimuli through the dentine. In *Sensory Mechanisms in Dentine* (Anderson DJ, ed.). Oxford: Pergamon Press, 1963; 73–79.
6. Brännström M. *Dentine and Pulp in Restorative Dentistry.* Nacka, Sweden: Dental Therapeutics AB, 1981.
    This book gives an extensive description of different aspects regarding the responses of the pulp–dentine complex to clinical procedures. Dentine sensitivity and dental pain in general are discussed in detail in relation to pulp tissue reactions and pulp diagnosis.
7. Byers MR. Dental sensory receptors. *Int. Rev. Neurobiol.* 1984; 25: 39–94.
    This is a review paper describing the structure of the dental innervation. The morphology of both pulpal and periodontal nerves and receptors is presented and discussed in relation to the functional aspects.
8. Byers MR. Effect of inflammation on dental sensory nerves and vice versa. *Proc. Finn. Dent. Soc.* 1992; 88 (Suppl. 1): 459–506.
9. Byers MR. Neuropeptide immunoreactivity in dental sensory nerves: variation related to primary odontoblast function and survival. In *Dentine/Pulp Complex* (Shimono M, Maeda T, Suda H, Takahashi K, eds). Tokyo, Japan: Quintessence, 1996; 124–9.
10. Byers MR, Närhi M. Dental injury models: experimental tools for understanding neuroinflammatory interactions and polymodal nociceptor function. *Crit. Rev. Oral Biol. Med.* 1999; 10: 4–39.
    This paper presents a comprehensive review on morphological and functional aspects of dental nociceptors. In particular,

neural responses to injury and inflammation are covered. The activation mechanisms and afferent functions of the intradental nerves in the mediation of nociceptive information to the brain are presented. The role of the nociceptors in regulation of the inflammatory and repair reactions in the pulp tissue is also described. In addition, the use of intradental nerve stimulation as a pain model and the application of the dental injury models to study the polymodal nociceptor function and neurogenic inflammatory reactions is discussed.

11. Byers MR, Taylor PE. Effect of sensory denervation on the response of rat molar pulp to exposure injury. *J. Dent. Res.* 1993; 72: 613–18.

12. Chattipakorn SC, Light AR, Willcockson HH, Närhi M, Maixner W. The effect of fentanyl on *c*-fos expression in the trigeminal brain stem complex produced by pulpal heat stimulation in the ferret. *Pain* 1999; 82: 207–15.

13. Coimbra F, Coimbra A. Dental noxious input reaches the subnucleus caudalis of the trigeminal complex in the rat, as shown by c-fos expression upon thermal or mechanical stimulation. *Neurosci. Lett.* 1994; 173: 201–4.

14. Davidson RM. Neural form of voltage-dependent sodium current in human cultured dental pulp cells. *Arch. Oral Biol.* 1994; 39: 613–20.

15. Edwall L, Olgart L. A new technique for recording of intradental sensory nerve activity in man. *Pain* 1977; 3: 121–6.
    This is the first report on intradental nerve recording in human subjects. The action potentials were recorded from dentine. The nerve responses to dental stimulation were related to pain responses reported by the subjects. The results show that intradental nerves are able to conduct nociceptive information.

16. Franco-Cereceda A, Henke H, Lundberg JM, Petermann JB, Hökfelt T, Fischer JA. Calcitonin gene-related peptide (CGRP) in capsaicin-sensitive substance P-immunoreactive sensory neurons in animals and man: distribution and release by capsaicin. *Peptides* 1987; 8: 399–410.

17. Guyton AC, Hall JE. *Textbook of Medical Physiology.* Philadelphia, PA: W. B. Saunders, 1996.

18. Gysi A. An attempt to explain the sensitiveness of dentine. *Br. J. Dent. Sci.* 1900; 43: 865–8.

19. Hirvonen TJ. A quantitative electron-microscopic analysis of the axons at the apex of the canine tooth pulp in the dog. *Acta Anat.* 1987; 128: 134–9.

20. Hirvonen T, Närhi M. The effect of dentinal stimulation on pulp nerve function and pulp morphology in the dog. *J. Dent. Res.* 1986; 65: 1290–3.

21. Holland GR. Odontoblasts and nerves; just friends. *Proc. Finn. Dent. Soc.* 1986; 82: 179–89.

22. Holland GR, Robinson PP. The number and size of axons at the apex of the cat's canine tooth. *Anat. Rec.* 1983; 205: 215–22.

23. Jyväsjärvi E, Kniffki K-D. Cold stimulation of teeth: a comparison between the responses of cat intradental A and C fibres and human sensation. *J. Physiol.* 1987; 391: 193–207.

24. Lawson SN. Peptides and cutaneous polymodal nociceptor neurones. *Progr. Brain Res.* 1996; 113: 369–86.

25. Lilja J. Sensory differences between crown and root dentin in human teeth. *Acta Odontol. Scand.* 1980; 38: 285–91.

26. Lilja J, Nordenvall K-J, Brännström M. Dentine sensitivity, odontoblasts and nerves under desiccated or infected experimental cavities. *Swed. Dent. J.* 1982; 6: 93–103.

27. Lundberg JM. Peptidergic control of the autonomic regulation system in the orofacial region. *Proc. Finn. Dent. Soc.* 1989; 85: 239–50.

28. Maggi CA, Meli A. The sensory-efferent function of capsaicin-sensitive sensory neurons. *Gen. Pharmacol.* 1988; 19: 1–43.

29. Magloire H, Vinard H, Joffre A. Electrophysiological properties of human dental pulp cells. *J. Biol. Bucc.* 1979; 7: 251–62.

30. Matthews B, Baxter J, Watts S. Sensory and reflex responses to tooth pulp stimulation in man. *Brain Res.* 1976; 113: 83–94.

31. Mumford JM, Bowsher D. Pain and prothopatic sensibility. A review with particular reference to teeth. *Pain* 1976; 2: 223–43.

32. Närhi MVO. The characteristics of intradental sensory units and their responses to stimulation. *J. Dent. Res.* 1985; 64: 564–71.

33. Närhi M, Kontturi-Närhi V. Sensitivity and surface condition of dentin–a SEM-replica study (abstract). *J. Dent Res.* 1994; 73: 122.

34. Närhi M, Kontturi-Närhi V, Hirvonen T, Ngassapa D. Neurophysiological mechanisms of dentin hypersensitivity. *Proc. Finn. Dent. Soc.* 1992; 88 (Suppl. 1): 15–22.

35. Närhi M, Jyväsjärvi E, Virtanen A, Huopaniemi T, Ngassapa D, Hirvonen T. Role of intradental A- and C-type nerve fibres in dental pain mechanisms. *Proc. Finn. Dent. Soc.* 1992; 88 (Suppl. 1): 507–16.

36. Närhi M, Yamamoto H, Ngassapa D. Function of intradental nociceptors in normal and inflamed teeth. In *Dentine/Pulp Complex* (Shimono M, Maeda T, Suda H, Takahashi K, eds). Tokyo, Japan: Quintessence Publishing, 1996; 136–140.

37. Olgart L. Excitation of intradental sensory units by pharmacological agents. *Acta Physiol. Scand.* 1974; 92: 48–55.

38. Olgart L. The role of local factors in dentin and pulp in intradental pain mechanisms. *J. Dent. Res.* 1985; 64: 572–8.

39. Olgart L. Neural control of pulpal blood flow. *Crit. Rev. Oral Biol. Med.* 1996; 7: 159–71.

40. Olgart L. Neurogenic components of pulp inflammation. In *Dentine/Pulp Complex* (Shimono M, Maeda T, Suda H, Takahashi K, eds). Tokyo, Japan: Quintessence Publishing, 1996; 169–75.
    The afferent nociceptive nerve fibers also have important efferent function in the neurogenic regulation of the inflammatory and repair reactions in their target tissues. This review paper describes these inflammatory mechanisms, including the mediators involved.

41. Olgart L, Gazelius B, Sundström F. Intradental nerve activity and jaw-opening reflex in response to mechanical deformation of cat teeth. *Acta Physiol. Scand.* 1988; 133: 399–406.

42. Pashley DH. Mechanisms of dentine sensitivity. *Dent. Clin. North Am.* 1990; 34: 449–73.

43. Scott D Jr, Tempel TR. A study in the excitation of dental pulp nerve fibres. In *Sensory Mechanisms in Dentine* (Anderson DJ, ed.). Oxford: Pergamon Press, 1963; 27–46.

44. Seltzer S, Bender IB, Ziontz M. The dynamics of pulp inflammation: correlations between diagnostic data and actual histopathological findings in the pulp. *Oral Surg. Oral Med. Oral Pathol.* 1963; 16: 969–77.
    In the early 1960s the research group of Dr Seltzer and Dr Bender definitely showed a poor correlation between the clinical pain symptoms and the actual histopathological condition of the pulp. The present paper is one of their significant series of studies regarding pulp diagnostics.

45. Sessle BJ. The neurobiology of facial and dental pain: present knowledge, future directions. *J. Dent. Res.* 1987; 66: 962–81.

46. Sigurdsson A, Maixner W. Effects of experimental clinical noxious counterirritants on pain perception. *Pain* 1994; 57: 265–75.

47. Stein C. Peripheral mechanisms of opioid analgesia. *Anesth. Analg.* 1993; 76: 182–91.
    It has been thought that opioids, e.g. morphine, have only central effects. This paper presents evidence that they can inhibit nociceptor activation in the peripheral tissues.

48. Torneck CD. Changes in the fine structure of human dental pulp subsequent to caries exposure. *J. Oral Pathol.* 1977; 6: 82–95.

49. Vongsavan N, Matthews B. The relationship between fluid flow in dentine and the discharge of intradental nerves. *Arch. Oral Biol.* 1994; 39: 140S.

50. Yamamoto H, Narhi M. Function of nerve fibres innervating different parts of dentine. *Arch. Oral Biol.* 1994; 39: 141S.

Chapter 5
The multidisciplinary nature of pain

Ilana Eli

Introduction

Pain is a complex experience of a multidisciplinary nature that is always subjective and associated with emotional and cognitive factors. Today it is widely accepted that the mere activity in the nociceptor and nociceptive pathways of the nervous system elicited by a noxious stimulus does not represent pain. Pain is always a psychological state and can be reported also in the absence of tissue damage or any likely pathophysiological cause.

Pain is often the primary motivator for patients to seek health care in general and dental treatment in particular. Dental treatment is closely associated with pain. Most dental patients expect to experience some degree of pain during dental treatment and dentists often use pain as a diagnostic tool. Self-reports of pain serve the practitioner to locate possible pathology and to arrive at conclusions regarding diagnosis and treatment, e.g. the use of tooth pulp stimulation as a diagnostic test for pulp vitality (50). However, pain is an unreliable indicator of pathology (24). In fact, little correlation exists between the amount of tissue destruction and the reported presence or absence of pain, whether derived pulpally, periodontally or periapically (54).

It is impossible to view pain as only a unique sensory reaction, therefore pain is defined as 'an unpleasant and emotional experience associated with actual or potential tissue damage, or described in terms of such damage' (26). Thus, pain is always subjective and unpleasant and not necessarily related to a stimulus or direct tissue damage. It is an emotional and cognitive experience affected by stress, anxiety, expectation, focus of attention, gender and culture, in other words, a multidisciplinary experience (Core concept 5.1).

Unlike many other sensations that are evoked by external events (seeing, hearing), pain can be classified among the bodily sensations that are evoked by internal events (so-called 'need states' such as hunger and thirst). Like other need states, pain is affected by distraction,

---

Core concept 5.1

Many people report pain in the absence of tissue damage or any likely pathophysiological cause. There is no way to distinguish this experience from that of tissue damage and it should therefore be accepted as pain. Activity induced in the nociceptor and nociceptive pathways by a noxious stimulus is not pain. Pain is always a psychological state.

---

suggestion, culture and learning and is associated with a predictable behavior.

In many acute pain situations, including pulpitis, anxiety may not only lower the pain threshold but may, in fact, lead to the perception that normally non-painful stimuli are painful. Although the explanation for such a phenomenon is not always fully understood, it is essential that the treating dentist accepts the fact that for the patient the experience is similar to that caused by drilling in a non-anesthetized tooth. In a similar manner, people differ in their pain perception and reaction according to their culture, social environment, gender and individual cognitive and emotional factors. Moreover, the same individual may react in a different manner to similar stimulations under different conditions (Core concept 5.2).

Pain may produce immediate behavioral manifestations, such as instantaneous withdrawal from the stimulus. It can also bring about long-term behavioral consequences, including the development of dental

---

Core concept 5.2

Pain research distinguishes between pain threshold and pain tolerance. Both are defined in terms of a subjective self-report:

- Pain threshold is the least recognizable pain experience.
- Pain tolerance is the greatest level of pain that one is prepared to endure.

---

anxiety and phobia, which in turn could lead to avoidance and severe neglect of dental care. Proper understanding of the pain phenomena enables the use of non-pharmacological modes for pain management and leads to better dental care and patient management in the immediate and long term. The various psychological factors that affect pain experience and their importance in dental treatment are addressed in this chapter.

Psychological factors affecting pain experience

Affective factors

Impact of stress, fear and anxiety

It is widely believed that anxiety is associated with increased pain report (9). A tense and anxious patient is more inclined to report pain during treatment than a relaxed one, because anxiety creates the expectancy for future pain. Therefore, an anxious patient who arrives for treatment with former pain memory is likely to expect pain during the treatment. This causes the patient to filter selectively any information given prior to treatment and to focus on stimuli that can resemble or be associated with pain. The slightest pressure on the tooth, for example, can be interpreted as pain and initiate a pain reaction. Arousal caused by anxiety may also lead to increased sympathetic activity and muscle tension, which may cause additional pain.

Dental anxiety is a prevalent obstacle that affects human behavior in the dental setting (15). Among all dental situations, the one causing the highest levels of stress and anxiety are oral surgical procedures and endodontic therapies (5, 17, 52, 60). Thus, there is a high probability that patients who arrive for endodontic treatment are anxious and expect to experience some degree of pain during treatment. This may prompt patients to report pain during treatment even when there is no pathophysiological basis for such a report (e.g. drilling in a tooth with non-vital pulp). Sometimes the achievement of proper local anesthesia is extremely difficult and the patient continues to complain of pain in spite of several attempts at anesthesia. Such situations are closely associated with patients' fear of dental treatment (27, 58).

Because pain by definition is always subjective, there is no way to distinguish between pain due to psychological reasons and pain originating from actual tissue stimulation. In both cases it is regarded and reported by the patient as pain and should be accepted and referred to as such (Key literature 5.1).

Key literature 5.1

In an extensive review regarding pain and anxiety in dental procedures, Litt (36) found that in acute pain situations, anxiety and pain may be indistinguishable. Anxiety not only lowers the pain threshold, but may actually lead to the perception that normally non-painful stimuli are painful (e.g. vibration of the drill felt on an anesthetized tooth).

Impact of mood

Mood, especially depression, influences pain perception and pain tolerance. There is a close relation between chronic pain states and depression (53). It has been hypothesized that chronic pain and depression are closely related, owing to similar neurochemical mechanisms in both disorders. Another reason for depressed mood is the way in which chronic pain interferes with important functioning in everyday life (e.g. decline in social activities and social rewards) (51).

Mood can affect pain perception also in short-term acute pain situations, such as dental treatment. For example, Weisenberg *et al.* (59) observed that acute pain perception was affected by a film-induced mood condition. In that study 200 subjects were exposed to three different types of films: humorous, a holocaust and a neutral. Before watching the film, immediately after and 30 min later, each subject was challenged with a trial of cold pressure pain. The results indicated that subjects who watched the humorous film tolerated the pain challenge better than any of the other subjects. This observation suggests that psychological approaches could have a significant effect on the sensory dimensions of pain and that pain tolerance in patients can be increased substantially with rather simple measures, including the showing of humorous films in the waiting room.

Cognitive factors

Pain is one of the most potent forms of stress. The experience of pain includes an actual confrontation with harm, which can be physical (e.g. injury), psychological (e.g. loss of control) or interpersonal (e.g. shame). As such, it is affected by both the potency of the stimulus and by the individual's ability to cope with the stressful event (49).

Attention versus distraction

Almost any situation that attracts a sufficient degree of intense, prolonged attention (e.g. sports, battle) can provide conditions for other stimulation to go unnoticed, including wounds that would cause considerable suffering under normal circumstances (39).

Broadly defined, distraction is directing one's attention from the sensations or emotional reactions produced by a noxious stimulus. Generally, distraction reduces pain compared with undistracted conditions (38).

Dentists can apply distraction techniques while treating their patients, e.g. by using background music or talking to the patient. Several advanced methods have been described as being effective in the dental clinic, such as mounting a television monitor near the ceiling and asking the patient to play a video game 'against the house' (8). Distraction techniques that require attentional capacity are effective in reducing pain-related distress, and even the simplest distraction technique is beneficial in reducing a patient's stress and pain perception.

Control

Research has shown that stress, coping mechanisms and reaction to pain are affected by the degree of control that patients feel they have over the stimuli that can induce pain (3, 35). For example, patients who were provided with information on N_2O analgesia showed higher pain tolerance thresholds to tooth pulp stimulation than patients who were not informed (13). Because the fear of uncontrolled, sudden, acute pain is a primary concern for most patients (33), continuous information regarding forthcoming procedures and the description of the likely sensations are important in order to provide patients with some sense of control or involvement. Thereby, anxiety and pain levels associated with dental procedures can be reduced (56).

Pain beliefs and expectations

Reaction to a stimulus, whether acute or chronic, is always affected by the meaning that the individual attaches to it. For example, the patient can interpret an episode of an unexpected and unexplained pain sensation during treatment as a sign of insufficient professional skill on the part of the dentist. This in turn can develop mistrust and make the patient assume that any further minor stimulus is a threat and evokes a pain reaction. Conversely, when mutual trust exists and when the patient has complete faith in the necessity of the treatment, such incidences are bearable and less traumatic.

In a classic experiment (1), subjects were requested to touch a vibrating surface for 1 s. Some were led to believe that the surface would cause pain, others that it would produce pleasure and the remainder were given no hint on what the vibrations would entail. As predicted, the 'pain subjects' usually reported the vibrations to be painful, the 'pleasure subjects' as pleasurable and the 'control subjects' as neutral sensations. This experiment shows that if a patient expects pain to occur during

---

> **Core concept 5.3**
>
> An ambiguous sensation can be perceived as either pleasurable or painful, based on individual cognitions and expectations. Therefore, patients' expectations influence the feeling of pain or no pain.

> **Key literature 5.2**
>
> In a study by Dworkin and Chen (12), subjects served as their own control when tooth pulp shocks were delivered either in a laboratory or in a clinical setting. A substantial decrease in the subjects' thresholds for sensation and pain, and in pain tolerance, was found when patients were challenged in the clinical setting. From this study it can be concluded that, in the dental office, patient's anticipation of threat and the associated anxiety are potent cognitive mediators of pain behavior. In other words, responses to pain stimuli change according to the situational context in which pain is experienced.

---

dental treatment, this increases the likelihood for pain to be perceived (Core concept 5.3).

In stressful situations, behavior, thoughts and emotional reactions are influenced not only by the stimulus as such but also by the individual's perception of 'self-efficacy', i.e. one's belief in having the relevant and necessary coping skills (2). If a patient believes that he or she can successfully cope with the anticipated pain, then this perception increases the pain tolerance, and vice versa. Generally, those who avoid dental care because of fear and anxiety perceive themselves as being reliably less able to tolerate pain. Such patients often claim to have an 'exceptionally low pain threshold' or report themselves as 'completely unable to endure pain'. Such a low self-efficacy further lowers their pain tolerance level during treatment and increases the probability that pain will be experienced (29, 30, Key literature 5.2).

Pain prediction and memory

Usually, memory for the general intensity of pain is good. However, the level of pain remembered by patients regarding previous dental treatments is more closely associated with their expectations of pain rather than to their real pain experience (28). Furthermore, mood and affective states influence the memory of pain (19).

When dental patients experience recurrent pain during treatment, their recall of the experience has an increased magnitude. This may lead to increased anxiety and increased pain perception. As time elapses, the painful experiences tend to gain negative impact, probably due to reconstruction of memories to make them consistent with the existing level of anxiety. The vicious circle is enhanced by feelings of shame due to the inability to cope with the situation. Other defensive adjustment mechanisms, such as suppression ('I don't even want to think of that'), denial ('There is nothing wrong with my teeth') or projection ('I simply hate dentists'), further contribute to the patient's inability to cope with the situation and increases the probability of pain during treatment (15).

Memory of past pain experience also depends on the intensity of the present pain. When the pain intensity is high, patients remember the levels of their prior pain as being more severe than originally recorded (14). This situation is occasionally seen among patients who experience postoperative pain after their first session of endodontic therapy. Postoperative pain causes patients to remember former treatment as more painful than in fact was originally experienced. This, in turn, leads to higher stress, higher expectation of pain and lower tolerance of pain in the next encounter with the dentist.

Environmental factors

Direct and indirect learning

Part of our behavior results from life experiences. The concepts and coping strategies of various life events (including pain) are continually affected by learning processes. For a learned behavior to develop, exposure to the stimulus in question must occur, resulting in a response pattern (conditioning). Further reinforcement of the response pattern (positive or negative) leads to the acquisition of new behaviors.

Unfortunately, the dental situation provides numerous opportunities for negative conditioning and the acquirement of maladaptive behaviors. The most common stimulus in this respect is pain. Although acute pain during dental treatment can be avoided in most cases, there are still many adults who have experienced it during treatment in the past. A dental practitioner who acts without perseverance toward an apprehensive patient serves to reinforce the negative behavior, thereby decreasing the patient's tolerance to pain. Reactions of impatience toward the 'difficult to handle' patient, associated with unconscious punishment (treatment applied in an impatient and harsh manner), reinforce the negative behavior of the patient and lowers his or her pain tolerance.

Numerous learned behaviors associated with pain are based on negative reinforcement – something uncomfortable or fearful that should be avoided. This type of learning includes escape and avoidance (to avoid or prevent the unpleasant situation before it occurs). One example is that of patients who react with symptoms

of pallor, nausea, sweating, dizziness or even fainting during administration of local anesthesia. In many instances, symptoms originate in the patient's fear of pain rather than being due to pathophysiological causes. The situation can result in significant stress to the dentist, who occasionally chooses to postpone treatment to the next appointment. Once the symptoms have served the patient as an adequate means to avoid the stressful situation, it may serve as a reinforcement to increase the probability of recurrence during subsequent confrontations. Patients develop a 'fainting prone' behavior that 'protects' them from the need to face treatment. The negative pattern is further reinforced by the dentist's reluctance to treat patients with such a medical history.

In some cases this maladaptive pattern is further reinforced by secondary gains, such as sympathy and attention from the environment, avoidance of unpleasant work or duties, etc. Reinforcement of pain behavior can also occur with pain medication. For some, the effects of pain medication reinforce pain behavior due to the development of physiological and psychological addiction. These individuals continue the pain behavior necessary and sufficient to lead to delivery of medication, even after the original nociceptive stimulus has resolved.

For learning to take place, patients do not have to have a direct experience. It can also be a result of observation (vicarious learning). This means that one sees what happens to another individual and assumes that one's own fate would be similar in nature. For example, a child who accompanies his or her parent to the dentist and watches a pain-related behavior may later, in a similar situation, imitate that behavior. Indeed, observing others respond to painful stimulation could either provoke or reduce the pain response of the observer (47).

Vicarious learning can also originate through identification (e.g. a parent who constantly complains about pain from a tooth or dental treatment) or through indirect suggestions. For a parent who brings his or her child to the dentist and reassures in a trembling voice that '. . . there is no reason to worry . . . it will not hurt at all . . .', the non-verbal suggestion may often be the reverse and cause increased pain sensitivity.

In conclusion, as with any other 'stressor', pain is also influenced by individually learned responses. Respondent and operant conditioning, indirect learning through modeling and suggestions, as well as social learning have a significant impact on the pain experience (6).

Social and cultural factors

The influence of social environmental factors and the level of approval given by different societies for the public expression of pain have a significant impact on pain behavior. A variety of studies in the 1950s and 1960s in the US found differences including denial of problems, social withdrawal and fewer complaints in cultural groups that tend to be more reserved, and more dramatic responses to pain, greater expressiveness and a need for social support in those cultural groups where expression of emotion is more accepted (61, 62, 63).

The cultural significance attributed to pain, symbols of pain and situations associated with pain make them acceptable or avoidable regardless of the actual intensity of the sensation. For example, acceptance of pain inflicted during the administration of local anesthesia as serving a positive purpose, rejection of pain caused by a needle puncture in the finger as symbolizing injury. The acceptance of pain does not mean that the feeling quality of the sensation has changed. The sensation is always unpleasant, but the unpleasantness is tolerated when cultural traditions call for its acceptance.

While ethnic groups differ with regard to factors that influence responses to pain, similarities exist in their report of the response. For example, a more recent study by Lipton (34) found that responses, attitudes and descriptions were relatively similar in facial pain patients from a wide variety of cultural backgrounds. Most of the items for which interethnic differences were found concerned emotions (stoicism vs expressiveness) in response to pain, and interference in daily functioning attributed to pain.

Further evidence exists that some dimensions of pain (time, intensity, location, quality, cause and curability) are universal, while others are culture-specific (40,41).

Gender and pain

Gender differences in response to pain stimuli are controversial. Some claim that women exhibit greater sensitivity to noxious stimuli than men (20), whereas others show only slight gender differences in ratings of chronic and experimental pain, pain-related illness behavior and personality (7).

In an extensive review concerning gender variation in clinical pain experience, Unruh (55) reports that women are more likely than men to experience a variety of recurrent pains. In most studies women report more severe levels of pain, more frequent pain and pain of longer duration than men. Women may be at greater risk of pain-related disability than men, but women also respond more aggressively to pain through health-related activities. Regarding psychosocial factors, the review shows that men may be more embarrassed by pain than women and that the meaning of pain may be

> **Key literature 5.3**
>
> Eli *et al.* (16) investigated the relationships of gender, anxiety and pain in the dental setting. In the study, 32 women and 32 men underwent diagnostic tooth pulp stimulation by an electric pulp tester. Although there was no direct impact of gender on the various pain measures (sensitivity threshold, pain threshold, pain tolerance), there were significant differences in the relationship between pain tolerance and the subjective evaluation of the painful experience by both genders. In women, the relationship was negative (the higher the one, the lower the other), whereas in men it was positive (the higher the one, the higher the other). It was concluded that women were affected more by the objective characteristics of the stimulus, whereas men were also affected by its psychological significance.
>
> Proper understanding of the variables that affect individual pain assessment in men and women is important, because it may produce emotional responses that can influence compliance.

affected by sociocultural factors and the perceived position of men and women in society. Embarrassment may cause men to minimize pain unless it increases in severity and interferes with work. Minimizing pain may be consistent with social and cultural norms that consider insensitivity to pain and pain endurance as attributes of virility.

There are considerable differences between types of clinical pain (22). Experimental pain, produced under controlled conditions by brief, noxious stimuli, differs from procedural and postsurgical pain. These kinds of pain have different meanings and make the study of pain more complex (Key literature 5.3).

Apparently, women and men make different assessments of procedural pain and may thus be affected differently by the experience. In a study regarding clinical pain in the dental office (18), it was shown that men expect to experience more pain preoperatively than women but remember less pain postoperatively. It was concluded that cognitive pain perception in clinical situations differs between genders, a fact that may originate in psychosocial factors such as expected gender roles.

Psychological approaches to pain management

Treatment strategies

Systematic attempts to treat pain have been closely aligned with how pain is conceptualized and evaluated (21). Traditionally, the focus in medicine (and dentistry) has been on the cause of the pain reported, with the assumption that there is a somatic basis for the pain and once it is identified the source can be blocked by medical or operative intervention. In the absence of physical basis, the situation was labeled as 'psychogenic pain'.

Today, it is widely accepted that such a dichotomous view is incomplete and inadequate. There is no question that physical factors contribute to pain symptoms, or that psychological factors play a part in pain reports. Therefore, an increasing range of psychologically based interventions is continuously incorporated in pain management.

Treatment of acute pain includes strategies based on information, distraction, relaxation and hypnosis. Generally, preparing the patient with coping skills such as information, distraction and relaxation helps to reduce the discomfort of potentially painful dental procedures. Patients who are properly prepared show less anxiety and present reports of low pain. Such non-pharmacological strategies facilitate acute pain management and are relatively easy to learn and perform. They should be part of the professional training of every dentist in general, as well as of specialties, especially in endodontics.

Effective treatment strategies for the management of prolonged chronic pain conditions (e.g. temporomandibular disease) include operant conditioning, cognitive–behavioral therapy, psychodynamic therapy, group therapy, biofeedback, relaxation and hypnosis.

Role of hypnosis as a mode for pain management in dental care

In spite of its ancient roots, hypnosis has been accepted only recently as a scientific and medical tool. Hypnosis has been surrounded by myths and mystery for so long that even today various popular misconceptions exist. There is no doubt that it is a powerful therapeutic tool (Core concept 5.4). From 1982 to 1985 alone, over 1000 articles were published on hypnosis (46), indicating an enduring willingness on the part of the scientific community to accept it as a legitimate topic for clinical and research investigation.

The use of hypnosis for anesthetic purposes dates back to the 19th century and is attributed to Recamier in 1821. In dentistry, Oudet used hypnosis as an anesthetic agent to extract a tooth in 1837 (48). Today, hypnosis has been described in the dental literature as having a dramatic effect when used as a sole anesthetic. Hilgard and Hilgard (23) summarized numerous case reports where procedures such as extractions, pulpotomies and pulpectomies were performed under hypnosis without other anesthetic agents.

Hypnosis is used in endodontic treatment (42–44) and in other dental procedures (32, 57) to allow treatment

without stress or pain. For example, it can reduce both the strength and unpleasantness of electrical tooth pulp stimulation (25). The use of hypnosis to induce local anesthesia is especially effective for medically compromised patients (37), for patients with specific fears (i.e. dental syringe, needle or injections) (4) and in treating patients with true (or suspected) hypersensitivity to local anesthetic agents (45).

Managing adverse reaction to local anesthesia

Occasionally, patients may present with a history of hypersensitivity to local anesthetic agents. The symptoms usually include immediate reactions to the injection procedure (dizziness, shortness of breath, tachycardia, etc.). Although the true incidence of local anesthetic allergy is low, such a history often involves both the patient's and the dentist's anxiety regarding the use of the drug in question. Hypnosis can play a major role in controlling pain and the associated distress. In many cases, adverse reactions to local anesthetic are psychogenic in nature. Fear of injection, or of dental treatment in general, could lead to some of the most frightening 'allergic' reactions – tachycardia and vasodepressor syncope. Even patients with a former diagnosis of allergy may not be allergic at all (10). Patients frightened by the use of local or general anesthesia, or those diagnosed as allergic, may suffer from severe adverse consequences. Patients correctly or incorrectly labeled as 'allergic' tend to postpone routine treatment until pain is intolerable, which causes deterioration of their dental condition (11). Again, hypnosis may be used as an efficient tool to induce analgesia/anesthesia and to enable routine dental care. Generally, the hypnotic response is easily achieved because of the patient's high motivation and because the method is solely used to achieve analgesia. Consequently, patients do not expect any 'psychological' intervention and therefore have less need to mobilize psychological defenses (31).

Core concept 5.4

Potential applications of hypnosis in dentistry include:

- Patients who suffer from dental fear, anxiety or phobia.
- Patients with excessive gagging reflex.
- Acute and chronic pain conditions.
- Enhancement of patient compliance with dental hygiene.
- Enhancement of patient adaptation to dentures.
- To induce local anesthesia in patients with specific fears and in treating patients with true (or suspected) hypersensitivity to local anesthetic agents.

Case study

Generally, anxiety increases the perception of noxious events as painful. Fear and anxiety are often encountered in the dental situation. Therefore, it could have a major effect on the patient's report of pain and concomitantly on the diagnosis (and treatment) of various dental pathologies, including endodontic lesions.

A 16-year-old girl suffering from dental phobia arrived at a dental clinic for a routine examination. Owing to high dental anxiety, the patient had previously received treatment under general anesthesia. On entering the clinic, she manifested a high degree of apprehension but agreed (with apparent stress) to undergo 'initial' examination.

Examination revealed a radiolucent lesion between the roots of teeth 12 and 13. Sensibility tests performed on the teeth adjacent to the lesion evoked a clear pain response, suggesting a non-endodontic etiology. To avoid possible misdiagnosis, the tests were repeated several times by two independent dentists with identical result. Contralateral teeth reacted in a similar manner. The patient was referred for further consultation to an Oral Surgery Clinic. Outcome of sensibility tests was consistent with previous results. Each time a cold or electrical stimulus was applied to the teeth in question, the patient reacted with pain coupled with apprehension.

It was decided to perform an excision biopsy of the lesion under general anesthesia. Owing to the proximity of the lesion to the apex of tooth 12, it was assumed that following the biopsy a possible devitalization of the tooth would occur. To avoid this complication and further trauma, preventive endodontic treatment was suggested prior to biopsy.

When the pulp of tooth 12 was opened, a non-vital, necrotic tissue was revealed. The canal was cleaned and sealed without further intervention. Six months later the lesion had resolved and no further treatment was necessary.

Comment

Pain is often a poor indicator of the cause of a condition. In this particular case, patient anxiety, stress and anticipation of pain may have led to subjective interpretation of the applied stimuli as painful and to a clinical reaction that suggested the presence of a vital pulp. In the diagnosis of endodontic pathology, pain often serves as an important parameter of evaluation. The high incidence of fear and anxiety among dental patients, and the influence of anxiety on the pain experience, call for a reserved frame of mind to individuals' report of pain.

References

1. Anderson DB, Pennebaker JW. Pain and pleasure: alternative interpretations for identical stimulation. *Eur. J. Soc. Psychol.* 1980; 10: 207–12.
2. Bandura A. Self-efficacy. Toward a unifying theory of behavior change. *Psychol. Rev.* 1977; 84: 191–215.
3. Bandura A. *Social Foundation of Thought and Action: a Social Cognitive Theory.* Englewood Cliffs, NJ: Prentice-Hall, 1986.
4. Bernick SM. Relaxation, suggestion and hypnosis in dentistry. *Pediatr. Dent.* 1972; 11: 72–5.
5. Brand HS, Gortzak RATh, Palmer-Bouva CCR, Abraham RE, Abraham-Inpijn L. Cardiovascular and neuroendocrine responses during acute stress induced by different types of dental treatment. *Int. Dent. J.* 1995; 45: 45–8.
6. Burdette BH, Gale EN. Pain as a learned response: a review of behavioral factors in chronic pain. *J. Am. Dent. Assoc.* 1988; 116: 881–5.
7. Bush FM, Harkins SW, Harrington WG, Price DD. Analysis of gender effects on pain perception and symptom presentation in temporo-mandibular pain. *Pain* 1993; 53: 73–80.
8. Corah NL, Gale EN, Illing SJ. Psychological stress reduction during dental procedures. *J. Dent. Res.* 1979; 58: 1347–51.
9. Craig KD. Emotional aspects of pain. In *Textbook of Pain* (2nd edn). (Wall PD, Melzack R, eds). London: Churchill Livingstone, 1989.
10. deShazo RD, Nelson HS. An approach to the patient with a history of local anesthetic hypersensitivity: experience with 90 patients. *J. Allergy Clin. Immunol.* 1979; 63: 387–94.
11. Doyle KA, Goepfred SJ. An allergy to local anesthetics? The consequences of a misdiagnosis. *J. Dent. Child.* 1989; 56: 103–6.
12. Dworkin SF, Chen AC. Pain in clinical and laboratory contexts. *J. Dent. Res.* 1982; 61: 772–4.
13. Dworkin SF, Chen ACN, Schubert MM, Clark DW. Cognitive modification of pain: information in combination with N_2O. *Pain* 1984; 19: 339–51.
14. Eich E, Reeves JL, Jaeger B, Graff-Radford SB. Memory of pain: relation between past and present pain intensity. *Pain* 1985; 23: 375–9.
15. Eli I. *Psychophysiology: Stress, Pain and Behavior in Dental Care.* Boca Raton, FL: CRC Press, 1992.

16. Eli I, Bar-Tal Y, Fuss Z. Korff E. Effect of biological sex differences on the perception of acute pain stimulation in the dental setting. *Pain Res. Manag.* 1996; 1: 201–6.

17. Eli I, Bar-Tal Y, Fuss Z, Silberg A. Effect of intended treatment on anxiety and on reaction to electric pulp stimulation in dental patients. *J. Endodont.* 1997; 23: 694–7.
Ninety-two patients who were about to undergo various dental treatments (calculus removal, filling, root canal treatment and extraction) were evaluated, comparing their dental anxiety and pain expectation from the intended treatment and their reaction to electrical tooth pulp stimulation. The data indicate that patients differ in their anxiety levels and their expectation to experience pain according to the following hierarchy: extraction, root canal treatment, filling, calculus removal. Dental anxiety decreased the sensation threshold of patients who expected easier treatments (calculus removal, filling) but increased the threshold of those who expected more stressful treatments (endodontic treatment, extraction).

18. Eli I, Baht R, Kozlovsky A, Simon H. Effect of gender on acute pain prediction and memory in periodontal surgery. *Eur. J. Oral Sci.* 2000; 108: 99–103.

19. Erskine A, Morley S, Pearce S. Memory for pain: a review. *Pain* 1990; 41: 255–65.

20. Fillingim RB, Maixner W. Gender differences in the responses to noxious stimuli. *Pain Forum* 1995; 4: 209–21.

21. Gatchel RJ, Turk DC. *Psychological Approaches to Pain Management*, New York: The Guilford Press, 1996.

22. Harkins SW. Discussion on 'Long term memory of acute post-surgical pain' by Sisk, A.L., *et al. J. Oral Maxillofac. Surg.* 1991; 49: 358–9.

23. Hilgard ER, Hilgard JR. *Hypnosis in the Relief of Pain.* Los Altos, CA: William Kaufmann Inc., 1975.

24. Horowitz LG, Kehoe L, Jacobe E. Multidisciplinary patient care in preventive dentistry: idiopathic dental pain reconsidered. *Clin. Prev. Dent.* 1991; 13: 23–9.

25. Houle M, McGrath PA, Moran G, Garret OJ. The efficacy of hypnosis and relaxation–induced analgesia on two dimensions of pain for cold pressor and electric tooth pulp stimulation. *Pain* 1988; 33: 241–51.
Twenty-eight subjects were submitted to tooth pulp stimulation and cold pressor stimulation of the forearm according to a specified protocol. The treatment conditions included progressive muscle relaxation and hypnotic induction with suggestions for analgesia. Both hypnosis and relaxation significantly reduced the strength and the unpleasantness of tooth pulp stimulation, but only the unpleasantness dimension of cold pressor pain. Authors conclude that the quality of the cognitive-based therapies used varies not only according to subject's characteristics and the efficacy of the intevention but also according to the nature of the noxious stimuli.

26. IASP Subcommittee on Taxonomy. Pain terms: a list with definitions and notes on usage. *Pain* 1979; 6: 249–52.

27. Kaufman E, Weinstein P, Milgrom P. Difficulties in achieving local anesthesia. *J. Am. Dent. Assoc.* 1984; 108: 205–8.

28. Kent G. Memory of dental pain. *Pain* 1985; 21: 187–94.
The possibility that patient memory for acute pain is reconstructed over time was tested by comparing the degree of pain remembered 3 months after a dental appointment with both expected and experienced pain, as reported immediately before and after the appointment. There was a closer association between remembered and expected pain than between remembered and experienced pain, particularly for patients with high dental anxiety.

29. Kent G. Self-efficacious control over reported physiological, cognitive and behavioural symptoms of dental anxiety. *Behav. Res. Ther.* 1987; 25: 341–7.

30. Kent G, Gibbons R. Self-efficacy and the control of anxious cognitions. *J. Behav. Ther. Exp. Psychiatry* 1987; 18: 33–40.

31. Kleinhauz M, Eli I. When pharmacologic anasthesia is precluded – the value of hypnosis as a slow anesthetic agent in dentistry. *Spec. Care Dentist* 1993; 13: 15–22.

32. Kleinhauz M, Eli I, Rubinstein Z. Treatment of dental and dental-related behavioral dysfunctions in a consultative outpatient clinic: a preliminary report. *Am. J. Clin. Hypn.* 1985; 28: 4–9.

33. Lindsay SJ, Humphris G, Barnby GJ. Expectations and preferences for routine dentistry in anxious adult patients. *Br. Dent. J.* 1987; 163: 120–24.

34. Lipton JA, Marbach JJ. Ethnicity and the pain experience. *Soc. Sci. Med.* 1984; 19: 1279–98.

35. Litt MD. Self efficacy and perceived control: cognitive mediators of pain tolerance. *J. Pers Soc. Psychol.* 1988; 54: 149–60.

36. Litt MD. A model of pain and anxiety associated with acute stressors: distress in dental procedures. *Behav. Res. Ther.* 1996; 34: 459–76.
This is an extensive review article that discusses the nature of pain and anxiety in the face of an acute stressor, and presents the dispositional and situational factors that contribute to the perception of an acute stressor as aversive. The article presents a model illustrating how the various factors interact.

37. Lu DP, Lu GP. Hypnosis and pharmacological sedation for medically compromised patients. *Compend. Contin. Educ. Dent.* 1996; 17: 32–40.

38. McCaul KD, Malott JM. Distraction and coping with pain. *Psychol. Bull.* 1984; 95: 516–33.

39. Melzack R. *The Puzzle of Pain.* New York: Basic Books, 1973.

40. Moore R, Miller ML, Weinstein P, Dworkin SF, Liou HH. Cultural perceptions of pain and pain coping among patients and dentists. *Commun. Dent. Oral Epidemiol.* 1986; 14: 327–33.

41. Moore RA, Dworkin SF. Ethnographic methodologic assessment of pain perceptions by verbal description. *Pain* 1988; 34: 195–204.

42. Morse DR. Hypnosis in the practice of endodontics. *J. Am. Soc. Psychosom. Dent. Med.* 1975; 22: 17–22.

43. Morse DR. Use of a meditative state for hypnotic induction in the practice of endodontics. *Oral Surg.* 1976; 41: 664–72.

44. Morse DR, Wilcko JM. Nonsurgical endodontic therapy for a vital tooth with meditation-hypnosis as the sole anesthetic: a case report. *Am. J. Clin. Hypn.* 1979; 21: 258–62.

45. Morse DR, Schoor RS, Cohen BB. Surgical and non-surgical dental treatments for a multi-allergic patient

with meditation-hypnosis as the sole anesthetic: case report. *Int. J. Psychosom.* 1984; 31: 27–33.

46. Nash MR. Twenty years of scientific hypnosis in dentistry, medicine, and psychology: a brief communication. *Int. J. Clin. Exp. Hypn.* 1988; 36: 198–205.

47. Neufeld RW, Davidson PO. The effects of vicarious and cognitive rehearsal on pain tolerance. *J. Psychosom. Res.* 1971; 15: 329–35.

48. Rosen H. *Hypnotherapy in Clinical Psychiatry.* New York: The Julian Press, 1953.

49. Roskies E, Lazarus RS. Coping theory and the teaching of coping skills. In *Behavioral Medicine: Changing Health Lifestyles* (Davidson PO, Davidson SM, eds). New York: Brunner/Mazel, 1980; 38.

50. Rowe AHR, Pitt Ford TR. The assessment of tooth vitality. *Int. Endodont. J.* 1990; 23: 77–83.

51. Rudy TE, Kerns RD, Turk DC. Chronic pain and depression: toward a cognitive–behavioral mediation model. *Pain* 1988; 35, 129–40.

52. Soh G, Yu P. Phases of dental fear for four treatment procedures among military personnel. *Mil. Med.* 1992; 157: 294–7.

53. Sternbach RA. *Pain Patients, Traits and Treatment.* New York: Academic Press, 1974.

54. Taintor JF, Langeland K, Valle GF, Krasny RM. Pain: a poor parameter of evaluation in dentistry. *Oral Surg.* 1981; 52: 299–303.

55. Unruh AM. Gender variations in clinical pain experience. *Pain* 1996; 65: 123–67.

56. Wardle J. Psychological management of anxiety and pain during dental treatment. *J. Psychosom. Res.* 1983; 27: 399–402.

57. Waxman D. *Hartland's Medical & Dental Hypnosis* (3rd edn). London: Bailliere Tindall, 1989.

58. Weinstein P, Milgrom P, Kaufman E, Fiset L, Ramsay D. Patient perceptions of failure to achieve optimal local anesthesia. *Gen. Dent.* 1985; 33: 218–20.

59. Weisenberg M, Raz T, Hener T. The influence of film-induced mood on pain perception. *Pain* 1998; 76: 365–75.

60. Wong M, Lytle WR. A comparison of anxiety levels associated with root canal therapy and oral surgery treatment. *J. Endodont.* 1991; 17: 461–5.

61. Zborowski M. Cultural components in responses to pain. *J. Soc. Issues* 1952; 8: 16–30.

62. Zborowski, M. *People in Pain.* San Francisco: Jossey-Bass, 1969.

63. Zola K. Culture and symptoms: an analysis of patient presenting complaints. *Am. Sociol. Rev.* 1966; 66: 615–30.

Chapter 6
Vital pulp therapies

Preben Hørsted-Bindslev and Gunnar Bergenholtz

Introduction

A multitude of harmful elements, alone or in combination, may under clinical conditions cause adverse reactions in the dental pulp (Fig. 6.1; see also Chapter 3). If not properly managed they may result in:

(1) Painful pulpitis.
(2) Pulpal tissue breakdown (pulpal necrosis).
(3) Root canal infection, leading to periapical inflammatory lesion (apical periodontitis).

These effects are the result of inflammation and associated tissue destruction. Tissue destruction *per se* is a necessary feature of inflammation in general and is required by the host to carry out an effective defense against foreign matter, including bacteria and bacterial elements. However, as far as the pulp is concerned it can be devastating and result in total breakdown of the tissue.

Infection and inflammation in the periapical tissue (see Chapter 9) frequently follow such an event, termed pulpal necrosis. Vital pulp therapy involves clinical procedures aimed at:

● Relieving painful symptoms of pulpitis.
● Preventing the development of a destructive course of pulpal inflammation.

In the current chapter the rationales for the clinical procedures employed and the techniques and materials applied to attain these objectives are described.

Clinical scenarios

Any direct exposure of the pulp to the oral environment involves the risk of destructive inflammatory breakdown (Fig. 6.2). It should be noted that a pulpal wound has little self-healing capacity unless properly treated. In contrast to the skin and mucosal tissues, where cuts or wounds normally heal within a short period of time, the pulp has no epithelia that can bridge the defect. This means that even a small exposure may present the bacterial flora of the oral cavity with the potential to cause a destructive and irreversible (non-healing) inflammatory condition.

Exposure of the pulp may result from caries, fracture, crack and inadvertent deep cavity and crown preparation. Although caries progresses at a fairly slow pace, the other injuries cause a sudden and immediate exposure of the tissue. This is significant from a therapeutic point of view. For example, after a longstanding exposure to caries the pulp may already be in a compromised state such that healing and repair are not possible, making it necessary for radical removal. On the other hand, on a recent fracture or deep cavity and crown preparation a fairly healthy pulpal tissue is challenged and the potential for a conservative tissue-saving procedure is often promising. This is especially true if the injury is treated without delay. If an exposure by crack, fracture or deep cavity is left untreated or undiagnosed, an acute inflammatory reaction ensues, which may result in a non-healing lesion.

Pulpal inflammatory lesions of a destructive nature may also appear without direct exposure of the tissue to the oral environment. Such cases can be seen in conjunction with a restorative treatment, which often is carried out within a fairly short period of time (weeks, months) prior to the debut of the symptoms. The cause may be related to the injury induced in the pulp by the restorative procedure and leakage of bacterial elements in gaps along the margins of the restoration (see Chapter 3).

Inflammatory changes of the pulp may or may not occur with pain. The pain symptoms vary and in their end stages prior to pulpal breakdown can be excruciating, requiring immediate attention. Symptoms suggestive of a more or less severe pulpal inflammatory involvement are summarized in Core concept 6.1.

Treatment options

In cases where the pulp has become directly exposed to the oral environment, the clinician may consider one of two treatment strategies. One approach is conservative and aims to preserve the pulp and re-establish non-painful and healthy conditions in the long term (Figs 6.3 and 6.4). The other is a procedure whereby the entire

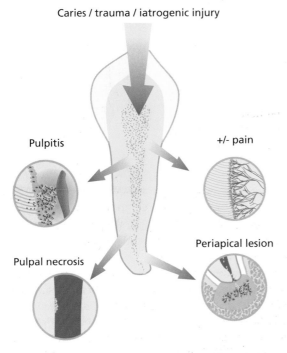

Caries / trauma / iatrogenic injury

Pulpitis

+/- pain

Pulpal necrosis

Periapical lesion

Fig. 6.1 Adverse pulpal reaction to caries, trauma or iatrogenic injury.

tissue is radically removed and replaced with a root canal filling (Fig. 6.5).

Prior to a definitive treatment, a preoperative emergency treatment may have to be carried out. Such a treatment is usually called for to alleviate a severely painful tooth or to maintain an accidental pulpal exposure until a definitive treatment can be carried out (see p. 85).

Vital pulp therapies include:

- *Indirect pulp capping*, which refers to a procedure whereby caries is excavated in a stepwise fashion in order to prevent iatrogenic pulpal exposure. This procedure may be used in situations of deep caries without signs of irreversible inflammatory changes in the pulp (see Chapter 7).
- *Direct pulp capping/partial pulpotomy.* These procedures are aimed at maintaining the pulp after it has become exposed to the oral environment (Fig. 6.3a). The open exposure is sealed off by the use of an appropriate wound dressing. The purpose of the seal is to prevent access of bacterial organisms in the oral cavity and to promote soft-tissue healing and hard-tissue repair of the exposed area. In pulp capping there is no removal of pulpal tissue, whereas in a partial pulpotomy some pulpal tissue is removed at the exposure site to a depth of 1–2 mm (Fig. 6.3b). This measure is carried out to clean the wound of infected tissue and to prepare a space for the wound dressing so that it can be applied securely (for a

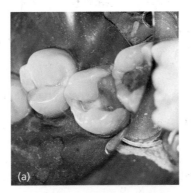

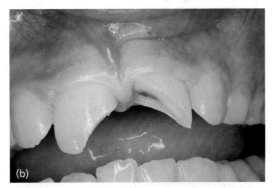

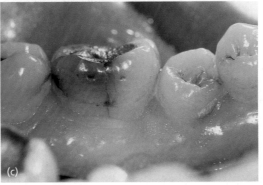

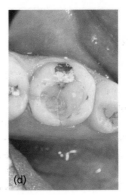

Fig. 6.2 Examples of clinical conditions requiring vital pulp therapy: (a) pulpal tissue directly exposed by caries; (b) pulpal tissue directly exposed by trauma; (c) non-exposed pulp but tooth presents with pain and there is a crack line on the lingual; (d) following removal of the filling, the crack seems to enter the pulp.

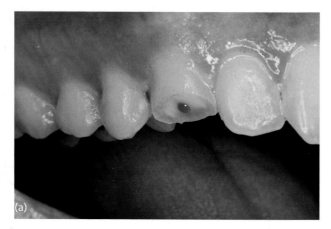

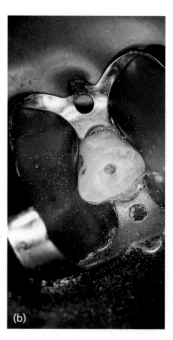

Fig. 6.3 (a) Clinical photograph of a pulp exposed to the oral cavity following a trauma. Pulp has been exposed for approximately 1 day. (b) The superficial portion of the pulp has been removed to prepare the site for a partial pulpotomy procedure.

Core concept 6.1

Pain symptoms commonly associated with a pulpal inflammatory lesion

- Increased sensitivity elicited by exposure to cold drinks, food and air or touch of an exposed dentine surface are early signs of pulpal inflammation. These symptoms are usually not suggestive of an advanced lesion. In the context of a recent restorative or periodontal treatment, such symptoms may emerge shortly after the procedure but often subside along with recovery of the tissue.
- Short, intermittent periods of lingering pain (seconds to minutes) by exposure to cold drinks, food and air may be signs of a pulpal inflammatory lesion in progress. Nevertheless, such symptoms may prevail for long periods of time (months, years) without resulting in pulpal necrosis.
- Longstanding (hours) severe pain, spontaneous or intermittently provoked by external stimuli, including hot food and drinks, is an alarming sign suggestive of an irreversible (non-healing) pulpal condition.

---

detailed description of the technique, see further below and Chapter 7).

- *Pulpotomy* is a term used for partial removal of diseased pulpal tissue. The procedure is often carried out in teeth with incomplete root formation, where pulpectomy for this reason cannot be carried out. Pulp is normally cut level with the canal orifices in two- and multi-rooted teeth, or as deep as necessary in teeth with a single root canal (Fig. 6.4). The remaining pulp tissue is covered with wound dressing. The aim of this procedure is to maintain the pulp

of the root portion vital and functioning so that root development can be completed (see also Chapter 7). The term apexogenesis is sometimes used for this procedure. In fully developed teeth, pulpotomy is often carried out as a temporary measure on an emergency basis until time is available for pulpectomy.

- *Pulpectomy* is an invasive procedure where the pulp tissue is removed in total by root canal instruments and subsequently replaced with a root filling (Fig. 6.5). A more detailed description of the procedures appears below.

Factors influencing choice of therapy

It is a most intricate task for a clinician to advocate the proper therapy when a pulp is exposed or when clinical signs and symptoms suggest a risk for pulpal necrosis. A conservative measure saves effort, time and money, whereas a pulpectomy, especially in the posterior tooth region, is often a technically demanding and time-consuming procedure. This is why direct pulp capping has enjoyed some popularity over the years for the management of pulpal exposures: it is non-invasive, easy to carry out and normally does not require an elaborate dental restoration afterwards. Nevertheless, a pulpectomy is the treatment of choice when the prognosis for pulpal survival is deemed questionable. If the pulp is assumed to be in an irreversible condition, a pulpectomy is always to be preferred in a fully developed tooth. The treatment is the most predictable and eliminates the risk for subsequent inflammatory breakdown of the tissue and associated infections and painful events. If a tooth

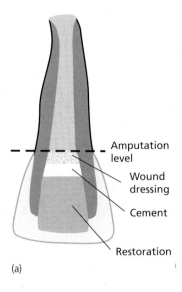
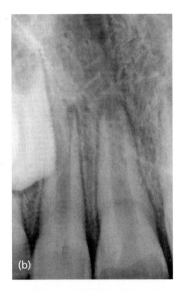

(a)   (b)

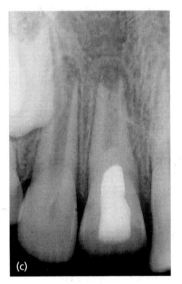
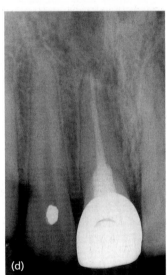

(c)   (d)

Fig. 6.4   Pulpotomy is a partial removal of pulpal tissue, also termed pulp amputation. The tissue is normally cut level with the root canal orifices in two- and multi-rooted teeth. In teeth with one root canal, tissue may be removed to the level of the cemento-enamel junction (a). Radiographs show: coronal fracture in tooth 11 with incomplete root formation (b); deposit of calcium hydroxide after removal of coronal pulp (c); root filling after completion of the root. In general, the pulpotomized tooth is followed radiographically and a root filling is not required unless excessive calcification occurs, or prosthodontic reconstruction is needed (d). (Courtesy of Dr M. Cvek.)

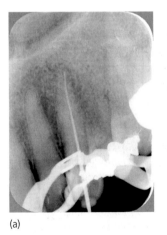
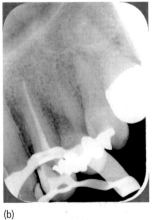

(a)   (b)

Fig. 6.5   Radiographs showing: (a) an instrument in the root canal of an upper lateral incisor in conjunction with a pulpectomy procedure; (b) the instrumented canal that has been filled.

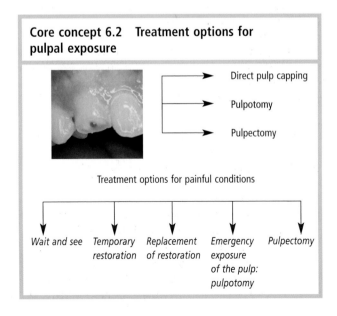

is incompletely developed, pulpectomy is precarious and pulpotomy serves as the alternative treatment (Fig. 6.4; Core concept 6.2).

In young individuals with incompletely developed roots, preservation of as much pulpal tissue as possible is essential. This makes way for continued development of the tooth structure. A pulpectomy, by eliminating the soft tissue of the pulp, prevents further growth and leaves a weakened tooth that is vulnerable to fracture. Cvek (13) reported that there is a close linear relationship between the degree of root closure in teeth where the pulp is lost and the rate of intra-alveolar fracture over time. In very immature roots the frequency of fracture was as high as 80% within 3–4 years after root canal therapy.

Pulpectomy not only eliminates the pulp but requires the sacrifice of hard tissue as well. Often the loss has to be larger than that initiated by the injury itself. This is because the treatment requires access to the root canal system and sufficient removal of the canal walls to allow proper filling. Inevitably this will reduce the resistance of the tooth to fracture by mastication forces (57). It also means that after completion of the procedure a rather extensive restoration is needed (see Chapter 12).

In conclusion, the time, effort, sacrifice of tooth structure and costs for a pulpectomy are greater than that for a pulp capping or partial pulpotomy procedure. Yet, critical to the choice of therapy is how the case presents itself and how that is deemed to affect the potential for pulpal survival upon a conservative tissue-saving measure. Therefore, the decision to carry out an invasive procedure or not must be based on a careful analysis of the clinical information that can be gained from the disease history and clinical examination of the patient.

Assessment of the preoperative condition of the pulp

Diagnostic criteria of an irreversibly injured pulp are by no means clear-cut. In fact, there are no objective means available, at present, by which the true condition of the pulp can be decided by, for example, a blood or tissue sample. Essentially there are two conditions that are used to guide the clinician:

(1) The presence and character of painful pulpal symptoms.
(2) The presence and type of pulpal exposure.

Core concept 6.1 summarizes the typical pain symptoms associated with pulpal inflammation. Although lingering pain, provoked by external stimuli, often is used to suggest an irreversible condition, studies have failed to find a strong correlation of such a symptom complex

---

Key literature 6.1

In his classical study Nyborg (40) prospectively followed a series of 225 cases that had been pulp capped due to pulpal exposure in conjunction with excavation of caries. The follow-up period varied from 10 months to 13 years. At follow-up, teeth were examined both clinically and radiographically for evidence of pulpal breakdown (painful symptoms of apical periodontitis and/or radiographic evidence of apical periodontitis). Eighty-one teeth were assessed histologically. Of the teeth that did not display painful symptoms at the time of treatment, the success rate was substantially higher (85%) than if patients had experienced pain prior to capping. Of the latter category, only 9 of 20 teeth were deemed to have a healthy pulp at the final follow-up. The study revealed that many teeth that were clinically without signs of pulpal pathology displayed severe inflammatory changes on histological examination.

---

with the true condition of the pulp (2, 59). In these studies pulps have been examined histologically after recording pain history and extraction of the teeth. It was found that report of severe pain was not necessarily associated with an advanced inflammatory breakdown of the pulp, and vice versa. Hence, a rather severe pulpal condition could have appeared without being accompanied by pain. Conversely, severe pulpal pain was sometimes present on rather modest tissue changes. Consequently, comparative studies have shown pain to be a rather weak predictor of the condition of the pulp, whether reversibly or irreversibly inflamed.

Nevertheless, the existence of a history of pain and the character of the pain presentation are crucial clinical manifestations because the mere presence of pain prompts a therapeutic decision. If combined with deep caries, cracked tooth, fracture or recent restorative procedure, a progressing inflammatory pulpal lesion may be imminent and an invasive therapy by pulpectomy would be required. This view is supported by the observation that pulp capping of carious exposures was less successful in patients displaying painful symptoms than in patients without pain at the time of treatment (40, Key literature 6.1).

A typical scenario suggestive of a progressing inflammatory condition of the pulp is when a tooth first becomes increasingly more sensitive to cold air or cold drinks and food products, which subsequently turns into shorter or longer periods of lingering pain elicited by the same stimuli. The intermittent character of the pain experience is a truly characteristic feature and is a differential diagnostic toward other painful conditions (see also Chapters 2 and 4). In the most severe cases, excruciating pain may linger for hours. Pain may occur spontaneously or be provoked by hot or cold drinks and

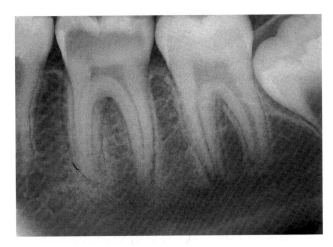

Fig. 6.6 Radiograph showing extensive caries in the crown of tooth 36. Although inflamed, the pulp is still vital and functioning. Periapically there are widened apical spaces at both roots and a sclerosis associated with the mesial root.

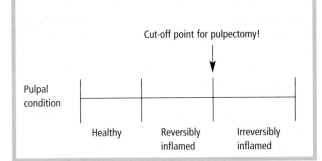

Core concept 6.3

- A pulpectomy procedure should be carried out when a pulpal condition is deemed irreversible.
- A pulp capping/partial pulpotomy procedure may be carried out when an exposed pulp is healthy or reversibly inflamed.
- Under clinical conditions the cut-off point between irreversibly inflamed and reversibly inflamed is often hard to identify.

food. In the end stages, prior to complete breakdown of the pulp, patients may find that cold water may alleviate the symptoms. The report of severe pain may be the only presenting symptom. Tenderness to percussion of the offending tooth and even of the neighboring teeth may or may not be observed in the final stages of pulpal inflammation.

Pulpal inflammatory lesions may cause the presentation in radiographs of loss of lamina dura, small periapical radiolucency and/or periapical sclerosis (Fig. 6.6). These findings in themselves are not necessarily indicative of an irreversible condition but can be helpful to identify the offending tooth in a painful case.

In conclusion, clinical and radiographic signs are less than decisive diagnostic measures to determine the spread of pulpal inflammation in a given case, and yet they are the only signs currently available for diagnosis in clinical practice. The decision to carry out an invasive procedure often has to be taken on the basis of the existence and the character of the pain symptoms (Core concept 6.3).

Management of exposed pulps by direct pulp capping/partial pulpotomy

Objective

Pulp capping and partial pulpotomy are procedures to consider when there is no history of lingering pain to external stimuli and when the pulp has been:

(1) Accidentally exposed to the oral environment by cavity preparation and traumatic injury.

(2) Exposed in conjunction with excavation of caries or hemisection in periodontal therapy.

Ultimately the procedures aim to preserve the vital functions of the pulp. Although not necessary for a successful outcome, it is considered advantageous that wound healing results in hard-tissue repair of the open exposure to enhance pulpal protection to secondary harmful events (Fig. 6.7).

Historical perspectives

In 1883 Hunter (26) claimed that 'Even though the pulp may be suppurating and the pus welling up in volumes, I shall save it' and he pressed a mixture of sparrow droppings onto the exposed pulp and achieved success 'fully equal to 98 per cent'.

Since Hunter so drastically introduced pulp capping, the treatment procedure has been vigorously disputed in the dental profession and is still a matter of controversy. The discussion often has been polarized, both as to when to do it, if at all, and as to what capping material should be preferred. The radicals have claimed that the long time perspective of the treatment is unpredictable and is doomed to failure, therefore the more invasive pulpotomy or pulpectomy must be carried out when the pulp is exposed. The conservatives, on the other hand, hold that success can be achieved, even when made in teeth following large and longstanding carious exposures, and they contend that pulp capping/partial pulpotomy indeed is worthwhile because if it fails then root canal therapy can be carried out.

The reason for the dispute has been the *de facto* uncertainty, already described, about the preoperative and

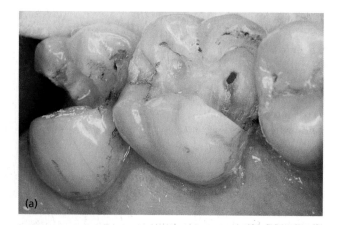

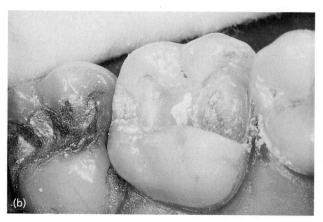

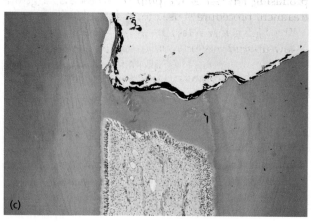

Fig. 6.7 Direct pulp capping: (a) exposure to bleeding pulp of a molar; (b) hard-tissue formation of the exposure (image courtesy of Dr B. Klaiber); (c) histological section showing hard-tissue formation 90 days following experimental pulp capping with a calcium hydroxide cement. Pulpal tissue displays a normal appearance.

postoperative diagnosis of the pulpal condition. Both are due to insufficient clinical measures to evaluate the true status of the pulp. Because major inflammatory changes may be present without concomitant clinical symptoms, a pulp-capped tooth may prevail for years without presenting clinical symptoms, even though there is extensive inflammatory breakdown (40; see also Key literature 6.2). A further reason has been a mediocre understanding of the healing potential of the pulp. Inflammation in the pulp is a dynamic process and for previously unaffected pulp that is housed in a large pulp chamber, especially in the young, the healing potential is substantial. Even after exposure to the oral environment for a period of time, healing is possible (6, 10, 24). Contrary to previous beliefs, inflammatory changes in one part of the pulp will not inevitably lead to pulpal necrosis and may heal if the proper measure is taken to sustain and optimize the healing potential.

Factors of importance for a successful outcome

As indicated in the text above, healing and repair of an exposed pulp depend initially on the preoperative condition of the tissue. Consequently, if inflammation has reached an irreversible state, no treatment can remedy the condition and a failure will show up as pulpal necrosis. This may or may not be preceded by painful events. Factors recognized as important for the long-term survival of the pulp to capping/partial pulpotomy are now deliberated upon.

Type of injury

An accidental pulpal exposure through intact dentine occurring during cavity and crown preparation has the greatest potential for a successful outcome. In this situation the pulp may be healthy and the bacterial contamination limited, therefore the immediate condition for healing is optimal.

In a traumatic injury, where the pulp has been exposed by a blow or fall, the healing conditions are favourable even though the pulpal wound may have been exposed to the oral environment for a period of time. Both clinical and experimental studies (6, 10, 11,

Key literature 6.2

Cvek (10) followed a series of 60 young teeth over 5 years that were treated with partial pulpotomy subsequent to pulpal exposure by trauma. Fifty-eight (97%) cappings were deemed successful, e.g. teeth were comfortable and without clinical or radiographic signs of pulpal breakdown. A further indication of pulpal vitality was completion of root development in teeth with incomplete root closure. In the study there was no difference in success rate, regardless of the time the pulp had been exposed to the oral environment (some teeth had received treatment first after several weeks), the size of exposure or the stage of root closure.

24) have demonstrated that bacterial contamination of the wound site becomes negligible (Key literature 6.2). Following proper disinfection and debridement, healing and hard-tissue repair have been shown to occur at a very high rate (10, 18, 38).

In exposures by caries, on the other hand, there may be a massive penetration of bacterial organisms to the tissue. This has usually resulted in a localized acute inflammation of the pulp, often as an abscess (see Chapter 3). The healing potential of such lesions is therefore unpredictable. The procedure of caries excavation, in addition, may exacerbate the lesion by forcing infected dentine chips into the tissue. Nevertheless, capping of carious exposures may be considered if symptoms of pulpitis are absent. It is generally agreed that the most favorable prognosis exists when perforation is made during the very final excavation of the deepest part of the caries lesion and when there is only a small exposure. An overall 5-year pulpal survival rate of 80% was found in 510 cases and no statistical differences were observed between carious and non-carious exposures (29). This finding is in accordance with the 93% success rate after 2 years reported for partial pulpotomy carried out in carious molars of teenagers (5, 38, 72).

Age

Although not consistently observed (3), it seems that the prognosis for capping and partial pulpotomy is better in young than old individuals (29, 72). The fact that the pulp of young teeth is rich in cells and blood vessels makes it prone to react favorably to microbiological and traumatic challenges. On the other hand, in an aged tooth and/or tooth exposed to previous injury the pulp is often poor in cells, fiber-rich and partly mineralized, therefore it is likely to be more vulnerable and less able to survive a capping procedure. The size of the pulpal space in an old tooth is also much smaller, thus providing a greater risk for pulpal breakdown upon destruc-

tive stimuli (4). In the study by Hörsted *et al.* (29), pulpal survival 5 years after pulp capping was 70% for 50–80-year-olds but 85% for 30–50-year-olds and 92% for 10–30-year-olds.

Size and location of the pulpal exposure

It has long been held that cappings should be considered only when there is exposure of an occlusal or incisal portion of the pulp, because capping of a more cervical exposure is thought to be less successful due to possible circulatory disturbances and necrosis of the coronally located portion of the tissue (21) (Fig. 6.8). Later, it was shown that cervical exposures may heal without compromising the rest of the pulp provided that a gentle treatment procedure is used (6, 7, 47).

The high success rate in clinical and radiographic follow-up studies after partial pulpotomy (10, 18, 38) has further put to question the relevance of exposure size as a significant parameter. It was once believed that cappings should be reserved only for pin-point exposures. Current knowledge suggests that the total volume of the pulp tissue in relation to the size of the exposure is more pertinent.

Clinical procedure

The procedure to carry out pulp capping/partial pulpotomy is simple. Success essentially depends on the

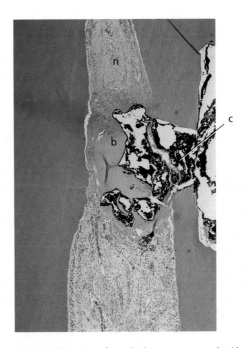

Fig. 6.8 Histological section of a pulpal exposure capped with calcium hydroxide cement. The capping material (c) has been pushed into the pulp, a major bleeding occurred (b) and the incisal pulp tissue became necrotic (n).

extent to which the wound site can be maintained free of bacterial provocations in both the short term and the long term (Clinical procedure 6.1).

Pulp capping is regarded as appropriate for immediate minor exposures, whereas partial pulpotomy is more apt for wounds that have been exposed to microbial challenges for a period of time, including large carious exposures. The recommendation is based on the results of experimental studies showing that after accidental exposure the infection remains superficial over the first 24 h (6, 11, 25). Over longer periods, infection usually has involved deeper areas of the pulp and therefore partial pulpotomy is advisable in these situations.

A partial pulpotomy offers the advantage that it removes the superficial and potentially infected layer of the pulp. Some surrounding dentine is removed as well, which creates a well-defined space for placement of the capping material (see Fig. 6.3b). The preparation should be carried out 1–2 mm deep with an end-cutting diamond burr in an air turbine under copious water irrigation in order to reduce the trauma on the tissue (see further Chapter 7). The operation is normally simple in a traumatized incisor but more demanding in a molar where, owing to the generally large wound cavity, bleeding may be difficult to stop.

A most critical step in pulp capping and pulpotomy procedures is to stop bleeding and to eliminate major blood clots prior to placement of the wound dressing. Blood clots serve as bacterial substrate and may support the growth of contaminating oral micro-organisms. If bleeding cannot be controlled properly, pulpectomy should be carried out. Another important consideration is to apply a gentle technique to avoid dilaceration and displacement of capping material to the deep portions of the pulp (27).

Integrity of the permanent restoration

Results of clinical studies and experiments in laboratory animals suggest that the integrity of the permanent restoration is of vital importance for the successful outcome of these procedures (3, 7, 29, 40). Even though the wound dressing may enhance hard-tissue repair of the exposure, the hard tissue often becomes porous and allows bacterial organisms to penetrate if gaining access to it (Fig. 6.9). In their experimental study, Cox *et al.* (7) observed that inflammatory pulpal lesions were frequent underneath repaired pulpal wounds and that these lesions correlated with the concomitant presence of bacteria in the newly formed hard tissue. The organisms conceivably originated from the oral environment after penetrating spaces at the margins of the permanent restoration.

Clinical procedure 6.1   Pulp capping

(1) Remove any blood clot with a sharp excavator in the case of timelag between exposure and treatment.

(2) Establish hemostasis by applying gentle pressure on the wound with a cotton pellet moistened with chlorhexidine, sterile saline or analgesic solution. Renew the cotton pellet if necessary and wait for complete hemostasis.

(3) Gently apply capping material to the wound without firm pressure.

(4) Cover the wound dressing with a hard-setting cement such as a glass ionomer cement.

(5) Restore and seal the cavity with a restoration.

(6) After 1 week, evaluate the presence or absence of symptoms.

(7) After 6 months, evaluate:
- symptoms
- reactions to thermal stimuli – absent, short, prolonged
- sensitivity to electric pulp testing – positive/negative
- periapical radiographic changes
- radiographically verified 'bridge' formation.

Based on the findings, continue recalls or do root canal treatment.

(8) Repeat (7) at yearly intervals.

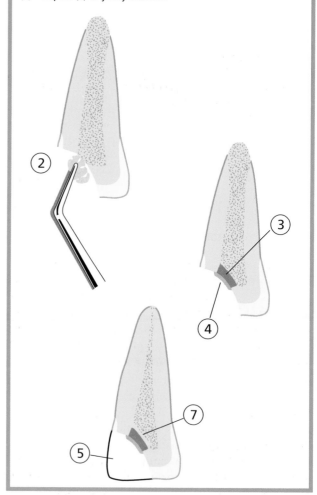

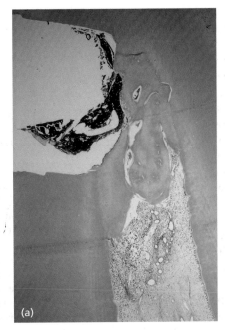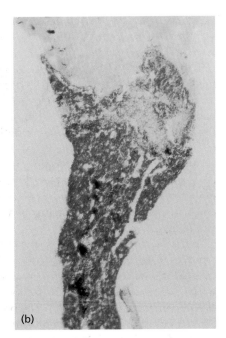

Fig. 6.9 Microphotographs from an experimental study carried out by Cox *et al.* (7), showing an inflammatory lesion underneath hard-tissue repair 13 months after pulp capping. (a) The porous nature of the hard tissue being formed is obvious. (b) Stainable bacterial organisms, seen as a purple mass, have penetrated the capping agent (black material), in this case a hard-setting calcium hydroxide compound.

Core concept 6.4

In selecting cases for pulp capping/partial pulpotomy, consider the factual conditions that prevail, i.e. whether they act in favor or against a successful outcome.

Critical factors are:

- Age of patient
- Degree of hemostasis that can be obtained
- The potential to provide a permanent restoration of long-term integrity.

The significance of the permanent restoration is also inferred by the observation of the declining rate of pulpal survival over time by Hörsted *et al.* (29) (Fig. 6.10). The use of adhesive techniques for the bonding of dental restorations to the tooth structure, or of any other restorative that results in a proper seal of its margins, should yield better long-term results (Core concept 6.4).

Capping materials and healing patterns

Calcium hydroxide

Since the 1930s calcium hydroxide water slurry and commercial hard-set compounds based on calcium hydroxide have been the prime materials for conservative treatment of pulpal wounds by pulp capping or pulpotomy. Calcium hydroxide suspensions and pastes are characterized by their inherent high pH. When applied to an exposed pulp, calcium hydroxide water slurry (pH 12.5) cauterizes the tissue and causes superficial necrosis. One would assume that such a treatment is detrimental to the pulp; it is detrimental, but only to a minor extent. Indeed, experience has shown that, in comparison with many other compounds, healing is predictable with this material (Fig. 6.11). It was even originally believed that the necrotic zone was a prerequisite for hard-tissue repair to be organized. Later studies have demonstrated that this is not necessarily so and that hard-tissue repair can develop in a less alkaline environment without a distinct zone of necrosis (16, 61, 63).

Hard-tissue repair of pulpal wounds is not unique to calcium hydroxide but can occur with a number of other materials (8, 12, 45) and with a variety of biologically active matrices and molecules (67). Even so, calcium hydroxide has remained the material of choice, primarily due to the solid clinical documentation. The material is likely to be important also from an antimicrobial point of view. Few oral micro-organisms survive in the high alkaline environment that this material provides, and therefore any microbes contaminating the wound site stand little chance of impairing healing (4).

Wound healing patterns to calcium hydroxide

Repair by hard tissue of a pulpal wound is a multifactorial process involving a wide range of cells, extracel-

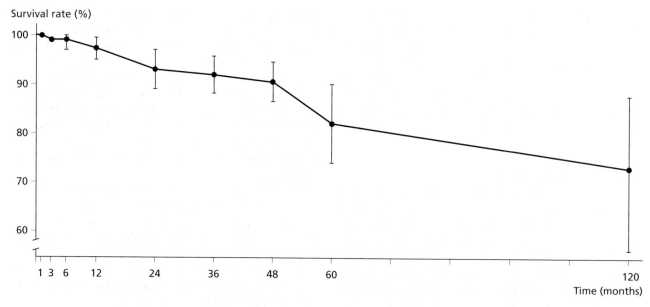

Survival rate (%)

Fig. 6.10 In a retrospective follow-up study of pulp cappings in 510 teeth by Hørsted *et al.* (29) it was found that, although the overall survival rate at 5 years was as high as 82%, the pulpal survival declined over time.

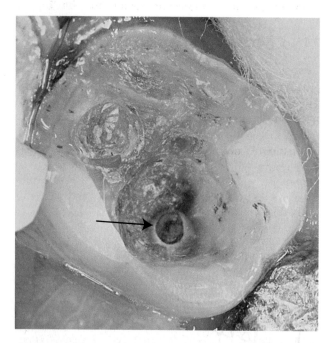

Fig. 6.11 Irregular hard-tissue repair of a pulp previously capped with calcium hydroxide (→). A crevice can be probed along the rim of the exposure, which may indicate that the hard tissue has been formed below a superficial layer of necrotic tissue.

lular molecules and physicochemical interactions (67). Although the exact mechanism by which calcium hydroxide initiates hard-tissue repair of a pulpal exposure is not fully understood, it is clear that in the process secondary odontoblasts are crucial (32, 71) (see Chapter

3). These cells are recruited from echtomesenchymal cells (stem cells) located in the pulp. Following a series of DNA replications, these cells migrate to the site of injury and differentiate into elongated and polarized odontoblast-like cells (17). The healing sequence following treatment of a wound in a healthy pulp and where pure calcium hydroxide or calcium-hydroxide-containing cements were applied with a gentle operative technique may be summarized as follows:

- One day after capping there will be a superficial layer of tissue necrosis and inflammatory cell infiltrates (55, 71). In response to calcium hydroxide cement, which provides lower pH, Fitzgerald (16) observed no necrosis but signs of bleeding and only a slight infiltrate of leukocytes.
- During the first few days thereafter, blood clots are resolved and the tissue is in a process of reorganization.
- The inflammatory reaction is gradually reduced and a collagen-rich matrix is formed in close relation to the necrotic zone or directly adjacent to the capping material.
- In the following week, mineralization of the amorphous tissue starts (Fig. 6.12).

The first mineralized tissue is irregular in nature and contains many cell inclusions. Subsequently a more dentine-like tissue with tubules is formed. Odontoblast-like cells line the tissue. It is a common feature that also the more regular-formed hard tissue contains cell inclusions and tunnel defects, rendering it permeable to noxious elements in the oral cavity (Fig. 6.9). A frequent term used for the hard-tissue repair is 'dentine bridge'. This designation is misleading, however, because the tissue often becomes highly permeable to bacteria and bacterial elements. In fact, it is often less able than primary dentine to protect the pulp from such elements. Hence, there will always be a risk for pulpal infection from possible surface seal breakdown.

Other materials for capping

Materials other than calcium hydroxide may also allow hard-tissue repair of pulpal wounds. This has given some strength to the theory that proper protection of the wound during the healing phase is just as, or more, important than the choice of a specific capping material. Accordingly, dentine bonding systems have recently been advocated for direct pulp cappings because the formation of a hybrid layer and subsequent restoration with resin composite is believed to result in leakage-free restoratives. In some reports the success rate has been similar to that with calcium hydroxide (9, 36). Other studies have shown that the use of a dentine bonding agent does not necessarily result in a permanent bacterial sealing of the cavity and 'bridging' of the wounded area (56). Pulpal inflammation and foreign body reactions against displaced resin particles have been described (14, 19, 23, 46, 66). Therefore dentine bonding materials should not be considered unless further documentation reveals results comparable to calcium hydroxide (4, 56).

Recent interest has focused further on the use of hydroxyapatite, tricalcium phosphate and mineral tri-oxide aggregate as potential capping materials (22, 48). However, if hard tissue subjacent to hydroxyapatite occurs, it has been described as irregular and incomplete and the use of tricalcium phosphate seems to be most effective if calcium hydroxide is added (31, 62). Mineral trioxide aggregate (MTA) material seems to produce a tissue response similar to that of calcium hydroxide (68) and offers, in addition, the advantage of setting hard with less risk of dissolution over time. So far, clinical documentation on the efficacy of this material is insignificant.

Bioactive molecules, known to be significant to the terminal differentiation of odontoblasts, have been proposed as an alternate way to achieve healing of pulpal wounds (53, 67) rather than caustic materials such as $Ca(OH)_2$ and MTA. Although promising in animal experiments, considerable research and development has to be carried out before bioactive molecules will find clinical applications.

In conclusion, solid experimental and clinical documentation accumulated over many years supports the use of calcium hydroxide in pulp capping and pulpotomy procedures. Predictable repair and healing of pulpal wounds can be expected provided that the treatment is undertaken on the basis of proper diagnosis and by the use of a proper technique (see Core concept 6.4). It is likely that calcium hydroxide will be replaced in the future by other less caustic materials that stimulate regeneration of dentine rather than repair with a porous hard tissue. Until further documentation is available, calcium-hydroxide-based compounds remain the materials of choice for direct capping and partial pulpotomy.

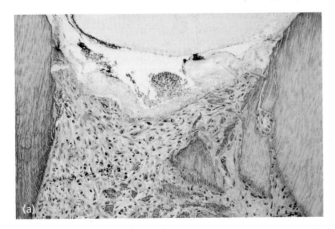 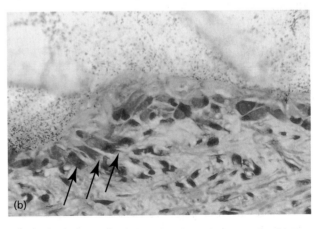

Fig. 6.12 Microphotographs from the study by Fitzgerald (16) showing tissue reorganization 5 days after capping of a healthy pulp in a monkey (a). Note the displacement of dentine chips. Unless not infected these chips do not impair but rather support the repair process and also become enclosed in it. Nine days after capping, new odontoblasts have appeared at the wound site and started to lay down a mineralizing matrix (arrows in b) (Courtesy of Dr M. Fitzgerald.)

Common reasons for pulpectomy

Painful pulpitis
Pulp exposure
Elective treatment in
  periodontal and
  prosthodontic therapy

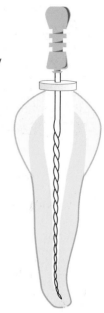

Fig. 6.13   Common reasons for pulpectomy.

Postoperative recall

Because of the inherent risk for pulpal infection and necrosis, direct pulp capping/partial pulpotomy should be followed clinically and radiographically. The postoperative control can be seen as a two-phase procedure: the initial phase entails an evaluation of whether healing and asymptomatic conditions have been attained; and the subsequent phase refers to the continued follow-up on a yearly basis. The latter is prompted by the prevailing risk of pulpal breakdown that may occur several years after treatment, due to infection along a defective restoration.

During the first weeks, minor sensations of spontaneous pain of short duration may occur. Such symptoms are expected to disappear. However, if symptoms get worse, indicating an irreversible inflammatory condition, pulpotomy or pulpectomy should be considered.

A 6-month recall is considered appropriate for the first follow-up. The tooth should be examined clinically according to the procedure outlined in Core concept 6.5. If there is no history of spontaneous pain, a positive reaction to electrical pulp testing and a normal periapical condition in radiographs, then treatment is considered successful. Apposition of hard tissue may or may not be seen radiographically. The restoration integrity should be checked for deficient margins, because marginal fractures or bulk fractures facilitate penetration of microorganisms to the wound site.

Pulpectomy

Pulpectomy is primarily carried out to prevent the development of a destructive course of pulpal inflammation, which may result in root canal infection and associated painful events (Fig. 6.13). This means that pulpectomy may be considered in any case where there are clinical signs indicating irreversible inflammatory changes in the pulp of a given tooth of the permanent dentition. A prerequisite is that root development is complete. Hence, the treatment may be performed regardless of whether the tissue is directly exposed to the oral environment or not. Pulpectomy is also the treatment of choice for any direct exposure of the tissue, when strict indications for direct pulp capping or partial pulpotomy are not fulfilled. Moreover, pulpectomy may be carried out following hemisection in periodontal therapy, and when retentive measures are needed in prosthodontic therapy. In these latter situations, the treatment is elective, which means that it is not prompted by a disease condition of the tissue.

Objective

Pulpectomy seeks to establish a condition where the tooth, following completion of treatment and after a follow-up period, is without clinical and radiographical signs of root canal infection (Fig. 6.14). In addition, the filling of the canal should be of such a quality that bacteria and bacterial elements in the oral environment are unable to penetrate the pulpal chamber and cause a periapical inflammatory lesion. The expectation is that such a healing result lasts permanently and for the duration of the patient's life. This objective is clearly attainable provided that treatment is carried out properly and

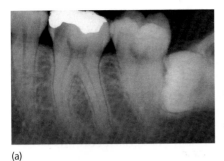 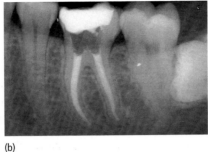 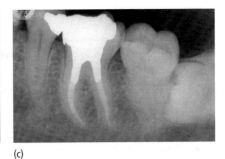

(a)   (b)   (c)

Fig. 6.14 Series of radiographs demonstrating a successful outcome of a pulpectomy in a lower molar: (a) deep caries mesially in tooth 36; (b) the final dense fill of the canal to proper length; (c) radiograph taken 4 years after completion of treatment. Tooth is asymptomatic and there are no radiographical signs of periapical inflammation indicating root canal infection. (Courtesy of Dr A. Gesi.)

with due consideration of the potential risk of bacterial contamination both during and after the procedure. It needs to be understood that although the treatment on many occasions involves removal of diseased and, to some extent, infected tissue, most of the tissue is not infected. This is particularly true for the apical portion of the pulp. An important objective of the treatment is therefore to maintain the sterile conditions of the root canal.

Critical procedural steps

Pulpectomy involves two principal steps:

(1) Removal of the connective tissue of the pulp in its entirety.
(2) Filling the root canal space thus obtained.

The tissue is removed by specially designed instruments that can be used to clean and widen the root canal space, both by hand and by rotary instrumentation. The various instruments and techniques by which they may be used in this context are comprehensively described in Chapter 16 and will not be dealt with here. The technique for filling instrumented root canals is presented in Chapter 18.

In order to achieve a predictable and successful outcome of pulpectomy, the following critical measures are considered in some detail:

● Anesthesia
● Aseptic technique
● Access and preparation of the root canal space
● Location and management of the apical wound.

Anesthesia

Pulpectomy is a highly painful procedure that should not be carried out without proper anesthesia. Routine procedures, including local infiltration or regional blocks, are to be followed and are most often sufficient.

However, pulpal anesthesia sometimes fails and one may find that the tissue can still be very sensitive and cannot be touched without causing intense pain, even if the injection has been given properly. This complication is more common in mandibular posterior teeth than in maxillary teeth, where infiltration anesthetics normally are effective (49). It is a common clinical finding, especially in patients with painful pulpitis, that complete anesthesia can be difficult to reach. Provided that the injection is given adequately and at the proper dosages, several mechanisms can be held responsible:

(1) Afferent nerve fibers deriving from inflamed tissue sites may have changed resting potentials and lowered excitability thresholds, which not only are restricted locally but extend throughout the affected nerve. Anesthetic agent is therefore unable to prevent total impulse transmission (35, 69).
(2) Patients under stress and anxiety have a lowered pain threshold (see Chapter 4).
(3) Accessory innervation, e.g. *nervus mylohyoideus*, may send branches to mandibular molars. The frequency has been estimated to be approximately 20% (58).

In the case of insufficient pulp anesthesia, one or several supplementary measures may be undertaken:

(1) Repeat injection and wait another 5–10 min.
(2) If not effective, combine regional block anesthesia with infiltration. For example, on mandibular blocks combine with infiltration at the bottom of the mouth distally to the tooth, to numb a potential extra nerve supply of *nervus mylohyoideus*. Combine infiltration of the maxillary incisor with a deposit deep into the nasopalatine duct to catch nerve branches.
(3) If still not effective, supplement with so-called periodontal ligament injection or intraosseous injection (Clinical procedure 6.2).

Clinical procedure 6.2

In the most headstrong cases where pulpal anesthesia is difficult to obtain, supplemental anesthesia of different modes may be attempted.

Intraligamentary injection

- Place short needle in the gingival sulcus, mesial or distal to the tooth.
- Advance into the periodontal ligament until resistance is met.
- Slowly inject 0.2 ml of anesthetic solution, which will penetrate the cancellous bone to the pulp.

This technique should not be used in teeth with marginal periodontitis.

Intraosseous injection

- Use infiltration anesthesia of soft tissue covering root apex and cortical bone.
- Perforate the periapical cortical bone with a solid needle driven by a contra-angle handpiece.
- Insert a short needle in the drilled canal.
- Inject 0.5 ml of non-vasopressor-containing, fast-penetrating anesthetic, e.g. articain, which is the anesthesia of choice (37, 39).

Intrapulpal injection

- Apply a cotton pellet saturated in anesthetic to the pulpal floor.
- Remove anesthetized dentine with a slow-speed handpiece. Repeat anaesthesia of dentine if necessary.
- Make a small perforation of the pulp, aiming at a snug fit of the needle in the perforation.
- Inject 0.5 ml of anesthetic into the pulp under firm pressure.
- Repeat procedure, if necessary, for each root canal following removal of the coronal pulp.

---

(4) As a final, desperate move one may be forced to give an injection directly into the pulp (intrapulpal injection) (Clinical procedure 6.2). It is important that such a measure is carried out only with full compliance of the patient. In an apprehensive or severely anxious patient the procedure should be avoided. It is then advisable to postpone treatment and reschedule the patient with a prescription for premedication. Different regimens may be practised, including a combination of oral administration of non-steroidal anti-inflammatory drugs and diazepam in proper dosages.

Formerly, when pain control could not be obtained in these extreme situations, pulpal devitalization was used. The procedure involved application onto the exposed pulp of a highly tissue toxic agent, e.g. formaldehyde.

Such a material would fix the tissue and render it necrotic within 1 week. Thereupon an endodontic procedure would ensue. This method is not used now because of the strong risk of leakage along the temporary filling to the marginal periodontium, where serious tissue destruction could result (see Case study).

Aseptic technique

Asepsis relates to measures undertaken during surgical operations to prevent the access of extraneous microorganisms to a given wound site. In endodontic therapies, including pulpectomy, potential sources of bacterial contamination of the pulpal chamber are from:

- Infected debris
- Saliva and gingival exudate
- Non-sterile instruments.

Hence, asepsis in endodontics involves procedures that are aimed to control these sources of infection.

Initially, prior to any attempt to enter root canals with instruments to extirpate the tissue, caries should be removed totally by careful excavation. Otherwise, there is an obvious risk that during canal instrumentation infected dentine is brought to the apical portion of the canal where it may induce and maintain an inflammatory lesion. Similarly, the tooth should be cleaned of any calculus and dental plaque. A defective filling is another source of bacterial contamination and should be eliminated and replaced before the initiation of treatment (Fig. 6.15a,b).

Proper asepsis in endodontics cannot be attained without the use of a rubber dam. Apart from providing an aseptic field of operation, a rubber dam facilitates the procedure and prevents instruments being dropped, which may be swallowed or aspirated into the lungs. Also, a rubber dam prevents leakage to the oral environment of tissue-irritating medicaments used during the treatment.

On intact teeth or teeth with only minor loss of tooth substance, a rubber dam normally can be applied without much effort. However, teeth with substantial substance loss may require different build-ups (Fig. 6.15b), including the placement of orthodontic or copper bands. Other measures to optimize rubber dam application include gingivectomy and crown-lengthening procedure.

Following the placement of a rubber dam it should be tested for leakage. This is best done with hydrogen peroxide (30%), which is carefully applied to the margins of the rubber dam. Leakage of saliva or gingival exudate will show up as a more or less intense foaming action (Fig. 6.16b).

To control leakage, the dam may be tightened to the tooth structure by dental tape. The technique is to

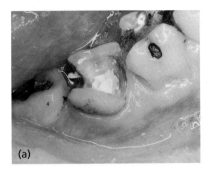
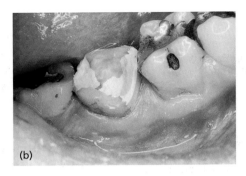
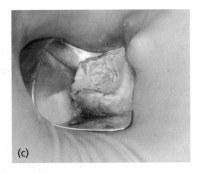

Fig. 6.15 Proper isolation of a tooth with a rubber dam is an absolute prerequisite to obtain an aseptic field of operation. Defective fillings should be eliminated first (a) and replaced with, for example, a glasionomer cement (b) or any other restorative that can prevent leakage of saliva and gingival exudate to the root canal during the procedure. (c) Rubber dam and clamp.

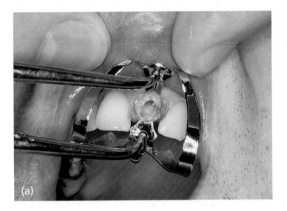
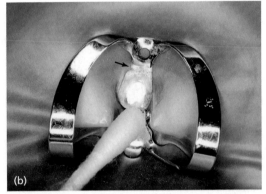
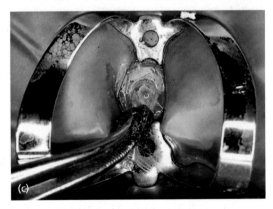

Fig. 6.16 Clinical photographs showing rubber dam application on upper incisor: (a) proper clamp is tested; (b) swab with hydrogen peroxide (30%) shows foaming action that needs attention (→); (c) disinfection with iodine tincture.

bring the tape through the tooth contacts and tie it underneath the clamp. Also, various forms of sealing agents may be used for the purpose of excluding oral fluid contamination. Finally the dam, the tooth and the pulpal wound should be disinfected with either an iodine tincture solution (5–10%) or chlorhexidine in alcohol (Fig. 6.16c).

An important step in the aseptic chain is to use sterile instruments. Instruments for root canal preparation are best maintained in boxes, which can be autoclaved (Fig. 6.17). During the operation, care should be exercised to avoid contamination of the part of the instrument that goes into the canal by, for example, finger touch or other non-sterile item.

Access and preparation of the root canal space

Technically, pulpectomy can be quite a demanding microsurgical operation. This is particularly true in posterior, multirooted teeth, where proper access to the root canal system often is difficult to attain. Pulpectomy also may be precarious in narrow and severely curved root canals. Other complications include:

- Overlooked root canals
- Incomplete elimination of pulpal tissue
- Lateral and apical overinstrumentation
- Incomplete filling of the root canal space.

It is obvious that under these conditions the prognosis for a successful outcome is lessened, because microbes either brought into the pulp chamber during the procedure or penetrating the pulp chamber after its completion may find conditions for growth and multiplication in the root canal system.

To optimize the conditions for a successful outcome, proper access to all root canals and thorough biome-

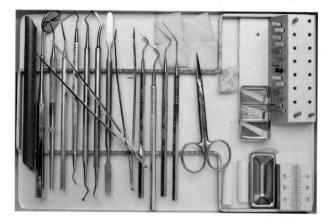

Fig. 6.17 Endodontic instruments arranged and sterilized in a cassette prior to use.

chanical instrumentation are critical. For a detailed account of the procedures associated with opening and instrumenting teeth for endodontic therapy, the reader is referred to Chapter 16.

To be completed successfully, a pulpectomy also requires sufficient time. It must not be rushed because of the imminent risk of leaving tissue elements behind (see Fig. 6.18). In other words, a pulpectomy should be completed in one and the same sitting and the canal then should be enlarged so that it can receive either a temporary or permanent root filling.

Location and management of the apical wound

Clinical, radiographic and histological studies have shown that containing instrumentation and root filling within 1–2 mm from the anatomical apex provide the best conditions for healing following pulpectomy, whereas apical overinstrumentation and overfilling have a negative effect on the result (50). Radiographic follow-up studies have also shown that leaving more than about 3 mm of the apical pulp reduces the chance of successful outcome (33, 34). Several points are strong arguments for the view that pulpectomy should be performed slightly short of the anatomical apex:

- The apical region of the root canal is reasonably well vascularized by virtue of its close relationship to the periapical tissue and to ramifications of the canal in the apical root structure. This provides sufficient conditions for healing, as opposed to a more coronal

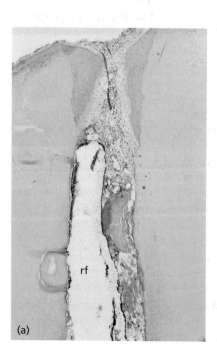
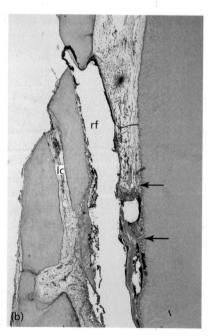

Fig. 6.18 It is important to recognize that non-instrumented tissue in overlooked canals and tissue remnants left on canal walls, in fins and in other canal irregularities, serve as potential sites for bacterial growth. In addition, tissue remnants prevent the establishment of a proper root filling that can seal off the instrumented canal. (a) Demineralized section of upper incisor. Root filling material (rf) is seen occupying the left part of the canal, and a mud of dentinal shavings and tissue remnants in the right part. Some inflammatory cells are located in the residual pulp tissue. (b) Demineralized section of upper incisor. The root filling (rf) is not following the main canal. Remnants of root filling material and pulpal tissue are seen in a lateral canal (lc). Inflammatory cells and dentinal shavings are seen lateral to the root filled main canal (←).

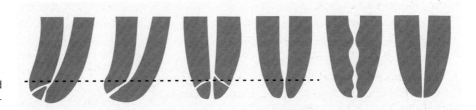

Fig. 6.19 The apical constriction (dotted line) and various configurations and locations of the apical foramen.

level of the root canal that is normally without collateral blood circulation (42).

- As the pulpal tissue and the dentine in this apical region most often are not infected, although it may be infiltrated with inflammatory cells, removal of the tissue and antimicrobial treatment are redundant.
- Instrumentation through the apical foramen may damage the root structure to the extent that a proper seal of the apical portion of the canal is jeopardized. Often an overinstrumented canal results in overfilling and a poor seal, to the detriment of a successful outcome. Root filling materials are not inert and overfilling may cause tissue destruction, inflammation and foreign body reaction in the periapical region (see Chapter 17). Ideally the apical wound should be slightly short of the apical foramen, where the canal is at its narrowest point. At this site many canals are almost circular and the wound surface can be kept to a minimum, leaving fair conditions for healing of the wound. This point is often termed the apical constriction. However, studies of the anatomy of the root apex have shown that the level of the apical constriction varies, although it is most often within 1 mm short of the apical foramen (15). In addition, the apical foramen often exists at a distance from the anatomical apex (Fig. 6.19). Because of these reasons it is logical to place the apical wound short of the anatomical apex and at a safety distance of about 1–2 mm from its level. The proper level is determined by placing an instrument in the canal to the assumed correct length and assessing the remaining distance to the anatomical apex in a radiograph. This procedure is termed working-length determination by the use of a trial file. Working-length determination can also be carried out electronically (see Chapter 16).
- Furthermore, confining the level of extirpation to 1–2 mm off the apex favors a shaping technique that is aimed at creating a step in the canal against which the root filling can be condensed. Accordingly, the chance of a tight fit between the filling and the canal walls increases, and the risk of overinstrumentation and displacement of the root filling material into the periapical tissue and bone decreases.

Permanent or temporary root filling after pulpectomy?

Provided that the extirpation procedure can be completed without complications, an immediate permanent canal filling is appropriate if there is sufficient time available for the filling procedure. If not, or if there is bleeding that is difficult to stop or concern about the technical outcome of the procedure in general, a temporary root filling is advocated. Leaving the canal unfilled is inappropriate because it may facilitate the growth of contaminating micro-organisms. Calcium hydroxide is then the material of choice. The rationale for its use is that:

(1) It fills up the canal space and prevents the multiplication of any contaminating bacterial organisms.
(2) It aids in stopping bleedings.
(3) It necrotizes any tissue remnants on the canal walls, which, upon a subsequent sitting, can be eliminated by instrumentation and the use of NaOCl irrigation (20).
(4) It favours the formation of hard tissue at the apical end of the root canal and at any cut lateral canals (60) (Fig. 6.20).

Wound healing after pulpectomy

The healing pattern following pulpectomy is characterized by an initial inflammatory reaction in the apical tissue due to the trauma induced by the cutting procedure. The residual pulp is often lacerated and may even be lost in the process (41). If, by accident, the root canal instrument has been pushed through the apical foramen during working-length determination or instrumentation of the canal, the apical termination of the preparation should still be confined to 1–2 mm from the anatomical apex to reduce the risk of periapical surplus of root filling material. In the absence of wound infection, reorganization soon occurs. This involves replacement of the injured tissue by connective tissue derived from the periapical region (28, 43). In the process, some internal or external root resorption may develop that later is repaired (Key literature 6.3).

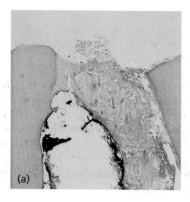
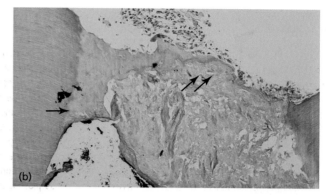

Fig. 6.20 (a) Microphotographs showing apical hard-tissue repair in tooth subjected to pulpectomy and filling with a calcium-hydroxide-containing cement 3 months earlier. (b) High magnification shows hard-tissue formation in relation to the root filling material (→) and dentinal shavings (⇉).

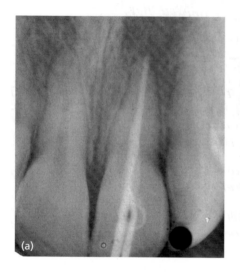
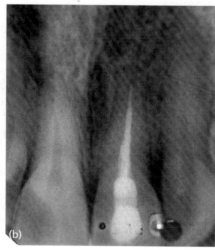

Fig. 6.21 Resorption of sealer: (a) root filling with gutta-percha points and a calcium hydroxide sealer after pulpectomy; (b) resorption or dissolution of the most apical part of the root filling after 10 months. (Courtesy of Dr A. Burhardt.)

Patients may experience some tenderness immediately following the procedure. These symptoms disappear in a few days' time, along with recovery of the apical tissue.

Materials used to fill root canals may compromise the normal healing pattern, owing to their irritating capacity, and result in a longstanding inflammatory lesion. In particular, this is the case when root filling material is extruded into the residual pulp and the periapical tissue, or into uninstrumented apical ramifications (51). Inflammatory cells accumulate close to the root filling material and remain for as long as toxic components are released. Eventually the material will be lined off by a fibrous connective tissue. These lesions usually go on unnoticed without causing much discomfort to the patient. On overfills extending into the periapical tissue, a radiolucent area can be found to circumscribe the material, thus reflecting the tissue irritation that is going on. The process of phagocytosis may eliminate the excess root filling material or occasionally also material inside the canal (Fig. 6.21). Hence, the responses to root filling material may remain for years and prevent complete healing, and yet root filling excesses do not cause extensive lesions and on more prominent lesions a bacterial etiology should be suspected.

It is not uncommon for dentine chips removed from the canal walls during the instrumentation to be displaced into or packed against the residual pulp (Fig. 6.22). Unless infected, this is usually regarded as beneficial because dentine chips:

(1) Separate the root filling material from the apical tissue
(2) Are instrumental in building up a hard tissue barrier (64).

It should be emphasized that neither the packed dentine chips nor the apposition of hard tissue onto displaced dentine chips is impermeable to bacteria and bacterial

Key literature 6.3

In an experimental study, deliberate apical overinstrumentation was performed by Hörsted and Nygaard-Östby (28) in 20 maxillary incisors and canines scheduled for extraction. The pulps were clinically healthy. The apical pulp tissue was removed or dilacerated and the indicator file was taken through the apical foramen (a).

To study the character of the subsequent tissue response, final shaping, filing and root filling was made substantially short of the radiographic foramen. After extracting the teeth 6–10 months later, histological examination revealed a cell-rich well-vascularized connective tissue within the apical part of the canal. This tissue bordered the root filling material and harbored only a few inflammatory

cells. Hard tissue was deposited on the canal walls in areas of previous internal root resorption (b).

The authors concluded that unintentional removal of the entire vital pulp to the periodontal membrane does not necessitate subsequent filling of the entire canal provided that strict asepsis is maintained during the treatment. Thus, if unintentional overinstrumentation is experienced, the root canal instrument should be withdrawn and further shaping and filing should be restricted to the original working length in order to facilitate a tight fit of the root filling and avoid surplus root filling material.

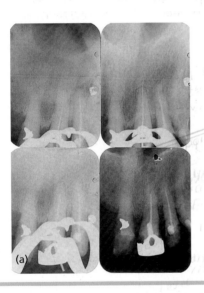

(a)

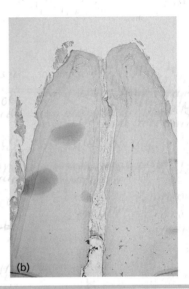

(b)

elements (54), therefore further treatment, e.g. a later access to the canal to prepare for a post space, must be performed under aseptic conditions.

Emergency treatment

Emergency treatment is primarily carried out to give relief from painful symptoms. It may also be driven by an unforeseen complication that is not associated with pain but that requires temporary treatment until a definitive treatment can be conducted. As for teeth with vital pulps, emergency treatment may occur due to:

(1) Painful pulpitis.
(2) Pulp exposure because of caries, iatrogenic injury or trauma in an otherwise non-painful tooth.
(3) Mid-treatment or post-treatment pain subsequent to pulpectomy.

Time often sets limits for what is possible to achieve. Time constraints may be due to unscheduled appoint-

ments in between regularly scheduled patients in the clinic, or because a complication occurred at the end of a scheduled treatment session. This means that an emergency treatment, by its very nature, often is a compromise. Nevertheless, the operation has to be carried out and should be directed to either alleviate or prevent the development of a painful condition or any other adverse sequel. This part of the chapter describes procedure that may be undertaken to meet such objectives as far as the vital pulp is concerned.

Painful pulpitis

In an emergency situation one may be faced with patients in different degrees of pain and thus of different urgency for treatment. Although severely discomforting to the patient, it may just be an enhanced sensitivity to thermal, osmotic and tactile stimuli, which disappears upon removal of the pain stimulus. In yet other cases the condition is severe and lingering and the urgency for treatment is high (see Core concept 6.1).

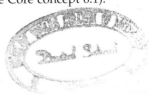

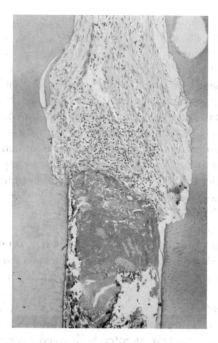

Fig. 6.22 Dentine chips removed from the canal walls during instrumentation are packed against the apical pulp tissue. About 2 months following root filling there is a slight inflammatory reaction of the tissue close to the dentine chips and resorption of the canal walls, but normal appearance of fibrous tissue and canal lumen further apically.

Also, the cause may vary. Most often teeth in pain are associated with a deep carious lesion or restoration penetrating either to the vicinity or straight to the pulp. There may also be a cracked or fractured tooth, where either large areas of dentine or a frank exposure of the pulp has emerged. Patients that more or less recently have been exposed to periodontal therapy may also present with episodic bursts of more or less lingering pain to external stimuli, indicating painful pulpitis.

Identifying the offending tooth is an important primary task and yet it may represent a most demanding diagnostic challenge (see also Chapter 2). The primary reason is that symptoms other than the patient's report of pain are rarely present. This means that if there is not an overt deep caries lesion, which is the most common cause of painful pulpitis, the clinician may be faced with the dilemma of assessing which one of several teeth is affected.

Management principles

Patients with pulpal pain may require a pulpectomy procedure but this decision should be taken only after careful consideration of the causes and the extent to which the pain condition can be alleviated by a more conservative approach. Determining the urgency for one

or the other mode of treatment is further complicated by the fact that patients in pain are often under great stress and may feel fear and anxiety for the treatment (see Chapter 5), therefore a condition may appear more severe than it actually is and thus prompt a more invasive procedure than is needed.

Cases where the pulp is not exposed and where the painful condition is about hypersensitivity or only short lingering pain to external stimuli are especially amenable to a conservative, or wait and see, kind of treatment. A recent restorative procedure or recent periodontal therapy belong to these cases. Often here the symptoms are of a temporary nature and will disappear over a few weeks without active treatment. If symptoms are pronounced or have persisted for some time, removal of the restoration and replacement of it with a new or temporary restoration may take care of the problem. However, root exposure subsequent to periodontal therapy or tooth wear is not managed as easily and requires some form of therapeutic agent that can block the permeability of the involved dentinal tubules so that the hydrodynamic mechanism for pain transmission along dentine is set off (see Chapter 4).

In cases where the condition of the pulp is deemed to be of an irreversible nature, the first step in the emergency treatment is to expose the pulp. If there is a caries lesion, all carious dentine should be excavated first and then several options are available, although time pressure often decides the choice of treatment. Several studies have indicated that pulpectomy with complete debridement of the root canals is the emergency treatment with the highest probability of pain relief (44, 65). However, sufficient time often is not available to comfort the acute patient by this procedure and therefore it should not be undertaken. An alternative faster treatment with a high rate of success is pulpotomy, where the coronal pulp is removed (21, 44) (Clinical procedure 6.3). The fastest and simplest treatment, but the least predictable, is to cover the pulpal exposure with a cotton

---

Clinical procedure 6.3 Emergency pulpotomy

(1) Prepare access opening to the pulp and remove the coronal pulp with a bur in an air-rotor.
(2) Irrigate with copious amounts of 0.1% chlorhexidine or 0.5% NaOCl.
(3) Control hemorrhage by pressure with sterile cotton pellets. In the case of profuse bleeding, soak pellets in 3% hydrogen peroxide or an aqueous mixture of Ca(OH)$_2$.
(4) Apply a small sterile cotton pellet to the pulpal wound at the canal orifices.
(5) Restore access cavity with a temporary filling.
(6) Perform pulpectomy as soon as possible.

pellet and a temporary filling. Where pulp is exposed after caries removal in an asymptomatic tooth, this procedure is normally sufficient until the patient can be scheduled for pulpectomy.

Special considerations

It was previously held that a sedative or antibacterial dressing such as eugenol, camphorated phenol or steroids was a necessary adjunct to obtain pain relief. Comparative studies have shown that there is no additional effect from using agents of this nature over what is gained by the placement of a sterile dry cotton pellet (21, 70). The cotton pellet also may be omitted because its function is merely to ease the location of the canal orifices at the next sitting upon removal of the temporary filling. The pellet must be small to permit a 4–5 mm thick layer of temporary filling material (e.g. zinc oxide–eugenol cement) to prevent microbiological leakage and contamination of the pulp between sittings.

Although pulpectomy has shown the highest success rate of pain relief, pulpotomy has given total or partial pain relief in about 95% of cases in clinical follow-ups (30, 44). In situations where pain relief is not accomplished by pulpotomy, pulpectomy should be performed and the patient should be made aware that some postoperative tenderness or a slight dull pain in the affected region is to be expected for a couple of days after the emergency procedure. If continuing to be severe, the patient should be advised to call and ask for a new appointment.

Pulpal exposure by trauma or caries in a non-painful tooth

In the case of pulp exposure of an asymptomatic pulp by trauma or caries, direct pulp capping or partial pulpotomy may be considered (see p. 71). Either treatment should be given as soon as possible following injury and then a permanent filling to preclude bacterial contamination should be carried out. If proper conditions for capping or pulpotomy do not exist, then pulpectomy is the treatment of choice and may be scheduled for a later appointment. In this case pulpal exposure should be managed by a temporary dressing as described above.

Mid-treatment or post-treatment emergency

A painful condition may remain after emergency pulpectomy or arise following pulpectomy of an initially non-painful tooth. The latter condition is termed endodontic flare-up. The cause is likely to be of bacterial origin combined with an inadequate technical procedure. Contamination due to not applying a rubber dam,

an unsatisfactory temporary restoration, displacement of carious dentine and bacterial plaque into the canal have been identified as key factors (1, 30, 52, 70). In combination with inappropriate intracanal medication, incomplete instrumentation, non-instrumented canals and apical overinstrumentation, it is easy to comprehend that conditions for bacterial multiplication are created in the root canal system. It should be emphasized that complications of this nature should be rare and only occur at a low rate in properly managed clinical practice (30, 65, Core concept 6.6). Cracked tooth substance and traumatic occlusion are other factors that should be taken into consideration when examining patients for causes of an endodontic flare-up.

To alleviate a painful condition after pulpectomy, the first step is to assess the need to carry out a re-entry procedure. This is particularly relevant if the tooth is already permanently filled. Many times the condition is self-healing and may be controlled simply by over-the-counter pain medication and a reduction of the functional cusps. If re-entry is deemed necessary, the endodontic procedure should follow the same strict routine as described above, which includes proper rubber dam application and disinfection. If necessary, the access opening should be adjusted to gain optimal entry to the root canal system. It is advantageous to enter without anesthesia for the control of any missed canals or incomplete removal of pulpal tissue. Of course, the control should be carried out with great care under gentle probing of potential canal orifices and root canals. Special notice should be given to the high frequency of maxillary molars with two mesial canals; the one that is most often missed is the mesiolingual canal. In lower molars the distal root may also harbor two canals. Copious irrigation and re-instrumentation of the canals should then follow, if necessary under local anesthesia. On carrying out the procedure, ensure proper working length and temporize the canal with a dressing of calcium hydroxide. In order to secure a bacteria-tight temporary filling of sufficient strength, a mix of a zinc oxide–eugenol cement or similar compound should be applied over the calcium hydroxide dressing, followed by a surface seal of hard-setting cement.

An endodontic flare-up may be associated also with an overfilled root canal. Normally, a small extrusion of

---

Core concept 6.6

Adherence to basic endodontic principles – including aseptic treatment, complete removal of accessible pulpal tissue and filling of canal to proper length – favors pain relief and precludes endodontic flare-ups.

root filling material does not cause more than slight tenderness, if at all, over a couple of days and subsides over the following days. However, if a severe pain condition has developed along with apical tenderness and some swelling, often there is a bacterial cause where, along with the root filling material, micro-organisms have been pushed into the periodontal tissues as well. Gross overfills may cause quite severe tissue responses due to a strong toxic reaction.

A rare but severe complication is associated with root filling material being forced into the mandibular canal. This is especially true if a paraform-releasing paste has been used (see Chapter 17). In such instances the patient may be numb for a few days, which later leads to a severe pain condition due to neuritis. Such a painful condition may last for weeks or months and cannot be cured by surgical intervention.

Case study

Sequelae following the use of toxic endodontic medicaments

A patient appeared in the dental clinic with pain and swelling related to the first right mandibular molar, a reduced capability of opening the mouth and paresthesia of the right lower lip. Root canal treatment had been initiated by another dentist some time previously and paraform used as a deposit between sittings. The intraoral examination revealed exposed cortical bone between the molar and the second premolar (a). Removal of a temporary filling in the molar released a strong smell of camphorated paramonochlorphenol from a cotton pellet and revealed devitalized pulp tissue and a mesial perforation of the pulp chamber.

The pulp chamber and the root canals were irrigated with copious amounts of sterile saline and the canals were further cleaned and shaped, followed by an intracanal deposit of a calcium hydroxide suspension. Antibiotics were prescribed.

Surgical removal of the necrotic tissue the following day revealed a mesial perforation of the molar (b).

The swelling was resolved and the paresthesia was reduced after 1 week.

One month later a bone sequester was removed and a deep periodontal pocket was probed mesially and in the furcation area (c, d), after which it was decided to extract the molar. Part (e) shows the mesial aspect of the extracted tooth, with perforation and apical remnants of the periodontal membrane. An implant was inserted later.

The case emphasizes the problematic use of highly toxic endodontic medicaments, which under adverse circumstances may leach to the surrounding periodontal tissues, resulting in serious destruction. (Courtesy of Dr K. Bröndum.)

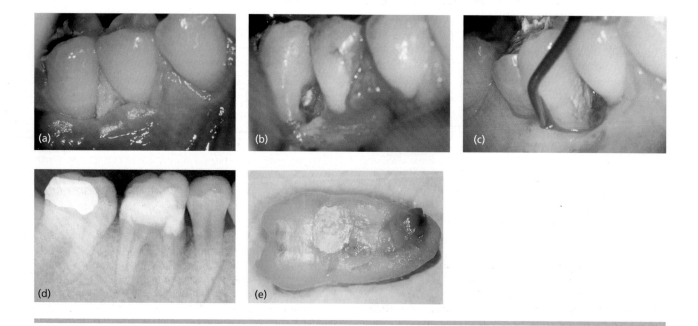

References

1. Abbott PV. Factors associated with continuing pain in endodontics. *Aust. Dent. J.* 1994; 39: 157–61.

2. Baume LJ. Diagnosis of diseases of the pulp. *Oral Surg.* 1980; 29: 102–16.

3. Baume LJ, Holz J. Long term clinical assessment of direct pulp capping. *Int. Dent. J.* 1981; 31: 251–60.

4. Bergenholtz G. Evidence for bacterial causation of adverse pulpal responses in resin-based dental restorations. *Crit. Rev. Oral Biol. Med.* 2000; 11: 467–80.

5. Caliskan MK. Pulpotomy of carious vital teeth with periapical involvement. *Int. Endodont J.* 1995; 28: 172–6.

6. Cox CF, Bergenholtz G, Fitzgerald M, Heys DR, Heys RJ, Avery JK. Capping of the dental pulp mechanically exposed to the oral microflora – a 5 week observation of wound healing in the monkey. *J. Oral Pathol.* 1982; 11: 327–39.

7. Cox CF, Bergenholtz G, Heys DR, Syed SA, Fitzgerald M, Heys RJ. Pulp capping of dental pulp mechanically exposed to oral microflora: a 1–2 year observation of wound healing in the monkey. *J. Oral Pathol.* 1985; 14: 156–68.

8. Cox CF, Keall Cl, Keall HJ, Ostro E, Bergenholtz G. Biocompatibility of surface-sealed dental materials against exposed pulps. *J. Prosthet. Dent.* 1987; 57: 1–8.

9. Cox CF, Hafez AA, Akimoto N, Otsuki M, Suzuki S, Tarim B. Biocompatibility of primer, adhesive and resin composite systems on non-exposed and exposed pulps of non-human primates. *Am. J. Dent.* 1998; 11: S56–63.

10. Cvek M. A clinical report on partial pulpotomy and capping with calcium hydroxide in permanent incisors with complicated crown fracture. *J. Endodont.* 1978; 4: 232–7.

11. Cvek M, Cleaton-Jones PE, Austin JC, Andreasen JO. Pulp reactions to exposure after experimental crown fractures on grinding in adult monkeys. *J. Endodont.* 1982; 9: 391–7.

12. Cvek M, Granath L, Cleaton-Jones P, Austin J. Hard tissue barrier formation in pulpotomized monkey teeth capped with cyanoacrylate or calcium hydroxide for 10 and 60 minutes. *J. Dent. Res.* 1987; 66: 1166–74.

13. Cvek M. Prognosis of luxated non-vital maxillary incisors treated with calcium hydroxide and filled with guttapercha. A retrospective clinical study. *Endodont. Dent. Traumatol.* 1992; 8: 45–55.

14. de Souza Costa CA, Lopes do Nascimento AB, Teixeira HM, Fontana UF. Response of human pulps capped with a self-etching adhesive system. *Dent. Mater.* 2001: 17: 230–40.

15. Dummer PM, McGinn JH, Rees DG. The position of topography of the apical canal constriction and apical foramen. *Int. Endodont. J.* 1984; 17: 192–8.

16. Fitzgerald M. Cellular mechanics of dentinal bridge repair using ^{3}H-thymidine. *J. Dent. Res.* 1979; 58: 2198–206.

17. Fitzgerald M, Chiego D, Heys DR. Autoradiographic analysis of odontoblast replacement following pulp exposure in primate teeth. *Arch. Oral Biol.* 1990; 35: 707–15.

18. Fuks AB, Gavra S, Chosack A. Long-term follow up of traumatized incisors treated by partial pulpotomy. *Pediatr. Dent.* 1993; 15: 334–6.

19. Gwinnet AJ, Tay FR. Early and intermediate time response of the dental pulp to an acid etch technique in vivo. *Am. J. Dent.* 1998; 11: S35–44.

20. Hasselgren G, Olsson B, Cvek M. Effects of calcium hydroxide and sodium hypochlorite on the dissolution of necrotic porcine muscle tissue. *J. Endodont.* 1988; 14: 125–7.

21. Hasselgren G, Reit C. Emergency pulpotomy: pain relieving effect with and without the use of sedative dressings. *J. Endodont.* 1989; 15: 254–6.
Seventy-three patients seeking emergency treatment because of acute pulpal pain were subjected to pulpotomies. After removal of the coronal portion of the pulp a cotton pellet moistened with camphorated phenol, eugenol, cresatin or isotonic saline, or simply a dry pellet, was placed on the remaining pulp tissue by random selection. Alternatively, zinc oxide–eugenol cement was placed directly on the pulpal tissue, which also was used for sealing the access cavities in the 73 teeth. Three of the patients returned for further treatment with pulpectomies after the anesthetic effect had disappeared. The residual 70 patients had no pain 1 day after the emergency treatment, irrespective of whether a medicament was used or not. The common use of sedative dressings seems thus to have no pain-relieving effect. The important part of the emergency treatment is removal of the irritants and the most inflamed part of the pulp tissue, followed by a bacteria-tight temporary filling.

22. Hayashi Y, Imai M, Yanagiguchi K, Viloria IL, Ikeda IL, Ikeda T. Hydroxyapatite applied as direct pulp capping medicine substitutes for osteodentin. *J. Endodont.* 1999; 25: 225–9.

23. Hebling J, Giro EMA, de Souza Costa CA. Biocompatibility of an adhesive system applied to exposed human dental pulp. *J. Endodont.* 1999; 25: 676–82.

24. Heide S, Kerekes K. Delayed partial pulpotomy in permanent incisors of monkeys. *Int. Endodont. J.* 1986; 19: 78–89.

25. Heide S, Mjör IA. Pulp reactions to experimental exposures in young permanent monkey teeth. *Int. Endodont. J.* 1983; 16: 11–19.

26. Hunter FA. Saving pulps. A queer process. *Items of Interest* 1883; 352.

27. Hørsted P, El Attar K, Langeland K. Capping of monkey pulps with Dycal and a Ca-eugenol cement. *Oral Surg.* 1981; 52: 531–53.

28. Hørsted P, Nygaard-Östby B. Tissue formation in the root canal after total pulpectomy and partial root filling. *Oral Surg.* 1978; 46: 275–82.

29. Hørsted P, Søndergaard B, Thylstrup A, El Attar K, Fejerskov O. A retrospective study of direct pulp capping with calcium hydroxide compounds. *Endodont. Dent. Traumatol.* 1985; 1: 29–34.

30. Imura N, Zuolo ML. Factors associated with endodontic flare-ups: a prospective study. *Int. Endodont. J.* 1995; 28: 261–5.

31. Jaber L, Mascrès C, Donohue WB. Electron microscope characteristics of dentin repair after hydroxyapatite direct pulp capping in rats. *J. Oral Pathol. Med.* 1991; 20: 502–8.

32. Kardos TB, Hunter AR, Hanlin SM, Kirk EEJ. Odontoblast differentiation: a response to environmental calcium? *Endodont. Dent. Traumatol.* 1998; 14: 105–11.

33. Kerekes K, Tronstad L. Long-term results of endodontic treatment performed with a standardized technique. *J. Endodont.* 1979; 5: 83–90.

34. Ketterl W. Kriterien für den Erfolg der Vitalexstirpation. *Dtsch. Zahnärztl. Z.* 1965; 20: 407–16.

35. Kimberly CL, Byers MR. Inflammation of rat molar pulp and periodontium causes increased calcitonin gene-related peptide and axonal sprouting. *Anat. Rec.* 1988; 222: 289–300.

36. Kitasako Y, Inokoshi S, Tagami J. Effects of direct resin pulp capping techniques on short-term response of mechanically exposed pulps. *J. Dent.* 1999; 27: 257–63.

37. Malamed S. *Handbook of Local Anethesia* (4th edn). St. Louis: Mosby, 1997.

38. Mejàre I, Cvek M. Partial pulpotomy in young permanent teeth with deep carious lesions. *Endodont. Dent. Traumatol.* 1993; 9: 238–42.

39. Myer SL. The efficacy of an intraosseous injection. System of delivering local anesthetic. *J. Am. Dent. Assoc.* 1995; 126: 81–6.

40. Nyborg H. Capping of the pulp. The processes involved and their outcome. A report of the follow-ups of a clinical series. *Odontol. Tidskr.* 1958; 66: 296–64.

41. Nyborg H, Tullin B. Healing processes after vital extirpation. An experimental study of 17 teeth. *Odontol. Tidskr.* 1965; 73: 430–46.

42. Nygaard-Östby B. *Introduction to Endodontics.* Oslo: Universitetsforlaget, 1971.

43. Nygaard-Östby B, Hjortdal O. Tissue formation in the root canal following pulp removal. *Scand. J. Dent. Res.* 1971; 79: 333–49.

44. Oguntebi BR, DeSchepper EJ, Taylor TS, White CL, Pink FE. Postoperative pain incidence related to the type of emergency treatment of symptomatic pulpitis. *Oral Surg.* 1992; 73: 479–83.

45. Oguntebi BR, Heaven T, Clark AE, Pink FE. Quantitative assessment of dentin bridge formation following pulp-capping miniature swine. *J. Endodont.* 1995; 21: 79–82.

46. Pameijer CH, Stanley HR. The disastrous effects of the 'Total Etch' technique in vital pulp capping in primates. *Am. J. Dent.* 1998; 11: S45–54.

47. Pereira JC, Stanley HR. Pulp capping: influence of the exposure site on pulp healing – histologic and radiographic study in dogs' pulp. *J. Endodont.* 1981; 7: 213–23.

48. Pitt Ford TR, Torabinejad M, Abedi HR, Bakland LK, Kariyawasam SP. Using mineral trioxide aggregate as a pulp-capping material. *J. Am. Dent. Assoc.* 1996; 127; 1491–8.

49. Potocnik I, Bajrovic F. Failure of inferior alveolar nerve block in endodontics. *Endodont. Dent. Traumatol.* 1999; 15: 247–51.

50. Ricucci D. Apical limit of root canal instrumentation and obturation, part 1. Literature review. *Int. Endodont. J.* 1998; 31: 384–93.

51. Ricucci D, Langeland K. Apical limit of root canal instrumentation and obturation, part 2. A histological study. *Int. Endodont. J.* 1998; 31: 394–409.
    Report presents histological observations of the apical and periapical tissue from 41 root filled human teeth. Inflammatory tissue reactions were seen many years after completion of root fillings in cases with extrusion of root filling material into the periapical tissue, whereas the most favorable histological conditions were observed when obturation remained at or short of the apical constriction.

52. Rosenberg PA, Babick PJ, Schertzer L, Leung A. The effect of occlusal reduction on pain after endodontic instrumentation. *J. Endodont.* 1998; 24: 492–6.

53. Rutherford B, Fitzgerald M. A new biological approach to vital pulp therapy. *Crit. Rev. Oral Biol. Med.* 1995; 6: 218–29.

54. Safavi K, Hørsted P, Pascon EA, Langeland K. Biological evaluation of the apical dentin chip plug. *J. Endodont.* 1985; 11: 18–24.

55. Schröder U. Effects of calcium hydroxide-containing pulp capping agents on pulp cell migration, proliferation, and differentiation. *J. Dent. Res.* 1985; 64: 541–8.

56. Schuurs AHB, Gruythuysen RJM, Wesselink PR. Pulp capping with adhesive resin-based composite versus calcium hydroxide: a review. *Endodont. Dent. Traumatol.* 2000; 16: 240–50.

57. Sedgley CM, Messer HH. Are endodontically treated teeth more brittle? *J. Endodont.* 1992; 18: 332–5.

58. Sillinpä M, Vuori V, Lehtinen R. The myohyoid nerve and mandibular anesthesia. *Int. J. Oral. Maxillofac. Surg.* 1988; 17: 206–7.

59. Seltzer S, Bender IB, Ziontz M. The dynamics of pulp inflammation: correlations between diagnostic data and actual histologic findings in the pulp. *Oral Surg.* 1963; 16: 846–71.

60. Spångberg L, Engström B. Studies on root canal medicaments II. Cytotoxic effect of medicaments used in root filling. *Acta Odontol. Scand.* 1967; 25: 183–6.

61. Stanley HR, Lundy T. Dycal therapy for pulp exposures. *Oral Surg.* 1972; 34: 818–27.

62. Sübay RK, Asci S. Human pulpal response to hydroxyapatite and a calcium hydroxide material as direct capping agents. *Oral Surg.* 1993; 76: 485–92.

63. Tronstad L. Reaction of the exposed pulp to Dycal treatment. *Oral Surg.* 1974; 38: 945–53.

64. Tronstad L. Tissue reactions following apical plugging of the root canal with dentin chips in monkey teeth subjected to pulpectomy. *Oral Surg.* 1978; 45: 297–304.

65. Trope M. Flare-up rate of single-visit endodontics. *Int. Endodont. J.* 1991; 24: 24–7.

66. Tsuneda Y, Hayakawa T, Yamamoto H, Ikemi T, Nemoto K. A histopathological study of direct pulp capping with adhesive resins. *Operat. Dent.* 1995; 20: 223–9.

67. Tziafas D, Smith AJ, Lesot H. Designing new treatment strategies in vital pulp therapy. *J. Dent.* 2000; 28: 77–92.

68. Tziafas D, Pantelidou O, Alvanou A, Belibasakis G, Papadimitriou. The dentinogenic activity of mineral trioxide (MTA) in short-term capping experiments. *Int. Endodont. J.* 2002; 35: 245–54.

69. Wallace JA, Michanowicz AE, Mundell RD, Wilson EG. A pilot study of the clinical problem of regionally anesthetizing the pulp of an acutely inflamed mandibular molar. *Oral Surg.* 1985; 59: 517–21.

70. Walton R, Fouad A. Endodontic interappointment flare-ups: a prospective study of incidence and related factors. *J. Endodont.* 1992; 18: 172–7.

71. Yoshiba K, Yoshiba N, Nakamura H, Iwaku M, Ozawa H. Immunolocalization of fibronectin during reparative dentinogenesis in human teeth after pulp capping with calcium hydroxide. *J. Dent. Res.* 1996; 75: 1590–97.

72. Zilberman U, Mass E, Sarnat H. Partial pulpotomy in carious permanent molars. *Am. J. Dent.* 1989; 2: 147–50.

Chapter 7
Endodontics in primary teeth

Ingegerd Mejàre

Introduction

The need for endodontic treatment in primary teeth is usually related to caries in molars, with the main objective being to maintain space in order to prevent crowding of the permanent teeth. Normally, the most important time period is before the first permanent molars have reached occlusion. The special features of the primary molar, such as the complicated root anatomy and close relation to the permanent tooth germ and its restricted time of function, make the treatment principles partly different from those of permanent teeth. These principles will be reviewed in this chapter.

The normal pulp

The histological appearance of the normal pulp in a primary tooth is no different from that of the permanent tooth. Physiological ageing occurs in both, although the time span during which this occurs is shorter in primary teeth. A common misunderstanding is that the primary tooth is not as sensible to pain as the permanent tooth and that operative treatment therefore would not require local anesthesia to the same extent. Even though it has been observed that the quantity of nerve fibers is smaller in the pulp of primary teeth (41), there is no proof that the primary tooth would not be equally sensible to pain. The only exception would be just before exfoliation, when the number of nerves within the pulp decreases.

Pulp inflammation

Even though there has been some controversy in the literature as to the capacity of the pulp of primary teeth to respond to caries by forming reparative dentine, several histological studies have demonstrated a frequent occurrence of reparative dentine in primary molars with deep caries (19, 39, 42, 51). Magnusson and Sundell (28) found

a significantly lower frequency of pulp exposure with a stepwise excavation procedure compared with direct complete excavation of deep caries in primary molars, suggesting that the pulp has good potential to produce reparative dentine.

The morphology of the primary molar implies that the clinical symptoms of pulp tissue reactions to damage may differ from those of permanent teeth (Core concept 7.1). Thus, owing to the relatively small distance from the coronal pulp floor to the bifurcation and the frequent presence of accessory canals through the pulpal floor, pulp inflammation by caries in primary molars more often results in pathological changes in the interradicular area. Fistula and abscesses due to pulp infection also are seen more often in primary teeth, probably because of the relatively thin buccal cortical bone in young children.

Internal root resorption is the most common sequel to inflammation after pulpotomy, the origin of which is not understood. It may be due to the different way in which the pulp tissue in primary teeth react to irritating agents. Thus, it has been shown that the physiological process of shedding occurs in areas lacking predentine, which has been shown to increase the risk of internal resorption (34, 55). By using calcium hydroxide as a dressing material after pulpotomy, the presence of a remaining blood clot between the dressing and the wound surface has been suggested to enhance the internal root resorption process (52).

Healing

A proper preoperative pulp diagnosis is decisive for successful endodontic treatment in primary teeth. Presupposing that the cause is removed, the extent to which inflammation can be present in the pulp while the pulp recovers and undergoes repair and healing is not known. In other words, the stage at which the inflammatory process is irreversible is uncertain but essential, because endodontic treatment in primary teeth focuses mainly on vital pulp therapy.

Core concept 7.1   Special features of the pulp and root morphology of primary molars in comparison with permanent molars

- The molar has practically no root socle.
- The coronal pulp chamber is comparatively large and wide and the distance to the surface of the tooth is small, both in the occlusal and approximal directions.
- The pulp horns are relatively large, both in the occlusal and approximal directions, making the tooth vulnerable to mechanical and carious exposure.
- The distance from the pulpal floor to the bifurcation is short and the area between the pulp floor and the bifurcation often contains accessory canals. Because of this and a possible less-well-mineralized dentine in this area, an interradicular widened periodontal membrane with loss of lamina dura or bone loss is a common radiographic sign of extensive inflammatory changes or necrosis of the pulp tissue.
- The roots are often flared and bent and then converging in the apical part and in close relation to the permanent tooth. In the coronal part the root canals are reasonably wide and accessible, whereas in the apical part they often show intricate morphology with narrow, ribbon-shaped and curved canals. Instrumentation may therefore be difficult, particularly in upper molars.

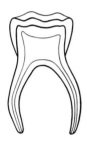 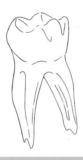

Results from recent clinical studies on direct or stepwise excavation of deep carious lesions in young permanent teeth and partial pulpotomy of cariously exposed pulps in both primary and young permanent teeth suggest that the pulp has good potential to recover once the irritants are removed (21, 26, 30, 49, 64). Thus, for example, a 100% clinical and radiographic success rate was observed after stepwise excavation in young permanent molars with deep carious lesions after observation periods of at least 2 years. Important prerequisites for a successful treatment were the absence of clinical and/or radiographic pathological symptoms.

The operative technique must be pointed out as an important factor for successful endodontic treatment. Thus, it has been shown that presumably infected dentine fragments unintentionally left behind in the pulp tissue cause widespread inflammatory reactions

(22). Therefore, meticulous cleansing of the exposed pulp is crucial, particularly when using capping techniques (21).

Repair and healing after pulpotomy, where the amputation site is situated at the orifices of the root canals, depend on whether or not preoperative inflammatory reactions also involve the root pulp, on the operative technique and on the characteristics of the wound dressing used. Furthermore, infection due to bacterial leakage is a prime threat to both repair and healing (4), and the importance of a bacteria-tight seal cannot be overemphasized.

Diagnosis

In order to assess the extent of pulp inflammation, two diagnostic terms are often used: *chronic partial pulpitis*, designated for teeth without preoperative clinical and/or radiographic symptoms of pulp inflammation; and *chronic total pulpitis*, designated for teeth with preoperative symptoms of pulp inflammation extending into the root pulp (7, 8, 51). For the sake of simplicity, the terms partial and total pulpitis will be used here.

Although essential for the outcome of the treatment, there is at present no means of precisely determining clinically the histological status of the pulp. Teeth judged to be without signs of total pulpitis might have profound pulpal inflammation. The proportion of correctly diagnosed pulps in histological terms judged from preoperative clinical findings has been investigated, with results varying from 56 to 81%. Most investigators have reported a poor correlation between clinical and histological findings (7, 8, 23, 39, 42), whereas others have found a relatively high agreement of about 80% (24, 51). Several of these studies suffer from a relatively small number of teeth and it is often not stated how the teeth were selected. Overall, it seems that, generally, the probability of arriving at a histologically correct pulp diagnosis based on clinical symptoms is rather poor.

In the clinic, it may be sufficient to know whether the pulp is treatable with vital pulp therapy or not, and it has been suggested that if the teeth are divided into two treatment categories only, i.e. 'treatable' (= partial pulpitis; vital pulp treatment) or 'not treatable' (= total pulpitis or necrosis; extraction), the agreement between clinical and histological findings will improve (8, 24). However, these studies also suffer from a small number of selected materials and in one (8), the difference between the two groups was not statistically significant. In the other (24), the basis for grouping the teeth focused on the character of the bleeding of the exposed pulp combined with the character of pain, a variable that is difficult to make unequivocal and reliable.

Core concept 7.2 Clinical signs of total pulpitis

- Radiographic pathological changes, such as widened peri-odontal membrane with loss of lamina dura, interradicular or periapical resorptive periodontitis (owing to superimposed structures, radiographic changes may be difficult to discover in maxillary molars).
- Abnormal tooth mobility.
- Spontaneous or persistent pain, particularly at night.
- Radiographic signs of calcifications in the pulp chamber.
- Dark-red and/or thick-viscous bleeding of the exposed pulp.
- Pulp exposed after removal of necrotic dentine – large pulp exposure.
- Profuse bleeding of the exposed pulp.
- Pain from percussion and/or pressure (often difficult to inter-pret, particularly in younger children).

Thus, although there are no clinical means to determine accurately the extent and severity of pulp inflammation, a number of clinical symptoms can be used to enhance the probability of arriving at a proper pulp diagnosis (Core concept 7.2). It has to be realized though, that teeth with deep carious lesions without any of these symptoms and accordingly classified as partial pulpitis may be classified correctly in histological terms in no more than 60–70% and at best in 80% of cases.

Importantly, it is less difficult to predict total pulpitis from clinical symptoms than it is to predict a healthy pulp or a pulp with partial pulpitis (7, 8, 23, 39), and the obvious presence of any of the listed symptoms (apart from pain from percussion and/or pressure, which is often difficult to interpret) indicates total pulpitis. Particular notice should be given to radiographic pathological changes such as widened and diffusely outlined lamina dura and the presence of spontaneous pain, particularly at night, both of which strongly suggest total pulpitis. Severe symptoms such as swelling, fistula or an abscess suggest pulp necrosis.

Wound dressings – characteristics and modes of action

The ideal dressing material for either unexposed or exposed vital pulps should be bactericidal, enhance the repair and healing of the pulp and promote the formation of reparative dentine or, in the case of an exposed pulp, the formation of a hard-tissue barrier. The dressing also should be biocompatible and not interfere with the physiological process of root resorption. Unfortunately, the ideal dressing is still to be discovered. Meanwhile, a variety of dressing materials are used. A detailed list of clinical success rates observed for different treatment procedures with different dressing materials is presented in Table 7.1.

Presented below are the most commonly used wound dressings: calcium hydroxide, formocresol (FC), glutaraldehyde, Ledermix®, zinc oxide–eugenol cement and ferric sulfate.

Calcium hydroxide

Calcium hydroxide, used as a dressing material on both unexposed and exposed pulps, is a strong alkaline compound with a pH of about 12 that causes a superficial necrosis of about 1.5–2 mm in the area underneath its placement. After the initial irritation of the underlying tissue, the pulp produces new collagen and thereafter a bone-like hard tissue. Avoidance of an extrapulpal blood clot is particularly essential when using calcium hydroxide as a wound dressing, because its presence may interfere with pulp healing (52). Therefore, it is important to use a gentle technique, implying cutting with high-speed equipment and diamond burs followed by irrigation with water or saline in order to achieve hemostasis.

The formation of a hard-tissue barrier, although seldom complete, protects the pulp mechanically and partially from bacterial infection (Fig. 7.1). It should be noted though that the presence of such a barrier, often considered a criterion of successful treatment, is no guarantee of a healthy residual pulp (37, 50).

Unsuccessful outcomes of pulpotomies using calcium hydroxide as a wound dressing have been attributed to a blood clot left behind between the dressing and wound surface (52). An *in vitro* laboratory study showed that blood and serum substantially lowered the pH of calcium hydroxide and thereby reduced its bactericidal effect (29). The presence of bacteria combined with a blood clot may therefore be an important cause of failure. Because the blood clot probably serves as a buffer, it also prevents calcium hydroxide from exerting its superficial necrotizing effect on the pulp tissue. Another reason for failure could be an incorrect pre-operative pulp diagnosis. Thus, it has been suggested that calcium hydroxide has no other effect besides promoting the formation of a hard-tissue barrier and therefore cannot be used successfully on an inflamed pulp tissue (52). The latter suggestion is, however, not consistent with recent reports on relatively high rates of successful treatments using partial pulpotomy in cariously exposed pulps (30, 49).

After pulpotomy with calcium hydroxide as a wound dressing, reported success rates vary between 31 and 59%. Using the same diagnostic criteria, the success rates are higher when calcium hydroxide is used as a dressing after partial pulpotomy (78–83%) (Table 7.1). As

Table 7.1 Reported clinical success rates of vital pulp treatment procedures of primary molars with deep carious lesions, along with type of wound dressing, number of teeth in the study and follow-up times.

Author (Ref.)	Treatment procedure	Wound dressing	Number of teeth	Follow-up time	Success rate (%)
Davies (5)	Direct pulp capping	Calcium hydroxide	71	23–36 mo	60
Pritz (38)	Direct pulp capping	Calcium hydroxide	20	2 yrs	57
Schröder (51)	Partial pulpotomy	Calcium hydroxide	93	1 yr	83
Jeppesen (21)	Partial pulpotomy	Calcium hydroxide	78	4 yrs	78
Schröder (50)	Pulpotomy	Calcium hydroxide	33	2 yrs	59
Via (62)	Pulpotomy	Calcium hydroxide	103	2 yrs	31
Hicks et al. (18)	Pulpotomy	FC[a], Buckley's formula	164	3.5 yrs	89
Mejàre (32)	Pulpotomy	FC, Buckley's formula	74	2.5 yrs	55[b]
Rölling and Thylstrup (47)	Pulpotomy	FC, Buckley's formula	98	3 yrs	70
Fuks and Bimstein (13)	Pulpotomy	FC, diluted to 1/5	77	2 yrs	94
Morawa et al. (35)	Pulpotomy	FC, diluted to 1/5	125	6–60 mo	98
Smith et al. (54)	Pulpotomy	Ferric sulfate	242	4–57 mo	74[c]
Fuks et al. (11)	Pulpotomy	Ferric sulfate	55	6–34 mo	93
Fei et al. (10)	Pulpotomy	Ferric sulfate	29	1 yr	97
Shumayrikh and Adenubi (53)	Pulpotomy	Glutaraldehyde, 2%	61	1 yr	74
Tsai et al. (60)	Pulpotomy	Glutaraldehyde, 2 or 5%	150	3 yrs	79
Fuks et al. (12)	Pulpotomy	Glutaraldehyde, 2%	53	2 yrs	82
Garcia-Godoy (14)	Pulpotomy	Glutaraldehyde, 2%	49	1.5–3.5 yrs	96
Gerdes et al. (15)	Pulpotomy	Ledermix®[d]	101	3 yrs	76[e]
Hansen et al. (16)	Pulpotomy	Ledermix®	14	1–42 mo	79
Magnusson (27)	Pulpotomy	Zinc oxide–eugenol	40	6–39 mo	55
Hansen et al. (16)	Pulpotomy	Zinc oxide–eugenol	14	1–42 mo	57

[a] FC = formocresol.
[b] 61% of the molars had obvious preoperative clinical signs of total pulpitis.
[c] The success rate after 2–3 years was 81% ($n = 57$) and after >3 years it was 74% ($n = 31$).
[d] Contains a synthetic corticosteroid and Ledermycin®.
[e] Successful is defined as functioning, i.e. teeth with radiographic evidence of internal root resorption were included in successful cases (15%).

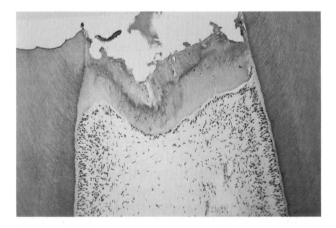

Fig. 7.1 Hard-tissue barrier in a primary molar formed after pulpotomy using calcium hydroxide as a wound dressing (H & E, ×40). (Courtesy of M. Cvek.)

judged from these studies, it seems that the partial pulpotomy technique is more favorable. However, prospective randomized studies comparing these two techniques are necessary to confirm this assumption.

Formocresol

Formocresol (FC) is used as a dressing material after pulpotomy. The original compound, Buckley's FC, contains concentrated formalin (19% formaldehyde), cresol (35%) and glycerol (7%) in an aqueous solution, the main active component being formaldehyde. Nowadays, Buckley's formula is often diluted to one-fifth of its original strength. Depending on the concentration and time of exposure to formaldehyde, part of the root pulp tissue is devitalized. Importantly, it has been shown that not even after prolonged application of the full concentration of FC was the entire pulp devitalized (33, 45).

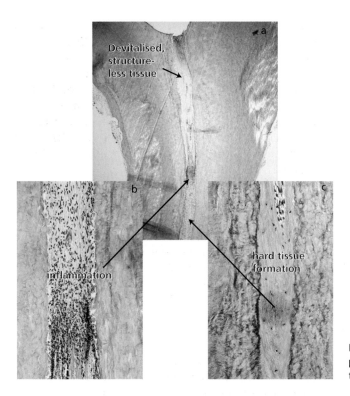

Fig. 7.2 Palatal root of upper second molar. Pulp tissue reactions after pulpotomy with Buckley's formocresol as dressing, 2.5 years postoperatively: (a) overview (H & E, ×25); (b, c) middle part of the root (H & E, ×60).

The most common histological appearance when using FC as a wound dressing is devitalized pulp tissue in the upper part of the root canal, inflammatory changes with internal root resorption and apposition of hard tissue in the middle section, with the most apical part usually showing normal pulp tissue (45) (Fig. 7.2). Thus, the use of FC does not result in repair and healing in histological terms, and a hard-tissue barrier underneath the dressing is not formed. This makes the tooth vulnerable to contamination from bacterial leakage and emphasizes the importance of a bacteria-tight seal when restoring the tooth.

As shown in Table 7.1, in most studies on pulpotomy the clinical success rates using Buckley's formula are higher than those obtained with calcium hydroxide as a dressing material (18, 25, 32, 47, 50, 62). Also, when diluted to 1:5, the clinical success rates of FC are considerably higher than that of calcium hydroxide (13, 35). Fuks and Bimstein (13), reporting a clinical success rate of 94% after 2 years of observation, recommended the use of the diluted formula of FC instead of Buckley's FC.

The most probable reason for the relatively high clinical success rate with FC as a dressing material is that, as long as the devitalized tissue does not become infected, the tooth usually stays asymptomatic. Furthermore, because of the more extensive devitalization of the pulp compared with calcium hydroxide, the use of FC is not as sensitive to a correct preoperative diagnosis of the inflammatory status of the root pulp as when calcium hydroxide is used. The clinical success rate when using Buckley's FC on molars with obvious clinical signs of total pulpitis amounted to 82% after 1.5 years of observation but dropped to 50% after 3 years (32).

Glutaraldehyde

Glutaraldehyde (GA) – a dialdehyde – has gained increasing attention as a possible substitute for FC as a wound dressing, the suggestion being less pulp devitalization but similar clinical results. Glutaraldehyde has not been produced commercially yet, the main reason being its instability, even when refrigerated.

Like FC, GA can cause allergic skin reactions, and hand dermatitis has been reported in dental assistants after using the disinfecting agent Cidex® (36). There are no unequivocal indications of mutagenic properties of GA. The cytotoxicities to human fibroblasts of the full concentration or a 1:5 dilution of FC were 2–3 times more toxic than 2.5% GA (20). In another study, however, little difference in the relative toxicities was observed between formaldehyde and GA when the data were calculated in terms of molar concentrations rather than dilution (58). Interestingly, GA appeared more toxic to rat nasal epithelium than FC (57). Owing to cross-linking, GA is less penetrative than formaldehyde and consequently causes less immediate damage to pulp tissue. However, in a study on monkeys GA did not result in repair and healing in histological terms (59) and it cannot be ruled out that, under a narrow zone of fixation, partial cell damage and/or a slow death of cells deeper within this zone may lead to chronic cell injury (58).

Studies reporting on the clinical success rate of GA as a wound dressing are listed in Table 7.1. Using 2 or 5% GA, the success rates vary from 74 to 96%, the periods of observation being between 1 and 3.5 years (1, 12, 14, 53, 60).

It has been suggested that the buffered GA solution is more effective than the unbuffered solution. The concentration and time of exposure to the tissue show a strong interaction (58), implying that GA needs a relatively long contact time with the pulp tissue to achieve optimal fixation. Whether this problem can be circumvented in the clinic by raising the concentration is debatable. Thus, the optimal strength of GA is yet uncertain and there are also varying opinions about whether it should be included in the permanent dressing of zinc oxide–eugenol cement or not. Additional studies on the possible optimal use of GA as a wound dressing therefore seem necessary.

Corticosteroids

The concept behind using corticosteroids as a wound dressing is to suppress and, ideally, reverse any inflammatory reactions in the pulp tissue. Ledermix® – the only commercially available dressing material for this purpose – is a synthetic glucocorticoid with some Ledermycin® (demethylchlortetracycline) added to it, mixed with calcium hydroxide, zinc oxide and eugenol.

There is a great deal of controversy associated with the efficacy of corticosteroids and their capacity, when used locally, to reverse pulp inflammation. Thus, Hansen (17) showed that the active component of Ledermix was decomposed after 18 days. It has been argued also that any anti-inflammatory effect is restricted to the contact area between the dressing and the pulp tissue (2). Furthermore, the dressing does not induce the formation of a hard-tissue barrier, a characteristic considered to be important in protecting the pulp of primary molars from bacterial leakage and subsequent infection. These factors may explain why Ledermix has not gained any widespread popularity as a dressing material.

Hansen *et al.* (16) compared zinc oxide–eugenol with Ledermix as a wound dressing after pulpotomy in cariously exposed pulps and found less severe internal root resorptions and inflammatory reactions in teeth where Ledermix was used. Although a lenient material without any observed side-effects, only a few studies report on the success rate with a corticosteroid as the wound dressing. In a small study of 30 molars and varying observation times, Hansen *et al.* (16) reported a success

rate of 79%. In a 3-year study with 101 molars, Gerdes *et al.* (15) reported a success rate of 76% (defined as functioning teeth and including 12 teeth with internal root resorptions and 4 teeth with radiographic and clinical symptoms). From these studies it might be expected that corticosteroids are superior to calcium hydroxide as a dressing material (see Table 7.1). However, because of the lack of randomized prospective clinical studies using different wound dressing materials, it is not possible to propose the best material.

Zinc oxide–eugenol cement

Zinc oxide–eugenol cement, probably not so often used today as a dressing material alone after pulpotomy, results in a high percentage of internal resorptions and reported clinical success rates are low (55–57%) (16, 27).

Ferric sulfate

Ferric sulfate ($Fe_2 (SO_4)_3$) in a 15.5% solution has been used as a coagulative and hemostatic agent in crown- and bridgework. Blood proteins agglutinate when they are exposed to the ferric and sulfate ions but the exact mechanisms of action are still debated.

When used as a wound dressing after pulpotomy, a metal–protein blood clot forms at the site of pulp exposure. Ferric sulfate mixed with zinc oxide–eugenol has been investigated as a possible alternative to FC (10, 11, 54). The reported clinical success rates are similar to that of diluted FC and vary from 74 to 97%. In the retrospective study by Smith *et al.* (54) the clinical success rate was 74% after 3 years of observation ($n = 242$); Fei *et al.* (10) reported a 97% success rate after 3–12 months ($n = 29$); and Fuks *et al.* (11) found a success rate of 93% after observation times varying from 6 to 34 months ($n = 55$). Overall, the reports are few, the number of teeth are small and most observation times are short. Therefore, it still remains uncertain whether ferric sulfate will replace FC as a more biological and equally clinically effective wound dressing.

Objectives of pulp treatment

Strictly, the objectives of pulp treatment are repair and healing of the residual pulp tissue in histological terms and a well-functioning tooth until normal exfoliation. At present, calcium hydroxide is the only dressing that, theoretically, has the potential to fulfil these criteria.

However, because of the low clinical success rate after pulpotomy using calcium hydroxide as a wound dressing and because of the restricted lifetime of the primary tooth, less strict criteria for the success of pulp treatment

Advanced concept 7.1 Concerns about the use of formocresol as a wound dressing in primary teeth

The use of formocresol (FC) as a wound dressing after pulpotomy in primary molars has been critically reviewed (40, 61). Besides its cytotoxicity, the main concerns are possible carcinogenicity, mutagenicity and the fact that formaldehyde is a potent allergen.

Formaldehyde (CH_2O), the main active agent of FC, is a small, highly reactive molecule that rapidly converts to water and carbon dioxide. It is cytotoxic and causes devitalization when applied to pulp tissue, the extent of which is dose- and time-dependent (33). Damage to the permanent successor due to possible diffusion of FC through the pulpal floor has not been observed, however (13, 44).

Animal studies have shown that formaldehyde has mutagenic and carcinogenic effects. Carcinoma in man due to formaldehyde exposure is, however, extremely rare (56) and the carcinogenic potential from a single application of FC to the pulp tissue of a primary tooth is negligible. If formaldehyde is a mutagen in humans, then we are in serious trouble, because most of us inhale formaldehyde daily, mainly from cars, wooden products, textiles, perfumes and other cosmetics and burning wood.

Any increase in positive reactions to patch tests in children who have had a previous FC pulpotomy could not be found (46), but allergic reactions to formaldehyde after root canal treatment have been observed in adults (6, 9). There are no known studies on a possible immune response from applying an antigen (allergen) directly to exposed pulp tissue. Although potential antigen-presenting cells mediating the immune response are present in pulp tissue, it seems very unlikely that a single dose of FC applied directly on pulp tissue would sensitize a person. Immunoglobulin E-mediated sensitivity to formaldehyde also seems to be rare (6). In contrast, contact allergy from the handling of the medicament is of major concern for dental personnel.

For the above-mentioned reasons and the lack of healing properties, FC is far from ideal as a wound dressing and efforts to find an efficient substitute for formaldehyde-containing wound-dressing materials in pediatric dentistry are important.

Key literature 7.1

In the study by Leksell et al. (26), the prevalence of pulp exposure after stepwise versus direct complete excavation of permanent posterior teeth with deep carious lesions was assessed in 127 teeth from 116 patients aged 6–16 years (mean = 10.2 years). Included were teeth with radiographs revealing carious lesions to such a depth that pulp exposure could be expected if direct complete excavation was performed, but teeth with clinical symptoms other than transient pain shortly before treatment were not accepted. The teeth were randomly selected for either treatment procedure.

Stepwise excavation implied removal of the bulk of carious tissue and application of calcium hydroxide, followed by sealing of the cavity with zinc oxide–eugenol cement. After a period of 8–24 weeks, the rest of the carious dentine was removed and the cavity sealed with calcium hydroxide, zinc oxide–eugenol and a restorative material. Direct complete excavation entailed removal of all carious dentine followed by sealing, as mentioned above. In the case of pulp exposure, a pulp treatment was performed.

The pulp was exposed in 40% of the teeth treated by direct complete excavation. The corresponding figure for those treated by stepwise excavation was 17.5%. The difference was statistically significant. The teeth with no pulp exposure after direct or stepwise excavation showed normal clinical and radiographic conditions at the last check-up (mean = 43 months).

In conclusion, stepwise excavation can prevent pulp exposure in teeth with deep carious lesions and the results indicate that this treatment procedure is successful provided that no preoperative symptoms of pulp inflammation are present.

are accepted in many countries, i.e. besides no general harm, no damage should be inflicted to the permanent tooth and the primary tooth should be symptomless until normal exfoliation. Formocresol is considered by many to meet these criteria and, owing to the comparatively high clinical success rate, is still a commonly used dressing material, although healing in histological terms does not occur (Advanced concept 7.1).

Operative treatment procedures

Indications and clinical success

Based on clinical and radiographic symptoms and other possible considerations for deciding the best therapy, the following operative treatment options are available (see Core concept 7.3):

- Stepwise excavation
- Pulp capping – direct, indirect
- Partial pulpotomy
- Pulpotomy
- Pulpectomy and root canal treatment
- Extraction.

Stepwise excavation

The purpose of stepwise excavation is to prevent pulp exposure by intermittent removal of carious dentine. By comparing the number of pulp exposures from stepwise excavation with those from direct complete excavation, it has been demonstrated both in primary and permanent molars that pulp exposures often can be prevented by stepwise excavation (26, 28, Key literature 7.1).

It has been assumed that by placing calcium hydroxide temporarily on the remaining innermost layer of carious dentine, the pulp tissue is stimulated to produce reparative dentine, allowing complete excavation without pulp exposure to be carried out at a subsequent treatment occasion. It is also possible that, by alleviating

Core concept 7.3 Deep carious lesions

Pulp treatment procedures and their indications	Indicated pulp status

Stepwise excavation

Indications: deep carious lesions, where the bulk of necrotized dentine has not yet reached the pulp; no clinical and/or radiographic signs of pathology, such as persistent pain, widened periodontal membrane or interradicular or periapical periodontitis.

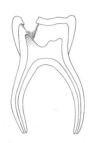

Indirect pulp capping

Indication: as for stepwise excavation (no clinical and/or radiographic signs of pathology), but differs in that the innermost layer of carious dentine is deliberately and permanently left behind. The indication is only when, for practical reasons, stepwise excavation cannot be performed.

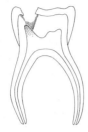

Direct pulp capping

Indication: accidental or pinpoint carious pulp exposure of a symptomless tooth.

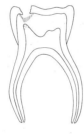

Partial pulpotomy

Indications: traumatic exposure or pulp exposure due to caries; no clinical or radiographic signs of pathology.

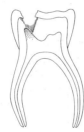

Pulpotomy

Indication: clinical and/or radiographic symptoms indicating coronal pulp inflammation.

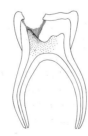

Pulpectomy/root canal treatment

Indications: inflammation extending into the root pulp, pulp necrosis and where special concern makes the tooth valuable.

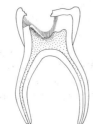

the bacterial load, pulpal healing and repair are facilitated. Other mechanisms such as remineralization of the remaining dentine may be involved but if and to what extent they contribute to the lower frequency of pulp exposures following stepwise excavation is not known.

Based on animal studies, Bergenholtz (3) suggested that the healing capacity of the pulp could be substantial once the irritating agents are removed. This assumption was confirmed by the favorable results of the >90% clinical success rate when stepwise excavation was used to treat deep carious lesions in young permanent posterior teeth (26). Although there are no clinical studies confirming the value of stepwise excavation in primary teeth, there is no reason to believe that this procedure should not be favorable also in primary molars. Stepwise excavation is therefore recommended for deep carious lesions in primary molars, presupposing that there are no or only minor preoperative subjective symptoms and no radiographic signs of pathology (i.e. no signs of irreversible pulp inflammation).

Indirect pulp capping

Indirect pulp capping is similar to stepwise excavation but differs in the sense that the innermost layer of carious dentine is deliberately and permanently left behind. This is not an ideal situation, because the amount of caries left behind will remain unknown, and the indication should therefore be when, for practical reasons, stepwise excavation cannot be performed.

Direct pulp capping

Direct pulp capping means that a minimal pulp exposure is just cleaned and covered with a wound dressing, preferably calcium hydroxide. Reported clinical success rates after direct pulp capping are low (5, 38) and the procedure should therefore be restricted to an accidental or pinpoint carious exposure.

Partial pulpotomy

Partial pulpotomy implies removal of only the most superficial part of the pulp tissue adjacent to the exposure, and is indicated for a traumatic pulp exposure or a pulp exposure from a deep carious lesion. Important prerequisites for a favorable result are the same as for stepwise excavation, i.e. no or only minor preoperative subjective symptoms, no radiographic signs of pathology and normal bleeding of the exposed pulp tissue. Two studies report on the clinical success rate in primary molars, varying from 78 to 83% after 1–4 years of observation (21, 49).

Pulpotomy

The indications for pulpotomy (implying removal of the entire coronal pulp) are the same as for partial pulpotomy, i.e. teeth with carious exposures with no or only minor preoperative subjective symptoms, no radiographic signs of pathology and normal bleeding of the exposed pulp tissue. Pulpotomy has been the most commonly used vital pulp therapy and numerous reports have been presented on the success rates. Depending on the status of the pulp, the operative technique, wound dressing and observation time, success rates vary between 31 and 98% (Table 7.1).

Although randomized prospective studies comparing partial pulpotomy and pulpotomy are lacking, the relatively high success rates reported for partial pulpotomy suggest that pulpotomy may be restricted to borderline cases, i.e. when clinical and/or radiographic findings are not easily interpreted and possibly indicate irreversible inflammation in the coronal pulp tissue.

Pulpectomy and root canal treatment

Usually, a primary tooth with clinical and/or radiographic symptoms indicating total pulpitis or pulp necrosis should be extracted. However, if the tooth is considered of special importance (e.g. when the permanent successor is missing) or if the child and the parents appreciate this type of service, pulpectomy or root canal treatment can be performed. The size and shape of the root canals are often considered a hindrance but root canal instrumentation might be performed if the canals are considered accessible. In order not to damage the underlying permanent tooth, broaches and files must be handled with extreme care and a resorbable medicament such as calcium hydroxide should be placed in the canals.

Extraction

Generally, clinical and/or radiographic signs of total pulpitis or pulp necrosis suggest extraction of the tooth. This is particularly important in a child with a history of severe acute or chronic illness, because the child should not be subjected to the possibility of further infection resulting from pulp therapy.

How to do it – procedures and important points

Stepwise excavation

Procedure: After local anesthesia, all peripheral caries, the bulk of necrotic and part of the demineralized dentine are removed. A layer of calcium hydroxide is placed on the remaining carious dentine and covered with zinc oxide–eugenol cement. After 6–8 weeks the rest of the carious dentine is removed and the bottom of the cavity is again covered with a calcium hydroxide layer. A layer of slow-setting zinc oxide–eugenol cement

or a fast-setting calcium-hydroxide-containing cement is placed and the cavity is permanently restored (see Case study 1). Alternatively, another intermediate excavation can be performed.

Partial pulpotomy

Procedure: Local anesthesia and a rubber dam are applied. All caries is removed and 1–1.5 mm of the exposed pulp tissue is removed with a spherical diamond bur and high-speed equipment (with water). It is not critical to use sterile saline but a coolant with ample flow is important. Remove all carious dentine adjacent to the pulp exposure before cutting the pulp tissue. Jeppesen (21) emphasized the importance of careful cleansing of possibly injected dentine chips from the area of amputation before applying the wound dressing. Bleeding is stopped by irrigation with sterile saline or water. Dry gently with sterile cotton pellets. A layer of calcium hydroxide is applied and gently pressed in contact with the wound surface. A layer of slow-setting zinc oxide–eugenol cement or a fast-setting calcium-hydroxide-containing cement is placed and the cavity restored.

Pulpotomy using calcium hydroxide

Procedure: Local anesthesia and a rubber dam are applied. Access to the pulp chamber is gained. The coronal pulp is removed with a spherical diamond bur and high-speed equipment. The wound surface is irrigated with saline or water. Bleeding is stopped by applying cotton pellets using slight pressure. After hemostasis, the wound surfaces at the orifices of the root canals are covered by a layer of gently pressed calcium hydroxide. A layer of slow-setting zinc oxide–eugenol cement covered with a fast-setting cement is placed and the cavity is restored. The restoration is crucial and a stainless-steel crown is probably the most effective for preventing bacterial leakage.

Pulpotomy using formocresol (FC)

Procedure: Local anesthesia and a rubber dam are applied. The coronal pulp is removed with a spherical bur and high-speed equipment. The wound surfaces at the orifices of the root canals are irrigated with saline or water. Bleeding is stopped by applying cotton pellets using slight pressure. After hemostasis, a cotton pellet soaked in FC is applied to each wound surface and left in place for 3–5 min. Full-strength FC (19% formaldehyde) is recommended if signs of total pulpitis are present, otherwise a one-fifth dilution is sufficient. The pellets are removed and a paste of one drop of FC mixed with zinc oxide–eugenol is placed on the wound surface. Avoid placing the pellets on the pulpal floor. A layer of slow-setting zinc oxide–eugenol cement covered with a fast-setting cement is placed and the cavity is restored (see Case study 2).

Pulpotomy using glutaraldehyde

Procedure: Local anesthesia and a rubber dam are applied. The operative procedure is in principle the same as for FC. Pellets soaked in a 2% buffered freshly prepared glutaraldehyde solution are placed on the wound surfaces and left in place for 3–5 min. The pellets are removed and a slow-setting zinc oxide–eugenol cement covered with a fast-setting cement is placed and the cavity restored.

Follow-up principles

Clinical and radiographic follow-ups should be done 6 months postoperatively and then at yearly intervals; in general, primary teeth subjected to endodontic treatment should be observed until exfoliation.

Long-term follow-ups are essential (21, 48). In most studies, success or failure has been judged from clinical and radiographic examinations only. However, in a study by Jeppesen (21) on partial pulpotomy, 43/76 clinically successful cases were judged histologically after 4 years of observation and were considered to be successful in 88%. This is of great importance from the view of follow-up procedures. Thus, after a follow-up of 4 years, the risk of additional failures was small but the potential for new failures was still present.

Table 7.1 gives an overall picture of pulpal survival assessed by clinical means subsequent to different treatment procedures of carious pulp exposures. Reported data differ in the diagnostic criteria for pulp treatment, with follow-up periods and criteria for successful treatment making direct comparisons impossible. It appears, however, that direct pulp capping and pulpotomy using calcium hydroxide or zinc oxide–eugenol as dressing materials result in the lowest clinical success rates. It is noteworthy that very few randomized studies have been performed with the aim of comparing different procedures and dressing materials.

Treatment failure

The clinical means for revealing an unsuccessful treatment include clinical inspection and radiographic examination. The earliest signs of failure are most often radiographically detected internal root resorption and/or interradicular bone loss, with subjective symptoms such as pain being unusual. Particularly in small children, electric pulp testing is often unreliable and instead careful inspection of the tooth and the surrounding oral mucosa should be made. Pathological tooth mobility, swelling or fistula constitute late and definite signs of an unsuccessful treatment.

As mentioned earlier, the formation of a hard-tissue barrier when using calcium hydroxide as a wound dressing is no proof of healing (37), but failure to produce hard tissue at the amputation site always means marked pathological changes histologically (21) (Fig. 7.3).

Radiographic signs of failure

Internal root resorption: This is the most common complication after pulpotomy in primary teeth, particularly after pulpotomy with zinc oxide–eugenol or calcium hydroxide as wound dressings. When zinc oxide–eugenol was used (27) it was observed in 18/40 (45%) teeth within a follow-up time of 3 years, whereas it was found in 11/33 (33%) after 2 years with calcium hydroxide as wound dressing (50). The prevalence was considerably lower when the partial pulpotomy technique was used – 4/93 (4%) (49) – although the follow-up time in that study was only 1 year. Jeppesen (21), also using the partial pulpotomy technique, did not report any failures due to internal root resorption after almost 4 years of observation. With calcium hydroxide as wound dressing, most internal root dentine resorptions were observed within the first year after pulpotomy (50).

Internal root dentine resorption occurs also after pulpotomy using FC, glutaraldehyde or Ledermix® as wound dressings (Fig. 7.4). In a study by Mejàre (32),

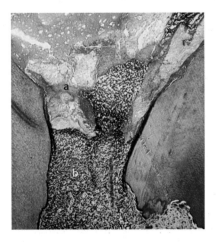

Fig. 7.3 Unsuccessful pulpotomy using calcium hydroxide as dressing material: (a) remnants of hard-tissue barrier; (b) heavy infiltration with inflammatory cells; (c) internal root resorption (H & E, ×40). (Courtesy of Ulla Schröder.)

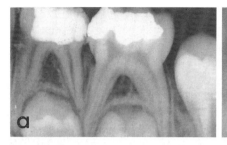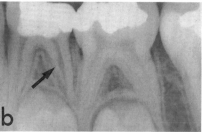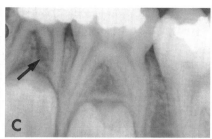

Fig. 7.4 Lower left first molar with radiographic evidence of internal root resorption after pulpotomy with Buckley's formocresol as dressing material: (a) at the time of treatment; (b) 18 months postoperatively; (c) 3 years postoperatively.

16/74 (22%) molars with FC as dressing showed internal root resorptions after 2.5 years of observation, whereas the prevalence was only 1/70 (1%) when the diluted formula of FC was used after 2 years of observation (13). With glutaraldehyde as a dressing, 6/50 (12%) showed internal root resorption after 2 years of observation (12). The use of Ledermix resulted in internal root resorptions in 18/101 (18%) after 3 years of observation (15).

As mentioned earlier, the reason for the emergence of internal root resorption after pulpotomy is not clear. Concerning calcium hydroxide, it has been suggested to be the result of either preoperative pulp inflammation in the root pulp or an extrapulpal blood clot left behind between the dressing and the remaining pulp tissue. Regarding FC or glutaraldehyde, the reason is probably the irritating effects of the medicaments.

Interradicular periodontitis: This was a common cause of failure after FC pulpotomies using Buckley's formula (32, 47) and was found in 29/74 (39%) teeth in a study by Mejàre (32) (Fig. 7.5). It should be noted, though, that in this study more than half of the teeth had obvious clinical signs of total pulpitis at the time of treatment, indicating a poor pulp condition and thus probably reducing the prerequisites for successful treatment. When using the one-fifth dilution of FC or glutaraldehyde, interradicular periodontitis has been less commonly observed: 3–4% (12, 13).

Periapical periodontitis: This was the most common reason for failure after partial pulpotomy and occurred in 10/93 (11%) teeth 1 year postoperatively in one study (49) but only in 2/78 (3%) teeth during a follow-up time of almost 4 years in another study (21). After 3 years of observation with Ledermix as a dressing, periapical periodontitis was observed in 9/101 molars (15).

Pulp obliteration: This has been observed mostly after pulpotomies using FC or glutaraldehyde as a wound

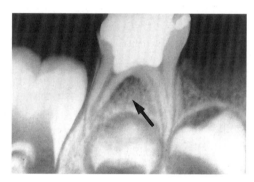

Fig. 7.5 Lower right second molar with radiographic evidence of interradicular osteitis 2.5 years after pulpotomy with Buckley's formocresol as dressing material.

dressing (Fig. 7.6). Thus, radiographic evidence of pulp obliteration was seen in 62–80% of molars pulpotomized using Buckley's formula of FC (18, 32, 47, 63). When the diluted formula was used (13), pulp obliteration was observed in 20/70 (29%) after 2 years of follow-up. With glutaraldehyde, pulp obliteration occurred in 20/50 (40%) after 2 years of observation (12), whereas Tsai *et al.* (60) reported a lower prevalence of 26/150 (17%) after 3 years of observation.

The reason for pulp obliteration is probably a response to the irritating effects of these agents, particularly the vascular damage inflicted upon the remaining vital pulp. Thus, it was shown that the formaldehyde component of FC is rapidly transported through the vascular system, causing severe thrombosis and hemorrhage at varying and seemingly unpredictable distances from the wound surface (31). As a consequence, remote parts of the original pulp tissue are damaged and may react by producing hard tissue. Similar reactions probably occur with glutaraldehyde as a wound dressing. It should be noted that this common reaction following FC and glutaraldehyde pulpotomies implies that vital tissue remains in the root canals. In most clinical studies this complication is not judged as a failure.

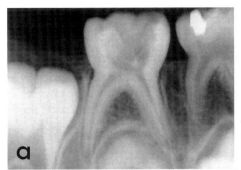 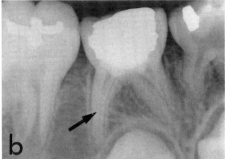

Fig. 7.6 Radiographic evidence of pulp obliteration in a lower right second molar following pulpotomy with Buckley's formocresol as dressing material: (a) preoperatively; (b) 2 years postoperatively.

Premature exfoliation: This complication is not considered as a failure but deserves to be mentioned. Thus, exfoliation of molars may occur faster than their antimeres both after FC and glutaraldehyde pulpotomies. It has been suggested that glutaraldehyde is superior to FC in this respect, because it resulted in a lower percentage of premature exfoliation: 15 versus 47% with Buckley's FC and 39% with the diluted formula (12). Although not properly evaluated, the clinical significance of a possible premature exfoliation of, at most, 6 months is probably of minor importance.

Indications and contraindications for pulp treatment in primary teeth

The most important reason for keeping a primary tooth until exfoliation is to preserve the space to prevent crowding in the permanent dentition. Concerning the molars, normally the most important time period is before the first permanent molars have reach occlusion. Other important reasons are to maintain masticatory functions, to prevent tongue habits and to preserve aesthetics. Furthermore, it might be important to keep the primary teeth for psychological reasons and the age and/or mental condition of the child may require special handling and considerations. When the permanent tooth is missing, the primary tooth may be important to keep for an extended period of time.

The following conditions generally contradict pulp treatment and the tooth should be extracted:

- Presence of clinical and/or radiographic symptoms indicating severe inflammatory reactions in the pulp, pulp necrosis, swelling, fistula or abscess.
- Medically compromised children, particularly those with a lowered resistance to infection, e.g. children with severe cardiac conditions.
- An unrestorable tooth or less than two-thirds of the root is present, i.e. the remaining function time of the tooth is short.

Advanced concept 7.2   New biological approaches to vital pulp therapy (from Rutherford and Fitzgerald (43))

Bone morphogenetic protein molecules

New techniques focus on biological approaches to vital pulp therapy. Based upon the nature of the wound dressing, biological agents – compounds synthesized in and by biological systems – are in contrast to calcium hydroxide for example, which can be looked upon as a non-biological material. At present, the most promising approach is within molecular biology, which provides opportunities to develop new strategies for the treatment of exposed pulps. Among the new agents, highly purified proteins have gained particular interest and a number of experimental studies suggest that *bone morphogenetic protein molecules* can induce reparative dentinogenesis in humans. Observations from animal experiments indicate that reliable therapeutic induction of reparative dentinogenesis and the preservation of pulp vitality would be possible even in diseased and damaged pulps.

Transdentinal treatment

The stepwise excavation procedure, where calcium hydroxide is used to induce reparative dentine, is an example of transdentinal treatment. The new transdentinal approach implies the use of biological agents to control pulp response through an existing layer of dentine. A layer of reparative dentine deep within the remaining dentine would provide extra protection from external irritants. The reduced permeability of this reparative dentine provides an additional protection of the pulp from thermal and mechanical challenges. A controlled amount of reparative dentine immediately following extensive dentine loss without pulp exposure would be a desirable clinical goal.

Although no materials are presently available to satisfy these criteria, there are indications that dentine matrix proteins are potentially capable of working in this direction.

Future directions

The degree and extent to which an existing pulp inflammation can be treated successfully using vital pulp therapy has still not been determined and there is no precise definition of what 'irreversible' pulp inflammation means. In order words, the capacity of the inflamed pulp to recover is largely unknown. Because endodontic treatment in primary teeth focuses on vital pulp therapy, this is an essential future research field. In this respect, prospective randomized studies where the partial pulpotomy technique is compared with the pulpotomy technique are of vital importance. Another important task is to find better assays for the clinician to decide the status of the pulp from clinical symptoms.

Furthermore, the fundamental biological processes leading to reparative dentinogenesis are not fully understood, nor is it clarified how the mechanisms behind tissue regeneration and healing work. This is essential in order to understand new efforts in biological approaches to vital pulp therapy (43) (Advanced concept 7.2).

Acknowledgement

The author would like to thank Nils Pyk for providing some of the illustrations for this chapter.

Case study 1

Stepwise excavation in a 5-year-old

History

A healthy 5-year-old boy presents with a deep carious lesion in the upper right second molar. There is no complaining of toothache other than sporadic pain in connection with meals and no visible pathological periapical changes.

Treatment

In order to avoid mesial drifting of the first permanent molar, it is important to keep the second primary molar at least until the first permanent molar has reached occlusion. Because there are no clinical or radiographic symptoms indicating irreversible pulp inflammation, the diagnosis is chronic partial pulpitis and stepwise excavation is the therapy of choice.

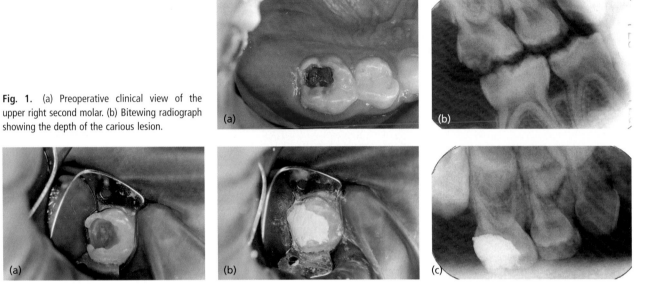

Fig. 1. (a) Preoperative clinical view of the upper right second molar. (b) Bitewing radiograph showing the depth of the carious lesion.

Fig. 2. (a) Clinical view after excavation of the bulk of necrotic dentine. (b) Calcium hydroxide was applied and the cavity was filled with a slow-setting zinc oxide–eugenol cement. (c) The radiograph shows no signs of periapical pathological changes.

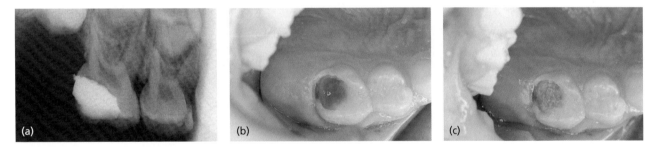

Fig. 3. At the second visit 8 weeks later, the tooth is without symptoms: (a) the radiograph shows no pathological changes; (b) the clinical view after reopening and removal of the temporary filling; (c) the clinical view after removal of the remaining carious dentine. A new layer of calcium hydroxide was applied to the deeper parts of the lesion, a layer of fast-setting calcium hydroxide was placed and the tooth was restored with glass ionomer cement.

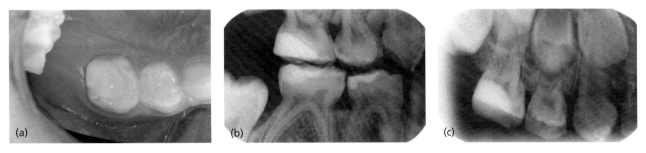

Fig. 4. One year later, the tooth is without symptoms: (a) clinical view; (b) bitewing radiograph showing the relation of the coronal pulp to the restoration; (c) periapical conditions according to the radiograph are without any pathological changes. Note that the first permanent molar is in a pre-eruptive position, in which the second primary molar plays an important role as a space maintainer.

Case study 2

Pulpotomy using formocresol in a 5-year-old

History

A healthy 5-year-old boy presents with a deep carious lesion in the lower right second primary molar. There is no history of pain other than occasionally after sweet food intake. There are no signs of swelling of the gingiva or fistula and the tooth mobility is normal. The radiograph reveals a deep carious lesion and the interradicular area shows a widened periodontal membrane and a diffusely outlined lamina dura. At caries excavation, necrotic dentine reaches the pulp chamber and the bleeding at pulp exposure is profuse and dark.

Treatment

In order to avoid mesial drifting of the first permanent molar it is important to keep the second primary molar at least until the first permanent molar has reached occlusion. In this case there are obvious signs of total pulpitis, such as necrotic dentine reaching the pulp tissue, dark profuse bleeding at exposure and periradicular pathological signs, as judged radiographically. With the pulp diagnosis being total pulpitis, the prognosis using calcium hydroxide as a wound dressing after pulpotomy would be poor. An alternative to extraction is to use formocresol as the wound dressing. In this case pulpotomy was carried out and full-strength formocresol was chosen as the wound dressing.

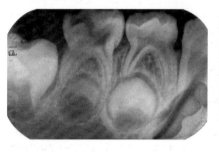

Fig. 1. Preoperative radiograph revealing a deep carious lesion in the lower right second primary molar. Note the position of the lower first permanent molar with its angled erupting direction.

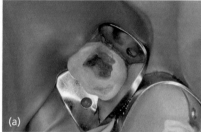 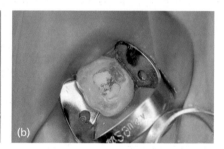

Fig. 2. (a) Formocresol has been applied to the root canal orifices for 5 minutes and the bleeding has stopped. (b) The formocresol-containing wound dressing has been applied to the root canal orifices. Note that the pulpal floor is not covered with the dressing.

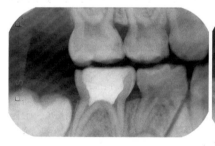 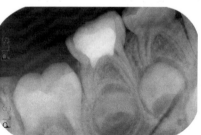

Fig. 3. Radiographs taken 6 months postoperatively. The right image shows the interradicular area towards the mesial root still shows a diffusely outlined lamina dura, although the picture is not easily interpreted. Otherwise the tooth is symptomless.

Fig. 4. Radiograph taken 2 years postoperatively. There are no obvious signs of periradicular pathology, the tooth is clinically symptomless and the first permanent molar has erupted and reached occlusion.

References

1. Araujo FB, Ely LB, Pergo AM, Pesce HF. A clinical evaluation of 2% buffered glutaraldehyde in pulpotomies of human deciduous teeth: 24 month study. *Braz. Dent. J.* 1995; 6: 41–4.
2. Baume LJ, Fiore-Donno G. The use of cortico-steroid-antibiotic preparation in endodontic therapy. In *Transactions of the Fourth International Conference on Endodontics* (Grossman LI, ed.). Philadelphia, PA: University of Pennsylvania, 1968; 62–82.
3. Bergenholtz G. Inflammatory response of the dental pulp to bacterial irritation. *J. Endodont.* 1981; 7: 100–104.
4. Bergenholtz G, Cox CF, Loesche WJ, Sved SA. Bacterial leakage around dental restorations: its effect on the dental pulp. *J. Oral. Pathol.* 1982; 11: 439–50.

5. Davies GN. Pulp therapy in primary teeth. *Aust. Dent. J.* 1962; 7: 111–20.

6. Ebner H, Kraft D. Formaldehyde-induced anaphylaxis after dental treatment? *Contact Dermat.* 1991; 24: 307–8.

7. Eidelman E, Ulmansky M, Michaeli Y. Histopathology of the pulp in primary incisors with deep dentinal caries. *Pediatr. Dent.* 1992; 14: 372–5.

8. Eidelman E, Touma B, Ulmansky M. Pulp pathology in deciduous teeth. Clinical and histological correlations. *Israel J. Med. Sci.* 1968; 4: 1244–8.

9. El Sayed F, Seite-Bellezza D, Sans B, Bayle-Lebey P, Marguery MC, Bazex J. Contact urticaria from formaldehyde in a root canal dental paste. *Contact Dermat.* 1995; 33: 353.

10. Fei AL, Udin RD, Johnson R. A clinical study of ferric sulfate as a pulpotomy agent in primary teeth. *Pediatr. Dent.* 1997; 19: 327–32.

11. Fuks AB, Holan G, Davis JM, Eidelman E. Ferric sulfate versus dilute formocresol in pulpotomized primary molars: long-term follow up. *Pediatr. Dent.* 1997; 19: 327–30.

12. Fuks AB, Bimstein E, Guelmann M, Klein H. Assessment of a 2 percent buffered glutaraldehyde solution in pulpotomized primary teeth of schoolchildren. *J. Dent. Child.* 1990; 57: 371–5.

13. Fuks A, Bimstein E. Clinical evaluation of diluted formocresol pulpotomies in primary teeth of school children. *Pediatr. Dent.* 1981; 3: 321–4.

14. Garcia-Godoy F. A 42-month clinical evaluation of glutaraldehyde pulpotomies in primary teeth. *J. Pedodont.* 1986; 10: 148–55.

15. Gerdes I, Ravn JJ, Lambjerg-Hansen H. Vital pulpotomy in primary molars with Ledermix® cement used as amputation material (in Danish, English summary). *Tandlægebladet* 1977; 81: 421–6.

16. Hansen HP. Ravn JJ, Ulrich D. Vital pulpotomy in primary molars. A clinical and histological investigation of the effect of zinc oxide-eugenol cement and Ledermix®. *Scand. J. Dent. Res.* 1971; 70: 13–23.

17. Hansen HP. Kortikoider i endodontin (in Danish). *Tandlægebladet* 1969; 73: 539–56.

18. Hicks MJ, Barr ES, Flaitz CM. Formocresol pulpotomies in primary molars: a radiographic study in a pediatric dentistry practice. *J. Pedodont.* 1986; 10: 331–9.

19. Ireland RL. Secondary dentin formation of deciduous teeth. *Am. Dent. J.* 1941; 28: 1626–32.

20. Jeng HW, Feigal RJ, Messer HH. Comparison of the cytotoxicity of formocresol, formaldehyde, cresol and glutaraldehyde using human pulp fibroblasts cultures. *Pediatr. Dent.* 1987; 9: 295–300.

21. Jeppesen K. Direct pulp capping on primary teeth – a long-term investigation. *J. Int. Assoc. Dent. Child.* 1971; 12: 10–19.

22. Kalnins V, Frisbie HE. Effect of dentine fragments on the healing of the exposed pulp. *Arch. Oral. Biol.* 1960; 2: 96–103.

23. Kisling E. Histologiske undersögelser af mælketændernes pulpae som grundlag for en klinisk diagnose (in Danish). *Dens Sapiens* 1957; 17: 52–61.

24. Koch G, Nyborg H. Correlation between clinical and his-tological indications for pulpotomy for deciduous teeth. *J. Int. Assoc. Dent. Child.* 1970; 1: 3–10.

25. Law DB. An evaluation of vital pulpotomy technique. *J. Dent. Child.* 1956; 23: 40–44.

26. Leksell E, Ridell K, Cvek M, Mejàre I. Pulp exposure after stepwise versus direct complete excavation of deep carious lesions in young permanent posterior teeth. *Endodont. Dent. Traumatol.* 1996; 12: 192–6.

27. Magnusson B. Therapeutic pulpotomy in primary molars – clinical and histological follow-up. Zinc oxide–eugenol as wound dressing. *Odontol. Rev.* 1971; 22: 45–54.

28. Magnusson BO, Sundell SO. Stepwise excavation of deep carious lesions in primary molars. *J. Int. Assoc. Dent. Child.* 1977; 8: 36–40.
The aim was to assess possible benefits (avoiding pulp exposure) of stepwise excavation of deep carious lesions in primary molars. A total of 110 molars with deep caries without symptoms of pulpitis were randomly selected for either immediate and complete excavation of all carious dentine or a stepwise excavation procedure whereby a thin layer of remaining caries close to the pulp was covered with calcium hydroxide and the cavity sealed with zinc oxide–eugenol cement. After 4–6 weeks the cavity was reopened and all remaining caries was removed. In the group immediately and completely excavated, the frequency of pulp exposures was 53% versus 15% for teeth excavated by the stepwise procedure. Two teeth in the stepwise excavation group developed pulpitis and were extracted. Three teeth in the immediate excavation group and one in the stepwise excavation group had necrotic pulps. The authors conclude that stepwise excavation can reduce the problems caused by the inadequacy of current methods of pulp treatment in primary teeth.

29. Mejàre B. Bactericidal effect of calcium hydroxide on enterococci in blood and serum. *J. Dent. Res.* 1986; 65: abstr. 12.

30. Mejàre I, Cvek M. Partial pulpotomy in young permanent teeth with deep carious lesions. *Endodont. Dent. Traumatol.* 1993; 9: 238–42.

31. Mejàre I, Larsson Å. Short-term reactions of human dental pulp to formocresol and its components. A clinical–experimental study. *Scand. J. Dent. Res.* 1979; 87: 331–45.

32. Mejàre I. Pulpotomy of primary molars with coronal or total pulpitis using formocresol technique. *Scand. J. Dent. Res.* 1979; 87: 208–16.

33. Mejàre I, Hasselgren G, Hammarström LE. Effect of formaldehyde-containing drugs on human dental pulp evaluated by enzyme histochemical technique. *Scand. J. Dent. Res.* 1976; 84: 29–36.

34. Mjör IA. Dentine and pulp. In *Reaction Patterns in Human Teeth* (Mjör IA, ed.). Boca Raton, FL: CRC Press, 1983; 101.

35. Morawa AP, Straffon HL, Han SS, Corpron RE. Clinical evaluation of pulpotomies using diluted formocresol. *ADC J. Dent. Child.* 1975; 42: 360–63.

36. Nethercott JR, Holness DL, Page E. Occupational contact dermatitis due to glutaraldehyde in health care workers. *Contact Dermat.* 1988; 18: 193.

37. Nyborg H. Capping of the pulp. *Odontol. Revy* 1958; 66: 296–364.

38. Pritz W. Erfahrungen mit Calxyl zur pulpenüberkappung. *Zahnärztl. Welt.* 1957; 58: 120–24.

39. Prophet AS, Miller J. The effect of caries on the deciduous pulp. *Br. Dent. J.* 1955; 99: 105.

40. Ranly DM. Formocresol toxicity. Current knowledge. *Acta Odontol. Pediatr.* 1984; 5: 93–8.

41. Rapp R, Avery K, Strachan DS. Possible role of acetyl-cholinesterase in neural conduction within the dental pulp. In *Biology of the Dental Pulp Organ: a Symposium* (Finn SB, ed.). Alabama: University of Alabama Press, 1968; 309–31.

42. Rayner JA, Southam JC. Pulp changes in deciduous teeth associated with deep carious lesions. *J. Dent.* 1979; 7: 39–42.

43. Rutherford B, Fitzgerald M. A new biological approach to vital pulp therapy. *Crit. Rev. Oral Biol. Med.* 1995; 6: 218–29.

44. Rölling I, Poulsen S. Formocresol pulpotomy of primary teeth and the occurrence of enamel defect on permanent successors. *Acta Odontol. Scand.* 1978; 36: 243–7.

45. Rölling I, Hasselgren G, Tronstad L. Morphologic and enzyme histochemical observations on the pulp of human primary molars 3 to 5 years after formocresol treatment. *Oral Surg.* 1976; 42: 518–28.

46. Rölling I, Thulin H. Allergy tests against formaldehyde, cresol and eugenol in children with formocresol pulpotomized primary teeth. *Scand. J. Dent. Res.* 1976; 84: 345–7.

47. Rölling I, Thylstrup. A 3-year clinical follow-up study of pulpotomized primary molars treated with the formocresol technique. *Scand. J. Dent. Res.* 1975; 83: 47–53.

48. Sawusch RH. Dycal capping of exposed pulps in primary teeth. *J. Dent. Child.* 1963; 30: 141–9.

49. Schröder U, Szpringer-Nodzak M, Janicha J, Wacinska M, Budny J, Mlosek K. A one-year follow-up of partial pulpotomy and calcium hydroxide capping in primary molars. *Endodont. Dent. Traumatol.* 1987; 3: 304–6.

50. Schröder U. A 2-year follow-up of primary molars, pulpotomized with a gentle technique and capped with calcium hydroxide. *Scand. J. Dent. Res.* 1978; 86: 173–8.

51. Schröder U. Agreement between clinical and histologic findings in chronic pulpitis in primary teeth. *Scand. J. Dent. Res.* 1977; 85: 583–7.

52. Schröder U. Effect of an extra-pulpal blood clot on healing following experimental pulpotomy and capping with calcium hydroxide. *Odontol. Revy* 1973; 24: 257–69.

53. Shumayrikh NM, Adenubi JO. Clinical evaluation of glutaraldehyde with calcium hydroxide and glutaraldehyde with zinc oxide eugenol in pulpotomy of primary molars. *Endodont. Dent. Traumatol.* 1999; 15: 259–64.

54. Smith NL, Sue Seale N, Nunn ME. Ferric sulfate in primary molars. A retrospective study. *Pediatr. Dent.* 2000; 22: 192–9.

55. Soskolne WA, Bimstein E. A histomorphological study of the shedding process of human deciduous teeth at various chronological stages. *Arch. Oral Biol.* 1977; 22: 331–5.

56. Squire RA, Cameron LL. An analysis of potential carcinogenic risk from formaldehyde. *Regul. Toxicol. Pharmacol.* 1984; 4: 107–29.

57. St Clair MB, Gross EA, Morgan KT. Pathology and cell proliferation induced by intra-nasal instillation of aldehydes in the rat: comparison of glutaraldehyde and formaldehyde. *Toxicol. Pathol.* 1990; 18: 353–61.

58. Sun HW, Feigal RJ, Messer HH. Cytotoxicity of glutaraldehyde and formaldehyde in relation to time of exposure and concentration. *Pediatr. Dent.* 1990; 12: 303–7.

59. Tagger E, Tagger M. Pulpal and periapical reactions to glutaraldehyde and paraformaldehyde pulpotomy dressing in monkeys. *J. Endodont.* 1984; 10: 364–71.

60. Tsai TP, Su HL, Tseng LH. Glutaraldehyde preparations and pulpotomy in primary molars. *Oral surg.* 1993; 76: 346–50.

61. Waterhouse PJ. Formocresol and alternative primary pulpotomy medicaments: a review. *Endodont. Dent. Traumatol.* 1995; 11: 157–62.

62. Via FW. Evaluation of deciduous molars treated by pulpotomy and calcium hydroxide. *J. Am. Dent. Assoc.* 1955; 50: 34–43.

63. Willard RM. Radiographic changes following formocresol pulpotomy in primary molars. *J. Dent. Child.* 1976; 43: 414–15.

64. Zilberman U, Mass E, Sarnat H. Partial pulpotomy in carious permanent molars. *Am. J. Dent.* 1989; 2: 147–50.

Part 3
THE NECROTIC PULP

Chapter 8
The microbiology of the necrotic pulp

Else Theilade

Historical background

Micro-organisms colonizing the necrotic pulp have long been established as the cause of acute and chronic periapical inflammation. The first observation of these micro-organisms was by Antony van Leeuwenhoek, whose home-made microscope also enabled him to make the first drawings of dental plaque bacteria in 1683. However, it took about 200 years before root canal micro-organisms came under biological investigation, namely by the father of oral microbiology, Willoughby D. Miller (1853–1907).

Miller in 1890 described the clinical effects of 'gangrenous tooth-pulps' as centers of infections varying from hardly perceptible periapical inflammation to severe local and general symptoms, sometimes even with fatal outcome (Key literature 8.1). He cultured and characterized bacteria from the necrotic pulp and studied their pathogenic potential in animal experiments (45).

With the publication in 1911 of William Hunter's book 'Oral Sepsis as a Cause of Disease' (cited in Ref. 15), interest centered around the theory of focal infection, the concept that infected teeth might cause infections in other parts of the body and also many other systemic diseases. Hunter accused dentists of producing masses of oral sepsis with their procedures for fillings, crowns and bridges, which often caused pulpitis, pulp necrosis and periodontal disease. A more suitable name for 'conservative dentistry' would be 'septic dentistry'. His publications (35) led to the view that all teeth suspected of infection should be extracted. This resulted in mass extractions and probably a delay in the development of endodontic therapy, but eventually also in biologically sound treatment principles, including the elimination of infection.

Essential role of micro-organisms in endodontic disease

Animal experiments

Some early authors suggested that decomposition of necrotic pulp tissue or stagnant tissue fluid might cause apical periodontitis even in the absence of bacteria. However, it was demonstrated that subcutaneous implantation in experimental animals of empty tubes or sterile dead tissue caused only a transient inflammation that did not prevent healing, whereas necrotic tissue contaminated with bacteria caused intense inflammation and often abscess formation (42, 72).

A classical study in germ-free and conventional rats in 1965 (36) demonstrated the essential role of micro-organisms in the pathogenesis of periapical lesions (Key literature 8-2). In agreement with this, aseptically necrotized pulps that were sealed and remained sterile for 6–7 months in experimental monkeys did not induce inflammatory reactions in the periapical tissues. In contrast, pulps lacerated by instrumentation and contaminated with oral flora caused clinical, radiographic and histological signs of periapical inflammation (48).

Human studies

Studies in humans have shown that periapical inflammation is connected with the presence of bacteria in the root canal. Demonstration of micro-organisms in root canals by culture has many pitfalls and older studies are not very reliable. It was greatly improved with the studies in 1966 (47) of Möller, who developed methods for sampling, transport and culture by taking into account the fastidious and often obligate anaerobic nature of the micro-organisms. Cultural studies of nonvital pulps of teeth with closed necrosis after trauma have demonstrated the absence of growth in cases without radiographic signs of periapical inflammation, trauma that severs its blood supply, will have excellent conditions for growth there. In the case of bacteria entering a vital pulp, their survival will depend on their number and virulence as opposed to the defense mechanisms of the pulp.

Dental caries

When a deep caries lesion reaches the pulp (Fig. 8.1), the massive bacterial invasion will cause pulpal inflammation followed by necrosis and periapical inflammation. In such cases the bacteria gaining access will be the complex microflora of deep caries dominated by anaerobic, Gram-positive bacteria (19, 33). It is generally accepted that bacteria do not normally reach the pulp in significant numbers as long as it is covered by clinically sound dentine. By microscopy and anaerobic culture, investigators have demonstrated bacteria in a few of the dentinal tubules in front of the carious lesion. Small numbers of bacteria can even enter unexposed, vital pulps from deep caries (34), but such bacteria normally will be eliminated by the immune system of the pulp.

Trauma

Pulp exposure due to trauma will give access to oral bacteria (Fig. 8.1). In humans, as in animal experiments (36, 48), this will cause bacterial invasion and pulpal inflammation followed by infected necrosis and periapical inflammation (Key literature 8.2). In addition, there is clinical evidence that bacteria may enter the pulp in cases of cracked-tooth syndrome, i.e. initial incomplete fracture (Fig. 8.2) (23). Laboratory experiments indicate that bacteria can enter through even minor cracks in enamel and dentine following trauma (41). Also, the dentinal tubules exposed by tooth fracture during cavity and crown preparation or under restorations with marginal leakage are a potential pathway (7). Furthermore,

whereas most cases with such lesions gave growth (9, 47, 63).

Entry of micro-organisms into the root canal

In some cases of infected necrotic pulp, a wide open pathway for the entry of bacteria is found clinically in the form of pulp exposure due to caries or fracture. On the other hand, infection and apical periodontitis occur also in cases of closed necrosis, even in apparently intact teeth. As reviewed below, several ways of entry seem possible and have been the subject of much research and even more speculation but few firm conclusions (Fig. 8.1) (for reviews, see Refs 11 and 50). Even a few bacteria entering a pulp that is necrotic, e.g. following a

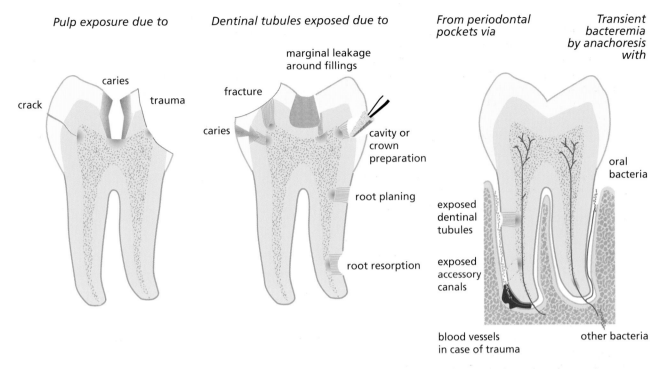

Pulp exposure due to *Dentinal tubules exposed due to* *From periodontal pockets via* *Transient bacteremia by anachoresis with*

Fig. 8.1 Drawing illustrating the pathways of entry for micro-organisms into the root canal. Obvious ways of entry are pulp exposures due to caries or trauma. Potential pathways are cracks in enamel and dentine due to trauma, and dentinal tubules exposed by caries, fracture, cavity or crown preparation, marginal leakage around fillings, root resorption or root planing. From periodontal pockets, potential pathways are via exposed accessory canals, via exposed dentinal tubules or via blood vessels in the case of trauma. During bacteremia, blood-borne bacteria may colonize an inflamed or necrotic pulp (anachoresis). (See text for details.)

if the periodontium is traumatized, bacteria from the gingival crevice or pocket may reach the pulp through severed blood vessels (27). Whether or not bacteria entering by these routes can survive and multiply depends on the state of the pulp. They will often be eliminated and further entry prevented by the dentine–pulp complex (10).

Periodontal disease

In the presence of periodontal pockets, several entry routes (Fig. 8.1) seem possible for the complex subgingival microflora, which are also well suited for growth in the necrotic pulp. The microflora (43, 61) are predominantly anaerobic and comprise many different Gram-negative rods, spirochetes and various Gram-positive rods and cocci, all of which are common in necrotic pulps. In fact, the similarity of the endodontic and periodontal microflora and even the presence of identical clones are important arguments for the entry of bacteria from deep pockets into non-vital pulps of non-carious teeth (26, 37).

From subgingival plaque, bacteria and their products can enter through accessory lateral and furcal canals, or ultimately through the apical foramen. Furthermore,

dentinal tubules exposed due to root caries, gaps in cementum formation in the cervical area or by removal of the cementum by root resorption or root planing could be a path of entry (1). Inflammatory reactions and sometimes even local necrosis have been demonstrated histologically in pulp tissue adjacent to such potential entry pathways (38, 55). However, in other histological studies no correlation beween periodontal disease and pulp tissue changes have been found (71). In a study of experimentally induced marginal periodontitis in monkeys (12), it was demonstrated that neither periodontal destruction (limited to the cervical half of the roots) nor plaque accumulation on exposed root dentine causes severe alterations in the pulp. As long as the pulp is vital and functioning the bacteria usually will be eliminated, followed by healing of the dentine–pulp complex (10), but they will become established if the pulp is necrotic.

Anachoresis

Anachoresis (Greek: retreating) is a phenomenon known for many years by which blood-borne bacteria or other materials are preferentially localized in areas of inflammation (Fig. 8.1) (for a review see Ref. 54). Animal exper-

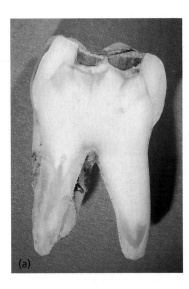
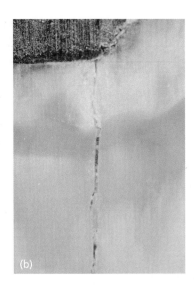

Fig. 8.2 Cracked-tooth syndrome: (a) incompletely fractured maxillary molar; (b) higher magnification of the crack. Beneath the amalgam restoration, the crack extends to the pulp. From: Geurtsen W. *Int. J. Periodont. Restor. Dent.* 1992; 12: 395–405 (23).

iments have shown that bacteria injected intravenously could be demonstrated in a large proportion of pulps that were inflamed due to the preparation of deep cavities and chemical irritation (14, 24, 54). It is a well-established fact that transient bacteremia is not uncommon in humans (see Chapter 10). Depending on the source of the bacteria, such bacteremias could bring non-oral as well as oral bacteria to the root canals. Oral bacteria from dental plaque or infected root canals can be retrieved from venous blood immediately after tooth extraction, periodontal surgery, scaling, endodontic treatment, toothbrushing and even chewing (8, 18, 31, 54). Anachoresis is therefore a possible explanation for the infection in some clinical cases of closed pulp necrosis, although bacteria are normally rapidly eliminated from the blood.

Conclusion

There are numerous possible pathways for entry of micro-organisms into the root canals, even in the absence of clinically obvious pulp exposure from caries or fracture (Fig. 8.1). Oral bacteria, mainly from carious lesions and periodontal pockets, can gain access through cracks in enamel and dentine, exposed dentinal tubules or accessory canals. Blood-borne oral as well as extra-oral bacteria may enter the canals in the case of bacteremia. No data are available concerning the relative frequency of these entry routes in the clinical situation. The intact dentine–pulp complex is a highly efficient defense system often capable of preventing entry and eliminating any entering micro-organisms. The necrotic pulp, on the other hand, gives excellent growth conditions for micro-organisms.

Location of micro-organisms in endodontic infections

The presence of micro-organisms is generally demonstrated by the culture of necrotic pulp tissue or fluid from the canal (see below). Special sampling techniques as well as histological and ultrastructural studies are needed to clarify the location of micro-organisms (Fig. 8.3), whether in the necrotic pulp, on the root canal wall, in the dentinal tubules, on the root cementum or in periapical soft-tissue lesions (for reviews, see Refs 50 and 64).

Necrotic pulp tissue is the major location of bacteria causing periapical lesions (Fig. 8.3). Necrotic tissue in root canals can support the growth of many microbial species. Mixed microbial masses consisting of cocci, rods, filamentous bacteria, spirochetes and yeasts have been demonstrated in necrotic pulps in studies using light microscopy of histological tissue sections, as well as by transmission electron microscopy of ultrathin sections and scanning electron microscopy of root fragments (2, 39, 49, 52, 57) (Fig. 8.4).

Generally, micro-organisms also adhere to some areas of the root canal walls, either as dense aggregates or as thin, single- or multilayered condensations (Figs 8.4–8.6). Such adherent masses can contain one or several morphological types, sometimes with filamentous forms and chains of cocci perpendicular to the canal wall—a biofilm rather similar to dental plaque in structure (49, 57). When the pulp is necrotic and infected, micro-organisms also grow into some of the dentinal tubules for a variable distance (Fig. 8.5), in one study measured to 10–150 µm (57) and usually confined to the inner third (39). In cases of periapical lesions, micro-

Location of microorganisms in endodontic infections

Extraradicular

Intraradicular

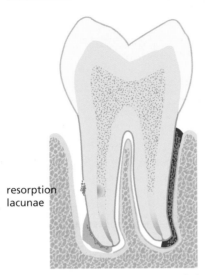

in dentinal
tubules

in necrotic
pulp tissue
(the major
site)

resorption
lacunae

periapical soft
tissue lesions

periodontal plaque
on the root surface

Fig. 8.3 Drawing illustrating the locations of endodontic micro-organisms. The major locations are intraradicular: in the necrotic pulp tissue, adhering to the root canal walls and in the inner part of dentinal tubules. Extraradicular micro-organisms may be present in periodontal plaque on the root surface, in resorption lacunae and in periapical soft tissue. (See Advanced concept 8.1 and the text.)

Advanced concept 8.1   Micro-organisms in periapical lesions

The long standing idea that solid granulomas and true radicular cysts do not generally harbor micro-organisms is still valid.

Extraradicular microbes may be found:

- In abscessed lesions (usually symptomatic)
- In periapical actinomycosis
- In infected radicular cysts, particularly those with cavities open to the root canal (periapical pocket cysts)
- On pieces of root dentine displaced into the periapex.

Nair PNR, 1997 (50)

There is evidence of bacterial presence in periradicular tissues in asymptomatic apical periodontitis persisting after root filling.

Sunde PT, et al., 2000 (62)
Gatti JJ, et al., 2000 (22)

---

organisms are always found in these intraradicular locations, often walled off by neutrophil granulocytes or an epithelial plug at the apical foramen (49).

Periapical bacterial plaque has been demonstrated by scanning electron microscopy as a coating of various microbial forms embedded in a structureless material on the outer root surface, generally near the main apical foramen (Fig. 8.7). In resorption lacunae bacteria and yeast cells sometimes could be detected (40, 50, 73). It is not clear how common such extraradicular micro-

organisms are. They have been demonstrated mainly in cases with acute symptoms or fistulae, or in cases not responding to previous endodontic treatment. Extraradicular micro-organisms are liable to removal by host defense mechanisms unless they find protection in a biofilm on a solid surface.

In ultrastructural studies, micro-organisms are generally not found in the soft-tissue lesion in cases of chronic apical periodontitis (apical granuloma) or in periapical true cysts (when the cavity is completely encased in an epithelial lining so that no communication to the root canal exists) (50). An exception to this rule is the occasional finding of typical actinomyces-containing colonies in granulomas and in radicular cysts and abscesses (29, 51). In cases of periapical abscess with or without sinus (fistula), various bacterial forms and yeasts may be present in the lesion, sometimes inside phagocytes (Fig. 8.3 and Advanced concept 8.1). Also, radicular cysts may contain micro-organisms, particularly those with the cyst cavity open to the root canal (Advanced concept 8.1) (50).

In contrast to the above statements, bacterial DNA could be demonstrated with a sensitive molecular genetic technique in periapical tissues removed during surgical treatment of asymptomatic apical periodontitis persisting after root filling (Advanced concept 8.1) (22, 62). The location of these (viable or non-viable) bacteria is not clear – it could be in the soft-tissue lesion or on the root surface – and the risk of sample contamination during the operation cannot be ruled out.

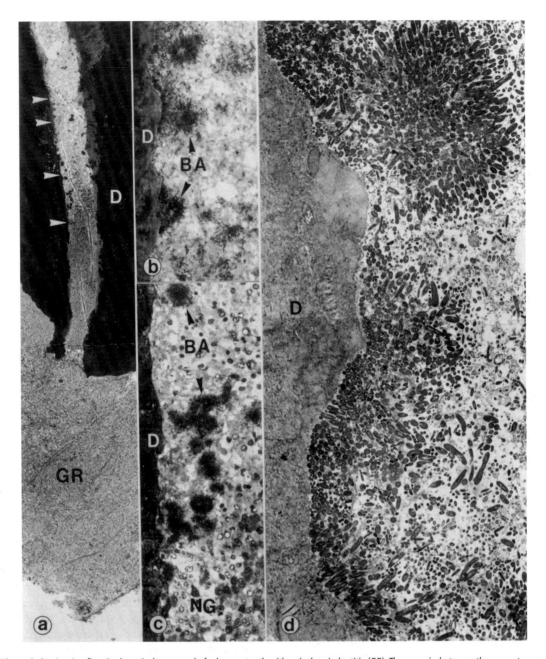

Fig. 8.4 The endodontic microflora in the apical root canal of a human tooth with apical periodontitis (GR). The areas in-between the upper two and the lower two arrowheads in (a) are magnified in (b) and (c), respectively. Note the dense bacterial aggregates (BA) sticking (in b) to the dentinal (D) wall and also remaining suspended among neutrophilic granulocytes (NG) in the fluid phase of the root canal content (in c). The neutrophilic granulocytes appear to form a defensive wall, against the advancing bacterial front. A transmission electron microscopic view (d) of the pulpodential interphase shows bacterial condensation on the surface of the dentinal wall, forming a thick layered plaque. Magnification: (a) ×46; (b) ×600; (c) ×370; (d) ×2350. From: Nair PNR. *Periodontology 2000* 1997; 13: 121–48 (50).

Methods to study the root canal microflora

The microflora of necrotic pulps have been studied for more than 100 years, mainly by direct microscopy and cultivation (45). Much knowledge has been gained through research into the composition, ecology and pathogenic potential of the microflora. In clinical practice, root canal cultures may be used to determine the microbiological status and to assess the efficacy of the treatment prior to root filling. In case of persistent infection after root filling, information on the micro-organisms and

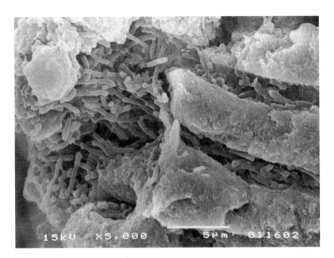

Fig. 8.5 A colony consisting of cocci and rods in an ecological niche on the root canal wall. The aggregated bacteria also show some penetration into the dentinal tubules. Scanning electron microscopy, magnification ×5000. From: Sen BH, Piskin B, Demirci T. *Endodont. Dent. Traumatol.* 1995; 11: 6–9 (57).

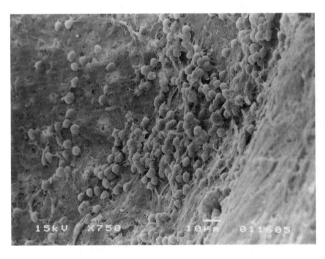

Fig. 8.6 Yeast cells along root canal wall in the middle third of the root. They form separate colonies in the root canal. Notice their attachments to the canal with filamentous structures. Scanning electron microscopy, magnification ×750. From: Sen BH, Piskin B, Demirci T. *Endodont. Dent. Traumatol.* 1995; 11: 6–9 (57).

their antibiotic sensitivity patterns may become useful. There are, however, several methodological problems in sampling and cultivation to overcome, owing to the location of the micro-organisms and the complexity of the microflora (Fig. 8.3, Core concept 8.1).

For many years, the methods for sampling, transport, cultivation and identification were rather inadequate for the many fastidious, often anaerobic micro-organisms present. Therefore, false-negative cultures (no growth in spite of micro-organisms living in the root canal) were common. False-positive cultures, i.e. growth of contami-

Core concept 8.1	Problems in root canal cultures
Sampling:	Inaccessible location
	contamination
Transport:	death of micro-organisms
	overgrowth of others
Cultivation:	media not adequate
	anaerobiosis not adequate
	'uncultivatable' organisms
Identification:	time-consuming
	expensive
	taxonomy not yet defined

Culture-independent, molecular genetic techniques can solve some of the problems.

nating micro-organisms not present in the root canal, were also a common event. Of course, optimal techniques to minimize such false results and to secure the growth of all members of the mixed microflora are essential (47, 63, 64). Methods for microbial identification with and without culturing are rapidly developing, and the names and taxonomic position of many bacteria change with the acquired knowledge (Core concept 8.1).

Sampling

For clinical indications and procedures for microbiological sampling, see Chapter 11. Strict asepsis is necessary during sampling to avoid contamination from teeth (plaque or caries), oral mucosa, saliva, fingers and instruments. Therefore, caries should be excavated, fillings, crowns, plaque and calculus removed, a rubber dam applied and the tooth and rubber dam disinfected. Sterile burs and instruments are used to gain access to the root canals, and samples are taken with sterile paper points. The canal may contain an inflammatory exudate, but if not it is necessary to introduce a small amount of sterile fluid. By slight instrumentation with a small file, necrotic tissue and material from the canal wall are dispersed in the fluid, which is then absorbed with a sufficient number of paper points to soak up all the fluid. The paper points should be transferred immediately to a tube of prereduced transport medium (47) designed to keep the organisms alive without growing (and without changing their proportions) during transport to the laboratory (Core concept 8.1).

Microscopy and cultivation

The micro-organisms must be dispersed in the fluid, e.g. by vigorous mixing with glass beads, before

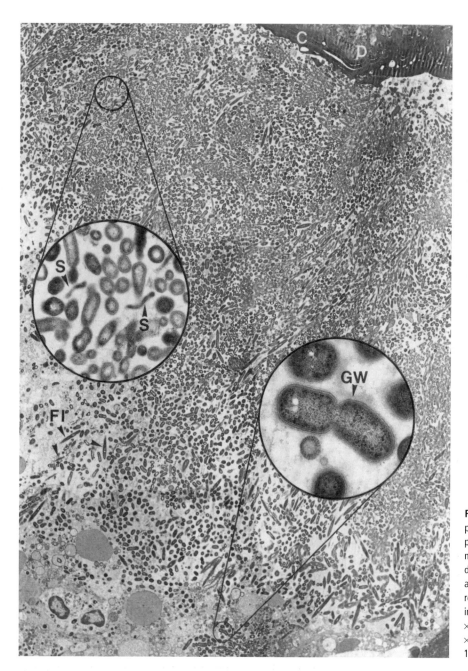

Fig. 8.7 Massive bacterial plaque at the periapex of a human tooth with acute apical periodontitis of endodontic origin. Note the mixed bacterial flora consisting of numerous dividing cocci, rods (lower inset), filaments (FI) and spirochetes (S, upper inset). Rods often reveal a Gram-negative cell wall (GW, lower inset). C, cementum; D, dentine. Magnification: ×2680; upper inset: ×19 200; lower inset: ×36 400. From: Nair PNR. *Periodontology 2000* 1997; 13: 121–48 (50).

cultivation and preparation of slides for microscopy. By direct observation with phase-contrast or dark-field microscopy, scanning electron microscopy or microscopy of Gram-stained smears, all morphological types present may be noticed but some of them (e.g. spirochetes) may not be recovered in cultures (17). The presence of specific bacteria may be assessed in smears stained with the indirect immunofluorescent technique (3).

For cultivation, dilutions of the dispersed sample are spread on agar media, which are then incubated long enough (10–14 days) to allow even slow growers to form colonies. In a broth culture, the fastest growing bacteria will overgrow the others and members of a mixed microflora will be missed (64). Non-selective agar media containing hemolyzed blood (Fig. 8.8) fulfill many special nutrient requirements and are best suited to culture the many bacterial types as well as yeasts (32). For scientific purposes, selective media may be included, e.g. Sabouraud agar for yeasts, mitis salivarius agar for streptococci, or Rogosa SL agar selective for lactobacilli. Special media are required for the growth of

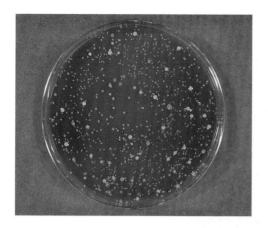

Fig. 8.8 Agar plate of non-selective medium containing hemolyzed blood inoculated with diluted suspension of paper point sample from root canal with necrotic pulp. After anaerobic incubation at 37°C for 10 days, several colony types are seen, indicating a mixed infection. (Courtesy of L. Kruse.)

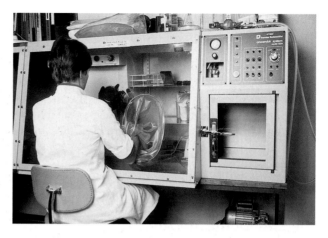

Fig. 8.9 Anaerobic box for processing of microbiological cultures in an oxygen-free atmosphere. (Courtesy of L. Kruse.)

mycoplasms and spirochetes, but only some of the latter are cultivatable even when special techniques are used (32) (Core concept 8.1).

The micro-organisms colonizing root canals are facultative and obligate anaerobes, therefore anaerobic techniques for handling and incubation of cultures are essential for accurate results (47, 63). This requirement can be fulfilled by incubation in anaerobic jars or, even better, by an anaerobic box in which work with samples and cultures as well as incubation are carried out in an oxygen-free atmosphere (Fig. 8.9). In order to facilitate the identification of facultative anaerobic and capnophilic (carbon dioxide-loving) bacteria, a set of agar plates is incubated in air supplemented with carbon dioxide. Generally, one or two colonies of each type are subcultured for identification. Because different bacteria may have similar colonies, for some purposes it is better to isolate a large number of colonies, e.g. 50, from a sample (79).

Methods for identification

Precise identification, at the species level, of endodontic isolates is very time-consuming and costly and sometimes not even possible because many members of the oral microflora are not yet sufficiently characterized. Some are even impossible to culture (Core concept 8.1). Detailed identification of micro-organisms is essential in research, e.g. concerning the etiology of different periapical disease states and the role of certain bacteria or microbial combinations in disease progression and treatment outcome.

Bacterial isolates can simply be grouped on the basis of characters such as colony morphology and pigmentation, cell morphology, motility or not, Gram-staining

reaction and facultative or obligate anaerobe. Genus or species identification in addition requires several biochemical tests for enzyme activities and end products, possibly by commercial test kits (13, 59, 63, 76). Unknown isolates must be compared with reference strains of defined species. In research, similarities between strains can be examined with advanced methods such as DNA–DNA homology analysis or protein profiles of cell extracts by polyacrylamide gel electrophoresis (4, 18).

Modern molecular genetic techniques (for a review, see Ref. 77) hold great promise also for examination of endodontic samples because they are 'heralding a new, culture-independent era of medical microbiology' (quoted from Ref. 74). Elimination of the need for culturing means that the (probably numerous) uncultivatable bacteria can be included. One such method (16) is a 16S rDNA-directed PCR (polymerase chain reaction) applicable at different levels (bacteria in general, bacterial order- or family-specific, species-specific and subspecies- or virulence factor-specific). As the 16S rRNA/DNA databanks acquire rapidly increasing numbers of reference sequences, such methods will become more useful.

In medical microbiology, diagnostic kits are commercially available for quick examination without culturing for some specific pathogens, e.g. for hemolytic streptococci in throat samples. Similar methods are developed to examine periodontal pockets for a few species deemed to be of special interest. Such tests can be based on specific antibodies applied in various ELISA (enzyme-linked immunosorbant assay) systems for bacterial antigen detection. The DNA–DNA hybridization techniques using DNA probes for specific bacteria are also applicable (for a review, see Ref. 77). With the 'checkerboard' DNA–DNA hybridization method, DNA extracted from endodontic samples has been reacted with DNA probes from up to 40 bacterial species, with results indicating the presence of many of these species (22, 58, 62). Such methods designed to detect specific bacteria are only reliable if appropriate specific DNA probes are available, and they seem less suitable for endodontic microbiology, where the presence of any of a large number of oral as well as non-oral species is of interest.

Composition of the endodontic microflora

The resident oral microflora comprise more than 300 species of cultivable bacteria and an unknown number of species that we cannot grow with present methods. Probably most of these can be present in the necrotic pulp, where also yeasts and several bacteria of extra-oral origin may be found (Core concept 8.2). The special environment in the root canal (and our methods of study), however, selects certain species to be found most frequently (13, 59, 64, 75, 76). Generally, a mixture of several (1–16) species has been cultured from samples taken from necrotic pulps at the start of treatment (25, 63, 76).

Oral bacteria in the necrotic pulp

In the field of oral bacteriology new species are continuously being described, and new knowledge leads to changes in classification and names. Therefore, the same bacteria may have different names in older and newer articles (43, 66). Although recent techniques allow very precise identification, e.g. based on DNA sequences, naming is far less reliable in older studies using a more or less extensive series of traditional tests.

The micro-organisms in root canal samples from deciduous as well as permanent teeth are predominantly the same bacteria as those found in dental plaque, periodontal pockets and carious lesions (19, 26, 33, 37, 43, 56, 61). The majority of isolates in initial cultures are obligate anaerobic bacteria. These constituted 91% of the isolates from closed necrosis (69), 90% of isolates from necrotic pulps of deciduous teeth (56) and 68% from the apical part of necrotic pulps in carious teeth (5). A large proportion of the anaerobes are asaccharolytic, peptide- and amino acid-degrading bacteria (56, 64).

The many genera and species currently identified in root canal samples comprise obligate anaerobic and facultative anaerobic oral bacteria (Table 8.1) (3, 4, 5, 9, 13, 17, 25, 69, 76, 78). Among the streptococci, species of the anginosus group (*S. anginosus, S. intermedius, S. con-*

> ### Core concept 8.2   The microflora of the necrotic pulp
>
> Usually a mixture of several oral bacterial species also found in dental plaque, periodontal pockets and carious lesions. Dominated by obligate anaerobes.
>
> Most frequently found are species of:
>
> - *Peptostreptococcus*
> - *Eubacterium*
> - *Prevotella*
> - *Porphyromonas*
> - *Fusobacterium*
> - *Streptococcus*
>
> Yeasts (most commonly *Candida albicans*) and bacteria of extra-oral origin (notably *Enterococcus faecalis*) also may be present initially but are more common in samples taken later during prolonged treatment, or in cases of retreatment of failed root fillings.

---

stellatus) and mitis group (*S. mitis, S. oralis, S. gordonii, S. sanguis, S. parasanguis*) are common, and in carious teeth also *S. mutans*. It was suggested (44) that *S. sanguis* and *S. salivarius* often occur in root canal cultures due to contamination with saliva or invasion through leaking temporary fillings. Lactobacilli are mainly found in teeth with caries. *Actinomyces israelii* (as well as other *Actinomyces* species) may be present, and sometimes actinomycotic periapical lesions develop (29, 51).

Black-pigmented bacteria of the genera *Porphyromonas* and *Prevotella* (previously classified in the genus *Bacteroides*) have attracted much attention as potential pathogens in endodontic as well as in periodontal microbiology (6, 28, 69). These anaerobic, Gram-negative rods are very common isolates from necrotic pulps before treatment, especially the *Prevotella* species *Pr. nigrescens, Pr. intermedia, Pr. tannerae, Pr. melaninogenica, Pr. denticola* and *Pr. buccae*, as well as the *Porphyromonas* species *P. endodontalis* and *P. gingivalis*. Other oral bacteria commonly found are species of *Peptostreptococcus, Eubacterium, Veillonella, Fusobacterium, Selenomonas, Campylobacter* (previously *Wolinella*), *Neisseria, Capnocytophaga, Eikenella* and *Treponema*, the latter generally demonstrated by direct microscopy. Some species such as *Treponema denticola* and *Bacteroides forsythus*, which are difficult to culture, have been demonstrated with DNA techniques applied directly to root canal samples (16, 58).

Oral yeasts in the necrotic pulp

Yeasts of the genus *Candida* and sometimes other fungi are common members of the resident oral microflora (43). Yeasts have also been observed by electron

Table 8.1 Common genera in infected root canals.

Obligate anaerobes	Facultative anaerobes
Gram-positive cocci	Gram-positive cocci
• *Streptococcus*	• *Streptococcus*
• *Peptostreptococcus*	• *Enterococcus*
Gram-positive rods	Gram-positive rods
• *Actinomyces*	• *Actinomyces*
• *Lactobacillus*	• *Lactobacillus*
• *Bifidobacterium*	
• *Propionibacterium*	
• *Eubacterium*	
Gram-negative cocci	Gram-negative cocci
• *Veillonella*	• *Neisseria*
Gram-negative rods	Gram-negative rods
• *Porphyromonas*	• *Capnocytophaga*
• *Prevotella*	• *Eikenella*
• *Fusobacterium*	
• *Selenomonas*	
• *Campylobacter*	
Spirochetes	Yeasts
• *Treponema*	• *Candida*

microscopy in root canals that had been exposed to the oral cavity (Fig. 8.6) (40, 57), and in biopsies from root filled teeth with therapy-resistant periapical lesions (52). In many older cultural studies, yeasts alone or together with bacteria are reported in up to 17% of cases (for a review, see Ref. 75). In a recent study of 967 samples cultured from unfilled root canals with therapy-resistant infection (75), yeasts were found in 7%, sometimes in pure culture but more often together with bacteria (Core concept 8.2). Most isolates were *Candida albicans* and the rest were identified as *C. glabrata*, *C. guilliermondii*, *C. inconspicua* and *Geotrichum candidum*. A surprisingly high prevalence (40%) of yeasts (in most cases together with bacteria) was demonstrated in pus from dentoalveolar abscesses from deciduous teeth in children with nursing bottle caries, a condition known to favor the growth of yeasts in the mouth (70).

Bacteria of extra-oral origin in the necrotic pulp

Facultatively anaerobic, enteric bacteria are frequently found in root canals, sometimes in initial samples but especially in samples taken later during treatment in the case of poor response or during retreatment of failed root fillings (5, 46, 53, 59, 66, 68, 79). By far the most common species in this group is *Enterococcus faecalis*

(formerly *Streptococcus faecalis*), which is the only isolate from many of these cases. Other enteric bacteria isolated comprise species of *Enterobacter*, *Acinetobacter*, *Proteus*, *Klebsiella* and *Pseudomonas*. It is not clear whether these bacteria are present initially to become predominant during treatment, or enter the canals later due to failures in aseptic technique and temporary seals (Core concept 8.2). *Staphylococcus* species are also among the bacteria occasionally present in root canal cultures, in some cases probably as a contaminant from the skin.

Ecology of the necrotic pulp and the root canal

Colonization of the root canal

Apical periodontitis is an inflammatory reaction to a polymicrobial infection of necrotic pulp tissue and root canal walls. Microbial communities generally comprising several species (Table 8.1) grow as dense aggregates in the necrotic tissue and, in addition, adhere to the dentinal walls in dense masses similar to dental plaque, invade dentinal tubules and sometimes colonize periapical cementum (Figs 8.4–8.7) (49, 57). The microfloras entering the root canal differ in their origin: from deep dentinal caries, predominantly Gram-positive obligate anaerobes; from periodontal pockets, many obligately anaerobic, Gram-negative rods and spirochetes in addition to Gram-positive cocci and rods; and from saliva and supragingival plaque, larger proportions of facultative anaerobes and sometimes yeasts and non-oral bacteria (33, 37, 43, 61). Bacteria of extra-oral origin could also enter from bacteremia originating from the intestinal tract, for example.

The ecological determinants deciding the success or failure of the growth of micro-organisms entering the root canal environment (Core concept 8.3) comprise microbial adhesion and coaggregation, low oxygen concentration and oxidation/reduction potential, nutrition available from the host and synergistic as well as antagonistic relations between the micro-organisms (see below). With time, a climax community is established of cooperating and competing micro-organisms in balance with each other and the local environment. The objective of endodontic treatment is to eliminate or at least disturb this community with mechanical debridement and antimicrobial agents. New micro-organisms may, however, enter the canals, mainly through leaking temporary fillings or due to failure of the aseptic technique.

The development over time of the microflora in necrotic pulps in human teeth is not known. Some indication may, however, be derived from experimental

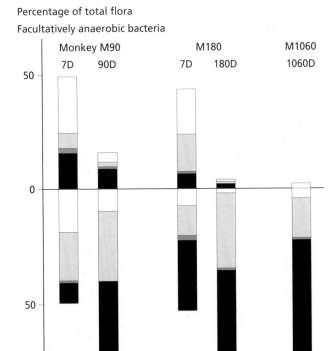

Percentage of total flora
Facultatively anaerobic bacteria

Obligately anaerobic bacteria

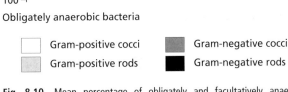

Gram-positive cocci   Gram-negative cocci
Gram-positive rods   Gram-negative rods

Fig. 8.10 Mean percentage of obligately and facultatively anaerobic bacteria in root canals in three experimental monkeys (M90, M180 and M1060) at different times (7, 90, 180 and 1060 days) after sealing the canals following mechanical removal of the pulp and exposure to the oral microflora for 1 week. From: Fabricius L, et al. Scand. J. Dent. Res. 1982; 90: 134–44 (20).

monkey studies (21, 48) where pulps were mechanically traumatized and exposed to the oral flora for 1 week and thereafter sealed for up to 3 years (Figs 8.10 and 8.11). Samples taken 7 days after sealing showed about 50% facultative and 50% obligate anaerobes, whereas the microflora cultured after 90, 180 and 1060 days had 85%, 95% and 98% obligate anaerobes, respectively, with increasing predominance of Gram-negative rods. When pure cultures of bacterial strains, singly or in combinations, were inoculated into traumatized pulps of monkeys (20) or mice (60), pure cultures of obligate anaerobes often failed to colonize, whereas mixtures of facultative and obligate anaerobes were more successful.

Inherent properties of the resident oral flora are the ability of some microbial species to adhere to host surfaces and the tendency of different species to form coaggregates (i.e. stick together), so that dense masses of adhering micro-organisms are formed (Core concept 8.3). These processes are essential for the colonization of oral mucosa and teeth. On the hard, non-shedding surfaces of teeth and dental materials they are responsible for the formation of dental plaque, i.e. a polymicrobial biofilm resistant to elimination (for reviews, see Refs 43 and 61). In root canals (Figs 8.4–8.7), micro-organisms are present not only as aggregates in the necrotic tissue but also adhering to the hard tissues as dense aggregates and single- or multilayered condensations on canal walls, in dentinal tubules and sometimes on periapical cementum (2, 39, 40, 49, 50, 52, 57, 73). This mode of colonization produces microbial communities where the members benefit from each other as well as compete (Core concept 8.3). It also hampers chemical and mechanical elimination of the endodontic microflora.

The predominantly obligately anaerobic microflora (Figs 8.10 and 8.11; Table 8.1), with only a few percent facultative anaerobes and rare occurrence of obligate aerobes, reflects the low oxygen tension and reduced redox potential in the necrotic pulp and the root canal microflora (Core concept 8.3). As in dental plaque, any oxygen entering, e.g. with saliva, will presumably be consumed by the facultative anaerobes and these have enzymes to remove toxic oxygen products. In the dense microbial aggregates, low oxygen levels and a low redox potential suitable for obligate anaerobes will prevail.

Nutrition of the endodontic microflora

The nutrients available for the endodontic microflora (Core concept 8.3) are derived from degradation of the

Percentage of total flora
Facultatively anaerobic bacteria

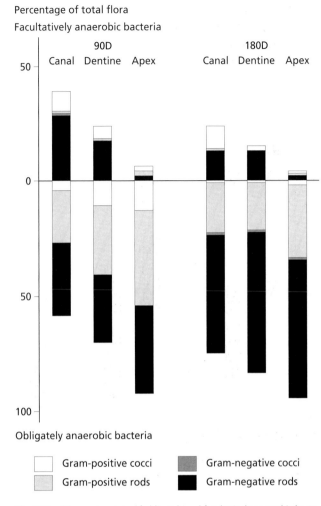

Obligately anaerobic bacteria

	Gram-positive cocci		Gram-negative cocci
	Gram-positive rods		Gram-negative rods

Fig. 8.11 Mean percentage of obligately and facultatively anaerobic bacteria from different parts of the root canal system in final samples in experimental monkeys (M90 and M180) 90 and 180 days after sealing the canals following mechanical removal of the pulp and exposure to the oral microflora for 1 week. From: Fabricius L, *et al. Scand. J. Dent. Res.* 1982; 90: 134–44 (20).

necrotic pulp tissue and by tissue fluid and inflammatory exudate entering from the periapical tissues (56, 64). These sources supply the necessary nutrients: not only the basic requirements of all bacteria for sources of carbon, energy, nitrogen and inorganic ions, but also many special requirements for glycoproteins, amino acids, fatty acids, vitamins, hemin, purines and pyrimidines of the various fastidious oral bacteria that are predominant members of the endodontic microflora. In this environment, growth of micro-organisms requiring carbohydrate for energy is limited, whereas asaccharolytic and protein- and amino acid-degrading bacteria are favored (56, 65). The nutrients available and the slightly alkaline pH resulting from the anaerobic degradation of amino acids promote the growth of *Peptostreptococcus*, *Eubacterium*, *Prevotella*, *Porphyromonas* and *Fusobacterium* species.

The degradation of large molecules such as glycoproteins occurs extracellularly, probably by the concerted action of enzymes from different species in the polymicrobial community, and the amino acids and small amounts of sugars liberated may serve as nutrients for all. In general the limited supply of nutrients restricts growth, especially in the deeper layers of the microbial aggregates. The situation in many respects is similar to that of plaque in periodontal pockets (for reviews, see Refs 43 and 61). For the micro-organisms in dental plaque there are many examples of intermicrobial food chains, where metabolic products (e.g. hemin, vitamin K, H_2, CO_2, NH_3, formate, acetate, succinate) of one species serve as essential nutrients for others.

Microbial synergism and antagonism

In addition to supplying nutrients, food chains are also useful for the removal of waste products that otherwise might inhibit microbial growth. Such food chains (or food webs comprising several species) also seem to be important for the nutrition of the microbial community in the root canal and the balance between its members (Core concept 8.4) (for reviews, see Refs 43, 64 and 65). All the inhabitants in the dense microbial aggregates colonizing root canals (Figs 8.4–8.7) may benefit also from the ability of some species to inactivate host resistance mechanisms by degrading antibodies and killing or inhibiting phagocytes. In thick biofilms the micro-organisms are also largely inaccessible to the antimicrobial agents applied in therapy.

Antagonistic relations also exist between the different populations present (Core concept 8.4). They are not only cooperating but also competing for nutrients, space and attachment sites. Some of their metabolic products (e.g. H_2O_2, fatty acids, sulfur compounds) may accumulate in concentrations that are inhibitory or toxic to other species. Bacteriocins are bactericidal compounds produced by some species that are active against other species or other clones of the same species, so that competing micro-organisms can be suppressed (43, 61). Such complex synergistic and antagonistic interactions between members play a role in the establishment and regulation of the climax community in an infected root canal.

Pathogenic potential of endodontic micro-organisms

Opportunistic pathogens

The resident oral microflora live in commensal association with the human mouth, usually coexisting peacefully with its host. There is a certain measure of mutualism (reciprocal benefit), e.g. the host benefits from the colonization resistance of the oral microflora against introduced pathogens and against overgrowth of micro-organisms normally present in small numbers. On the other hand, the relation may also turn into parasitism when the micro-organisms under certain conditions become harmful for the host and cause disease. In other words, the oral micro-organisms are opportunistic (potential) pathogens. They will always cause disease if they colonize a location such as a root canal, which is normally sterile. When the pulp is necrotic the micro-organisms are located in the necrotic tissue, on the canal walls and in the dentinal tubules (Fig. 8.3). In this situation the host defenses are severely compromised and unable to eliminate the micro-organisms growing outside their reach, and even forming dense aggregates and impermeable biofilms on hard-tissue surfaces (Figs 8.4–8.6). Any micro-organisms that invade or are introduced into the periapical connective tissue may cause clinical symptoms of acute inflammation (Core concept 8.5). They will, on the other hand, generally be killed and removed by the innate and adaptive immune systems operating in the inflammatory process unless they form a biofilm on a solid surface (Fig. 8.7).

Virulence factors

Any microflora succeeding in colonizing the root canal seem to produce more or less severe disease. There is no single or unique pathogen. The presence of different complex mixtures of micro-organisms in the root canals is typical of periapical disease. The sum of several virulence factors produced by the consortia of micro-organisms present will determine the degree of patho-

genicity of the endodontic microflora (Advanced concept 8.2). Information on virulence factors is limited to examples in certain oral species that have attracted attention, mainly as potential pathogens in periodontal disease (43, 61). Some of these are also common in endodontic samples and similar pathogenic mechanisms are likely to be active in periapical disease (64–66).

Host defense mechanisms are unable to remove micro-organisms located outside their reach in the necrotic pulp and on the walls of the root canal (Figs 8.4–8.7). In addition, some micro-organisms can impair host defense, with enzymes degrading plasma proteins such as immunoglobulins, complement factors, proteinase inhibitors and proteins involved in the clotting, fibrinolytic and kinin systems (43, 66). Such enzymes have been demonstrated in *Porphyromonas* and *Prevotella* species and may offer protection to the whole microbial community, not only to the producers. Phagocytosis is of paramount importance in host defense. Although leukotoxin-producing (phagocyte-killing) bacteria are rare in the endodontic microflora, several of the bacteria commonly found can evade phagocytosis or resist intracellular killing in various ways. One such mechanism is the above-mentioned degradation of plasma proteins essential for opsonization, and another is the presence of a capsule around some bacteria (61, 66).

Direct damage to the periapical connective tissue and bone may be caused by extracellular bacterial enzymes such as proteases, collagenase, hyaluronidase and chondroitin sulfatase. Such enzymes are produced by several species isolated from root canals, notably *Prevotella*, *Porphyromonas*, *Peptostreptococcus*, *Eubacterium* and *Treponema* species (30). The endodontic microflora also produce cytotoxic metabolites, which may damage the tissues and cause inflammation: ammonia, amines, indole, hydrogen sulfide, methyl mercaptan, butyrate, propionate, succinate and others (43, 61, 64, 66). Another group of cytotoxic substances are the lipopolysaccharide endotoxins of Gram-negative bacteria. They act as anti-

---

Advanced concept 8.2   Some microbial virulence factors implicated in periapical disease

Colonization of root canal

- Surface components for adhesion and coaggregation
- Enzymes to get nutrients
- Microbial food chains

Evasion of host defenses

- Location
- Immunoglobulin-degrading proteases
- Complement-degrading proteases
- Capsules
- Inhibition of phagocytes

Direct tissue damage

- Proteases and other enzymes
- Cytotoxic metabolic products
- Lipopolysaccharide endotoxins

Indirect tissue damage due to inflammatory response to the micro-organisms

- Cytokines
- Proteases and other enzymes from host cells

Table 8.2 Occurrence of symptoms in 31 cases of apical periodontitis in which black-pigmented bacteria (37 strains) were isolated from the root canal[a]. From: Haapasalo et al., 1986 (28).

Species	No. with symptoms	No. without symptoms
Porphyromonas gingivalis	6[b]	
Porphyromonas endodontalis	2	
Prevotella intermedia/nigrescens	10[b]	5
Prevotella denticola	3	9
Prevotella loescheii	1	1
Black-pigmented bacteria present[c]	9	22
No black-pigmented bacteria[c]	2	29

[a] Black-pigmented bacteria were cultured from 31 of 62 teeth.
[b] In three cases Po. gingivalis was found together with Pr. intermedia/nigrescens.
[c] Occurrence of symptoms 1 week after initial treatment while the bacteria were isolated at start.

Core concept 8.6   Association of signs and symptoms with specific bacteria

There is no absolute correlation between the presence of specific bacteria and signs and symptoms of acute inflammation.

There is, however, an increased incidence of pain, swelling and abscess in cases with mixed infection comprising many anaerobic species, especially in the presence of certain species of Porphyromonas, Prevotella, and/or Peptostreptococcus.

---

genic and toxic compounds, which cause inflammation and induce bone resorption.

Many virulence factors of the endodontic microflora can induce inflammation, and this will lead indirectly to host tissue damaging itself (Advanced concept 8.2). Although the inflammatory process is protective for the host, aiming at elimination of the micro-organisms and their products, it also causes degradation of periapical connective tissue fibers and extracellular matrix, and osteoclasts are activated to bone resorption. In addition, dormant epithelial rests may be stimulated to proliferate (50). In these intricate processes many cell types participate, notably neutrophil granulocytes, macrophages, lymphocytes, plasma cells and tissue cells. Among the many biologically active substances are cytokines released by inflammatory cells and tissue cells, complement factors, antibodies, and enzymes released from neutrophils, macrophages and tissue cells.

Association of signs and symptoms with specific bacteria

Although periapical inflammation is usually chronic with no subjective symptoms, it can also become acute with symptoms such as tenderness to pressure on the tooth, exudate in the canal, spontaneous pain, swelling,

abscess formation, and sometimes spread of the infection with fever. It is logical to assume that some micro-organisms (Table 8.1) and certain mixtures are more virulent than others and therefore more likely to cause acute symptoms, and there is in fact some evidence for this hypothesis. However, the large individual variation and the small number of cases studied prevent firm conclusions, and no absolute correlations have been established (6, 20, 25, 28, 30, 60, 63, 67, 69, 79). The risk of acute symptoms is increased in case of large quantities of micro-organisms in the canal and in the presence of mixtures of several, mainly anaerobic species. Furthermore, in some studies Porphyromonas, Prevotella, Peptostreptococcus, Fusobacterium and Eubacterium species were associated with an increased incidence of symptoms (Table 8.2; Core concept 8.6) (25, 28, 63, 69, 79).

The Porphyromonas and Prevotella species forming black colonies on blood agar (previously called black-pigmented Bacteroides or bpb) have attracted special attention in endodontic as well as periodontal microbiology. The important role of bpb in mixed anaerobic infections has been known for more than 35 years and for some of them was confirmed in a study of experimental infections induced in guinea pigs by subcutaneous injections of combinations of root canal bacteria (67). Persistent abscesses and transmissible infections could only be produced with mixtures comprising *Po. endodontalis* or *Pr. intermedia/nigrescens*. (These studies were before 'Bacteroides intermedius' was divided into *Pr. intermedia* and *Pr. nigrescens*.)

Studies of black-pigmented bacteria in cases of periapical inflammation with and without acute symptoms (28, 69) suggest that the presence of *Po. endodontalis*, *Po. gingivalis* or *Pr. intermedia/nigrescens* in the mixed microflora increases the risk of clinical symptoms and abscess formation. In one of these studies of 62 cases of apical periodontitis (35 acute and 27 clinically asymptomatic cases), 37 strains of 'black-pigmented *Bacteroides*' were isolated from 31 (50%) of the teeth, always in a mixed anaerobic microflora (28). These bacteria were cultured from both symptomatic and asymptomatic teeth, and there were also several symptomatic cases from which they were not isolated. However, the proteolytic species *Po. gingivalis* and *Po. endodontalis* were present only in acute infections, whereas *Pr. intermedia/nigrescens* was found in both symptomatic and asymptomatic cases and *Pr. denticola* occurred mostly in asymptomatic root canals (Table 8.2). Especially if the canal contains black-pigmented bacteria, the method of canal instrumentation is an important determinant also in the development of post-treatment abscess because these bacteria are likely to cause acute symptoms if pushed out apically.

One study (25) suggests that statistically significant associations exist between individual endodontic symptoms and particular combinations of specific bacteria. Thus, pain was associated with mixtures of anaerobes comprising *Peptostreptococcus* and *Prevotella* species. Swelling was particularly associated with isolation of *Eubacterium*, *Peptostreptococcus* or *Prevotella* species, and even more strongly with a combination of *Peptostreptococcus* and *Prevotella* species. Exudate in the canal was significantly associated with combinations of *Prevotella/Eubacterium* species and *Peptostreptococcus/Eubacterium* species.

In some cases the root canal infection seems resistant to treatment, as indicated by persisting exudate in the canal and/or other symptoms. Cultures from such cases after several treatment sessions often show streptococci, enterobacteria and yeasts. These may have been present from the start and be relatively resistant to treatment. It seems, however, as if their presence is often due to contamination of canals left open or inadequately sealed, or to other failures in aseptic technique (59, 75). In studies of root filled teeth retreated due to persisting periapical lesions, the microflora cultured differed markedly from that of untreated teeth. It consisted mostly of one or two species of mainly Gram-positive bacteria, and the most common isolate was *Enterococcus faecalis* (46, 68).

Conclusion

Research into the microbiology of apical periodontitis has demonstrated the essential role of micro-organisms in the necrotic pulp and the root canal for the development of periapical inflammation. The microflora is generally a mixture of several oral species dominated by obligate anaerobic bacteria with smaller proportions of facultative anaerobes. Oral yeasts and enteric bacteria may also be present; these often become predominant during prolonged treatment in cases of persistent infection, and they are common in retreated cases due to failure of previous root fillings. Information on the endodontic microflora is an important part of the scientific basis for the development of modern treatment principles. The treatment aims at elimination of micro-organisms located not only in the necrotic pulp tissue but also on the root canal walls and inside the dentinal tubules. This requires mechanical instrumentation and locally applied antimicrobial agents under the maintenance of aseptic techniques, as well as an adequate seal to prevent contamination during and between treatment sessions.

References

1. Adriaens PA, De Boever JA, Loesche WJ. Bacterial invasion in root cementum and radicular dentin of periodontally diseased teeth in humans: a reservoir of periodontopathic bacteria. *J. Periodont.* 1988; 59: 222–30.
2. Andreasen JO, Rud J. A histobacteriologic study of dental and periapical structures after endodontic surgery. *Int. J. Oral Surg.* 1972; 1: 272–81.
3. Assed S, Ito IY, Leonardo MR, Silva LAB, Lopatin DE. Anaerobic micro-organisms in root canals of human teeth with chronic apical periodontitis detected by indirect immunofluorescence. *Endodont. Dent. Traumatol.* 1996; 12: 66–9.
4. Bae K-S, Baumgartner JC, Shearer TR, David LL. Occurrence of *Prevotella nigrescens* and *Prevotella intermedia* in infections of endodontic origin. *J. Endodont.* 1997; 23: 620–3.
5. Baumgartner JC, Falkler WA. Bacteria in the apical 5 mm of infected root canals. *J. Endodont.* 1991; 17: 380–3.
6. Baumgartner JC, Watkins BJ, Bae K-S, Xia T. Association of black-pigmented bacteria with endodontic infections. *J. Endodont.* 1999; 25: 413–15.
7. Bender IB, Seltzer S, Kaufman IJ. Infectibility of the dental pulp by way of dental tubules. *J. Am. Dent. Assoc.* 1959; 59: 466–71.

8. Bender IB, Naidorf IJ, Garvey GJ. Bacterial endocarditis: a consideration for physician and dentist. *J. Am. Dent. Assoc.* 1984; 109: 415–20.

9. Bergenholtz G. Micro-organisms from necrotic pulp of traumatized teeth. *Odontol. Revy* 1974; 25: 347–58.

10. Bergenholtz G. Pathogenic mechanisms in pulpal disease. *J. Endodont.* 1990; 16: 98–101.

11. Bergenholtz G, Hasselgren G. Endodontics and periodontics. In *Clinical Periodontology and Implant Dentistry* (3rd edn) (Lindhe J, Karring T, Lang NP, eds). Copenhagen: Munksgaard, 1997; 296–331.

12. Bergenholtz G, Lindhe J. Effect of experimentally induced marginal periodontitis and periodontal scaling on the dental pulp. *J. Clin. Periodont.* 1978; 5: 59–73.

13. Brauner AW, Conrads G. Studies into the microbial spectrum of apical periodontitis. *Int. Endodont. J.* 1995; 28: 244–8.

14. Burke GW, Knighton HT. The localization of micro-organisms in inflamed dental pulps of rats following bacteremia. *J. Dent. Res.* 1960; 39: 205–14.

15. Burnett GW, Scherp HW. *Oral Microbiology and Infectious Disease* (3rd edn) Baltimore: Williams & Wilkins, 1968; 27–31, 467, 485.

16. Conrads G, Gharbia SE, Gulabivala K, Lampert F, Shah HN. The use of a 16S rDNA directed PCR for the detection of endodontopathogenic bacteria. *J. Endodont.* 1997; 23: 433–8.

17. Dahle UR, Tronstad L, Olsen I. Observation of an unusually large spirochete in endodontic infection. *Oral Microbiol. Immunol.* 1993; 8: 251–3.

18. Debelian GJ, Olsen I, Tronstad L. Anaerobic bacteremia and fungemia in patients undergoing endodontic therapy: an overview. *Ann. Periodont.* 1998; 3: 281–7.

19. Edwardsson S. Bacteriological studies on deep areas of carious dentine. *Odontol. Revy* 1974; 25: Suppl. 32.

20. Fabricius L, Dahlén G, Holm SE, Möller ÅJR. Influence of combinations of oral bacteria on periapical tissues of monkeys. *Scand. J. Dent. Res.* 1982; 90: 200–6.

21. Fabricius L, Dahlén G, Öhman AE, Möller ÅJR. Predominant indigenous oral bacteria isolated from infected root canals after varied times of closure. *Scand. J. Dent. Res.* 1982; 90: 134–44.

22. Gatti JJ, Dobeck JM, Smith C, White RR, Socransky SS, Skobe Z. Bacteria of asymptomatic periradicular endodontic lesions identified by DNA-DNA hybridization. *Endodont. Dent. Traumatol.* 2000; 16: 197–204.

23. Geurtsen W. The cracked-tooth syndrome: clinical features and case reports. *Int. J. Periodont. Restor. Dent.* 1992; 12: 395–405.

24. Gier RE, Mitchell DF. Anachoretic effect of pulpitis. *J. Dent. Res.* 1968; 47: 564–70.

25. Gomes BPFA, Lilley JD, Drucker DB. Associations of endodontic symptoms and signs with particular combinations of specific bacteria. *Int. Endodont. J.* 1996; 29: 69–75.

26. Goncalves RB, Robitaille M, Mouton C. Identical clonal types of *Porphyromonas gingivalis* or *Prevotella nigrescens* recovered from infected root canals and subgingival plaque. *Oral Microbiol. Immunol.* 1999; 14: 197–200.

27. Grossman LI. Origin of micro-organisms in traumatized, pulpless, sound teeth. *J. Dent. Res.* 1967; 46: 551–3.

28. Haapasalo M, Ranta H, Ranta K, Shah H. Black-pigmented *Bacteroides* spp. in human apical periodontitis. *Infect. Immun.* 1986; 53: 149–53.

29. Happonen, R-P, Söderling E, Viander M, Linko-Kettunen L, Pelliniemi LJ. Immunocytochemical demonstration of *Actinomyces* species and *Arachnia propionica* in periapical infections. *J. Oral Pathol.* 1985; 14: 405–13.

30. Hashioka K, Suzuki K, Yoshida T, Nakane A, Horiba N, Nakamura H. Relationship between clinical symptoms and enzyme-producing bacteria isolated from infected root canals. *J. Endodont.* 1994; 20: 75–7.

31. Heimdahl A, Hall G, Hedberg M, Sandberg H, Söder P-Ö, Tunér K, Nord CE. Detection and quantitation by lysis-filtration of bacteremia after different oral surgical procedures. *J. Clin. Microbiol.* 1990; 28: 2205–9.

32. Holdeman LV, Cato EP, Moore WEC. *Anaerobe Laboratory Manual* (4th edn). Blacksburg VA: Anaerobe Laboratory, Virginia Polytechnic Institute and State University, 1977.

33. Hoshino E. Predominant obligate anaerobes in human carious dentin. *J. Dent. Res.* 1985; 64: 1195–8.

34. Hoshino E, Ando N, Sato M, Kota K. Bacterial invasion in non-exposed dental pulp. *Int. Endodont. J.* 1992; 25: 2–5.

35. Hunter W. The role of sepsis and of antisepsis in medicine. *Dent. Cosmos* 1918; 60: 585–602.

36. Kakehashi S, Stanley HR, Fitzgerald RJ. The effects of surgical exposures of dental pulps in germ-free and conventional laboratory rats. *Oral Surg.* 1965; 20: 340–9.

37. Kobayashi T, Hayashi A, Yoshikawa R, Okuda K, Hara K. The microbial flora from root canals and periodontal pockets of non-vital teeth with advanced periodontitis. *Int. Endodont. J.* 1990; 23: 100–6.

38. Langeland K, Rodrigues H, Dowden W. Periodontal disease, bacteria, and pulpal histopathology. *Oral Surg.* 1974; 37: 257–70.

39. Lin L, Langeland K. Light and electron microscopic study of teeth with carious pulp exposures. *Oral Surg.* 1981; 31: 292–316.

40. Lomcali G, Sen BH, Cankaya H. Scanning electron microscopic observations of apical root surfaces of teeth with apical periodontitis. *Endodont. Dent. Traumatol.* 1996; 12: 70–6.

41. Love RM. Bacterial penetration of the root canal of intact incisor teeth after a simulated traumatic injury. *Endodont. Dent. Traumatol.* 1996; 12: 289–93.

42. Makkes PC, Thoden van Velzen SK, Wesselink PR. Reactions of the living organism to dead and fixed dead tissue. *J. Endodont.* 1978; 4: 17–21.

43. Marsh P, Martin M. *Oral Microbiology* (4th edn). Oxford: Wright, 1999; 10–15, 17–32, 41–6, 58–80, 91–2, 106–17, 127–36.

44. Mejàre B. The incidence and significance of *Streptococcus sanguis*, *Streptococcus mutans* and *Streptococcus salivarius* in root canal cultures from human teeth. *Odontol. Revy* 1974; 25: 359–78.

45. Miller WD. *The Micro-Organisms of the Human Mouth* (unaltered reprint of the original work published in 1890 in Philadelphia). Basel: S. Karger, 1973; 96–9, 285–95.

46. Molander A, Reit C, Dahlén G, Kvist T. Microbiological status of root filled teeth with apical periodontitis. *Int. Endodont. J.* 1998; 31: 1–7.

47. Möller ÅJR. *Microbiological Examination of Root Canals and Periapical Tissues of Human Teeth. Methodological Studies.* Göteborg: Akademiförlaget, 1966.

48. Möller ÅJR, Fabricius L, Dahlén G, Öhman AE, Heyden G. Influence on periapical tissues of indigenous oral bacteria and necrotic pulp tissue in monkeys. *Scand. J. Dent. Res.* 1981; 89: 475–84.
   The pulps were aseptically necrotized. In 26 teeth they were kept sterile by sealing and 52 were infected with oral flora. After 6–7 months, the teeth and periapical tissues were examined. The non-infected root canals were all sterile and the necrotic tissue did not induce periapical inflammation. The teeth with infected necrotic tissue showed inflammation clinically (12/52 teeth) and radiographically (47/52 teeth). All infected teeth examined histologically showed strong periapical inflammation.

49. Nair PNR. Light and electron microscopic studies of root canal flora and periapical lesions. *J. Endodont.* 1987; 13: 29–39.

50. Nair PNR. Apical periodontitis: a dynamic encounter between root canal infection and host response. *Periodontology 2000* 1997; 13: 121–48.

51. Nair PNR, Schroeder HE. Periapical actinomycosis. *J. Endodont.* 1984; 10: 567–70.

52. Nair PNR, Sjögren U, Krey G, Kahnberg K-E, Sundqvist G. Intracanal bacteria and fungi in root filled, asymptomatic human teeth with therapy-resistant periapical lesions: a long-term light and electron microscopic follow-up study. *J. Endodont.* 1990; 16: 580–8.
   Light and electron microscopy were used to analyze nine therapy-resistant and asymptomatic human periapical lesions, which were removed as block biopsies during surgical treatment. The findings suggest that in the majority of root filled teeth with therapy-resistant periapical lesions, micro-organisms persist in the apical root canal and may play a significant role in endodontic treatment failures.

53. Peciuliene V, Balciuniene I, Eriksen HM, Haapasalo M. Isolation of *Enterococcus faecalis* in previously root filled canals in a Lithuanian population. *J. Endodont.* 2000; 26: 593–5.

54. Robinson HBG, Boling LR. The anachoretic effect in pulpitis. I. Bacteriologic studies. *J. Am. Dent. Assoc.* 1941; 28: 268–82.

55. Rubach WC, Mitchell DF. Periodontal disease, accessory canals and pulp pathosis. *J. Periodont.* 1965; 36: 34–8.

56. Sato T, Hoshino E, Uematsu H, Noda T. Predominantly obligate anaerobes in necrotic pulps of human deciduous teeth. *Microb. Ecol. Health Dis.* 1993; 6: 269–75.

57. Sen BH, Piskin B, Demirci T. Observation of bacteria and fungi in infected root canals and dentinal tubules by SEM. *Endodont. Dent. Traumatol.* 1995; 11: 6–9.

58. Siqueira JF, Rocas IN, Souto R, de Uzeda M, Colombo AP. Checkerboard DNA–DNA hybridization analysis of endodontic infections. *Oral Surg.* 2000; 89: 744–8.

59. Sirén EK, Haapasalo MPP, Ranta K, Salmi P, Kerosuo ENJ. Microbiological findings and clinical treatment procedures in endodontic cases selected for microbiological investigation. *Int. Endodont. J.* 1997; 30: 91–5.

60. Sobrinho APR, Barros MHM, Nicoli JR. *et al.* Experimental root canal infections in conventional and germ-free mice. *J. Endodont.* 1998; 24, 405–8.

61. Socransky SS, Haffajee D. Microbiology of periodontal disease. In *Clinical Periodontology and Implant Dentistry* (3rd edn). (Lindhe J, Karring T, Lang NP, eds) Copenhagen: Munksgaard, 1997; 138–88.

62. Sunde PT, Tronstad L, Eribe ER, Lind PO, Olsen I. Assessment of periradicular microbiota by DNA–DNA hybridization. *Endodont. Dent. Traumatol.* 2000; 16: 191–6.

63. Sundqvist G. *Bacteriological Studies of Necrotic Dental Pulps.* Umeå, Sweden: Umeå University Odontological Dissertations, 1976; no. 7.
   Teeth with intact crowns were selected and strict precautions against contamination taken. Anaerobic conditions were maintained for sampling, transport and cultivation. No bacteria could be isolated from any samples from 13 teeth free from periapical destruction. From 18/19 teeth with periapical osteitis, 1–12 strains of bacteria were cultured, the majority being anaerobes. Teeth with acute symptoms had a complex anaerobic flora comprising 'Bacteroides melaninogenicus'.

64. Sundqvist G. Endodontic microbiology. In *Experimental Endodontics* (Spångberg LSW, ed). Boca Raton, FL: CRC Press, 1990; 131–53.

65. Sundqvist G. Associations between microbial species in dental root canal infections. *Oral Microbiol. Immunol.* 1992; 7: 257–62.

66. Sundqvist G. Taxonomy, ecology and pathogenicity of the root canal flora. *Oral Surg.* 1994; 78: 522–30.

67. Sundqvist G, Eckerbom MI, Larsson ÅP, Sjögren UT. Capacity of anaerobic bacteria from necrotic dental pulps to induce purulent infections. *Infect. Immun.* 1979; 25: 685–93.

68. Sundqvist G, Figdor D, Persson S, Sjögren S. Microbiological analysis of teeth with failed endodontic treatment and outcome of conservative re-treatment. *Oral Surg.* 1998; 85: 86–93.
   Fifty-four root filled teeth with persisting periapical lesions were selected for retreatment. After removal of the root filling, canals were sampled by means of advanced microbiological techniques. The microflora were mainly single species of predominantly Gram-positive organisms. Enterococcus faecalis was the species most commonly recovered. The success rate of retreatment was 74% : 80% for cases with negative culture prior to filling versus 33% for cases with positive culture.

69. Sundqvist G, Johansson E, Sjögren U. Prevalence of black-pigmented *Bacteroides* species in root canal infections. *J. Endodont.* 1989; 15: 13–19.

70. Terheyden H, Knospe HJ, Dunsche A, Meunier D. Keimspektrum odontogener Abszesse im Milchgebiss. *Dtsch. Zahnärztl. Z.* 1997; 52: 124–5.

71. Torabinejad M, Kiger RD. A histologic evaluation of dental pulp tissue of a patient with periodontal disease. *Oral Surg.* 1985; 59: 198–200.

72. Torneck CD. Reaction of rat connective tissue to polyethylene tube implants. Part II. *Oral Surg.* 1967; 24: 674–83.

73. Tronstad L, Barnett F, Cervone F. Periapical bacterial plaque in teeth refractory to endodontic treatment. *Endodont. Dent. Traumatol.* 1990; 6: 73–7.

74. Wade WG, Spratt DA, Dymock D, Weightman AJ. Molecular detection of novel anaerobic species in dentoalveolar abscesses. *Clin. Infect. Dis.* 1997; 25 (Suppl. 2): S235–6.

75. Waltimo TMT, Sirén EK, Torkko HLK, Olsen I, Haapasalo MPP. Fungi in therapy-resistant apical periodontitis. *Int. Endodont. J.* 1997; 30: 96–101.

    Among 967 microbiological samples taken by general practitioners from persistent endodontic infections, 692 gave growth and yeasts were isolated from 47 (7%) of these. The yeasts were found in pure culture in 6 (13%) and together with bacteria in 41 (87%) of these samples. The accompanying bacteria were mostly streptocooci and other Gram-positive facultative anaerobes. In some cases, obligate anaerobes were found in addition.

76. Weiger R, Manncke B, Werner H, Löst C. Microbial flora of sinus tracts and root canals of non-vital teeth. *Endodont. Dent. Traumatol.* 1995; 11: 15–19.

77. Williams RC, Paquette DW. Detection of putative pathogens. In *Clinical Periodontology and Implant Dentistry* (3rd edn) (Lindhe J, Karring T, Lang NP, eds). Copenhagen: Munksgaard, 1997; 403–7.

78. Xia T, Baumgartner JC, David LL. Isolation and identification of *Prevotella tannerae* from endodontic infections. *Oral Microbiol. Immunol.* 2000; 15: 273–5.

79. Yoshida M, Fukushima H, Yamamoto K, Ogawa K, Toda T, Sagawa H. Correlation between clinical symptoms and micro-organisms isolated from root canals of teeth with periapical pathosis. *J. Endodont.* 1987; 13: 24–8.

Chapter 9
Apical periodontitis

Risto-Pekka Happonen and Gunnar Bergenholtz

Introduction

In the process of pulpal necrosis, bacteria, bacterial products and inflammatory mediators accumulate in the root canal system and may spread beyond apical foramina and elicit lesions in the periodontal tissues. Because these lesions typically are inflammatory in nature and most often located near the tip of roots, collectively they are termed apical periodontitis. Periodontal lesions of endodontic origin may also develop in a juxtaposition along the lateral aspects of the roots. In these instances the causative agents are released along lateral or accessory canals (Fig. 9.1). Proper terms for these lesions would be juxtaradicular or lateral periodontitis. In this text we use the terms apical periodontitis and endodontic lesion to describe the inflammatory processes of the periodontal tissues that are initiated and maintained by an endodontic source of irritants.

Apical periodontitis serves an important protective function and seeks to prevent the spread of bacteria and bacterial elements to other body compartments. Yet, the process occasionally may be associated with severe clinical symptoms and may also, although rare, be a life-threatening condition. Pain, tenderness and swellings often bring the patient to the dentist (Figs 9.2a and 9.2b). For the most part, apical periodontitis stays asymptomatic and is thus largely inconspicuous to the patient, to be revealed only by routine radiographic examination (Fig. 9.2c). The microbial load and the state of the host defense are important parameters that determine the clinical presentation. In this chapter the pathogenesis and the various clinical and microscopic features of apical periodontitis are dealt with (Core concept 9.1).

Etiological factors

Apical periodontitis primarily evolves as a response to a bacterial challenge emanating from an infected, necrotic pulp. Bacteria infect pulps subsequent to injury,

most commonly by caries, dental trauma or iatrogenic injury (see further in Chapter 3). It needs to be recognized that as early as during the advancement of pulpal inflammation, e.g. in response to a carious exposure, periapical tissue responses emerge. Sometimes these early responses manifest themselves radiographically by the loss of lamina dura and the development of a small radiolucent area, but overt lesions as presented in Fig. 9.2 are invariably not clinically evident unless there is a necrotic pulp where bacteria have invaded the pulp chamber and multiplied into large numbers.

Apical periodontitis may also appear or prevail after endodontic therapy, due to treatment failing to prevent bacteria from infecting the root canal system or failing to rid an already established infection (see Chapters 6 and 11).

In conjunction with endodontic therapy, apical periodontitis may be initiated by iatrogenic injury. *Iatrogenic injury* is an injury caused by the dentist. Inadvertent extrusion of cytotoxic or allergenic medicaments and root filling materials is one example of iatrogenic injury. This often causes a cytotoxic response but may also result in hypersensitivity or foreign body reactions (13, 34, 35; Chapter 17). Root perforation – an artificial communication between the root canal space and the periodontal tissues – is another example that may occur during instrumentation of root canals in endodontic therapy or in conjunction with preparation for a post space in prosthodontic therapy. Such a communication may serve as a pathway for bacterial elements to enter the periodontal tissue and sustain an endodontic lesion.

Core concept 9.2 summarizes the factors associated with apical periodontitis.

Whereas medicaments and root filling materials often cause clinical lesions of limited duration, bacterially induced lesions prevail and remain as a non-self-healing process. The reason for non-healing is that the host defense is unable to reach sufficiently far into the root canal space to kill the bacterial invaders. Consequently, an untreated root canal infection, once established, remains as a chronic process and exposes the organism continuously to bacterial elements.

Specific features of the infecting microbiota

In an untreated tooth microbial infection is an absolute prerequisite for apical periodontitis (16, 28). It needs to be emphasized that necrotic pulpal tissue alone is unable to sustain frank inflammation and only initiates a phagocytic response. However, repair is seldom pos-

sible because the opening of the apical foramen is often too small to allow periodontal tissue to replace the necrotic tissue. Therefore, if not infected concomitantly or shortly after the injury, a necrotic pulp remains a target for microbial colonization. Studies have shown that this will occur sooner or later (2, 42) because necrotic tissue serves as an attractive substrate for certain oral micro-organisms (Chapter 8).

The course and the severity of the tissue response to root canal infection depend on the state of the

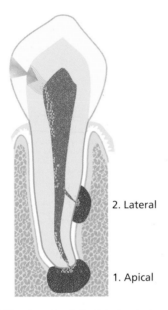

2. Lateral

1. Apical

Fig. 9.1 Potential locations of endodontic lesions in the periodontium.

> ### Core concept 9.1
>
> Even though apical periodontitis may cause severe clinical reactions, it basically serves a protective function because it is set up at least to confine, if not to kill, the infection to the root canal space and prevent it from spreading. Therefore apical periodontitis, although often referred to as a lesion, should be regarded as an important protective, inflammatory buffer zone (39).

> ### Core concept 9.2
>
> Apical periodontitis may be associated with:
>
> (1) Extensive inflammatory lesion of a vital pulp.
> (2) Infected pulp necrosis.
> (3) Failed endodontic treatment.
> (4) Iatrogenic injury from extrusion of medicaments and root-filling material.

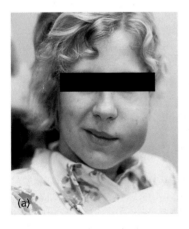
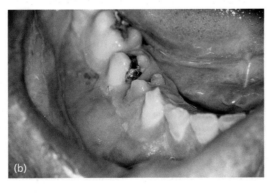
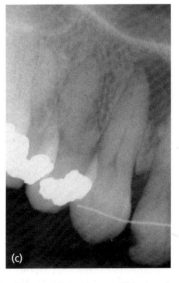

Fig. 9.2 Different clinical presentations of apical periodontitis due to an infected, necrotic pulp: (a) extra-oral swelling in the right cheek region; (b) intra-oral, vestibular swelling (associated with the severely broken lower premolar); (c) apically positioned radiolucent area (upper right, canine incisor).

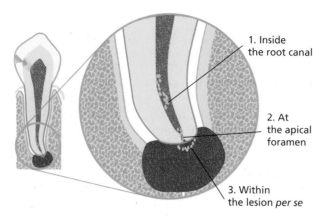

Fig. 9.3 Potential positions of the bacterial front in a necrotic pulp: (1) inside the root canal at a small distance from the apical foramen; (2) at the apical foramen; (3) within the lesion *per se*.

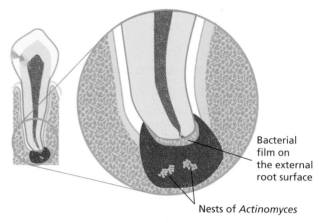

Fig. 9.4 Bacterial may occur in the lesion as either a film on the external root surface or as nests, as in this example.

individual's defense potential and the quality and the number of micro-organisms of the infecting microbiota. Thus, a lesion may become severe and detrimental in an individual with a poor general health condition. Acute and severe lesions may nevertheless develop in healthy individuals and often do so at early stages where micro-organisms have rapidly increased in numbers and where the local tissue defense is not yet fully organized. The presence of certain, particularly pathogenic, organisms also seems to play an important role. Thus, organisms belonging to the genera of *Porphyromonas*, *Prevotella*, *Fusobacterium* and *Peptostreptococcus* are more often associated with symptomatic and painful lesions than are other types of organisms (7, 8, 42–44). Nevertheless, all bacteria that colonize root canals are considered pathogens but most of them are associated with silent lesions.

Bacteria responsible for apical periodontitis are not normally able to establish themselves in the lesion *per se* (29). The reason is that bacteria attempting to invade the tissue effectively are held back and are eliminated by the host defense. Therefore, apical periodontitis is normally initiated and maintained by the release of bacterial elements produced during growth and disintegration of bacteria within the confines of the root canal space (Fig. 9.3), but there are exceptions.

In purulent lesions (periapical abscesses) bacteria may be found within the exudate. This can be confirmed either by direct microscopy of smears or by culture of pus (50). Once the acute phase has subsided, the host defense normally eliminates these organisms. Occasionally such lesions continue and are clinically discernible by a periodic release of pus into the oral environment along a fistulous tract (see below).

Certain bacteria in root canal infections may invade and survive long term within the lesion site and may compromise the potential for a successful outcome of endodontic treatment. There are two possibilities for this kind of infection (Fig. 9.4):

(1) In spite of the host defense, bacteria may proliferate from the root canal space and form a bacterial film on the external root surface (48).

(2) Various *Actinomyces*-related species, especially *Actinomyces israeli* and *Propionibacterium propionicum*, may invade the lesion site and produce colonies of bacterial masses or nests that escape phagocytosis and destruction (9). Such lesions are designated *periapical actinomycosis* and are characterized by the radial arrangement of these Gram-positive filamentous organisms. The history of such lesions is usually associated with clinical exacerbations and poor responses to endodontic treatment. *Exacerbation* is a term often used to denote the sudden change from a silent to an acute lesion with overt clinical symptoms of pain and swellings. At surgery, yellowish sulfur granules characteristic of actinomycotic infections often can be found within the soft-tissue lesion.

Tissue responses and reaction patterns

The temporal events of the neurovascular and cellular responses in apical periodontitis are not vastly different from those of inflammatory processes in connective tissue and bone tissue elsewhere. Its chronic nature and specific location in a bone tissue compartment nevertheless necessitate an account of the organization of the tissue lesion at both early and established stages. Similar to periodontal disease, the inflammatory process is not in response to a single bacterial organism but to a

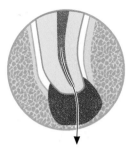

- periapical abscess
- periapical granuloma
- radicular cyst
- osteomyelitis

Fig. 9.5 Overview of periapical tissue responses to root canal infection.

large variety of combinations of different organisms. This means that, depending on the pathogenecity of the microbiota, the tissue lesion may have a different clinical presentation in terms of extent and severity.

The response of the periodontal tissues to the bacterial challenge involves different phases (Fig. 9.5). The early stage of apical periodontitis shows a distinct acute character and is rapidly expanding. The most conspicuous feature is bone resorption, which gives space for an inflammatory soft-tissue lesion at the root end. In this early stage of the process, frank clinical presentation may or may not appear. On very rare occasions the infection may take an adverse course and spread far into the adjacent bone to cause osteomyelitis (see below).

After termination of the acute phase, the process enters into a balanced host–tissue response. The condition is then characterized by a continuous combat of bacterial invaders at the same time as the host attempts to reorganize and repair the tissue damage. Owing to the consistent release of bacterial elements, healing cannot occur and the defense reaction continues and enters into a chronic stage of inflammation that may last for years. A common term for this condition is periapical granuloma, which refers to the granulation tissue that is formed in the process. It needs to be recognized that apical periodontitis is not an autonomic process because it is entirely dependent on the constant release of bacterial elements from the root canal space.

On a long-term basis a periapical granuloma may eventually develop into a radicular cyst. A radicular cyst is a closed, fluid-filled sac that is lined with epithelium. It expands and may eventually cause considerable destruction of alveolar bone (see below).

Early events

As in any inflammatory reaction to microbial infection, early events in apical periodontitis include:

- Neurovascular responses.
- Migration and accumulation of inflammatory cells of both the innate and the adaptive immune system.
- Tissue destruction.

To provide sufficient space for the inflammatory lesion, the periodontal ligament and the adjacent alveolar bone are initially broken down. Several local and systemic factors in a concerted action participate in this process and include both bacterially derived components and pro-inflammatory host-derived substances. The latter refer to arachidonic acid derivatives, components of the kallikrein–kinin system, cytokines, free radicals, metalloproteinase enzymes, as well as antigen–antibody complex formations and associated complement activation (21, 24, 32, 39). Although bacterial components such as enzymes and cell wall constituents can stimulate tissue destruction (including bone resorption) directly, it is their indirect stimulation through host-derived mediators that is likely to be the most significant mechanism (24).

The process of bone resorption is carried out by osteoclasts (Fig. 9.6). Resorptive cytokines (e.g. interleukin 1) and prostaglandins stimulate these cells. In the early phases of apical periodontitis, osteoclasts are abundant and outperform bone-forming osteoblasts. Consequently, the net result is loss of bone tissue within a limited area, which will remain for as long as the inflammatory lesion prevails. This results in an important diagnostic feature, because apical periodontitis in radiographs will show up as a radiolucent area (see Fig. 9.2c and Chapter 15).

Along with the process of bone resorption, some apical parts of the root will be lost as well. However, root resorption will be much less pronounced and is often visible only in microscopic sections, seldom in radiographs (20). Yet, root tips may sometimes be foreshortened to the extent that the original configuration of the apical canal anatomy is altered.

Of the inflammatory cells that appear initially, the polymorphonuclear leukocyte (the neotrophil) plays a central role and forms the first line of defense. These cells meet the bacterial front and hold it back through phagocytosis and intracellular killing. Thereby, the spreading of bacterial organisms is most often prevented. The bacterial front is then kept inside the root canal or at the foramen (Fig. 9.3). Effective neutrophils furthermore help to limit the disease process (Key literature 9.1). Yet, when caused to accumulate in large numbers, an acute abscess is formed that, under pres-

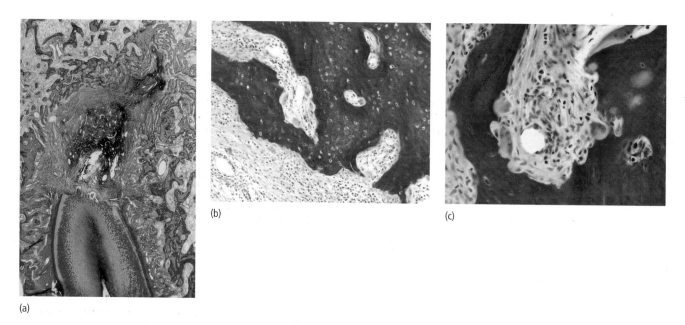

(a)

(b)

(c)

Fig. 9.6 Bone resorption is an important feature of the early inflammatory response in apical periodontitis. In the case shown in (a), bone is resorbed within a fairly large area outside the root tip where the inflammatory lesion appears to be spreading. This case also displays foreshortening of the root tip due to resorption. Osteoclastic activities are seen within a bone marrow spaces in (b) and (c) near the root tip of a tooth with progressing apical periodontitis. Microphotographs are from unpublished experimental material in non-human primates.

Key literature 9.1

In an experimental study Stashenko *et al.* (40) induced endodontic lesions in rats by leaving bur exposures of pulp uncovered to the oral environment for up to 20 days. A group of animals received both before and periodically after the injury a biological response modifier (PGG glucan), which upregulates host defense mechanisms. This drug enhances primarily the number of circulating neutrophils and monocytes, as well as their phagocytic capability. There were significantly less teeth with complete pulpal necrosis in PGG-treated animals compared with control animals. Also, these animals had less alveolar bone destruction and periapical soft-tissue lesion, implicating the significant role of neutrophils and monocytes in limiting the disease process.

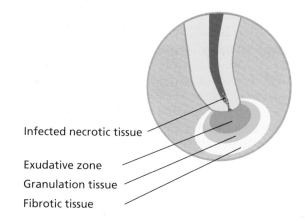

Infected necrotic tissue

Exudative zone

Granulation tissue

Fibrotic tissue

Fig. 9.7 In response to root canal infection, the tissue lesion presents different features at various distances from the root tip.

---

sure, will create pathways for drainage into either the oral cavity or the maxillary sinuses and also, but rarely, extra-orally (see further below).

The character of the tissue lesion changes over time and with distance from the root end. Although neutrophils will dominate the lesion site next to the bacterial front, macrophages and other mononuclear leukocytes (i.e. macrophages and T- and B-cells) with distinct immunological functions come to predominate in more peripheral areas and operate to resist further the spread of bacterial elements (Advanced concept 9.1). Mixed to a various extent with the inflammatory cells are fibrovascular elements representing attempts to repair. This area of the lesion is often referred to as the exudative zone (Fig. 9.7). More peripherally a much stronger expression of tissue repair develops where there is fibroblastic activity and the formation of new vessels. This area of the lesion appears similar to the granulation tissue that is formed prior to normal tissue repair. However, repair will not be completed as long as there is egress of bacterial substances from the root canal system.

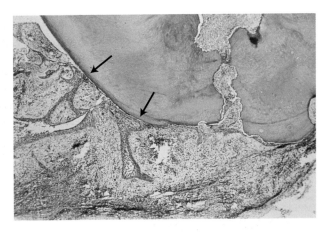

Fig. 9.8 Epithelial strands in a periapical granuloma that seem to attach to the root tip (arrows).

Advanced concept 9.1   Recruitment of inflammatory cells in developing apical periodontitis

The complement system, a component of the innate immunity, is important for the recruitment of neutrophils to the lesion site. As a first line of defense it is activated directly by microbial elements without the presence of antibodies, which later becomes an important defense mechanism. Activation of complement results in the formation of C3b binding to the surface of bacteria, which leads to opsonization and lysis. Complement activation also generates chemotactic factors, e.g. C3a and C5a anaphylatoxins, which stimulate the migration of neutrophils.

Dendritic cells (DCs) and some macrophages (see Chapter 3) present in the tissue are activated after making contact with the bacterial elements. Within hours they produce a variety of cytokines, including chemokines, which attract neutrophils, macrophages, T-cells and mature DCs to the lesion site. Thus, DCs and macrophages serve an important role as gatekeepers and amplifiers of the innate and adaptive immunity.

Mature DCs regulate the specific immune responses occurring during the initial phases of apical periodontitis. The activation phase includes cloning in regional lymph nodes of antigen-specific lymphocytes (T-cells), which soon appear at the lesion site and later become a dominant cell type in the lesion (41). During the early active phase, helper T-cells (CD4+) predominate over cytotoxic T-cells (CD8+), whereas in the more established chronic phase the situation is reversed (41). This feature suggests that helper T-cells are active during expansion of the inflammatory process. Thus, they are likely to be involved in the bone resorptive process by activating macrophages to produce bone-resorptive mediators.

B-cells are less abundant than T-cells in the early events but become an important constituent in the established lesion. Activated B-cells become plasma cells and produce a variety of immunoglobulins, of which IgG is the most dominant class (35). Recent observations suggest that antibody-mediated mechanisms by a variety of actions, including opsonization and activation of the complement system, are of great importance in confining the root canal infection and prevent it from spreading (14).

At increasing distances from the root tip there are decreasing numbers of inflammatory cells. Conversely, the volume of fibroblasts, ground substance and collagen is increased. Yet, clusters of mononuclear inflammatory cells may prevail in bone marrow spaces next to the soft-tissue lesion.

Dense, collagen-rich tissue usually becomes prominent at the very periphery of the process and separates the soft-tissue lesion from the surrounding alveolar bone. This tissue response seems to be yet another means by which the process is localized (19).

In conclusion, the tissue lesion in apical periodontitis, which on a molecular and cellular level consists of a complex series of events, balances tissue destruction with protective elements to limit the bacterial exposure of the host organism.

Epithelial proliferation

Occasionally strands of epithelial cells are encountered within the lesion site (Fig. 9.8). These cells are thought to originate from the rests of Malassez in the periodontal ligament. During the process of periapical inflammation, cytokines and growth factors are released that bring these epithelial cells to divide and proliferate. Yet, not every lesion will contain epithelial strands: it has been estimated that no more than ca. 50% of longstanding lesions contain epithelium (31, 32).

On observing tissue sections, epithelial cells seem to take a random course through the lesion. Sometimes they appear to attach to the root surface (Fig. 9.8). In other instances epithelium may block the exit of the root canal, thus appearing to form another defense barrier against the bacterial mass in the root canal space (33). In the mass of epithelial cells, neutrophils frequently appear (12).

Radicular cyst

Radicular cyst develops as a sequel to apical periodontitis and is the most common of all cysts in the jaws and the oral tissue. A cyst is a cavity with epithelial lining filled by fluid or semisolid material surrounded by a dense connective tissue (Fig. 9.9).

Radicular cysts can locate at any tooth-bearing area of the jaws, but the anterior maxilla appears to be a predilection site. They are asymptomatic unless secondarily infected or so large that they become clinically discernible from their expansion (Fig. 9.10). They may perforate the cortical bone and on palpation will be

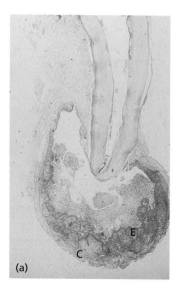

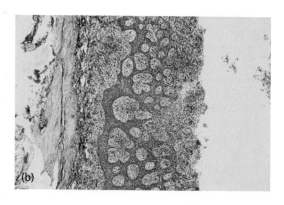

Fig. 9.9 (a) A radicular cyst attached to the apical end of an extracted root is seen. Epithelium (E) and a connective tissue capsule (C) surround the cyst lumen. (b) Proliferating cyst epithelium in a typical arcade-like configuration accompanied by intense inflammatory cell infiltrates.

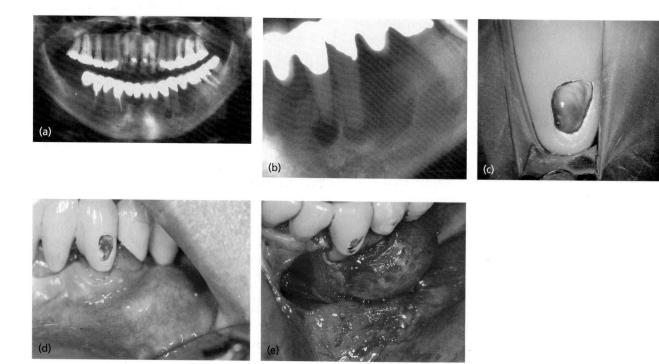

Fig. 9.10 Different clinical presentations of radical cysts are displayed. Radiographs (a) and (b) demonstrate two separate radiolucent areas. One is associated with tooth 33 and one larger lesion is associated with tooth 34 and has expanded in a distal–coronal direction. Although the size and shape of a lesion are not definitive criteria for cyst formation, there are other features suggestive of radicular cyst. On opening tooth 33 for endodontic treatment, clear exudates drew off from the root canal (c). It was not possible to stop exudation and thus completion of conventional endodontic therapy was prevented. At the buccal and distal aspects of tooth 34 there was a distinct prominence that was hard and non-tender to palpation (d). On raising a flap for enucleation, the expansive process is more clearly visible (e). Thin bone tissue limited the fluid-filled process at the surface. Histological examination of a tissue specimen confirmed the diagnosis.

noticeable as a fluctuating though not particularly painful area. Some individuals appear to be more prone than others to develop radicular cysts on root canal infection, for reasons that have yet to be established.

The epithelial lining of radicular cysts derives from the proliferation of the epithelial rests of Malassez and is regarded as being a direct effect of the inflammatory process (45, 49). On the basis of histological serial

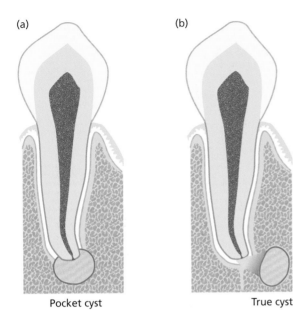

(a)   (b)

Pocket cyst   True cyst

Fig. 9.11 Radicular cysts may appear in two configurations: a *pocket cyst* (a) where there is direct communication between the cyst cavity and the root canal space; and a *true cyst* (b) where no such communication exists.

sections taken through cystic lesions, a proposal has been made for the subdivision of radicular cysts into true cysts and pocket cysts (31). In a pocket cyst there is a direct continuity between the cyst cavity and the root canal space, whereas no such direct communication is present with the true cyst (Fig. 9.11).

A radicular cyst may remain within the bone after extraction of the tooth (teeth) involved. Such a cyst is termed a residual cyst. Residual cysts may remain stationary or slowly expand over time.

In microscopic examinations, non-cornifying stratified squamous epithelium of varying thickness is typically seen on the inner surface of the cyst cavity (see Fig. 9.9). The epithelial lining often shows a folded, arcade-like configuration. Both the cyst epithelium and the outer connective tissue capsule variably are infiltrated by mononuclear leukocytes and neutrophils. The epithelium may be disrupted or even completely missing as a result of secondary infection of the cyst wall. Sometimes mucous cells or ciliated cells can be noted on the surface of the epithelial lining.

Given the pathogenesis of radicular cysts (Advanced concept 9.2, Key literature 9.2), epithelial growth ceases when the stimulating factors are eliminated. Subsequently the epithelium lining becomes thin, as is often the case in a residual cyst. Inflammatory infiltrates of the cyst wall also become scanty.

Other histological features of radicular cysts include the presence of Rushton's hyaline bodies and cholesterol

---

Advanced concept 9.2   Pathogenesis and growth of radicular cysts

The factors that initiate proliferation of the epithelial rests of Malassez are not well known. Both bacterial endotoxins as well as cytokines of inflammatory cells have been implicated (26). There is also evidence that epidermal growth factors are involved in this process (22, 23, 47). Once started, epithelial proliferation will continue for as long as stimulating factors are present.

The mechanism behind the development of the cyst cavity has been the focus of much speculation. Two hypotheses still prevail (32). One states that when the epithelial mass increases in size, the central cells will undergo degeneration and necrosis due to lack of nutritional supply. The necrotic material in turn attracts neutrophils, which, together with tissue exudate, result in the formation of microcavities that eventually coalesce to form a radicular cyst. Another theory is built on the assumption that epithelial cells grow to form an epithelial lining on the inner aspect of an abscess cavity.

Also, the exact mechanism for the subsequent slow increase in the size of the radicular cysts has not received its final explanation. Some believe that increased osmotic pressure in the cyst cavity is a key element (38). Increased osmosis leading to the passage of fluid from the surrounding tissue into the cyst lumen is likely to occur due to breakdown of epithelial and inflammatory cells. Furthermore, cyst expansion is related to the release of bone-resorbing factors from mononuclear leukocytes present in the cyst wall, including interleukin, mast cell tryptase and prostaglandins (10, 25, 6, 46).

Key literature 9.2

In a classic experiment in primates, Valderhaug (49) removed the pulp tissue in teeth and left the root canals open to the oral environment for up to 360 days.

Although initially severe inflammatory lesions, including migration of epithelial cells, were seen in the apical area, it took more than 200 days before cyst formation developed. The observation suggests that the inflammatory process in the apical periodontium is capable of inducing proliferation of the epithelial rests of Malassez and that radicular cysts may result if apical periodontitis is left untreated for a long period of time.

---

crystals. Rushton's bodies are circular or polycylic bodies often consisting of concentric amorphous lamellae. Although their source so far remains obscure, they have been proposed to be either of hematogenous or odontogenic epithelial origin (3, 27).

Often, but far from always, both the cyst capsule and the cyst cavity contain cholesterol, which forms sharp needle-like crystals. In tissue sections they are not seen but appear as typical tissue clefts from the dissolution of the cholesterol during tissue processing. The crystals are formed in the connective tissue of the cyst capsule and

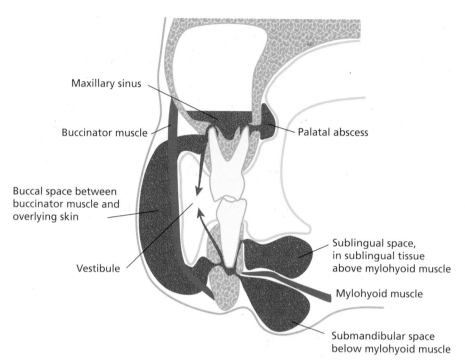

Maxillary sinus

Buccinator muscle

Palatal abscess

Buccal space between
buccinator muscle and
overlying skin

Vestibule

Sublingual space,
in sublingual tissue
above mylohyoid muscle

Mylohyoid muscle

Submandibular space
below mylohyoid muscle

Fig. 9.12 Common pathways of a periapical abscess. The route depends on the location of the roots in relation to the surrounding anatomical structures: (1) sublingual space, in the sublingual tissue above the mylohyoid muscle; (2) submandibular space below the mylohyoid muscle; (3) palatal abscess; (4) buccal space between buccinator muscle and overlying skin; (5) maxillary sinus; (6) vestibule.

are gradually moved towards and into the cyst cavity. They attract multinuclear giant cells of the foreign body type and thus elicit a foreign body response in the connective tissue (30). The crystals are thought to derive from disintegrating red blood cells dying in large numbers in apical periodontitis in stagnant vessels of the lesion. Inflammatory cells dying in large numbers in apical periodontitis and circulating plasma lipids are other proposed sources (1, 37).

Periapical abscess

Hyperemia, edema and the aggregation of inflammatory cells in the periapical area may lead to the formation of a periapical abscess. Such a lesion is commonly associated with severe pain and swellings and may occur as a direct sequel to the infection and breakdown of a vital pulp before the periapical tissue defense is fully organized. Periapical abscesses may also develop following exacerbation of an established, clinically silent lesion. The cause then is often related to an endodontic treatment. In conjunction with treatment, bacteria and bacterial elements may have been forced inadvertently outside the apical foramen. It may also be that particularly virulent micro-organisms were favored by the procedure, e.g. by apical overinstrumentation that enhanced their nutritional supply. Such a lesion is known as an endodontic flare-up (see further in Chapter 11).

Microscopically, a periapical abscess is characterized by tissue necrosis and an abundance of dead and active neutrophils in the center. At the periphery there

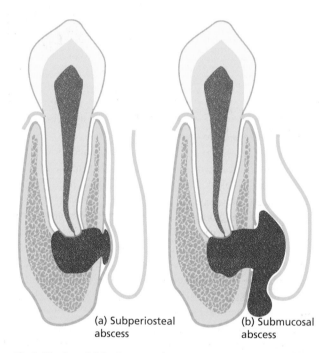

(a) Subperiosteal
abscess

(b) Submucosal
abscess

Fig. 9.13 Potential developments of a periapical abscess. In a subperiosteal abscess, pus has assembled underneath the periosteum (a). In a submucosal abscess (b), pus has broken through the periosteum and accumulated in the mucosal tissue. The latter is often associated with a distinct extra-oral tissue swelling.

are delicate bundles of collagen and bone resorption is ongoing (Fig. 9.6). Here, the inflammatory infiltrate becomes more mononuclear in nature. As bone resorption advances, pus collected within the periapical tissue

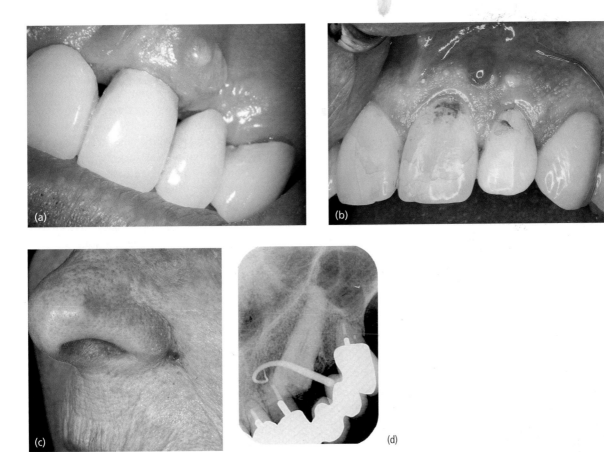

Fig. 9.14 Clinical photographs demonstrating different presentations of fistulous tracts: (a) and (b) show typical intra-oral fistulations. In (c) there is an extra-oral fistulation at the angle of the nose. By tracing the pathway with a gutta-percha cone, the origin was determined by radiography to the lateral upper incisor (d). Images (c) and (d) courtesy of Dr F. Frisk.

compartment may penetrate surrounding bone and seek its way further along the anatomical pathways and through the anatomical structures with the least resistance (Fig. 9.12). This will result in the development of a localized abscess in the adjacent soft tissue. Cellulitis is a feature seen in this context, representing diffuse dissemination of inflammatory exudate in the soft tissue. **Cellulitis** is a term that refers to an acute diffuse spreading of inflammation within the tissue and should be distinguished from a swelling due to an abscess, which represents a localized collection of pus.

Usually abscesses manifest themselves as a tender swelling that may have accumulated either under the periosteum – a subperiosteal abscess (Fig. 9.13a) – or in the mucosa after breakthrough of the periosteum (Fig. 9.13b). On palpation the latter lesion fluctuates, whereas a subperiosteal abscess often feels hard and very tender.

In its most severe forms the patient may have trismus, fever and difficulties in swallowing. Because this can be a life-threatening condition, prompt referral to an oral and maxillofacial surgeon for proper diagnosis and treatment is necessary. Any untreated periapical abscess with overt clinical manifestations should be considered a potential health threat that, in any given circumstance, may lead to a serious condition including orofacial abscesses, cellulitis, deep cervical infections and cavernous sinus thrombosis.

A much less severe manifestation of a periapical abscess is a sinus tract or fistula (Fig. 9.14). A sinus tract is defined as a passage of pus from an abscess cavity to an external environment through a tissue membrane such as the oral mucosa or the skin (Fig. 9.15). Depending on the anatomical location of the tooth apex, fistulous tracts may spread not only to the oral cavity or skin but also to maxillary sinuses and cause odontogenic sinusitis. Except for sinus infections, these lesions are not normally associated with severe symptoms of pain or swellings but may cause tenderness and patient discomfort. A most conspicuous feature is that they recur and release pus periodically.

Osteomyelitis

Osteomyelitis is a diffuse inflammatory process that expands within bone tissue. In the jaws, osteomyelitis may arise from odontogenic infections or any type of trauma such as bone fracture and surgical procedure (18). The condition is rare but more common in the mandible than in the maxilla. Systemic disease such as immunological and nutritional deficiencies, as well as impaired blood circulation in bone, predisposes to osteomyelitis.

Osteomyelitis occurs in acute and chronic forms. A periapical abscess where the root canal infection has not been confined is the most common cause of acute osteomyelitis of the jaws. Often a mixed infection but also single organisms such as *Staphylococcus aureus* and enterobacteria may be associated with this condition. In chronic forms, including chronic suppurative osteomyelitis, a causative organism is often hard to establish. The diagnosis and treatment of acute and chronic forms of osteomyelitis should be left to specialists in oral and maxillofacial surgery. Treatment varies depending on the clinical features and may include long-term antibiotic therapy, surgical treatment and hyperbaric oxygen therapy (15).

Condensing osteitis

Condensing osteitis is also known as focal sclerosing osteomyelitis (Fig. 9.16). This is a condition that does not pose much of a threat to patients and does not require treatment. Typically these lesions are asymptomatic and are seen as radiopaque masses often affecting molars of the mandibular region. The lesion consists of dense sclerotic bone formed in the response to a longstanding, low-grade inflammatory process, e.g. a pulpal lesion (4). Inflammatory cells are usually scanty. These lesions may or may not disappear after endodontic therapy or tooth extraction (11).

Epidemiology

Periapical inflammatory lesions are frequent manifestations. Although epidemiological data are limited, it is obvious that lesions are common in populations where caries is prevalent. There is also a link to age. The elderly, who frequently have suffered dental injuries by caries or restorative procedures, show 5–10% of their teeth to be affected (5, 17, 51). Population studies have also found that endodontic treatments of less than optimal quality

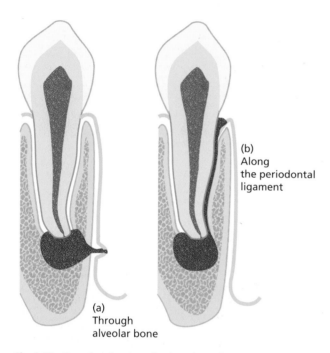

(b)
Along
the periodontal
ligament

(a)
Through
alveolar bone

Fig. 9.15 Examples of various directions that a fistulous tract may take: (a) through alveolar bone to the oral environment; (b) along the periodontal ligament to the oral environment.

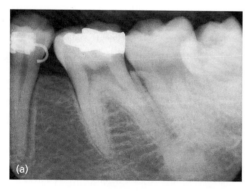
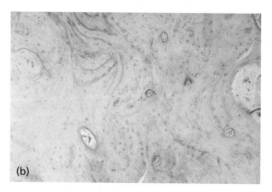

Fig. 9.16 (a) A large sclerotic bone reaction is associated with the distal root of a mandibular molar. The tooth is asymptomatic and responds to pulp vitality tests. (b) Dense sclerotic bone devoid of inflammatory cells is a typical histological finding in condensing osteitis.

present with higher frequencies of lesions than those where endodontics was adequately performed (50, 5, 17; see also Chapter 14).

The prevalence of radicular cysts has been estimated from biopsy specimens after periapical surgeries as well as from sections of soft-tissue lesions that have been recovered in conjunction with extraction. Data from numerous studies vary considerably and reported incidences among apical inflammatory lesions subjected to analysis vary from 5 to 55%. Variation most likely depends on the criteria used for the designation of cysts and the population in focus for the study. When very strict criteria were used Nair *et al.* (31) reported an incidence of 15%, of which true apical cysts made up the majority.

Case study 1

The radiograph in (a) is from a 37-year-old woman who was referred for treatment because of occasional pain episodes on the left mandibular area. On clinical examination, a fluctuating swelling was found lingually. Radiological examination revealed a round cystic lesion associated with the first premolar tooth. Endodontic treatment had been given several years earlier to the tooth that was clinically mobile. The cyst and the tooth were removed surgically in one piece.

A cyst associated with the apical area of the root is confirmed on histological examination (b).

Higher magnification shows that the cyst is not directly in contact with the apex of the root (c). A chronic inflammatory cell infiltrate is seen in the cyst capsule on the right side of the root.

Thin cyst epithelium has a corrugated orthokeratinized surface (d).

Diagnosis: Keratocyst, orthokeratinized variant.

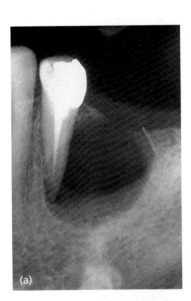

(a)

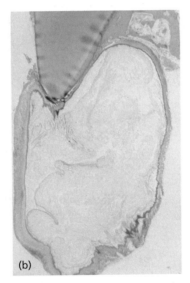

(b)

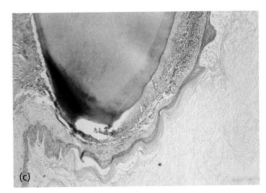

(c)

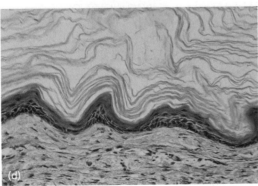

(d)

Case study 2

A 41-year-old woman suffering from diabetes mellitus, Meniere's disease, chronic pyelonephritis resulting in renal failure and secondary hyperparathyroidism displayed multiple periapical radiolucent lesions (teeth 37, 36, 34, 33, 32, 43, 44, and 47) on orthopantomographic examination (a). The patient was dialysis dependent. There were no clinical symptoms. All the teeth except for tooth 47 were found to respond as vital on sensibility testing. The lesions were considered to be associated with secondary hyperparathyroidism. No treatment was given.

Radiographic examination 3 years later shows complete resolution of the periapical lesions (b). Kidney transplantation had been performed 1 year earlier, resulting in improvement of imbalance in the calcium metabolism.

Diagnosis: Bone destruction due to secondary hyperparathyroidism.

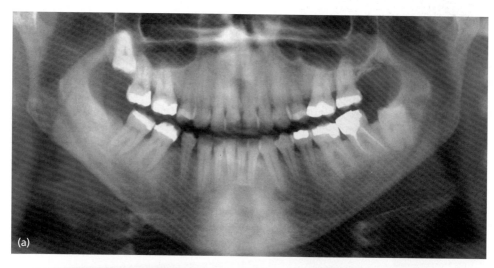

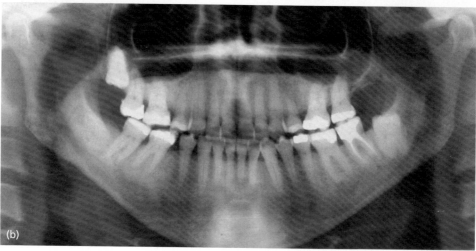

Case study 3

An asymptomatic cystic lesion was found in radiological examination at the periapical area of mandibular front teeth in a 31-year-old woman (a). The pulps of the teeth involved were found to be vital. The lesion was removed surgically.

Histopathological examination revealed poorly organized bone tissue and cementum particles within a cellular connective tissue stroma (b).

Diagnosis: Periapical cemental dysplasia.

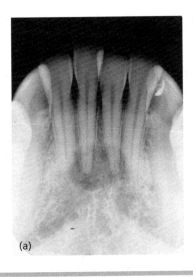

(a)

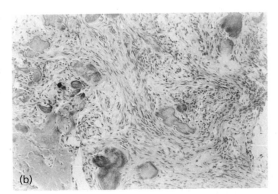

(b)

References

1. Arwill T, Heyden G. Histochemical studies on cholesterol formation in odontogenic cysts and granulomas. *Scand. J. Dent. Res.* 1973; 81: 406–10.

2. Bergenholtz G. Micro-organisms from necrotic pulp in traumatized teeth. *Odontol. Revy* 1974; 25: 347–58.

3. Browne R , Matthews JB. Intra-epithelial hyaline bodies in odontogenic cysts: an immunoperoxidase study. *J. Oral Pathol.* 1985; 14: 422–8.

4. Douglas GD, Trowbridge HO. Chronic focal sclerosing osteomyelitis associated with a cracked tooth. Report of a case. *Oral Surg.* 1993; 76: 351–5.

5. Eriksen HM, Bjertness E. Prevalence of apical periodontitis and results of endodontic treatment in middle-aged adults in Norway. *Endodont. Dent. Traumatol.* 1991; 7: 1–4.

6. Formigli L, Orlandini SZ, Tonelli P, Giannelli M, Martini M, Brandi ML, Bergamini M, Orlandini GE. Osteolytic processes in human radicular cysts: morphological and biochemical results. *J. Oral Pathol. Med.* 1995; 24: 216–20.

7. Gomes BPFA, Drucker DB, Lilly JD. Association of specific bacteria with some signs and symptoms. *Int. Endodont. J.* 1994; 27: 291–8.

8. Haapasalo M. *Bacteroides* spp in dental root canal infections. *Endodont. Dent. Traumatol.* 1989; 3: 83–5.

9. Happonen R-P. Immunocytochemical diagnosis of cervico-facial actinomycosis with special emphasis on periapical inflammatory lesions. *Thesis.* University of Turku, Finland, 1986.

10. Harris M, Jenkins MV, Bennett A, Wills MR. Prostaglandin production and bone resorption by dental cysts. *Nature* 1973; 245: 213–15.

11. Hedin M, Polhagen L. Follow-up study of periradicular bone condensation. *Scand. J. Dent. Res.* 1971; 79: 436–40.

12. Hill T. Experimental dental granulomas in dogs. *J. Am. Dent. Assoc.* 1934; 19: 1389–98.

13. Holland GR. A histological comparison of periapical inflammatory and neural responses to two endodontic sealers in the ferret. *Arch. Oral Biol.* 1994; 39: 539–44.

14. Hou L, Sasakj H, Stashenko P. B-cell deficiency predisposes mice to disseminating anaerobic infections: protection by passive antibody transfer. *Infect. Immun.* 2000; 68: 5645–51.

15. Hudson JW. Osteomyelitis of the jaws: a 50-year perspective. *J. Oral Maxillofac. Surg.* 1993; 51: 1294–301.

16. Kakehashi S, Stanley HR, Fitzgerald RJ. The effects of surgical exposures of dental pulps in germfree and conventional laboratory rats. *Oral Surg.* 1965; 20: 340–4.

17. Kirkevang LL, Ørstavik D, Hörsted-Bindslev P, Wenzel A. Periapical status and quality of root fillings and coronal restorations in a Danish population. *Int. Endodont. J.* 2001; 33: 509–15.

18. Koorbush GF, Fotos P, Goll KT. Retrospective assessment of osteomyelitis. Etiology, demographics, risk factors, and management in 35 cases. *Oral Surg.* 1992; 74: 149–54.

19. Larjava H, Sandberg M, Happonen R-P, Vourio E. Differential localization of type I and type III procollagen messenger ribonucleic acids in inflamed periodontal and periapical connective tissues by in situ hybridization. *Lab Invest.* 1990; 62: 96–103.

20. Laux M, Abbott PV, Pajarola G, Nair PN. Apical inflammatory root resorption: a correlative radiographic and histological assessment. *Int. Endodont. J.* 2000; 33: 483–93.

21. Lerner UH. Regulation of bone metabolism by the kallikrein–kinin system, the coagulation cascade, and the acute phase reactants. *Oral Surg.* 1994; 78: 481–93.

22. Li T, Browne RM, Matthews JB. Immunocytochemical expression of growth factors by odontogenetic jaw cysts. *Mol. Pathol.* 1997; 50: 21–7.

23. Lin LM, Wang S, Wu-Wang C, Chang K, Leung C. Detection of epidermal growth factor receptor in inflammatory periapical lesions. *Int. Endodont. J.* 1996; 29: 179–84.

24. Marton IJ, Kiss C. Protective and destructive immune reactions in apical periodontitis. *Oral Microbiol. Immunol.* 2000; 15: 139–50.

25. Meghji S, Harvey W, Harris M. Interleukin 1-like activity in cystic lesions of the jaw. *Br. J. Oral Maxillofac. Surg.* 1989; 27: 1–11.

26. Meghji S, Qureshi W, Henderson B, Harris M. The role of endotoxin and cytokines in the pathogenesis of odontogenic cysts. *Arch. Oral Biol.* 1996; 41: 523–31.

27. Morgan PR, Johnson NW. Histological, histochemical and ultrastructural studies on the nature of hyalin bodies in odontogenic cysts. *J. Oral Pathol.* 1974; 3: 127–47.

28. Möller ÅJ, Fabricius L, Dahlén G, Öhman AE, Heyden G. Influence on periapical tissue of indigenous oral bacteria and necrotic pulp tissue in monkeys. *Scand. J. Dent. Res.* 1981; 89: 475–84.

29. Nair PNR. Light and electron microscopic studies of root canal flora and periapical lesions. *J. Endodont.* 1987; 13: 29–39.

30. Nair PNR, Sjögren U, Sundqvist G. Cholesterol crystals as an etiologic factor in non-resolving chronic inflammation: an experimental study in guinea pigs. *Eur. J. Oral Sci.* 1998; 106: 644–50.

31. Nair PNR, Pajarola G, Schroeder HE. Types and incidence of human periapical lesions obtained with extracted teeth. *Oral Surg.* 1996; 81: 93–102.

32. Nair PNR. Apical periodontitis: a dynamic encounter between root canal infection and host response. *Periodontology 2000* 1997; 13: 121–48.

33. Nair PNR, Schroeder HE. Epithelial attachment at diseased human tooth-apex. *J. Periodontal Res.* 1985; 20: 293–300.

34. Pascon EA, Leonardo MR, Safavi K, Langeland K. Tissue reaction to endodontic materials: methods, criteria, assessment, and observations. *Oral Surg.* 1991; 72: 222–37.

35. Pulver WH, Taubman MA, Smith DJ. Immune components in human dental periapical lesions. *Arch. Oral Biol.* 1977; 23: 435–43.

36. Sjögren U, Sundqvist G, Nair PNR. Tissue reaction to gutta-percha particles of various sizes when implanted subcutaneously in guinea pigs. *Eur. J. Oral Sci.* 1995; 103: 313–21.

37. Skaug N. Lipoproteins in fluid from non-keratinizing jaw cysts. *Scand. J. Dent. Res.* 1976; 84: 98–105.

38. Skaug N. Soluble proteins in fluid from non-keratinizing jaw cysts in man. *Int. J. Oral Surg.* 1977; 6: 107–21.

39. Stashenko P. The role of immune cytokines in the pathogenesis of periapical lesions. *Endodont. Dent. Traumatol.* 1990; 6: 89–96.

40. Stashenko P, Wang CY, Riley E, Wu Y, Ostroff G, Niederman R. Reduction of infection-stimulated periapical bone resorption by the biological response modifier PGG glucan. *J. Dent. Res.* 1995; 74: 323–30.

41. Stashenko P, Teles R, D'Souza R. Periapical inflammatory responses and their modulation. *Crit. Rev. Oral Biol. Med.* 1998; 9: 498–521.

42. Sundqvist G. Bacteriological studies of necrotic dental pulps. *Thesis.* Umeå University, Umeå, Sweden, 1976.

43. Sundqvist G. Associations between microbial species in dental root canal infections. *Oral Microbiol. Immunol.* 1992; 7: 257–62.

44. Sundqvist G. Taxonomy, etiology, and pathogenicity of the root canal flora. *Oral Surg.* 1994; 78: 522–30.

45. Ten Cate AR. The epithelial cell rests of Malassez and the genesis of the dental cyst. *Oral Surg.* 1972; 34: 956–64.

46. Teronen O, Hietanen J, Lindqvist C, Salo T, Sorsa T, Eklund KK, Sommerhoff CP, Ylipaavalniemi P, Kontinen Y. Mast cell-derived tryptase in odontogenic cysts. *J. Oral Pathol. Med.* 1996; 25: 376–81.

47. Thesleff I. Epithelial cell rests of Malassez bind epidermal growth factor intensly. *J. Periodont. Res.* 1987; 22: 419–21.

48. Tronstad L, Barnett F, Riso K, Slots J. Extraradicular endodontic infections. *Endodont. Dent. Traumatol.* 1987; 3: 86–90.

49. Valderhaug J. Experimentally induced periapical inflammation in permanent and primary teeth of monkeys. *Thesis*, University of Oslo, Norway, 1974.

50. van Winkelhoff AJ, Carlee AW, deGraaf J. *Bacteroides endodontalis* and other black-pigmented *Bacteroides* species in odontogenic abscesses. *Infect. Immun.* 1985; 49: 494–7.

51. Ödesjö B, Helldén L, Salonen L, Langeland K. Prevalence of previous endodontic treatment, technical standard and occurrence of periapical lesions in a randomly selected adult, general population. *Endodont. Dent. Traumatol.* 1990; 6: 265–72.

Chapter 10
Systemic complications of endodontic infections

Nils Skaug

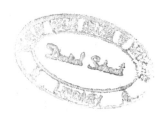

Introduction

Infectious processes associated with the root canal system of teeth may give rise to various complications that not only result in local manifestations but may also produce lesions in other body sites. As outlined in Fig. 10.1, there are three means by which a root canal infection may cause metastatic infections:

(1) Through an acute periapical abscess whereby pus, micro-organisms and their products are spread.
(2) By an endodontic treatment procedure where micro-organisms are disseminated to other body compartments along the circulatory system.
(3) By the release of bacterial products and pro-inflammatory mediators from a chronic periapical inflammatory lesion.

The clinical significance of these spreading mechanisms as well as the measures to be undertaken to prevent systemic complications in otherwise healthy patients or patients compromised by a systemic disease are discussed in this chapter.

Acute periapical infections as origin of metastatic infections

Acute manifestations of endodontic lesions involve the formation of abscesses in the periapical tissues. Although these lesions most often become confined to the oral region, they may extend to both nearby and distant body compartments along anatomical pathways (facial planes and spaces). Hence, a periapical abscess may spread and reach the maxillary sinuses, the brain, the cavernous sinus, the eye or the mediastinum. Needless to say, some of these conditions are truly life threatening. In addition to the direct spread of pus and bacterial elements, brain and lung abscesses also may be caused by septic emboli. Furthermore, oral bacteria involved in endodontic infections may be aspirated into the lung and cause serious infections. Acute osteomyelitis is yet another condition that can arise from an endodontic infection (see Chapter 9). Before the antibiotic era, all these non-oral infections caused by disseminating oral bacteria were often fatal. In contrast to the status in developing countries, complications of this nature are now rare in the industrialized world. Yet, when occurring, they still represent a threatening situation that demands proper dental and medical attention.

Spread of oral micro-organisms by the circulation

Invasion of the circulation by bacteria and their dissemination by the bloodstream throughout the body is called bacteremia. Bacteremias may occur as a result of surgical and other invasive procedures. They are generally asymptomatic and transient (duration <15–30 min) because the number of bacterial cells in the blood usually becomes low (<10 colony-forming units per ml). The host's reticuloendothelial system and the humoral immune response, furthermore, readily eliminate the organisms. Therefore, in healthy individuals transient bacteremias are usually of no clinical significance and asymptomatic. However, in individuals who lack normal protection against infections (compromised hosts) the bacteria may start to multiply in the blood resulting in sepsis, a serious infection, local or bacteremic, that is accompanied by systemic manifestations of inflammation. In compromised hosts (e.g. patients with cancer, unregulated diabetes or immunodeficiency), sepsis may proceed to a general fatal infection.

Oral micro-organisms may gain access to the blood after loss of oral mucosal integrity from trauma or manipulation. In connection with endodontic treatment procedures, for example, the placement of a rubber dam clamp often causes transient bacteremia. Bacteremias may also follow instrumentation of root canals (see below). Bacteremia can occur spontaneously as well as in conjunction with various types of professional dental treatments and other oral manipulations, including oral health procedures and mastication (Table 10.1).

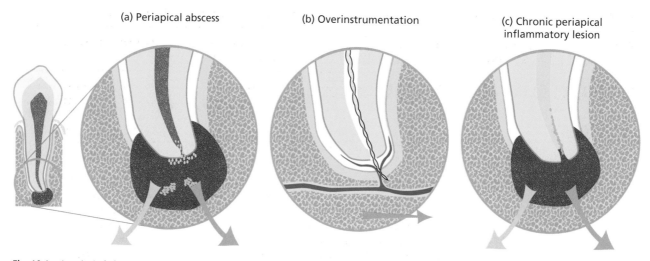

(a) Periapical abscess   (b) Overinstrumentation   (c) Chronic periapical inflammatory lesion

Fig. 10.1 A periapical abscess at a root tip (a), a root canal overinstrumentation (b) and an established periapical inflammatory lesion (c).

Table 10.1 Frequency of treatment-induced and self-induced transient bacteremias.

Dental procedure	Frequency of bacteremias	Reference
Intraligamental anesthetic injections in children	16–97	45
Tooth extractions	10–94	28
Periodontal surgery	36–88	18
Gingival scaling	8–80	18
	25–61	3
Endodontics	31–54	15
	0–5	5
Ultrasonic scaling	53	42
Periodontal probing	43	13
Prophylaxis	0–40	18
Matrix band with wedge placement	32	44
Subgingival irrigation	30	30
Rubber dam clamp placement	29	44
Polishing teeth	24	44
Suture removal	11–16	10
Routine daily oral activities		
Dental flossing	0–58	18
Chewing	17–51	18
Water irrigation device	7–50	18
Oral rinsing	50	19
Toothpicks	20–40	9
Tooth brushing	0–26	18

It is important to note that bacteremia occurs frequently from routine daily oral activities. In fact, bacteremias are 1000–8000 times more likely to be caused by daily oral manipulations than by dental treatment procedures (41). The incidence and magnitude of bacteremias of oral origin have been found to be directly proportional to the degree of oral inflammation and infection (40, 9) and occur more frequently in persons with high dental plaque scores and gingivitis than in individuals practising adequate oral hygiene (46).

Bacteremia and endodontic treatment

The actual number of micro-organisms induced in the bloodstream depends upon the size of the apical foramen, the degree of infection of the root canal and the method of root canal treatment (3). A variety of oral bacteria, and species that are found in infective endocarditis, have been isolated from infected root canals and periapical lesions (25), yet there are relatively few reports in the literature describing how often bacteremia occurs following endodontic therapy and few provide bacteriological findings (Table 10.2).

Studies performed during the 1960s were not able to demonstrate positive blood cultures even if the root canal system had been instrumented vigorously in the presence of saliva. However, when canals were instrumented beyond the root apex, there was a 25–30% incidence of bacteremia (8). Baumgartner *et al.* (5) used an aseptic technique to culture the blood of 20 patients and registered bacteremia in only one case when a root canal had been overinstrumented. Debelian *et al.* (14), on the other hand, found a comparatively high frequency of bacteremias subsequent to endodontic therapy (42%), particularly so in cases where the endodontic instrumentation had been deliberately carried out beyond the apical foramen (7/13 versus 4/13 for non-overinstrumented cases). In this latter study anaerobes were frequently isolated from the positive blood cultures, as opposed to previous studies where facultative

Table 10.2 Studies showing bacteria isolated from blood samples obtained in conjunction with non-surgical or surgical endodontic therapy.

Author (Ref.)	No. of teeth/ patients studied	Procedure	Frequency of positive blood samples	Number of isolates (n)
Rahn et al. (43)	56/56	Peripheral blood samples were obtained aseptically prior to apicoectomy and 3, 6 and 9 min postoperatively. Blood samples were cultivated aerobically and anaerobically	6/56 (10%)	*Streptococcus viridans* (n = 1) *Corynebacterium* sp. (n = 1) *Micrococcus* sp. (n = 1) *Staphylococcus* (n = 1) (coagulase-negative) *Lactobacillus fermentum* (n = 1) *Peptostreptococcus* sp. (n = 1)
Heimdahl et al. (24)	4/20	Blood samples were obtained aseptically in Vacutainer® tubes before, during and after intracanal endodontic instrumentation. After lysis-filtration, the blood samples were incubated anaerobically for 10 days	4/20 (20%)	*Micrococcus* spp. (n = 1) *Streptococcus* spp. (n = 1) *Corynebacterium hofmanii* (n = 1) *Neisseria* spp. (n = 1) Viridans group streptococci (n = 4) Anaerobic streptococci (n = 1)
Debelian et al. (14)	26/26	Blood samples were obtained aseptically during and after the endodontic procedure. See further Heimdahl et al. (24)	11/26 (42%)	*Prevotella intermedia* (n = 3) *Fusobacterium nucleatum* (n = 1) *Propionibacterium acnes* (n = 3) *Streptococcus intermedius* (n = 1) *Streptococcus sanguis* (n = 1) *Actinobacillus israelii* (n = 1) *Saccharomyces cerevisiae* (n = 1) (fungus)

organisms had predominated. These authors later verified that, for each patient in which a positive blood culture had been found, there was phenotypic and genotypic homology between the bacteria isolated from the root canal and the blood, suggesting that the blood bacteria originated from the treated root canals (15). Interestingly, in one patient the fungus *Saccharomyces cerevisiae* was recovered from both the root canal and the blood sample. (Advanced concept 10.1.)

Infective endocarditis

Bacteremia is considered a risk factor for the development of endocarditis. Bacterial endocarditis is a bacterial infection of the heart valves and the epithelial lining (endocardium) of the heart. The term infective endocarditis has recently been proposed to emphasize the fact that microbes other than bacteria also may cause endocarditis (23). According to new terminology, infective endocarditis is named after the infective microorganism, e.g. streptococcal endocarditis, staphylococcal endocarditis or fungal endocarditis (Table 10.3). Although currently termed infective endocarditis, bacterial endocarditis is still used by many authors in the dental and medical literature.

Infective endocarditis results from a complex interaction between the endocardium, local hydrodynamic

Table 10.3 Relative frequency of oral viridans streptococci associated with infective endocarditis at the New York Hospital from 1944 to 1983 (48).

Species	Frequency (%)
Streptococcus mitis	33–41
Streptococcus sanguis	31–47
Streptococcus anginosus	5–8
Streptococcus mutans	3–10
Streptococcus salivarius	1–2
Nutritionally variant	6–7
Unspeciated	1–3

effects, circulating micro-organisms and local and systemic host defense factors. In many countries it is a relatively uncommon life-threatening disease (approximately 50 cases are officially registered in Norway and 300 in Denmark per year). Infective endocarditis usually occurs in individuals with underlying congenital or acquired structural cardiac defects who develop bacteremia with bacteria prone to causing endocarditis. Symptoms of endocarditis generally start within 2 weeks of the incited bacteremia, although the time to diagnosis may be shorter or longer (48). A longer incubation period than 2 weeks between the invasive

Advanced concept 10.1 Accuracy of testing blood samples for bacterial presence

When drawing blood by venipuncture for culturing circulating oral bacteria, there is always a risk of contaminating the blood sample with skin commensals. The presence in blood cultures of typical skin bacteria, such as coagulase-negative staphylococci, corynebacteria or propionibacteria, indicates contamination from the skin. Recently it was shown that skin disinfection with alcoholic chlorhexidine is more efficacious than skin preparation with aqueous providone–iodine in reducing contamination of blood cultures (36). However, bacteria known as skin commensals also may be present in the oral microbiota, therefore it has been hard to tell whether such bacteria, when present in blood cultures, originate from the skin or the oral cavity. Recently developed molecular identification techniques may overcome this problem (15). A recent study (45) on bacteremias following local anesthetic injections in children showed blood culture with bacterial growth in 8% of the children prior to the injections. Both coagulase-negative staphylococci (a dominant member of the constant skin flora) and the oral bacterium *Streptococcus sanguis* were isolated from these preinjection blood cultures. Brown *et al.* (10) eliminated from their bacteremia study patients who demonstrated blood cultures positive for coagulase-negative staphylococci, corynebacteria and propionibacteria because they were thought to be indicative of skin contamination. In the study by Debelian *et al.* (15), homology was found between *Propionibacterium acnes* isolated in both the blood samples and the root canal samples, suggesting that in these cases the organism was not a skin contaminant.

The volume of blood used for culturing, the concentration of bacteria in the blood, the type of blood culturing system and the identification procedure employed determine the frequency of positive blood cultures with respect to type and number of species. With improved blood culture procedures and improvements in the isolation of anaerobic and fastidious microorganisms from blood, recovery of microorganisms from transient bacteremias has markedly increased during recent years. Therefore, not only higher frequencies of bacteremia but also more species and a higher number of microorganisms are expected when the results of more recent studies are compared with those of studies performed decades ago.

procedure and the onset of symptoms significantly lessens the likelihood of the procedure to be the proximate cause (29).

The symptoms are non-specific and include fever, malaise, anorexia, cardiac murmurs, splenomegaly, anemia and weight loss. Before the antibiotic era the mortality of bacterial endocarditis was 100%, and it still is if not treated adequately. Presently, the death rate is less than 10% for viridans (alfa-hemolytic) streptococcal endocarditis (51, 20) and 30% for staphylococcal endocarditis (20).

The organism(s) in the circulation causing the disease adheres to and forms vegetations in a focal area of the heart valves. A prerequisite is often a prior injury where fibrin and platelets have been released, which can capture circulating microbes. Multiplication within the vegetations leads to discharges of the infecting organism(s) back to the circulation, producing a constant bacteremia that gives multiple positive blood cultures. The clinical symptoms, including embolization to organs, are a direct result of this mechanism.

A wide variety of bacteria have been isolated from blood of patients with infective endocarditis. Viridans streptococci are the most common (50–63%) followed by staphylococci (25–26%) (20, 50). Various other microorganisms account for less than 10% (33). Among the oral viridans streptococci associated with infective endocarditis, *Streptococcus mitis* and *Streptococcus sanguis* dominate and account for more than two-thirds of the registered cases.

The reason why viridans streptococci are more likely than other types of streptococci to cause endocarditis relates to their release of extracellular polysaccharides, which provides them with an exceptional adhesion mechanism. Other adhesins like lipoteichoic acid, fibrinogen-binding protein, fibronectin-binding protein and platelet-interactive molecules are putative virulence factors of bacteria associated with endocarditis (20). It was suggested recently that the majority of infected root canals contain bacteria that may have the potential to cause bacterial infective endocarditis (4).

Staphylococcus aureus is another important pathogen that may originate from the oral cavity, although there is no convincing evidence that oral staphylococci can cause infective endocarditis (54). This organism is capable of infecting even structurally normal heart valves and is the most commonly isolated organism in infective endocarditis of intravenous drug abusers (50).

It needs to be recognized that oral micro-organisms presumed to cause infective endocarditis in a given case are not normally specific to the oral cavity only. Furthermore, the incubation period (the time between a procedure resulting in bacteremia and the onset of symptoms) is often well outside the accepted time frame, which should be within 10–14 days, depending on the causative organism (29). This means that it is often hard to establish the origin of a given heart infection.

Cardiac conditions and dental treatment procedures as risk factors for infective endocarditis

Certain cardiac conditions are thought to predispose individuals for infective endocarditis more often than others. Most at risk are those patients with a prior history of infective endocarditis and those with a prosthetic heart valve. In line with this knowledge, the American Heart Association (AHA) (12) has defined high risk and moderate risk categories for infective endocarditis (Core concept 10.1). This body has also defined dental and oral treatment procedures that are likely to cause hazardous bacteremia in these two infective endocarditis categories (Core concept 10.2). Hence, a variety of invasive dental procedures are felt to pose a risk for infective endocarditis, although the associations have never been firmly documented. Yet, endodontic surgery, including incision and drainage of abscesses and instrumentation beyond the tooth apex, belong to the dental procedures that, according to the AHA,

should be regarded as dangerous to individuals with cardiac conditions.

About 40% of all infective endocarditis cases occur in patients without previously identified risk factors. It has been estimated that 20% of cases can be related to dental treatment procedures or infections (20) but the vast majority are due to oral organisms and are not related to dental procedures (40).

Even if the oral focal infection theory (see below) no longer enjoys widespread acceptance, it has retained its position when it comes to the etiology of infective endocarditis. This is in spite of the lack of firm evidence for a cause–effect relationship. Therefore, to determine the cause of a given case of endocarditis, physicians often ask patients if they have received dental treatment in recent months. If the answer is yes, the dental treatment is usually blamed for the condition (51). Yet, there are only two well-controlled studies of dental risk factors for infective endocarditis (26, 49). One study found no increased risk associated with dental procedures in the preceding 90 days (26), although borderline increased risks were noted for endodontic treatment and dental scaling. In another large, population-based, case–control study (49) none of the dental procedures that were observed, except possibly for tooth extraction, was found to be a risk factor. This was true even in cases where there were underlying cardiac valvular abnormalities (prosthetic valves, previous history of endocarditis). The study did confirm, however, the importance of these heart abnormalities as risk factors for infective endocarditis.

Very recently the AHA issued the following statement

'Good oral health is important in reducing the risk for acute cardiovascular disease such as bacterial endocarditis. There is limited and inconclusive evidence that oral bacteria may play a role in chronic cardiovascular disorders such as coronary artery disease. Whether this relationship will eventually prove to be significant, as one of the many factors in the development of cardiovascular disease, or of no significance is presently unknown. Regular professional and home dental care can reduce acute cardiovascular risk from oral micro-organisms; neither routine nor extraordinary dental treatment procedures have been documented to prevent chronic coronary heart disease. The 1997 American Heart Association guidelines for the prevention of bacterial endocarditis in at-risk dental patients remain in effect as recommended.'

Therefore, even if dental procedures have not been confirmed as risk factors for infective endocarditis, cases are often infected with micro-organisms common to the oral microbiota (49) and transient bacteremias due to dental treatment procedures cannot be excluded as causative factors. Consequently, dentists must always be obser-

---

Core concept 10.1   Current definitions of the American Heart Association as to conditions representing high or moderate risk of infective endocarditis in combination with dental risk treatment involving bacteremia

High-risk category

- Prosthetic cardiac valves, including biprosthetic and homograft valves.
- Previous bacterial endocarditis.
- Complex cyanotic congenital heart disease (e.g. single ventricle states, transposition of the great arteries, tetralogy of Fallot).
- Surgically constructed systemic pulmonary shunts or conducts.

Moderate-risk category

- Congenital cardiac malformations other than those mentioned above.
- Acquired valvar dysfunction (e.g. rheumatic heart disease).
- Hypertrophic cardiomyopathy.
- Mitral valve prolapse with valvular regurgitation and/or thickened leaflets.

Core concept 10.2

The American Heart Association recommends antibiotic prophylaxis in cardiac patients at high and moderate risk for infective endocarditis when undergoing the following dental risk treatments:

- Dental extractions.
- Periodontal procedures, including surgery, scaling and root planing, probing and recall maintenance.
- Dental implant placement and reimplantation of avulsed teeth.
- Endodontic (root canal) instrumentation (only when beyond the apex) and surgery.
- Subgingival placement of antibiotic fibers and strips.
- Initial placement of orthodontic bands but not brackets.
- Intraligamentary local anesthetic injections.
- Prophylactic cleaning of teeth or implants where bleeding is anticipated.

vant of the potential risk of dental infections and dental procedures, and follow established guidelines for prevention.

Preventive measures

Current recommendations on antibiotic prevention of bacteremia sequelae

The AHA has issued widely accepted recommendations stating that antibiotics should be given to prevent endocarditis when a patient is undergoing dental risk treatment and when qualifying for the moderate or high risk category (Core concept 10.1). Dental risk treatment is defined as a treatment procedure that is known to produce bacteremia, which includes endodontic surgery and root canal instrumentation (Core concept 10.2). Certain procedures that are not recommended for antibiotic prophylaxis may nevertheless cause significant bleeding in patients with poor oral hygiene. In such cases prophylaxis is also appropriate. Consequently, the dentist is always responsible for the final decision as to whether antibiotic prophylaxis should be instituted. See Core concept 10.3 for guidelines on antibiotic prophylaxis and risk assessment of patients.

Prophylaxis is most effective when given preoperatively in doses that are sufficient to ensure adequate antibiotic concentrations in the blood during and 10 h after the procedure. To minimize the risk of anaphylactic reactions and antibiotic resistance, the AHA recommends oral regimens as the standard route. A single dose of 2 g (AHA) or 3 g (British Society of Antimicrobial Therapy, BSAC) (2, 27) amoxicillin in adults should then be given orally 1 h before the dental treatment. In the case of penicillin allergy, preferentially 600 mg of clindamycin is recommended as an alternative. Amoxicillin when given in the recommended doses is preferred to other penicillins because it ensures adequate antibiotic concentrations in the serum for 10 h postoperatively. For patients who are unable to take or absorb oral medication, 2 g of ampicillin sodium administered intramuscularly or intravenously within 30 min of the procedure is preferred.

If the patient has forgotten to take the prescribed antibiotic prior to the treatment, the medication can still be effective if given in conjunction with the procedure, but not later than 2 h after it was started. The rationale is that the antimicrobial effect primarily is due to inhibition of bacterial growth on the damaged heart valves and not, as thought before, to the colonization *per se* or to the killing of micro-organisms in the bloodstream (22).

It is well documented that antibiotic prophylaxis, according to the recommended regimens, may select for micro-organisms that are resistant to the drug. Resis-

tance is likely not to persist for more than 9–14 days after termination of prophylactic treatment, therefore dental treatments requiring an antibiotic umbrella should be scheduled with at least 14-day intervals. If a shorter interval is needed, an alternative antibiotic should be selected (Table 10.4). If a situation were to emerge where antibiotic prophylaxis is required twice within a short time interval (12–24 h), it is unlikely that a significant selection of resistant micro-organisms has occurred. In such instances the use of the same prophylactic regimen is acceptable.

Core concept 10.3   Risk assessments and antibiotic prophylaxis

Patients

- Oral bacteremias are transient, occur frequently and represent a negligible risk for infective endocarditis or metastatic infections in healthy individuals.
- Bacteremias following certain dental treatment procedures can provoke infective endocarditis in moderate- and high-risk individuals. Antibiotic prophylaxis therefore should be instituted.
- Immunocompromised patients (individuals with granulocyte count <3500, leukemic patients, bone marrow transplant patients with leukemia) are at high risk of bacteremia-induced infections. Antibiotic prophylaxis is needed and should be determined in consultation with the patient's physician because universal guidelines are not available.
- Recipients of organ transplants and cancer patients, although at increased susceptibility to infections, do not normally require routine antibiotic prophylaxis in conjunction with dental treatment.

Dental procedures

- The vast majority of infective endocarditis cases are not associated with dental treatment procedures.
- Placement of rubber dam clamps, root canal instrumentation beyond the apical foramen and endodontic surgery are associated with transient bacteremias and require antibiotic prophylaxis in patients at risk of infective endocarditis.

Preventive measures

- Any use of antibiotic prophylaxis must take into consideration the adverse effects of antibiotic toxicity and allergy, selection of resistant microorganisms, superinfections and effects on the microbial ecology.
- Under any circumstance, the dentist is ultimately responsible for the final decision as to whether antibiotic prophylaxis should be instituted and the selection of drug.

Failure to give proper antibiotic prophylaxis may generate malpractice claims.

Table 10.4 The American Heart Association's recommendations of 1997 on antimicrobial prophylaxis in patients at moderate and high risk of infective endocarditis undergoing dental treatment known to give high-level bacteremia.

Clinical situation	Agent	Regimen
Standard general prophylaxis	Amoxicillin	Adults: 2.0 g; children: 50 mg/kg orally 1 h before procedure
Unable to take oral medications	Ampicillin	Adults: 2.0 g intramuscularly (IM) or intravenously (IV); children: 50 mg/kg IM or IV within 30 min before procedure
Allergic to penicillin	Clindamycin	Adults: 600 mg; children: 20 mg/kg orally 1 h before procedure
	or	
	Cephalexin[a] or Cefadroxil[a]	Adults: 2.0 g; children: 50 mg/kg orally 1 h before procedure
	or	
	Azithromycin or Clarithromycin	Adults: 500 mg; children: 15 mg/kg orally 1 h before procedure
Allergic to penicillin and unable to take oral medications	Clindamycin	Adults: 600 mg; children: 20 mg/kg IV within 30 min before procedure
	or	
	Cephazolin[a]	Adults: 1.0 g; children: 25 mg/kg IM or IV within 30 min before procedure

[a] Cephalosporins should not be used in individuals with immediate-type hypersensitivity reactions to penicillins (e.g. urticaria, angioedema or anaphylaxis).

Antibiotic prophylaxis in compromised hosts

The antibiotic prophylaxis regimens of the AHA and BSAC seem to be appropriate for the prevention of bacteremia in cancer chemotherapy patients but might be inappropriate in patients with suppressed granulocyte count (<3500 per mm[3] blood), leukemic patients or bone marrow transplant patients. In the latter category of patients more effective agents against Gram-negative organisms are required (40). This is because the oral flora of such immunocompromised patients can be different from that of normal individuals and includes Gram-negative bacteria (e.g. *Klebsiella pneumoniae, Enterobacter cloacae, Escherichia coli*) that are highly resistant to the beta-lactam antibiotics, aminoglycosides, vancomycin and fluoroquinolenes. The most obvious risk for bone marrow transplant patients with leukemia is, however, septic shock caused by viridans streptococci (40). Hence, the latter authors recommend that dental patients with low granulocyte counts should be treated only on an emergency (non-elective) basis. Because of significant interindividual differences in the oral microflora of immunocompromised patients and the lack of controlled clinical studies, antibiotic prophylaxis in these patients should be based on microbiological evaluation and in collaboration with the patient's physician.

Patients in need of organ (e.g. heart, kidney, liver) transplantation should have a pretransplant dental evaluation. All required endodontic treatment should be completed in due time prior to the transplantation because of the increased risk of infection that these patients will be exposed to due to the immunosuppression. Antibiotic prophylaxis in such patients still has an empirical base and no guidelines have been issued so far. Root canal instrumentation beyond the tooth apex should always be avoided and any antibiotic prophylaxis prior to periapical surgery should be determined in consultation with the patient's physician.

An expert panel of dentists, orthopedic surgeons and infectious disease specialists recently concluded that antibiotic prophylaxis is not routinely indicated for most dental patients with total joint replacements, nor is it recommended for dental patients with pins, plates and screws (1). Antibiotic prophylaxis for the prevention of systemic infections is not recommended in hemodialysis patients, heart transplant patients or splenectomized patients, nor to prevent brain abscess (40).

Surgical intervention in an infected area is sometimes necessary. In addition to the risk for bacteremia, local spread of micro-organisms will always occur and may present a risk for metastatic infection. Yet, surgical antibiotic prophylaxis is only justified in immunocompromised patients and should begin 2 h before and be terminated when the surgery is finished and no later than 24–48 h after the surgery (for references, see Ref. 40).

It needs to be recognized that in order to achieve a satisfactory risk–benefit ratio any use of antibiotic prophylaxis must take into consideration the adverse effects of antibiotic toxicity and allergy, the selection of resistant micro-organisms, superinfections and effects on the microbial ecology (40).

Are the current antibiotic prophylaxis recommendations appropriate?

The most important rationale for antibiotic prophylaxis has been to prevent infective endocarditis because this disease carries high morbidity and mortality. Studies in experimental animals have indeed demonstrated that antibiotics can prevent infective endocarditis (16) and that penicillin is the drug of choice in the case of viridans streptococcal bacteremia. Yet, the effectiveness of antibiotics to prevent infective endocarditis in humans has not been proven and probably never will be because it is a rare disease and controlled studies cannot be conducted for ethical reasons (16). In the Strom *et al.* (49) study, a minority (<10%) of the cases had received antibiotic prophylaxis but the risk for infective endocarditis remained the same regardless of whether prophylactic antibiotics had been taken or not.

The lack of firm evidence that dental treatment is a frequent cause of infective endocarditis, the report of well-documented cases where antibiotic prophylaxis has failed to prevent infective endocarditis (29), the low compliance with the current guidelines for antibiotic prophylaxis, the unfavorable cost–benefit and risk–benefit relationships and the risk for selection of antibiotic resistance have initiated qualified questions as to the appropriateness of the current guidelines for prophylaxis against infective endocarditis before dental treatment. It has been proposed that antibiotic prophylaxis should be given only to patients with prosthethic heart valves or previous history of endocarditis and only in conjunction with procedures giving high-level bacteremias (extractions and gingival surgery, including implant surgery) (17). However, dentists should continue to follow the 1997 AHA guidelines until a revised document has been issued. Because infective endocarditis of oral origin is more likely to be due to poor oral health and hygiene than dental treatment *per se*, patients with cardiac abnormalities should be encouraged to maintain a high level of oral health (29).

The significance of the contribution of acute oral infections to prosthetic joint infections has been discussed for years. The current view is that it is likely that bacteremias associated with such infections can, and do, cause implant infection. Therefore, elimination of the source of infection (e.g. endodontic therapy or tooth extraction) is required in these patients (1).

Chronic periapical infections as origin of metastatic infections

Systemic effects of chronic dental infections

From 'oral sepsis' to 'focal infection'

'Gold fillings, gold caps, gold bridges, gold crowns, fixed dentures, built in, on, and around diseased teeth, form a veritable mausoleum of gold over a mass of sepsis to which there is no parallel in the whole realm of medicine or surgery.'

It is therefore not a matter of teeth and dentistry, it is an all important matter of sepsis and antisepsis.'

Sir William Hunter, 1861–1937

The belief that infected teeth are the cause of certain systemic diseases (e.g. arthritis) emerged at the beginning of the 19th century, but the notion may be tracked back to ancient times and Hippocrates (39). On the basis of his studies of the oral microbiota, the American dentist W. D. Miller drew attention to the possible interrelationship between oral infections and systemic diseases (34, 35). At the turn of the century the English physician W. Hunter introduced the term oral sepsis. It implied that in addition to dissemination of bacteria from the oral cavity, particularly from long-term oral infections of low grade, oral bacteria act specifically and selectively on different target organs by liberating toxins, thereby producing adverse systemic effects (41). According to Hunter's theory, the mouth was the most important septic focus and oral sepsis the most common source of sepsis. He alleged that conservative dentistry was synonymous with septic dentistry.

In 1912 the American physician F. Billings replaced the term oral sepsis with focal infection (39, 41). Focal infection occurs when micro-organisms disseminate from a localized area of infection (focus of infection) and establish themselves elsewhere in the body as a secondary infection. When an oral infection is the source of focal infection, the term oral focal infection is used. Dental focal infection implies that an infected tooth is the focus.

Figure 10.2 shows how dental infection was once thought to be responsible for dental sepsis and various connected systemic conditions. Common to these conditions, at that time, was that no cause other than oral

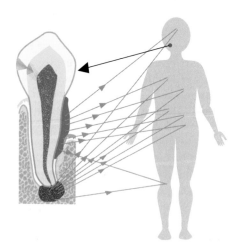

Fig. 10.2 According to the dental focal infection theory, a variety of systemic diseases affecting the brain, eyes, lung, heart, liver, joints and the skin are caused by dental sepsis, involving dissemination of bacteria and bacterial products from chronic periapical and marginal periodontitis.

focal infection could be found. Therefore, even the extraction of healthy teeth became justified to prevent systemic infections and diseases. As a consequence, endodontic therapy nearly disappeared in the USA for many years (11). Fellow colleagues even maintained that dentists who performed root canal therapy should be considered criminals and be sentenced to 6 months of hard labour (41). Later, the true etiology of many of the infectious conditions that were associated with oral foci was disclosed. It became obvious that over the years many healthy teeth had been removed for no good reason. The dental focal infection theory therefore gradually lost its influence. However, owing to the continued release of new case reports with claims that patients had been cured for arthritis or other chronic diseases after extraction of their infected or root filled teeth, and in spite of lack of scientific evidence, the dental focal infection theory never died (39, 41).

Potential mechanisms by which a chronic inflammatory periapical lesion may cause adverse systemic effects

The dental focal infection theory acquired a new dimension when immunopathological mechanisms were added to disseminated bacteria and microbial toxins as causative factors of systemic diseases (Fig. 10.3). Recent data suggest that chronic subclinical infections (e.g. chronic periodontal infections), as indicated by raised values within the normal range of C-reactive protein (33) and other acute-phase proteins (53), may induce systemic inflammation leading to such conditions as atherosclerosis, cardiovascular disease, cerebrovascular disease or preterm low-birthweight delivery. These observations have led to a paradigm shift in our understanding of the pathobiology of these complex associations. It is now realized that oral bacteria and their

products, particularly lipopolysaccharides and pro-inflammatory cytokines, induced locally in response to oral infections, enter the bloodstream and may subsequently activate systemic responses in certain susceptible individuals. It is not yet known whether these relationships are causal or consequential.

Deliberations in recent years

Spurred by epidemiological findings in large patient populations, a renewed interest has emerged in recent years on the role of chronic oral infections in certain systemic diseases such as coronary heart disease. Data from Finland, for example, have demonstrated a significant association in male patients to dental infections (31, 32, 47) and primarily to periodontal disease (21). Evidence from the literature also suggests that there is an association between severe periodontal infections and spontaneous preterm birth (52). It is now believed that systemic inflammations have common biological triggering mechanisms (IL-1β, IL-6, TNF-α, PGE2) and that they occur more frequently in individuals with hyperinflammatory monocyte phenotype (MØ+) than in individuals with normal monocyte phenotype. The monocytes of the former phenotype secrete three to tenfold greater amounts of these mediators in response to lipopolysaccharides than those of the normal monocyte phenotype (6, 7). Demonstration of DNA from *Actinobacillus actinomycetemcomitans*, *Porphyromonas gingivalis* and *Prevotella intermedia* in atheromas strongly indicates a role for these oral bacteria in atherosclerosis (6). Although they are known as periodontal pathogens, they are also involved in endodontic infections. Activated macrophages in periapical infections produce the pro-inflammatory cytokines (IL-1β and TNF-α) (38). Whether there is a relationship between the MØ+ monocyte phenotype, chronic periapical infection and systemic inflammation is currently not known (37). The latest review papers concerning possible relationships between periodontal disease, tooth loss and cardiovascular disease conclude that there is no such scientific evidence today, and that the previously demonstrated periodontitis-systemic disease associations are, in part, confounded by smoking.

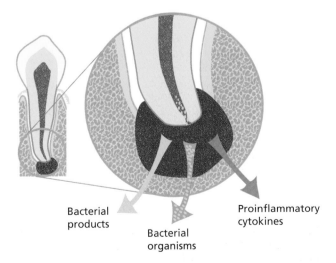

Bacterial products

Bacterial organisms

Proinflammatory cytokines

Fig. 10.3 Potential mechanisms of focal infection.

References

1. Advisory Statement. Antibiotic prophylaxis for dental patients with total joint replacements. *J. Am. Dent. Assoc.* 1997; 128: 1004–8.
2. Antibiotic prophylaxis of infective endocarditis. Recommendations from the Endocarditis Working Party of the British Society for Antimicrobial Chemotherapy. *Lancet* 1990; 335: 88–9.

3. Baltch AL, Schaffer C, Mark RDH, Hammer MS, Suthpen NT, Smith RP, *et al.* Bacteremia following dental cleaning in patients with and without penicillin prophylaxis. *Am. Heart J.* 1982; 104: 1335–9.

4. Bate AL, Ma JK-C, Pitt Ford TR. Detection of bacterial virulence genes associated with infective endocarditis in infected root canals. *Int. Endodont. J.* 2000; 33: 194–203.

5. Baumgartner CJ, Heggers P, Harrison JW. The incidence of bacteremias related to endodontic procedures. I. Non-surgical endodontics. *J. Endodont.* 1976; 2: 135–40.

6. Beck JD, Offenbacher S. Oral health and systemic disease: periodontitis and cardiovascular disease. *J. Dent. Educ.* 1998; 62: 859–70.

7. Beck JD, Slade G, Offenbacher S. Oral disease, cardiovascular disease and systemic inflammation. *Periodontology 2000* 2000; 23: 110–20.

8. Bender IB, Seltzer S, Tashman S, Meloff G. Dental procedures in patients with rheumatic heart disease. *Oral Surg.* 1963; 16: 466.

9. Bender IB, Naidorf IJ, Garvey GJ. Bacterial endocarditis: a consideration for physicians and dentists. *J. Am. Dent. Assoc.* 1984; 109: 415–20.

10. Brown AR, Christopher J, Schultz P, Theisen FC, Schultz RE. Bacteremia and intraoral suture removal: can an antimicrobial rinse help? *J. Am. Dent. Assoc.* 1998; 129: 1455–61.

11. Bellizzi R, Cruse WP. A historic review of endodontics, 1689–1963. Part 3. *J. Endodont.* 1980; 6: 576–80.

12. Dajani AS, Taubert KA, Wilson W, Bolger AS, Bayer A, Ferrieri P, *et al.* Prevention of bacterial endocarditis: recommendations by the American Heart Association. *J. Am. Dent. Assoc.* 1998; 128: 1142–51.

13. Daly C, Mitchell D, Grossberg D, Highfield J, Stewart D. Bacteremia caused by periodontal probing. *Aust. Dent. J.* 1997; 42: 77–80.

14. Debelian GJ, Olsen I, Tronstad L. Bacteremia in conjunction with endodontic therapy. *Endodont. Dent. Traumatol.* 1995; 11: 142–9.

15. Debelian GJ, Olsen I, Tronstad L. Anaerobic bacteremia and fungemia in patients undergoing endodontic therapy: an overview. *Ann. Periodontol.* 1998; 3: 281–7.

16. Durack DT. Prevention of infective endocarditis. *N. Engl. J. Med.* 1995; 332: 38–44.

17. Durack DT. Antibiotics for prevention of endocarditis during dentistry: time to scale back? *Ann. Int. Med.* 1998; 129: 829–31.

18. Epstein JP. Infective endocarditis: dental implications and new guidelines for antibiotic prophylaxis. *J. Can. Dent. Assoc.* 1998; 64: 281–92.

19. Felix C, Rosen S, App G. Detection of bacteremia after use of oral irrigation device in subjects with periodontitis. *J. Periodontol.* 1971; 42: 785–7.

20. Franklin C. Infective endocarditis: a review of the etiology, epidemiology and pathogenesis. In *Clinical Oral Science* (1st edn) (Harris M, Edgar M, Meghji S, eds). Bristol: Wright, 1998; 213–21.

21. Grau AJ, Buggle F, Ziegler C, Schwarz W, Meuser J, Tasman A-J, *et al.* Association between acute cerebrovascular ischemia and chronic and recurrent infection. *Stroke* 1997; 28: 1724–9.

22. Hall G, Heimdahl A, Nord CE. Bacteremia after oral surgery and antibiotic prophylaxis for endocarditis. *Clin. Infect. Dis.* 1999; 29: 1–8.

23. Harris SA. Definitions and demographic characteristics. In *Infective Endocarditis* (1st edn) (Kaye D, ed.). New York: Raven Press, 1992; 1–18.

24. Heimdahl A, Hall G, Hedberg M, Sandberg H, Söder P-Ö, Tunér K, Nord CE *et al.* Detection and quantitation by lysis-filtration of bacteremia after different oral surgical procedures. *J. Clin. Microbiol.* 1990; 28: 2205–9.

25. Kettering JD, Torabinejad M. Microbiology and immunology. In *Pathways of the Pulp* (7th edn) (Cohen S, Burns RC, eds). St. Louis, MO: Mosby, 1998; 463–75.

26. Lacassin F, Hoen B, Leport C, Selton-Suty C, Delahaye F, Goulet V, *et al.* Procedures accociated with infective endocarditis in adults. A case control study. *Eur. Heart J.* 1995; 16: 1869–974.

27. Littler WA, McGovan DA, Shanson DC. Changes in recommendations about amoxycillin prophylaxis for prevention of endocarditis. British Society for Antimicrobial Chemotherapy Endocarditis Working Party. *Lancet* 1997; 350: 1100.

28. Lockhart PB. An analysis of bacteremias during dental extractions. *Arch. Int. Med.* 1996; 156: 513–20.

29. Lockhart PB. The risk for endocarditis in dental practice. *Periodontology 2000* 2000; 23: 127–35.

30. Lofthus JE, Waki MY, Jolkovsky DL, Otomo-Corgel J, Newman N, Flemming T. Bacteremia following subgingival irrigation and scaling and root planing. *J. Periodontol.* 1991; 62: 602–7.

31. Mattila K, Nieminen MS, Voltonen VV, Rasi VP, Käsaniemi YA, Syrjälä SL, *et al.* Association between dental health and acute myocardial infection. *Br. Med. J.* 1989; 298: 779–81. *Designed a cumulative score system based upon the number of carious lesions, the extent of periodontal pocketing, the presence and magnitude of periapical lesions and the presence or absence of pericoronitis for correlation to coronary heart disease.*

32. Mattila KJ, Vantonen VV, Nieminen M, Huttunen JK. Dental infection and the risk of new coronary events: prospective study of patients with documented coronary artery disease. *Clin. Infect. Dis.* 1995; 20: 588–92.

33. Mendall M, Patel P, Ballam L, Strachan D, Northfield T. C reactive protein and its relation to cardiovascular risk factors: a population based cross sectional study. *Br. Med. J.* 1996; 312: 1061–5.

34. Miller WD. The human mouth as a focus of infection. *Dent. Cosmos* 1891; 33: 689–95.

35. Miller WD. *The Micro-organisms in the Human Mouth. The Local and General Diseases Which are Caused by Them.* Philadelphia, PA: S. S. White, 1890; 274–341.

36. Mimoz O, Karim A, Mercat A, Cosseron M, Falissard B, Parker F, *et al.* Chlorhexidine compared with providone-iodine as skin preparation before blood culture. A randomized, controlled trial. *Ann. Intern. Med.* 1999; 131: 834–7.

37. Murray CA, Saunders WP. Root canal treatment and general health: a review of the literature. *Int. Endodont. J.* 2000; 33: 1–18.

38. Nair PNR. Apical periodontitis: a dynamic encounter between root canal infection and host response. *Periodontology 2000* 1997; 13: 121–48.

39. O'Reilly PG, Claffey NM. A history of oral sepsis as a cause of disease. *Periodontology 2000* 2000; 23: 13–18.

40. Pallasch TJ, Slots J. Antibiotic prophylaxis and the medically compromised patient. *Periodontology 2000* 1996; 10: 107–38.
    Describing the principles of antibiotic prophylaxis, reviewing bacteremia, discussing various aspects of infective endocarditis, including dentist and physician compliance, and indicating proper use of antibiotic prophylaxis in patients with severely impaired resistance to infections.

41. Pallasch TJ. The focal infection theory: appraisal and reappraisal. *Calif. Dent. Assoc. J.* 2000; 28: 194–200.

42. Reinhardt R, Bolton R, Hlava G. Effect of non sterile versus sterile water irrigation with ultrasonic scaling and postoperative bacteremias. *J. Periodontol.* 1982; 53: 96–9.

43. Rahn R, Shah PM, Scäfer V, Frenkel G, Seibold K. Bakteriämie nach chirurgish endodontischen Eingriffen. *ZWR* 1987; 96: 903–7.

44. Roberts GJ, Holzel HS, Sury MR, Simmons NA, Gardner P, Longhurst P. Dental bacteremia in children. *Pediatr. Cardiol.* 1997; 18: 24–7.

45. Roberts, GJ, Simmons NB, Longhurst P, Hewitt PB. Bacteremia following local anesthetic injections in children. *Br. Dent. J.* 1998; 185: 295–8.

46. Sconyers JR, Crawford JJ, Moriarty JD. Relationship of bacteremia to toothbrushing in patients with periodontitis. *J. Am. Dent. Assoc.* 1973; 87: 616–22.

47. Seymour RA, Steele JG. Is there a link between periodontal disease and coronary heart disease? *Br. Dent. J.* 1998; 184: 33–8.

48. Starkebaum M, Durack D, Beeson P. The 'incubation period' of bacterial endocarditis. *Yale J. Biol. Med.* 1977; 50: 49–58.

49. Strom BL, Abrutyn E, Berlin JA, Kinman JL, Seldman RS, Stolley PD, *et al*. Dental and cardiac risk factors for infective endocarditis. A population-based, case–control study. *Ann. Intern. Med.* 1998; 129: 761–9.
    This population-based, case–control study concludes that dental treatment seems not to be a risk factor for infective endocarditis, even in patients with valvular abnormalities. Consequently, the policies for antibiotic prophylaxis in such patients should be reconsidered.

50. Tunkel AR, Mandell GL. Infecting micro-organisms. In: *Infective Endocarditis.* (Kaye D, ed.). New York: Raven Press, 1992; 85–97.

51. Wahl MJ. Myths of dental-induced endocarditis. *Comp. Cont. Educ. Dent.* 1994; 15: 1100–119.

52. Williams CECS, Davenport ES, Sterne JAC, Sivapathasundaram V, Fearne JM, Curtis MA. Mechanisms of risk in preterm low-birthweight infants. *Periodontology 2000* 2000; 23: 142–50.

53. Williams RC, Offenbacher S. Periodontal medicine: the emergence of a new branch of periodontology. *Periodontology 2000* 2000; 23: 9–12.

54. Younessi OJ, Walker DM, Ellis P, Dwyer DE. Fatal *Staphylococcus aureus* infective endocarditis. The dental implications. *Oral Surg. Endodont.* 1998; 85: 168–72.

Chapter 11
Treatment of the necrotic pulp

Paul Wesselink and Gunnar Bergenholtz

Introduction

This chapter details the procedures employed to carry out conservative root canal therapy (RCT) of teeth with necrotic pulps. The treatment may be performed regardless of whether the root canal system is infected or not. If not infected, the rationale for the treatment is to prevent microbial colonization and multiplication in the pulpal space and subsequent symptomatic or non-symptomatic presentations of apical periodontitis (4, 46) (Chapter 9). In most instances, however, RCT is curative and initiated to eliminate a root canal infection, thereby remedying periapical inflammatory tissue lesions (Fig. 11.1a, b). Treatment is also essential to impede the spread of root canal bacteria to distant organs (Chapter 10). Although extraction of the tooth in question solves the infection problem, it is a radical procedure not usually acceptable to patients. Thus RCT offers a realistic alternative, provided that the tooth is restorable. Hence, if properly conducted, RCT of teeth with infected pulp necrosis enjoys a high rate of success and can be expected to result in complete resolution of apical periodontitis in four out of five cases (22, 43).

Objectives and general treatment strategies

The overall objective of RCT is to exclude the root canal system as a source of bacterial exposure of the organism. Therefore a primary task includes efforts to rid bacteria resident in the root canal system (Fig. 11.2a–d). A second charge is to provide measures to ensure that root canal infection will not recur. The procedure includes several phases, of which cleaning with root canal instruments (Chapter 13) and disinfection are critical. To prevent reinfection, a filling is subsequently placed in the instrumented root canal(s) (Fig. 11.1b).

If successfully conducted, teeth with clinical symptoms of apical periodontitis (tenderness, pain, swelling, fistulae) become non-symptomatic. Successful treatment also demands that any radiographic evidence of apical periodontitis that existed prior to treatment should resolve and result in complete reorganization of the periapical tissue (Fig. 11.3).

Historical perspective

Over the years, different approaches to combat endodontic infections have been in vogue. In the beginning of the last century, following the discovery of the role that bacteria play in disease processes in general and apical periodontitis in particular, emphasis was placed on the use of strong antiseptics. Such agents were phenol derivatives and their mixtures, e.g. methylacresylacetate and camphorated monochlorophenol, and formaldehyde and its derivatives, e.g. formocresol and paraformaldehyde (10). Antiseptic agents were to be administered either to the orifice or to the interior of root canals in paste or liquid form. By evaporation, bacterial organisms would be killed without a cleaning procedure or filling of the root canal system (53). In yet other modes of treatment strong antiseptics were combined with mechanical instrumentation, followed by filling the instrumented canal(s) with a paste containing a strong antiseptic agent. By incorporating antiseptics in the root filling material, it was felt that where bacteria were not killed by the intracanal procedure a continuous release of antiseptic would prevent survival and regrowth of the remaining organisms. Indeed, such treatment approaches gained great popularity and are practised even today in many countries. However, the use of strong antiseptics in endodontics entails several serious concerns:

(1) Although they are effective against microbes, strong antiseptics cause substantial cell and tissue damage, particularly if being extruded to the periapical tissue environment (45) (see also Chapter 17).
(2) These disinfectants, also in diluted form, have the disadvantage of sensibilization and hypersensitivity responses (Chapter 17). Some chemicals even carry carcinogenic and mutagenic risks (24).

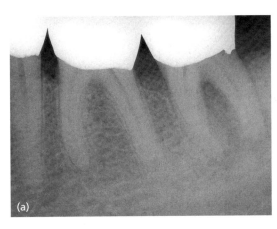
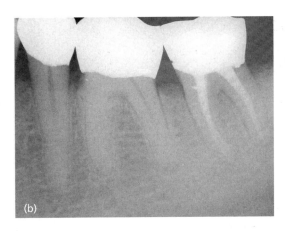

Fig. 11.1 The reason for carrying out root canal therapy is either preventive or curative. Radiograph (a) shows a lower second molar with periapical radiolucency associated with both roots, indicating an infected pulp necrosis and apical periodontitis. Radiograph (b) shows the permanently filled root canals following root canal therapy.

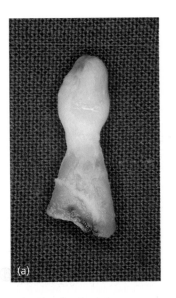
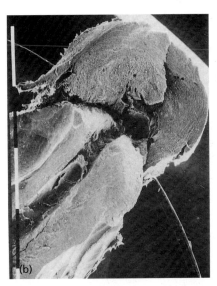

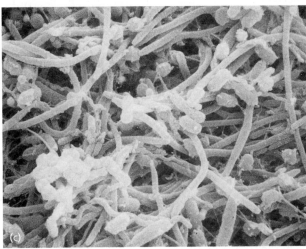
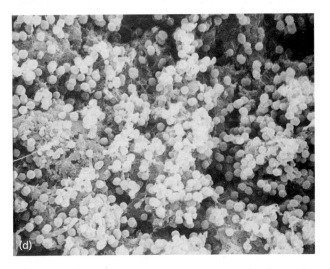

Fig. 11.2 (a) An extracted tooth with attached inflammatory soft-tissue lesion. On cracking the tooth open (b) and observing the interior (c, d) in the scanning electron microscope, various forms of bacterial morphotypes may be identified on the root canal walls, including filaments, spirochetes, rods and cocci. This kind of infection is the target for root canal therapy. Figures (b)–(d) are from Molven *et al.* (27) and published with permission of Munksgaard. (Courtesy of Dr O. Molven.)

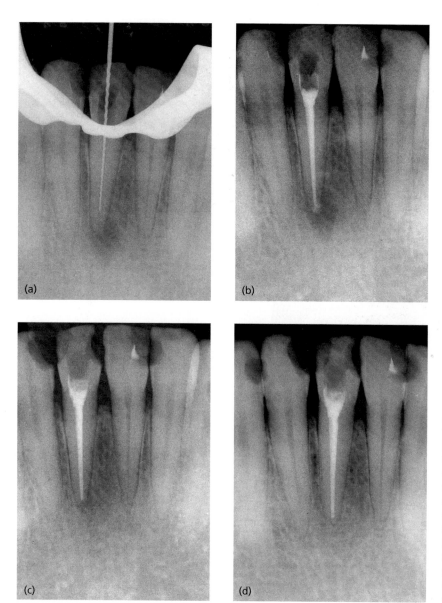

Fig. 11.3 A series of radiographs demonstrating the successful outcome of root canal therapy in a lower incisor. (a) A root canal instrument placed in the canal, which is used to clean the canal and determine the length of instrumentation in relation to the radiographic apex. Note the apical radiolucency, indicating apical periodontitis. (b) The instrumented canal has received a slightly overextended root filling. (c) A radiograph taken 2 years later. (d) Radiograph taken 6 years later, showing complete resolution of the previous lesion. The tooth now rests on a healthy periodontium and there are no symptoms (tenderness, pain, swellings) suggesting ongoing root canal infection.

(3) In liquid forms, chemicals are rapidly inactivated by inflammatory exudate and therefore provide antibacterial effects only of a short duration, thus becoming inactive within hours or a few days (13).

(4) Antiseptics included in root filling materials can cause tissue irritation and they eventually lose their antibacterial activity (17). If canals were improperly filled and/or poorly sealed coronally, infection can reappear.

In recent decades the treatment strategy for necrotic and infected pulps has changed in the move to find methods that are biocompatible. Thorough biomechanical instrumentation with the use of minimally toxic and allergenic disinfectants is now emphasized and will be detailed here.

Scheme for a routine procedure in RCT

To achieve an optimal result, several critical steps in RCT can be identified:

(1) Assessing, prior to treatment, the technical difficulties that may be encountered during the procedure in terms of being able to negotiate the canal anatomy (see Chapter 13).

(2) Opening the tooth to be treated in order to localize all canals, so-called access opening preparation (Fig. 11.4a).

(3) Providing an aseptic field of operation (Fig. 11.4b).

(4) Carrying out mechanical instrumentation of the canal interior (Figs 11.3a, 11.4c).

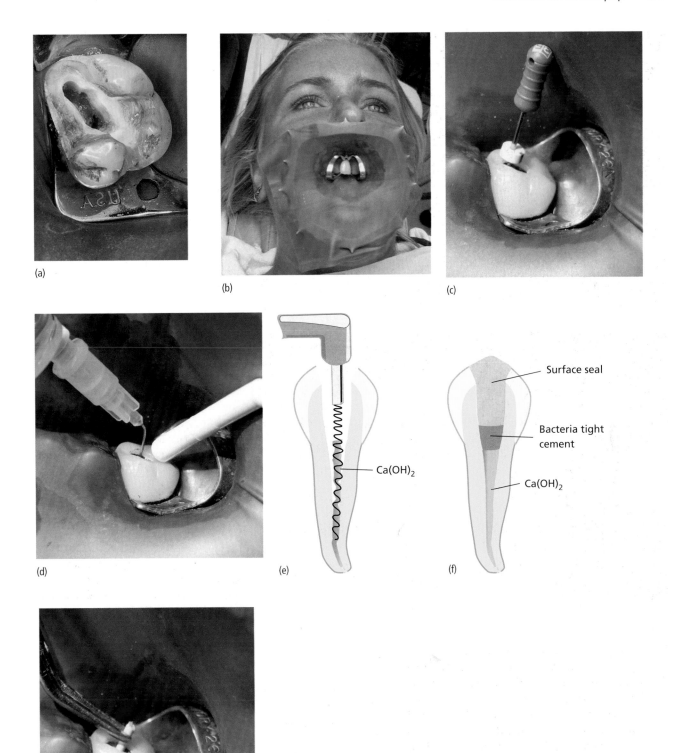

Fig.11.4 A routine procedure for combating infection in root canal therapy involves several important steps: (a) access to the root canal system; (b) rubber dam isolation and disinfection; (c) biomechanical preparation; (d) irrigation; (e) antimicrobial dressing; (f) temporary restoration between appointments; (g) root canal filling.

(5) Irrigating the canal system to remove debris and provide chemical disinfection (Fig. 11.4d).

(6) Placing an antimicrobial dressing until the next appointment (Fig. 11.4e).

(7) Closing the root canal system between appointments (Fig. 11.4f).

(8) Assessing the result of the initial treatment.

(9) Carrying out root canal filling (Figs 11.1b, 11.3b, 11.4g).

(10) Recalling the patient in 6–12 months to assess long-term outcome (Fig. 11.3c,d).

Access opening (Fig. 11.4a)

Once a decision for treatment has been taken and the difficulties assessed as to the presence of canal obstacles, length of canals and extent of curvatures, an access opening should be prepared. The purpose of such a step is to uncover all the canal orifices present to be able to carry out an unobstructed mechanical preparation of each root canal (see further Chapter 13). It is often advantageous to enter the tooth interior prior to the placement of a rubber dam to reduce the risk of going in the wrong direction and cause a perforation to the periodontal ligament space. Aligning the direction of the bur to the long axis of the tooth facilitates the procedure. This is particularly important in the teeth of elderly patients, where the pulpal chamber often is reduced by pulpal mineralizations and is then difficult to find.

Aseptic technique (Fig. 11.4b)

Even though teeth with necrotic pulps most often are infected, RCT requires an aseptic technique of operation. Asepsis is maintained first of all to exclude contamination with organisms that have greater resistance to treatment than members of the root canal microbiota. Common contaminants, difficult to manage, belong to the facultative Gram-positive segment, most notably enterococci. But other enteric bacteria and yeasts may be brought into the canal system due to the failure to maintain proper asepsis. Other sources of contaminating organisms are along leaky temporary restorations applied between sessions and by leaving canals open to the oral cavity for drainage (41, 51). Therefore elimination of micro-organisms from root canals naturally requires the prevention of oral contamination. As stated in Chapter 6, procedures in this context include removal of plaque and calculus, defective fillings and crowns and carious dentine prior to the initiation of treatment. For the subsequent RCT, proper rubber dam application is indispensable and also the use of sterile burs and instruments.

Mechanical instrumentation (Fig. 11.4c)

Cleaning the canal interior with hand and rotary instruments is a most important tool to remove the major bulk of the infecting bacterial mass and its nutritional supply. The instrumentation, if possible, should be carried out throughout the entire extension of each root canal and ideally end at its exit or slightly short of the apical foramen. The procedure aims to:

- Physically remove as much as possible of the bacterial mass.
- Remove sources of substrate for bacterial regrowth and multiplication, including necrotic tissue and tissue-breakdown products.
- Remove the inner portion of the root canal walls, where dentine is most heavily infected.
- Provide access for irrigation solutions to all parts of the root canal system for cleaning and chemical disinfection.
- Create a clean and properly shaped canal that facilitates the insertion of a well-sealing root filling.

The task is not an easy one. Not only are micro-organisms located in the main canal(s) (Fig. 11.2) but they will also enter any space and ramification available to them, including dentinal tubules (33), isthmuses and lateral canals (Fig. 11.5). This makes the cleaning and disinfection procedure precarious as well as demanding. In this context it needs to be recognized that crevices and lateral areas of oval-shaped canals (Fig. 11.5) are especially difficult to reach. If untouched by the instruments, both substrate and bacterial organisms may remain in such locations and if allowed a pathway to the apical environment a failure may ensue. In fact, studies examining the extent to which root canals are rendered clean after instrumentation often find remnants of necrotic tissue and debris on the canal walls, especially in oval-shaped canals (56). Bacteria lodged in dentinal tubules also may remain unaffected.

Narrow, partially blocked canals and canals in severely curved roots further complicate the instrumentation procedure (Fig. 11.6a,b). Instrumentation is also a demanding task where canals are extremely wide, e.g. in young immature teeth (Fig. 11.6c). One reason for this is that the armamentarium normally is designed for teeth with complete root development. Another is that instrumentation in such cases has to be limited owing to the already thin root structure. Therefore, the combat of infection in such root canals has to rely more on chemical disinfection and proper root filling than the mechanical instrumentation *per se*. However, the filling of incompletely developed roots, due to the open foramen, is a formidable task and it is often not possible

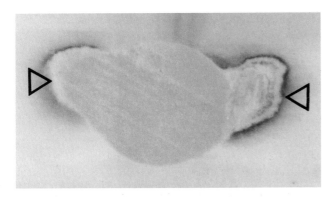

Fig. 11.5 Cross-sectional cut through a root canal partly filled with gutta-percha. Note the unfilled lateral extensions (arrow heads), which may provide space for bacterial growth and leakage of bacterial elements to the periapical tissue environment.

to attain an acceptable result unless an apical block is first created.

Yet, the instrumentation procedure is a highly important phase of RCT. By enlarging and preparing canals and giving them shape for access to chemical disinfectants and filling, the major bulk of the infecting microbiota is physically removed (5–8). Therefore the time spent in cleaning and shaping root canals according to the principles described in Chapter 13 is well worthwhile.

Considerations in routine cases

The instrumentation technique in routine cases, i.e. when the canal anatomy is within a fairly normal range in terms of width, length and curvature (Fig. 11.1), is no different to that carried out in conjunction with pulpectomy (Chapter 6). Yet, there are certain precautions that need to be undertaken to avoid primarily three complications:

(1) Blocking the canal patency.
(2) Causing an endodontic flare-up.
(3) Overextending the apical foramen.

Blocking the canal patency can occur by fracturing an instrument or by causing a ledge. Both complications are particularly common in narrow and curved canals and are often the result of improper technique. Obviously, effective removal of the infecting microbiota is hampered by such errors, therefore it is important that the instrumentation procedure follows a well-proven scheme of steps (see further Chapter 13).

To reduce the risk of causing an *endodontic flare-up* and *overextension of the apical foramen*, proper determination of the length of instrumentation (working length) carries special importance in RCT (Core concept 11.1). This

---

Core concept 11.1

Working length is a term used for the length of mechanical instrumentation in relation to the anatomical apex in a given root canal. Two methods are currently in use to determine this length: radiographic assessment by inserting a trial file into the canal to the vicinity of the apex (see Fig. 11.3a); and using an electronic device (see Chapter 13).

Core concept 11.2

Overextension of the apical foramen in conjunction with RCT is a serious complication because:

● Bacterial organisms and infected debris may be extruded into the periapical tissue and cause a flare-up of a non-painful lesion, aggravate a painful lesion and/or perpetuate apical periodontitis on a long-term basis.
● It may result in enhanced nutritional supply of any remaining organisms and boost their growth to cause endodontic flare-ups and/or long-term failure.
● It enhances the risk of overfilling.
● The potential to carry out a permanent root filling, which seals the apical portion bacterial-tight, often is impaired.

---

measure is undertaken primarily to ensure that the entire length of each canal is treated, if possible. If instrumentation is carried out too short, substantial amounts of bacterial organisms may be left behind and continue to sustain apical periodontitis. Indeed, this is one major cause of failure in RCT (22, 43).

Careful working length determination is also important to prevent instrumentation beyond the apical foramen, otherwise a set of complications may ensue (Core concept 11.2). One complication relates to the risk of extruding bacteria and infected dentine debris into the periapical tissue. If especially virulent, such organisms may aggravate a periapical inflammatory condition and cause the development of painful symptoms, including an apical abscess (endodontic flare-up). Extruded infected debris may also perpetuate apical periodontitis, despite complete elimination of bacterial organisms in the canal system *per se*.

Overinstrumentation also extends the apical foramen and promotes entry to the canal of inflammatory exudate. Owing to its content of serum proteins, the growth of proteolytic organisms is likely to be boosted. This latter mechanism may also lead to an endodontic flare-up.

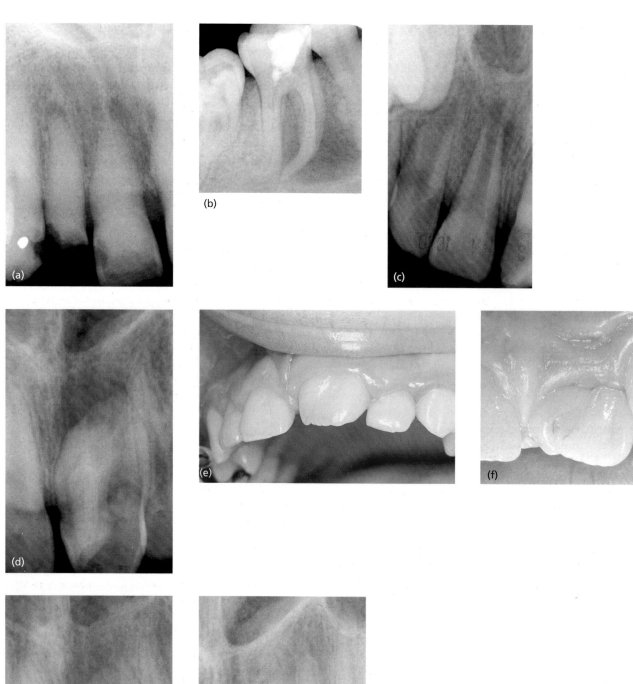
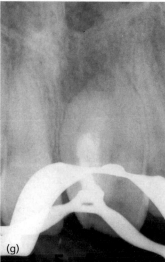
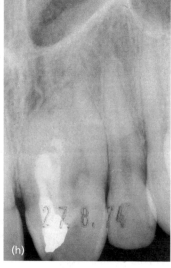

Fig. 11.6 Examples of cases displaying various degrees of difficulty: (a) a partially blocked canal due to previous mineralization processes in the pulp; (b) a tooth with severly curved root canal anatomy, especially the mesial root; (c) a tooth with incomplete root development; (d) a supernumerary tooth with a *dense invaginatus* fused to the permanent incisor; (e) buccal aspect; (f) lingual aspect. Following instrumentation and filling of the invagination only (g), the periapical lesion resolved (h). The tooth responded to an electric pulp tester and cold, indicating that the other portion had a vital pulp.

Another grave complication of overpreparation is so-called apical zipping (Chapter 13). This is when the canal orifice has been not only enlarged but also transported in a lateral direction. Similar to an incompletely developed root, such canals are extremely difficult to fill properly. Except for the risk of overfilling, often the root filling is unable to provide an apical seal (55). In fact, unfilled spaces (pockets) often remain along the apical portion of the root filling, where bacteria may continue to grow and maintain apical periodontitis (29).

Controlling pain during instrumentation

Usually treatment of a necrotic pulp does not require anesthesia. However, even in the presence of a radiolucency, functional sensory nerve fibers may prevail in the apical portion of the canal (25). Once canal instruments touch these fibers, a pain response is initiated. Thus, for completion of treatment, anesthesia may be required. Some patients may allow the necessary instrumentation without anesthesia, but this should not be conducted unless complete agreement with the patient has been sought. Usually after instrumentation with one or two file sizes, pain is gone.

It should be recognized that a pain response during instrumentation of a necrotic pulp may indicate that the foramen has been inadvertently pierced and that the working length should be reassessed. This should be carried out in spite of what appears to be a correctly recorded working length. Distinction between nerve fiber remnants and overpreparation is not always obvious and to ensure proper length of instrumentation one may:

(1) Take a control radiograph under a 20° distal or mesial angle with a file in place to obtain a good image of the buccal or lingual aspect of the root (such a radiograph shows more clearly than an orthogonal picture if the tip of the file extends into the periodontium).
(2) Carry out additional electrical measurements.
(3) Insert paper points to the presumed working length and observe whether moisture (bleeding or exudation) is picked up.

Hence, because of the sometimes-deviant exit of the apical foramen into the periodontium, it is advantageous to carry out RCT in the absence of anesthesia because this draws attention to the risk of overinstrumenting the canal. However, the comfort of the patient should be given the highest priority.

Irrigation and chemical disinfection (Fig. 11.4d)

Mechanical instrumentation of root canals needs to be supported by frequent irrigation. There are several important purposes of such a measure, primarily to clean out debris and dentinal shavings and to keep canals moist so that instruments can be run smoothly. It is also considered critical that the irrigating solution exerts antibacterial effects. Such a view is supported by clinical trials where bacteria frequently were recovered from teeth treated with mechanical instrumentation and water irrigation alone (5). To augment the efficacy of the instrumentation procedure, an irrigating solution for root canals should also be able to dissolve necrotic tissue remnants, especially in areas where mechanical instrumentation cannot reach, including crevices, invaginations and accessory canals. Low surface tension is thereby a desirable quality because it promotes the flow of fluid into such areas. To be able to dissolve the smear layer is yet another desirable property. Finally, the agent should cause minimal tissue damage and thus be minimally reactive in case it is extruded into the periapical tissue environment. However, care should be taken when using irrigants in order to prevent complications arising from their extrusion beyond the apical foramen (Clinical procedure 11.1).

A number of irrigating solutions are available, but none can be said to satisfy these requirements. Therefore, during RCT two or more agents may be combined.

Clinical procedure 11.1   Prevention and treatment of complications due to extrusion of irrigating solutions beyond the apical foramen

To prevent extrusion

- Use a small-diameter needle (0.4 mm) and insert no longer than 2 mm short of the working length. Apply a rubber stop on the needle for length control.
- Ensure that the needle is never locked into the canal.
- Use no excessive pressure to flow the fluid out of the syringe.

Sequelae to extrusion

- Immediate pain response, which may or may not be followed by edema.
- Within a few hours extensive swelling may occur in lip and eyelid.
- After some days there may be an extra-oral hematoma and some local soft-tissue necrosis.

Treatment of severe sequelae

- Administer strong analgesics. Local anesthetic may be administered but no vasoconstriction should be used in order to prevent the development of further tissue necrosis.
- Cold compresses during the first 6 h may be given for some relief.

Sodium hypochlorite

The most commonly employed solution for endodontic irrigation is sodium hypochlorite (NaOCl), which unites three important qualities essential to RCT:

(1) It dissolves organic material.
(2) It is a potent disinfectant.
(3) It is minimally tissue irritating in low concentrations.

The tissue-dissolving capacity of NaOCl is well established (2, 28). Both vital and necrotic tissue are affected and dissolved in excess of NaOCl. The speed of tissue dissolution is dependent on the extent of contact between active solution and tissue. Thus, stirring or the use of ultrasound, for example, will speed up the tissue-dissolving process considerably (28).

The effect of NaOCl is quickly inactivated in the presence of oxidizable material, such as dentine debris and organic material, because it dissociates into Na^+ and Cl^- ions (19, 28). Therefore, during RCT, the solution has to be replenished consistently. Although NaOCl breaks down collagen, it hardly affects the canal walls (18, 39). The addition of surfactant or hydrogen peroxide to NaOCl has not been proven to provide significant therapeutic effects (48).

Sodium hypochlorite is a strong and fast-acting disinfectant with a low tissue-irritating potential at low concentrations (0.5–1%) (43). It is a potent tissue irritant in higher concentrations (2.5–5%) (23, 3, 20, 35), so high concentrations should be either avoided or used with great care so that no solution is dropped into the eyes of the patient or extruded beyond the apical foramen, which may cause severe tissue irritation (see Clinical procedure 11.1). The risk–benefit ratio of the use of high concentrations of NaOCl can be questioned further on the basis of the limited gain in antibacterial effect found in clinical trials (8).

Ethylenediaminetetraacetic acid

Ethylenediaminetetraacetic acid (EDTA) is a calcium binder (chelator) that aids in removal of the smear layer. The smear layer is mainly composed of dentine particles embedded in an amorphous mass of organic material that forms on the inner root canal walls during the instrumentation procedure. Sodium hypochlorite is unable to dissolve this debris, which often contains bacterial organisms. Some contend that it is advantageous to leave the smear layer intact because it acts as a physical barrier for bacteria lodged in dentinal tubules and thereby locks them in. On the other hand, the smear layer counteracts disinfectants and blocks the penetration of medicaments into the dentinal tubules. Also, it interferes with adhesion and penetration of root filling material. Therefore, interchangeable irrigation with NaOCl and the dentine softener EDTA has been advocated (37).

Other irrigants

A variety of other disinfectants have found application in RCT, including detergents, chemotherapeutics, acids and combinations thereof. Brief comments are given here only on the use of chlorhexidine and antibiotics.

Chlorhexidine is of interest because of its extensive use in other medical and dental contexts. It is biocompatible and adheres to hydroxyapatite, which provides extended antimicrobial activity (19). So far the agent has only gained little acceptance in endodontics, most likely because of its lack of tissue-dissolving capacity (34).

It could be reasoned that an irrigant containing antibiotics is logical to combat root canal infections. Considering the limited effectiveness found in clinical trials, combined with the risk for sensitization and induction of bacterial resistance, the local use of antibiotics as an endodontic irrigant is not considered to be appropriate.

Interappointment dressing (Fig. 11.4e)

Mechanical instrumentation and irrigation with an antimicrobial solution (*biomechanical preparation*) has been found to render root canals free of cultivable organisms in approximately 50–80% of treated cases (5–8, 42, 38, 32). In teeth where bacteria were still recovered the number was nonetheless greatly reduced, showing that biomechanical preparation, if carefully conducted, is quite an effective means of bacterial removal in RCT. Yet, if given space and nutrition, regrowth to original numbers may soon occur.

In principle, there are two approaches to render the low number of remaining bacteria harmless:

(1) To further enhance bacterial elimination before the permanent root filling by applying a disinfectant in the instrumented canal(s) between two treatment sessions. This procedure is often referred to as an *interappointment dressing*.
(2) To entomb the remaining bacteria in the permanently filled root canal space. Root filling is then carried out after completion of the biomechanical preparation in the very same visit. It is expected that the antibacterial activity of the root canal sealer, in its unset stage, kills the organisms and/or they become deprived of nutritional supply and space for regrowth if pathways from and to the periapical tissue are effectively blocked.

Completion of treatment with a permanent root filling in the same session as the biomechanical instrumentation (*one-appointment endodontics*) may not always be conducted.

Core concept 11.3   Reasons for holding the root filling until a later appointment are:

(1) To observe the direct effect of the treatment on prevailing clinical symptoms, including pain, swellings and fistulae, and on lesions where the prognosis is regarded to be doubtful (if not resolving, renewed treatment can be carried out without having to remove the permanent root filling).
(2) To control apical suppuration, exudation or bleeding.
(3) To ensure that sufficient time is available for completion of the biomechanical preparation.

In straightforward, non-symptomatic teeth, where treatment can be carried out without complications and within a reasonable time span, a case can certainly be made for completion of RCT in one session. A one-visit treatment saves time and further offers the advantage that the peculiarities of the canal anatomy (e.g. curvatures, irregularities) are current to the operator and canals are therefore likely to be easier to fill than at a second appointment a week(s) or months later. Furthermore, any residual organisms in fins and crevices of the canal or in dentinal tubules, or both, may be enclosed by the root filling, thus offsetting their pathogenetic potential. Against this approach it can be argued that root fillings do not invariably seal root canals hermetically and any residual organisms may find both space and nutritional supply for regrowth, which may result in an endodontic failure. Indeed, Sjögren *et al.* (44), in a clinical follow-up, observed that the outcome of RCT of teeth with apical periodontitis was significantly less successful if cultivatable bacterial organisms were recovered at the time of filling rather than if not. Although several studies support the view that root canals after biomechanical preparation and before the permanent filling should be medicated with an antibacterial dressing to a second treatment session (5–8, 50), conflicting data exist as to the merit of such a measure (32, 54). Nonetheless, RCT should never be rushed at the expense of proper instrumentation and chemical disinfection in order to finish it in one session. Furthermore, awaiting the disappearance of clinical signs of ongoing infection is another strong argument for postponing permanent root filling to a later apppointment. For these reasons, RCT over two sessions is, for most cases, advocated as a routine procedure (Core concept 11.3).

Selecting an intracanal dressing

Over the years a multitude of antimicrobial agents have been used for intracanal dressing in RCT, including pastes, various forms of tinctures and aqueous solutions (10, 14). Iodine potassium in iodide (IKI, 5% and 10%) is an example of an aqueous solution with appealing properties. It is a potent disinfectant (30) because iodine evaporates to reach far into the dentinal tubules, crevices and fins of root canals (36, 30). Furthermore, its cytotoxic potential is low (45). However, in root canals the antimicrobial activity is of short duration and IKI is therefore unsuitable for use over extended periods of time. In fact, this applies to any liquid medicament because such agents are rapidly inactivated in root canals, particularly when there is seepage of exudate from an apical inflammatory process. As a consequence, regrowth of bacteria is likely to occur in the interim phase (7, 8). If liquid medicaments are to be used they should ideally be applied only for 5–10 min in an attempt to kill organisms in spaces inaccessible to instrumentation. Consequently, as an interappointment dressing, a substance should be selected that is not easily replaced by tissue fluid and that can remain physically intact over weeks or months.

In recent years, a water-slurry of calcium hydroxide $(Ca(OH)_2)$ has gained considerable acceptance as an interappointment dressing in endodontic therapies because it combines several attractive features (40, 14). It is a strong alkaline substance (pH 12.5) that in aqueous solution dissociates into calcium and hydroxyl ions, the latter providing antimicrobial effects (7) (Advanced concept 11.1) and tissue-dissolving capacity (21). With its fairly low solubility and mere physical presence, it is used as an intracanal dressing over long periods of time (Fig. 11.7). Its most essential function is then to obstruct bacterial regrowth, which may occur by:

(1) Eliminating space for bacterial growth.
(2) Blocking nutritional supply of inflammatory exudates deriving from the apical lesion.
(3) Releasing bactericidal hydroxyl ions.

It needs to be recognized that because of its low solubility the antibacterial capacity of $Ca(OH)_2$ is limited to the near vicinity of the micro-organisms. Therefore one cannot expect that it effectively kills organisms in non-instrumented parts of the root canal or bacteria lodged in dentinal tubules (30, 40) (see also Advanced concept 11.2). Yet, $Ca(OH)_2$ serves as an ideal intracanal dressing for follow-ups of treatment effects and thus offers convenient scheduling of the patients. Thereby, ample time can be reserved for observation of tissue healing in progress, e.g. for large lesions, symptomatic lesions or when prognosis for a successful outcome in any other respect appears questionable (Fig. 11.7).

In RCT, $Ca(OH)_2$ also serves an important function in controling seepage of inflammatory exudates into root canals. This type of leakage is especially a problem in conjunction with symptomatic periapical lesions, where suppurations hamper effective disinfection and adhesion of root filling material to the canal walls. In such instances permanent root filling is contraindicated. By blocking the canal space for bacterial multiplication and the associated release of inflammatogenic substances to the periapical tissue, healing of the acute phase of the lesion is promoted. Normally this will occur within 1 week and RCT subsequently can be continued.

Closing the root canal system between appointments (Fig. 11.4f)

To exclude bacterial contamination in endodontics, adequate temporary seals between appointments are required. Furthermore, canals should never be left open to the oral cavity for any extended period of time because of the risk of introducing oral organisms that are difficult to get rid of.

The first step is to fill the entire root canal space with Ca(OH)₂. Application can be done following mixing of Ca(OH)₂ powder and sterile water to a creamy paste, which is spiralled into the canal with a Lentulo spiral. This instrument is made of a fine, flexible wire spiralled in the shape of a reverse auger. It should be turned in a clockwise direction in a handpiece at slow speed and brought to the vicinity of the working length. Applying light pressure with a small cotton pellet at the canal orifice ensures that the entire canal is filled. A disadvantage of this method is the risk of extruding Ca(OH)₂ beyond the apical foramen, and care should be taken particularly when filling lower molars, which are close to the mandibular canal. Devices exist for injection of

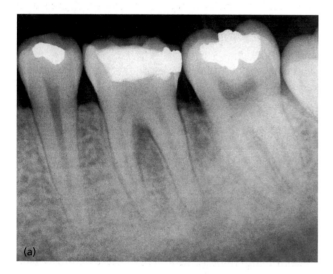
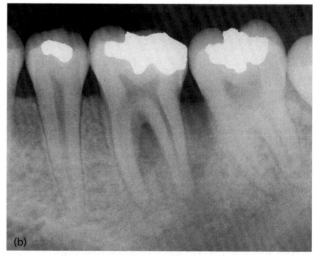

Fig. 11.7 (a) Successful treatment of tooth 36 in an adult patient following instrumentation and Ca(OH)₂ dressing, where the prognosis was deemed questionable *a priori* due to a large distal lesion and a lesion in the furcal region (b). The follow-up radiograph in (a) was taken 6 months after initiation of treatment. The lesions have resolved almost completely. (Courtesy of Dr C. Reit.)

Advanced concept 11.2   The use of bacteriological sampling in RCT

There are situations when bacterial sampling of root canals is a valuable tool. One is when RCT does not result in elimination of clinical symptoms. Such problems may be associated with the presence of unusual pathogens, i.e. *Pseudomonas*, *Proteus* and *Staphylococcus aureus*. In yet other instances, the lack of therapeutic effect may be due to a severe contamination problem. In medically compromised patients set on immunosuppressive therapy and in patients at very high risk of endocarditis or with multiple heart valve prostheses, a sample at the initial appointment is warranted to determine antimicrobial susceptibility in case a flare-up or a systemic complication ensues. This precaution may be undertaken in spite of the fact that patients are prescribed antimicrobial prophylaxis and because not all microorganisms may be susceptible to the prescription given (see further Chapter 10). If possible, it is normally wise to refer the latter kind of patient to an endodontic specialist.

Collecting a sample from root canals requires access to a laboratory that can process it. Some dental schools and large hospitals offer a mail-in service and provide culture materials, including sampling fluid and transport media.

Taking a sample requires effective rubber dam isolation and proper disinfection to avoid inclusion of contaminating organisms. This precaution is absolutely essential, otherwise the information is worthless. In line with these measures, all subsequent procedures must be undertaken with sterile instruments and proper aseptic technique. Prior to sampling, canals should have been emptied of paste medicaments for several days to allow the accumulation of a sufficient number of organisms to be collected. Liquid medicaments usually have lost their antimicrobial effect within a few days. Following the opening of the canal, any exudate present is first collected onto an absorbent point. The point is then transferred to a vial containing transport medium. If the canal is dry, sampling fluid is added and a root canal instrument, preferably a Hedström file, is used to shave off dentine debris from the root canal walls along the canal length. Paper points are used to transfer the suspension of dentine filings and sampling fluid to the transport medium. The sample, along with a filled-in referral form, should be mailed to the laboratory within 1 day. The result can usually be received within 1 week.

Core concept 11.4   Evaluation criteria

Root canal therapy is considered successful when there is absence of:

- Pain to apical palpation
- Pain or tenderness to percussion
- Sinus tract
- Swelling
- Radiographic signs of bone destruction
- Continuous root resorption.

$Ca(OH)_2$, e.g. by means of a commercially available syringe filled with $Ca(OH)_2$.

After application, the excess material in the pulp chamber should be removed and blotted dry with the end of a paper point or cotton pellet. The canal orifice and adjacent part of the pulp chamber should then be sealed with a soft temporary cement (e.g. Cavit, zinc oxide–eugenol) followed by a more rigid temporary filling that withstands the wear and pressure by occlusal forces (e.g. thick mixes of zinc phosphate cement, IRM, glassionomer). The first layer of soft cement ensures that a bacterial-tight seal is established until the second visit. An ultrasonic scaler or spoon excavator can then easily remove the cement without running the risk of damaging the tooth structure.

Root filling (Fig. 11.4g)

Permanent root filling of teeth with an infected necrotic pulp should not be carried out unless the biomechanical preparation is complete and no exudation exists in the canal that prevents adherence of the filling to the root canal walls. It is also regarded good clinical practice to postpone permanent root filling until the tooth is free from pain and other clinical symptoms of root canal infection. An objective means by which the clinician is assisted to decide when bacterial elimination is complete is not readily available. It was once believed that a bacterial sample would be able to provide guidance in this respect. Hence, a positive sample taken after biomechanical preparation would indicate that it should be continued, whereas a negative culture would signal successful disinfection (Advanced concept 11.2). However, the methodology has lost popularity in recent years and is practised only to a limited degree as a treatment control.

Recall

Patients subjected to RCT should be asked to return for a recall appointment within a period of 6–12 months (12). The purpose of that appointment is to ensure, by clinical and radiographic means, that healing is in progress. Signs of a successful outcome are that no clinical symptoms (pain, fistulae, tenderness and swellings) prevail or have appeared (Core concept 11.4). Inspection, palpation and percussion tests and examination of periodontal pocket probing depths (to search for fistulae along the periodontal ligament) can confirm such a condition.

The radiographic control reveals the extent to which a preoperative radiolucency has disappeared (Fig. 11.3). Already by 4–6 months, radiographic examination may reveal signs of bone healing in progress. Although some

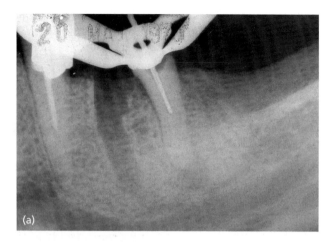 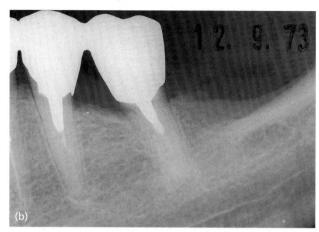

Fig. 11.8   Instrumentation was not possible over the entire length of the distal root in a lower molar due to obliteration (a). At recall 2 years later the lesion has reduced in size (b). Clinically, the tooth remained without inflammatory symptoms.

lesions take longer to heal, most healing lesions are likely to resolve with complete bone fill within 1 year (see further Chapter 14). In cases with a large lesion, where a self-sustaining and expanding cyst or other pathological lesion may be suspected, it is recommended to carry out the recall by 4–6 months. If healing is obviously not in progress, a surgical procedure may be considered (Chapter 14).

Considerations in advanced cases

Canal anatomy may be such that cleaning and disinfection of the root canal system can be conducted only with great difficulty. Root canals also may be partly or totally obstructed by mineralization within the pulpal chamber, e.g. as a result of inflammation or previous injury by trauma or operative procedure (Fig. 11.6a,b). There may also be developmental anomalies (Fig. 11.6d). It is highly important to identify carefully any potential difficulties prior to initiation of RCT (Fig. 11.8). Referral to an endodontic specialist or experienced colleague also may be considered.

Nevertheless, conservative management of what appears to be a hopeless case may still be successful by conventional RCT (1) (Fig. 11.8). Yet, the prognosis should be guarded. If a permanent cast restoration is to be carried out, restoration should be postponed until there are clear signs of healing in progress.

Effects of RCT on the intracanal microbiota

As described in Chapter 8, the microbiota of infected necrotic pulps is normally dominated by anaerobes, whereas facultatives usually occupy a minor portion of the root canal flora. However, there is great variation and a large number of individual species and combinations of species can be associated with the development and continuance of apical periodontitis (Chapter 8). Therefore, one has found little support for treatment approaches that selectively focus on specific organisms. Yet, findings of a dominance of facultatives, especially therapy-resilient enterococci in retreatment cases (cases where lesions have appeared or failed to heal subsequent to endodontic therapy; 26, 47), suggest that RCT normally is effective in combating the anaerobes. On this basis, one may speculate that RCT, if not properly conducted, may select the most robust segment of the root canal microbiota. Consequently, it can be regarded as important that the best possible effort to eradicate microorganisms should be taken at the initial treatment session. It seems reasonable, therefore, to caution against a procedure whereby instrumentation and chemical disinfection is carried out only half-way, and to postpone completion of biomechanical instrumentation to a later session. One may even elect to refrain from entering infected root canals if sufficient time is not available for completion of the biomechanical preparation in the first sitting.

Management of symptomatic lesions

Most lesions associated with an infected necrosis of the pulp prevail without acute signs of inflammation (pain, tenderness, fistulae, swellings). Nevertheless symptomatic lesions may develop spontaneously or be initiated in conjunction with RCT (Fig. 11.9). This section of the chapter is devoted to measures to be undertaken in such cases.

Painful cases prior to RCT

Symptomatic lesions may be associated with or without a distinct soft-tissue swelling. In some of these lesions, cellulitis or a periapical abscess may have already matured and manifested itself as a subperiosteal or submucosal abscess with distinct intra-oral or extra-oral swellings, or both (see further Chapter 9). To alleviate the condition, RCT is still the treatment of choice. However, in these instances patients often seek the dentist on an unscheduled appointment, and time therefore may set limits for what it is possible to do. There may also be a variety of other circumstances that make proper RCT impossible to carry out at the time the patient seeks the dentist. Some of these are technically related and include the presence of obstructions in the root canal that require substantial time to remove before the rest of the canal(s) can be accessed. Examples are

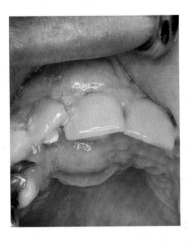

Fig. 11.9 A case with both buccal and palatal swellings due to an acute flare-up of an apical periodontitis.

hard-tissue obliterations, previous root fillings and crowns with posts. Thus, by its very nature, emergency treatment will often have to be a compromise, where the primary objective is to get the patient out of pain. Consequently, although a complete instrumentation and medication of the tooth is highly desirable to combat the infecting microbiota, it is only a secondary objective at this point and may have to be put on hold until the patient can be seen at a regularly scheduled appointment.

General procedure

An emergency procedure includes several critical steps:

(1) Establishment of a correct diagnosis of the condition.
(2) Assessment of the severity and a decision as to whether an invasive RCT and/or incision and drainage procedure is needed or if the condition can be managed by analgesics.
(3) Emergency treatment.
(4) Rescheduling for completion of RCT or endodontic surgery, if needed.

Any emergency treatment must take into account the management of both the root canal system and the periapex. If canals are accessible, opening the root canal(s) gives an opportunity to obtain drainage of exudate or pus (see further below) and to combat the infecting microbiota by biomechanical instrumentation (RCT). The emergency procedure also may include an attempt to drain off an abscess by surgical incision (Fig. 11.10). If canals are not accessible and if drainage by incision is not deemed possible, the emergency treatment may have to be limited to prescription of a strong analgesic and postponement of further measures until a more suitable time is available within a couple of days.

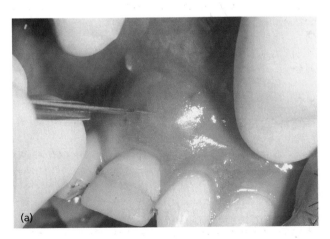
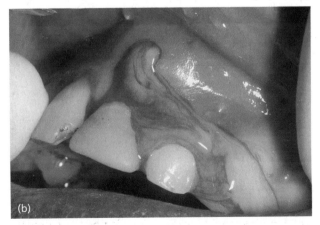

Fig. 11.10 Drainage of submucosal abscess is obtained by the use of a scalpel (a), by which pus is released (b). Images courtesy of the Department of Endodontics, University of North Carolina at Chapel Hill.

Emergency RCT

In teeth that hurt because of a painful manifestation of apical periodontitis, even the slightest pressure may cause pain and therefore the root canals of such teeth should be accessed with high-speed burs and light pressure. Occasionally it may be necessary to give local anesthesia, but in all other aspects the RCT is no different to that used in routine non-symptomatic cases.

On spreading inflammatory processes (cellulitis, subperiosteal abscess), drainage of exudate or pus under pressure may be possible along the root canal space. Sometimes it occurs directly in conjunction with access to the pulpal chamber (Fig. 11.11), but in other instances drainage may be obtained by careful bypassing of the apical foramen using a thin root canal instrument. If such drainage does occur, there is often immediate pain relief. It is highly important that the apical foramen is not pierced with instruments of more than ISO sizes 10–20, otherwise one runs the risk of causing an apical overpreparation and zipping of the apical foramen, thus making subsequent RCT precarious (see above). In the following, it is sufficient to clean the root canal system properly and close it up with a dressing of Ca(OH)$_2$ and temporary cement in the access opening.

With an abundant drainage of pus that does not halt immediately, it is advisable to let the patient sit for a while before closing the canal system, in order to equilibrate the apical tissue pressure. One should not leave canals open to the oral environment because this may cause a severe contamination problem. Hence, leaving root canals open without a surface seal may contribute to the establishment of a microflora, including enteric bacteria and yeasts, which subsequently are very difficult to get rid of (26, 47, 51).

If drainage of an abscess can be obtained by either root canal instrumentation or incision and drainage, prescribing antibiotics is redundant and undesirable.

If there is a lack of time and there is no drainage on careful piercing of the apical foramen after making the access, one has to close the canal system and postpone further biomechanical instrumentation until a more suitable occasion can be found. On many occasions pain relief can be obtained simply by such a measure, yet pain may not be alleviated immediately following emergency RCT, and the patient must be made aware of this (Core concept 11.5).

Pulp necrosis with a localized fluctuant swelling

With a localized, fluctuant, soft-tissue swelling indicating a submucosal abscess, an incision and drainage procedure should be attempted (Fig. 11.10). It is not possible to state categorically whether this should be done before or after accessing the root canal system, but as a rule of thumb it is recommended to carry out the procedure first, if there is an obvious fluctuation.

With a non-fluctuant tissue swelling it is advised not to incise the tissue because concern exists as to the possibility of worsening the condition and causing the spread of micro-organisms. Controlling the pain with analgesics until fluctuation occurs is probably the best choice of treatment because the administration of antibiotics may not be effective (see below).

Occasionally, localized intra-oral swellings are accompanied by some extra-oral distension resulting in an elevated cheek, swollen lips and sometimes even swollen eyelids. Usually, these symptoms do not require additional treatment or medication unless the swelling rapidly diffuses.

Pulp necrosis with diffuse swelling

In the presence of diffuse swelling that has rapidly progressed and is accompanied by systemic signs including fever (>39°C) and general malaise, patients should be referred to a hospital where intravenous antibiotics usually are given. In these cases it is not advised to try to control the infection by oral antibiotics prescribed by the general practitioner.

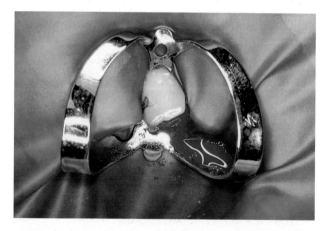

Fig. 11.11 Drainage of pus and blood along the root canal upon access of an upper lateral incisor with a necrotic pulp and painful apical periodontitis.

Core concept 11.5   Pain relief after emergency RCT

Pain may not disappear immediately after emergency RCT, therefore it is essential to:

- explain the situation to the patient
- adjust the occlusal contacts
- prescribe a suitable analgesic
- be available to the patient if severe pain continues

Use of antimicrobials (antibiotics)

In general the systemic use of antibiotics is a valuable adjunct to the treatment of infectious diseases. However, the risk of causing bacterial resistance makes it necessary to restrict their use in endodontics to those cases in absolute need. Such cases are primarily those where symptoms of endodontic infection suggest marked progression or systemic involvement, or both. The purpose of an antibiotic prescription is then to help to contain the process and to avoid possible serious systemic consequences (see also Chapter 10). This means that antibiotic therapy is not appropriate for the treatment of localized swellings where drainage and debridement can be successfully carried out.

In the exceptional case when antibiotics are to be prescribed, an adequate drug and accurate dosage should be given. Because there is no way of knowing which specific organisms are causing the lesion, the prescription must be initiated on an empirical basis. Thus, seeing the patient on a daily basis until the infectious process is contained should carefully monitor the result of therapy. If a satisfactory response is absent within the next few days, one may consider changing the antimicrobial. For drug selection, a careful history of allergy and drug reaction is necessary and one may consult the proper background literature for possible side-effects. Chapter 10 lists the various antimicrobials.

Management of postoperative pain – endodontic flare-up

Although painful conditions normally are prevented or cured by RCT, the RCT may also cause pain and swellings. This may occur even in teeth that were free of pain prior to treatment. The incidence of such conditions has been reported to be as high as 20–40% of treated cases (15), whereas the incidence of severe pain conditions appears to be <5% (20, 49, 52).

The primary cause is to be sought in the treatment procedure, whereby bacteria and bacterial elements have been extruded into the periapical tissue compartment and caused an exacerbation of the inflammatory lesion. An exacerbation may also follow by inadvertent extension of the apical foramen, which allows an enhanced nutritional supply to any bacterial organisms that survived the initial treatment. Normally these so-called endodontic flare-ups have a sudden onset and may not emerge until 1–2 days after the procedure. Improper use of irrigants and root canal dressings may also cause irritation to the extent that a painful condition emerges. However, if used correctly, root canal dressings and irrigation do not cause any more postoperative pain than the use of saline as an irrigant (20).

Key literature 11.1

Genet et al. (16) carried out a clinical follow-up study of 443 teeth in 443 patients, reporting the association between preoperative and operative factors and the incidence of postoperative factors after the first visit. Postoperative pain occurred in 27% of the cases, of which 5% were severe. A positive correlation was seen between the incidence of postoperative pain and: the presence of preoperative pain in cases of teeth with necrotic pulps; the presence of a radiolucency >5 mm in diameter; and the number of root canals treated. Women more frequently reported pain than men. When each of these factors was analysed independently they remained statistically significant, suggesting that the effects were cumulative.

Management

Research has shown that in over 50% of patients who experience pain after treatment the pain disappears within 1 day. After 2 days 90% were relieved of pain, whereas for only 3% pain lasted for longer than 1 week (16, Key literature 11.1). This means that most painful conditions do not need active treatment and can be managed by analgesics, although a number of patients experience severe pain and need to be seen again for assessment or active treatment.

If the pain is not severe (can be suppressed with a mild analgesic) it is best to abstain from further treatment, reassure the patient and prescribe a mild analgesic if no analgesic is being used already. Adjustment of occlusion also provides comfort. If pain is severe, the therapy depends on whether or not the previous canal preparation was complete or if the canal was permanently filled:

- If pain develops after *incomplete instrumentation*, then opening the canal and completing the RCT is appropriate.
- If pain persists or occurs in spite of *complete biomechanical preparation*, then reopening the tooth to attempt to drain off pus or exudates may alleviate the condition. After proper isolation with a rubber dam, gently instrument the canal with an ISO 20 instrument. If pus is discharged, then usually the pain is greatly reduced or disappears. Leave the tooth alone until pus stops discharging and then irrigate, dry and close up the access opening. The problem invariably may not resolve by such a measure, particularly if no pus is noticed, therefore a decision to reopen a properly instrumented and medicated root canal should be taken after careful assessment of the case and consideration of prescribing strong analgesics instead (11). The patient should be informed that the pain is expected to subside within the next few days. If the condition continues to be severe, a surgical procedure may have to be carried out.

- Filling of the root canal seldom results in postoperative pain (50, 20). If, *after root canal filling*, a painful condition appears, the case is best managed by pain medication, because the root canal is blocked for possible drainage. Furthermore, removal of the root canal filling may cause extrusion of root filling material and inadvertent overpreparation of the foramen. In the case of subperiosteal or submucous abscess, an incision may give the necessary drainage. Apical surgery or extraction may have to be carried out if the condition persists. An experienced colleague or endodontic specialist may be consulted prior to deciding on a possible unnecessary removal of the tooth.

Concluding remark

Patients may be greatly upset or concerned about the development or continuance of pain after RCT, especially when they have not received proper prior information that such complications may emerge. It is crucial that patients be told that a tooth treated for an infected pulp necrosis may become sensitive or even painful. It is also necessary to advise the patient about which measures to undertake, e.g. to call and get an emergency appointment. Good explanation and advice prevent considerable concern and may make pain more tolerable (9).

References

1. Åkerblom A, Hasselgren G. The prognosis for endodontic treatment of obliterated root canals. *J. Endodont.* 1988; 14: 565–7.
    Clinical follow-up study of cases not possible to instrument further than one-third of the root length. It was reported that complete periapical healing occurred in 10/16 teeth with preoperative periapical radiolucency.
2. Baumgartner JC, Cuenin PR. Efficacy of several concentrations of sodium hypochlorite for root canal irrigation. *J. Endodont.* 1992; 18: 605–12.
3. Becking AG. Complications in the use of sodium hypochlorite during endodontic treatment. *Oral Surg. Oral Med. Oral Pathol.* 1991; 71: 346–8.
4. Bergenholtz G. Micro-organisms from necrotic pulp of traumatized teeth. *Odontol. Revy* 1974; 25: 347–58.
5. Byström A, Sundqvist G. Bacteriologic evaluation of the efficacy of mechanical root canal instrumentation in endodontic therapy. *Scand. J. Dent. Res.* 1981; 89: 321–8.
6. Byström A, Sundqvist G. Bacteriologic evaluation of the effect of 0.5 per cent sodium hypochlorite in endodontic therapy. *Oral Surg. Oral Med. Oral Pathol.* 1983; 55: 307–12.
7. Byström A, Claesson R, Sundqvist G. The antibacterial effect of camphorated paramonochlorophenol, camphorated phenol and calcium hydroxide in the treatment of infected root canals. *Endodont. Dent. Traumatol.* 1985; 1: 170–75.
8. Byström A, Sundqvist G. The antibacterial action of sodium hypochlorite and EDTA in 60 cases of endodontic therapy. *Int. Endodont. J.* 1985; 18: 35–40.
9. Chapman CR. New directions in understanding and management of pain. *Soc. Sci. Med.* 1984; 19: 1261–77.
10. Chong BS, Pitt Ford TR. The role of intracanal medication in root canal treatment. *Int. Endodont. J.* 1992; 25: 97–106.
11. Cooper SA. Treating acute pain: do's and don'ts, pros and cons. *J. Endodont.* 1990; 16: 85–91.
12. European Society of Endodontology. Consensus report of the European Society of Endodontology on quality guidelines for endodontic treatment. *Int. Endodont. J.* 1994; 27: 115–24.
13. Fager FK, Messer HH. Systemic distribution of camphorated monochlorophenol from cotton pellets sealed in pulp chambers. *J. Endodont.* 1986; 12: 225–30.
14. Fava LR, Saunders WP. Calcium hydroxide pastes: classification and clinical indications. *Int. Endodont. J.* 1999; 32: 257–82.
15. Genet JM, Wesselink PR, Thoden van Velzen SK. The incidence of preoperative and postoperative pain in endodontic therapy. *Int. Endodont. J.* 1986; 19: 221–9.
16. Genet JM, Hart AAM, Wesselink PR, Thoden van Velzen SK. Preoperative and operative factors associated with pain after the first endodontic visit. *Int. Endodont. J.* 1987; 20: 53–64.
17. Gilbert DB, Germaine GR, Jensen JR. Inactivation by saliva and serum of the antimicrobial activity of some commonly used root canal sealer cements. *J. Endodont.* 1978; 4: 100–5.
18. Goldman LB, Goldman M, Kronman JH, Lin PS. The efficacy of several irrigating solutions for endodontics: a scanning electron microscopic study. *Oral Surg. Oral Med. Oral Pathol.* 1981; 52: 197–204.
19. Haapasalo HK, Sirén EK, Waltimo TM, Ørstavik D, Haapasalo MP. Inactivation of local root canal medicaments by dentine: an in vitro study. *Int. Endodont. J.* 2000; 33: 126–31.
20. Harrison JW, Baumgartner JC, Zielke DR. Analysis of interappointment pain associated with the combined use of endodontic irrigants and medicaments. *J. Endodont.* 1981; 7: 272–6.
21. Hasselgren G, Olsson B, Cvek M. Effects of calcium hydroxide and sodium hypochlorite on the dissolution of necrotic porcine muscle tissue. *J. Endodont.* 1988; 14: 125–7.
22. Kerekes K, Tronstad L. Long-term results of endodontic treatment performed with a standardized technique. *J. Endodont.* 1979; 5: 83–90.
    Clinical and radiographic follow-up study of patients treated by undergraduate students. Of 241 roots treated for a necrotic pulp, an overall success rate was attained in 89% over 5 years of observation.
23. Lamers AC, Van Mullem PJ, Simon M. Tissue reactions to sodium hypochlorite and iodine potassium iodide under clinical conditions in monkeys' teeth. *J. Endodont.* 1980; 6: 788–92.
24. Lewis B. Formaldehyde in dentistry: a review for the millennium. *J. Clin. Pediatr. Dent.* 1998; 22: 167–77.

25. Lin L, Langeland K. Innervation of the inflammatory periapical lesions. *Oral Surg. Oral Med. Pathol.* 1981; 51: 535–43.

26. Molander A, Reit C, Dahlén G, Kvist T. Microbiological status of root filled teeth with apical periodontitis. *Int. Endodont. J.* 1998; 31: 1–7.

27. Molven O, Olsen I, Kerekes K. Scanning electron microscopy of bacteria in the apical part of root canals in permanent teeth with periapical lesions. *Endodont. Dent. Traumatol.* 1991; 7: 226–9.

28. Moorer WR, Wesselink PR. Factors promoting the tissue dissolving capability of sodium hypochlorite. *Int. Endodont. J.* 1982; 15: 187–96.

29. Nair PNR, Sjögren U, Krey G, Kahnberg K-E, Sundqvist G. Intraradicular bacteria and fungi in root filled, asymptomatic human teeth with therapy-resistant periapical lesions: a long-term light and electron microscopic follow-up study. *J. Endodont.* 1990; 16: 580–88.

30. Ørstavik D, Haapasalo M. Disinfection by endodontic irrigants and dressings of experimentally infected dentinal tubules. *Endodont. Dent. Traumatol.* 1990; 6: 142–9.

31. Ørstavik D, Kerekes K, Molven O. Effects of extensive apical reaming and calcium hydroxide dressing on bacterial infection during treatment of apical periodontitis: a pilot study. *Int. Endodont. J.* 1991; 24: 1–7.

32. Peters LB, Wesselink PR. Periapical healing of endodontically treated teeth in one and two visits obturated in the presence or absence of bacteria in the root canal. *Int. Endodont. J.* 2002; 35: 660–67.

33. Peters LB, Wesselink PR, Buijs JF, van Winkelhoff AJ. Viable bacteria in root dentinal tubules of teeth with apical periodontitis. *J. Endodont.* 2001; 27: 76–81.

34. Ringel AM, Patterson SS, Newton CW, Miller CH, Mulhern JM. In vivo evaluation of chlorhexidine gluconate solution and sodium hypochlorite solution as root canal irrigants. *J. Endodont.* 1982; 8: 200–204.

35. Rosenfeld EF, James GA, Burch BS. Vital pulp tissue response to sodium hypochlorite. *J. Endodont.* 1978; 4: 140–46.

36. Safavi KE, Spångberg LS, Langeland K. Root canal dentinal tubule disinfection. *J. Endodont.* 1990; 16: 207–10.

37. Sen BH, Wesselink PR, Türkün M. The smear layer: a phenomenon in root canal therapy. *Int. Endodont. J.* 1995; 28: 141–8.

38. Shuping GB, Ørstavik D, Sigurdsson A, Trope M. Reduction of intracanal bacteria using nickel–titanium rotary instrumentation and various medications. *J. Endodont.* 2000; 26: 751–5.

39. Sim TPC, Knowles JC, Ng Y-L, Shelton J, Gulabivala K. Effect of sodium hypochlorite on mechanical properties of dentine and tooth surface strain. *Int. Endodont. J.* 2001; 34: 120–32.

40. Siqueira Junior JF, Lopes HP. Mechanisms of antimicrobial activity of calcium hydroxide: a critical review. *Int. Endodont. J.* 1999; 32: 361–9.

41. Sirén EK, Haapasalo MP, Ranta K, Salmi P, Kerosuo EN. Microbiological findings and clinical treatment procedures in endodontic cases selected for microbiological investigation. *Int. Endodont. J.* 1997; 30: 91–5.

42. Sjögren U, Sundqvist G. Bacteriologic evaluation of ultrasonic root canal instrumentation. *Oral Surg.* 1987; 63: 366–70.

43. Sjögren U, Hägglund B, Sundqvist G, Wing K. Factors affecting the long-term results of endodontic treatment. *J. Endodont.* 1990; 16: 498–504.

44. Sjögren U, Figdor D, Persson S, Sundqvist G. Influence of infection at the time of root filling on the outcome of endodontic treatment of teeth with apical periodontitis. *Int. Endodont. J.* 1997; 30: 297–306.

45. Spångberg L, Rutberg M, Rydinge E. Biologic effect of endodontic antimicrobial agents. *J. Endodont.* 1979; 5: 166–75.

46. Sundqvist G. *Bacteriological Studies of Necrotic Dental Pulps*, Odontological Dissertation No. 7, University of Umeå, 1976.
    Classical research paper. Advanced sampling, cultivation technique and taxonomic analysis were carried out to examine teeth with necrotic pulps injured by accidental trauma. The complexity of the root canal microbiota and its dominance of anaerobes were demonstrated. The study also showed a strong association between bacterial presence and occurrence of periapical lesion and, in contrast, with no bacterial presence the periapical tissue presented no radiolucency.

47. Sundqvist G, Figdor D, Persson S, Sjögren U. Microbiologic analysis of teeth with failed endodontic treatment and the outcome of conservative re-treatment. *Oral Surg.* 1998; 85: 86–93.

48. Svec TA, Harrison JW. The effect of effervescence on debridement of the apical regions of root canals in single-rooted teeth. *J. Endodont.* 1981; 7: 335–40.

49. Trope M. Flare-up rate of single-visit endodontics. *Int. Endodont. J.* 1991; 24: 24–6.

50. Trope M, Delano EO, Ørstavik D. Endodontic treatment of teeth with apical periodontitis: single vs. multivisit treatment. *J. Endodont.* 1999; 25: 345–50.

51. Waltimo TM, Sirén EK, Torkko HL, Olsen I, Haapasalo MP. Fungi in therapy-resistant apical periodontitis. *Int. Endodont. J.* 1997; 30: 96–101.

52. Walton R, Fouad A. Endodontic interappointment flare-ups: a prospective study of incidence and related factors. *J. Endodont.* 1992; 18: 172–7.

53. Wang ZG, Wang JD. A clinical observation on extensive periapical lesions of posterior teeth and their treatment with resinifying therapy. *Quintess. Int.* 1989; 20: 143–7.

54. Weiger R, Rosendahl R, Löst C. Influence of calcium hydroxide intracanal dressings on the prognosis of teeth with endodontically induced periapical lesions. *Int. Endodont. J.* 2000; 33: 219–26.

55. Wu M-K, Fan B, Wesselink PR. Leakage along apical root fillings in curved root canals. Part 1: effects of apical transportation on seal of root fillings. *J. Endodont.* 2000; 26: 210–16.

56. Wu M-K, Wesselink PR. A primary observation on the preparation and obturation of oval canals. *Int. Endodont. J.* 2001; 34: 137–41.

Part 4
THE ROOT FILLED TOOTH

Chapter 12
The root filled tooth in prosthodontic reconstruction

Eckehard Kostka and Jean-François Roulet

Introduction

After endodontic therapy a tooth must be restored to functional and esthetic demands. Teeth serving as abutments in prosthodontic reconstructions must be judged carefully regarding their ability to carry a load higher than the physiological one on a single tooth (Core concept 12.1; Fig. 12.1). In most cases the remaining tooth structure will be less than in vital teeth because the most frequently occurring reason for endodontic treatment needs is deep caries. Additionally, a further loss of tooth structure takes place during the preparation of the access cavity and the canal. The amount of coronal tooth structure is the most important factor in the decision for the kind of reconstruction. It is responsible for the retention of the restoration and the fracture susceptibility. When the remaining tooth structure does not provide enough retention for a core build-up, the root canal can support the retention by use of a post. Thus, in a single-rooted tooth with substantial loss of coronal tooth structure, post and cores are often needed.

There is evidence for changes in receptor properties in teeth with non-vital pulp leading to higher bite forces than in vital teeth (33). This must be considered by estimating the fracture susceptibility of a root filled tooth, especially within a prosthodontic reconstruction substituting some more teeth (Key literature 12.1).

Problems associated with root filled teeth as abutments

In order to achieve long-term clinical success in the prosthodontic restoration of root filled teeth it is essential to know the reasons for clinical failures. Some of these reasons, such as recurrent caries or periodontal breakdown, are the same as in vital teeth. One major difference to a vital tooth is the absence of a vital pulp with its potential of inflammatory reaction causing symptoms that act as a first indicator for the patient. To avoid caries and periodontal disease a proper recall regimen should be established to ensure adequate prophylaxis.

The loss of retention of a crown is possible in non-vital as well as in vital abutments, but in the latter early symptoms are warning the patient, rather than in a root filled-tooth. The following paragraphs discuss the problems associated with the prosthodontic reconstruction of root filled teeth.

Loss of retention

Retention loss is a failure of the connection between two parts of the restoration or the tooth respectively. A fracture within one of the materials may result clinically in a loss of retention as well, but its cause must be distinguished.

When the retention is lost at one abutment, either the complete prosthodontic reconstruction will feel loose, causing only slight symptoms in a tooth with non-vital pulp, or it will still be functioning satisfactorily and the partially lost retention remains undetected by the patient. In these cases the diagnosis of the retention loss is difficult but important. A gap between crown and tooth gives access to bacteria, possibly causing caries or periapical inflammation, depending on the location of the gap and the seal of the remaining barrier between the gap and the apex. Furthermore, the forces acting on the remaining reconstruction are higher, with an increasing risk of fracture or subsequent loss of retention of the other abutments. Therefore, it is of the utmost importance not to omit the minute check of the fit of every single abutment in a prosthodontic reconstruction at every recall examination.

The marginal fit is checked with a suitable explorer by trying to penetrate between the tooth and the restoration margin from an apical direction. If a gap cannot be felt, the movement of the restoration can be checked by applying a rocking and a push–pull motion with the fingers. In the case of a loose restoration, a movement of saliva along the cavo surface margin may be observed during this action. Movement at the margin should be

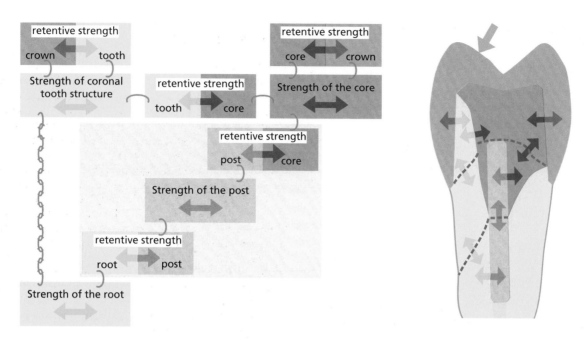

Fig. 12.1   Parts of a restored abutment tooth, with the weak points that have to withstand the acting forces compared with a system of chains.

Core concept 12.1

From a mechanical point of view in a prosthodontic reconstruction all parts of the restored abutment tooth and their junctions must resist the forces that act upon them. The strength of the complete reconstruction can be compared with a chain in which every link is one of the separate parts of the reconstruction, of the biological structures or their connections. Each chain is only as strong as its weakest link. In the case of two parallel chains, the overall strength is as high as the sum of the strengths of both chains, so when one is strong enough there is no need for the other one.

The term 'strength' means both the internal (tensile) strength of part of the reconstruction as well as the retentive (bond) strength between two parts.

In the case of an abutment tooth restored with a post and core, the links of the chains are as shown in Fig. 12.1.

Key literature 12.1

In 1986 Randow and Glantz (33) carried out a clinical experiment of exceptional design: in teeth of test persons they cemented crowns with extension bars to the buccal temporarily on matched pairs of neighboring or contralateral teeth, one being vital and one root-filled, supported with an individual cast post and core. Weights were applied at different lever arm positions until the test persons experienced pain. The pain loading level of the root filled teeth was more than twice as high as in the vital teeth. The experiment was repeated under local anesthesia but terminated at a loading level exceeding 125% of the root filled tooth without anesthesia. Under these conditions no difference in the reaction levels within the pair of teeth was observed, but in one root filled tooth a coronal dentine fracture occurred and the cemented post lost its retention.

These results show that root-treated teeth behave differently to vital teeth with regard to their tactile reactivity.

---

viewed using a magnifying glass. In the case of a subgingival margin, this examination is done with a suitable explorer.

Factors influencing retention

Retention of a crown

Factors influencing the retention of a crown on a prepared tooth are:

- Length of the prepared tooth
- Convergence angle
- Roughness of the preparation
- Roughness of the inner surface of the restoration
- Cementing agent.

Retention of a core build-up

The more the retention of the crown takes place on the build-up, the more important is its retention at the tooth. The build-up is attached to the tooth mechanically and/or chemically, depending on the material used. A plastic filling material can be condensed or syringed into undercuts, retention grooves or into the cervical part of the root canal. Additionally, it can be fixed by means of intradental pins or a post.

Retention of a post

The retention of a post depends on:

- Its design (tapered, parallel, individual)
- Insertion depth
- Macroretentions (thread, serrations)
- Microretentions (surface roughness)
- Cementing agent in combination with pretreatment of the dentine surface.

Fractures

Cohesive failure within a material occurs as a fracture.

Fractures of the superstructure

A fracture within the superstructure of a prosthesis does not depend on the endodontic treatment and can happen in a vital abutment as well, with the only difference that the reflective control of bite forces is reduced (33) due to the loss of receptors in the pulp or a change in the mechanoreceptor function in the periodontal membrane.

Core/post fractures

Core: The fracture susceptibility of a core build-up depends mostly on its dimensions, the material's strength and the forces acting upon it. Regarding these forces, there are major differences between anterior and posterior teeth in the amount and direction of force, the ratio between length and diameter and the area of the bonded surface. When a post is used, its coronal end can weaken the core build-up and exert stress, depending on its size and shape.

Post: A post often is the most retentive link in the chain of retention so will be more likely to cause fracture in the case of overload. Either it breaks itself or it fractures the root, depending on the strength of both. The fracture susceptibility of a post depends on the diameter, the material and the manufacturing process. It makes a great difference to the strength of the metal structure whether it is cast or wrought.

Tooth fractures

Factors influencing fracture risk

(1) *Mechanical properties of non-vital dentine.* For a long time endodontically treated teeth were thought to be more brittle due to a loss of moisture content. Several studies have investigated the mechanical properties of dentine in vital versus non-vital teeth

---

> ### Key literature 12.2
>
> Sedgley and Messer (38) investigated the dentine in vital versus root-filled teeth: 23 matched pairs of contralateral teeth freshly extracted for prosthodontic reasons were subjected to different mechanical tests. One of the corresponding teeth was vital and the other was endodontically treated 1–25 years ago (mean 10.1 years). Into two slices of dentine 0.3 mm thick cut from the necks of the teeth, holes of 1 mm diameter were punched in a universal testing machine and the shear strength and toughness were calculated from the stress–strain curve. Additionally, in one of the slices the Vickers hardness was determined midway between the root canal and the periphery. The coronal root canal openings of the remaining roots were prepared as a seat for a cone-shaped steel rod, followed by loading the teeth until fracture in an axial direction.
>
> Neither the punch shear strength or toughness nor the load to fracture differed significantly between vital and root-filled teeth. The hardness of the cervical dentine was 3.5% lower in endodontically treated teeth.
>
> These findings indicate that teeth do not become more brittle following endodontic treatment.

(Key literature 12.2). Although the moisture content did vary significantly, the compression strength and tensile strength did not show any significant difference (14). Other factors may be more responsible for the increased fracture susceptibility of endodontically treated teeth.

(2) *Amount of remaining tooth structure.* The loss of internal tooth structure in an endodontically treated tooth will be more responsible for its higher susceptibility to fracture than changes in its mechanical properties. Teeth with intact marginal ridges with only a small access preparation are most resistant against fracture and are not significantly weaker than intact teeth without any preparation (2, 10, 30, 34, 44). From a prosthodontic point of view, a maximum of internal tooth structure should be preserved to minimize the fracture risk. Thus, desirably the access would be minimal, i.e. just large enough to gain access to the canal. From this point of view the preparation of the canal, especially in the cervical area, should be as small as possible. This prosthodontic desire stands in contrast to modern endodontic concepts, where the direct straight access to the canal with a wide access opening for good overview is a general demand and good cervical flaring is recommended to ensure an optimal apical preparation, especially in curved canals. In more demanding root canal treatment it might be necessary to sacrifice sound tooth structure. In nearly straight canals the preservation of tooth structure can be the primary goal. The

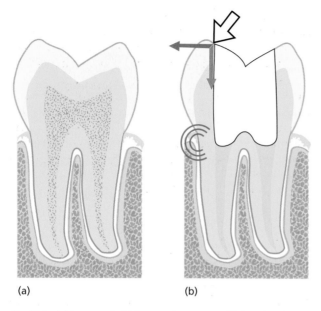

Fig. 12.2 (a) Intact tooth. (b) Forces acting on a root-filled tooth and resulting stress peak.

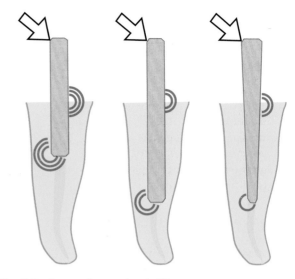

Fig. 12.3 Stress peaks at teeth with different posts.

prosthodontic reconstruction determines the forces acting on the tooth. The amount of tooth structure left after preparation determines its ability to carry loads. Which type of reconstruction is best suited for the remaining tooth structure needs to be judged at the very beginning of treatment.

When one or both of the proximal walls are lost, the tooth is substantially weakened as the support of the circumferential marginal ridges (and the roof of the pulp chamber) is lost and a horizontal force on a cusp acts over a long lever-arm on the weakest part in the cervical area, normally just above the alveolar crest. When a force acts on the oblique inner slopes of the cusps it will be divided into a vertical and a horizontal component, the latter exerting high stresses in the weak cervical portion (Fig. 12.2). Therefore an effective bonding or cuspal coverage is necessary whenever a proximal wall is lost and the cusps are not flat due to abrasion or anatomical form.

The (tensile) bond strength of any material to dentine is always weaker than the (tensile) strength of dentine. Therefore, the preservation of a maximum amount of dentine bulk should be the aim in endodontic therapy of an abutment tooth.

(3) *Type of post*. The type of post determines the amount of stress. Tapered posts, in contrast to parallel posts, lead to radial forces when loaded that are comparable to those of a wedge, and sharp edges (at the end of a post or at a tap) will induce stress, increasing the risk of root fracture (29, 42, 45).

(4) *Length of post*. The longer a post, the better the distribution of stresses, resulting in reduced stress at the apical end of the post because of leverage (Fig. 12.3) (15, 43). Extending the length to two-thirds of the root length results in a superior fracture resistance compared with short posts (16).

There is a lack of clinical data regarding the length of posts in relation to the level of alveolar bone, but it seems more favorable to extend the post below the alveolar crest when a post cannot be avoided.

(5) *Post diameter*. The thicker a post, the thinner and weaker will be the remaining tooth structure, leading to increased risk of fracture. On the other hand, a post must be thick and stiff enough to transmit lateral forces to the root uniformly. Normally, depending on the diameter of the root, the post diameter should not exceed 1.5 mm and in fragile roots this is less.

Perforations

Invaginations of the external root surface – stripping perforations

Roots are seldom round and often show curves, invaginations, flutes or other varieties in shape. The distal root of a mandibular molar is kidney-shaped in its cross-section, so care must be taken not to place the post preparation in the middle of the canal but in the bulkiest part of the root, i.e. the buccal or lingual edge (Fig. 12.4).

The mesial root of a lower molar and the mesiobuccal root of an upper molar are mostly curved in the distal direction. The most cervical parts of the canals go mostly

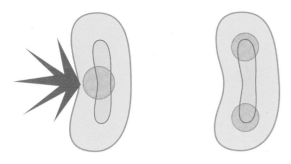

Fig. 12.4 Wrong and right placement of post in distal root of lower molar.

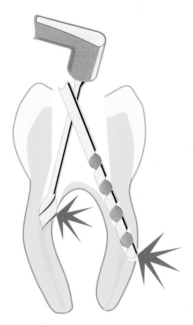

Fig. 12.5 Danger of perforation in curved canals.

in the mesial direction, so when this initial curve is not removed during the access preparation there is great danger of stripping perforation into the interradicular space or in the mesial direction (Fig. 12.5). Proper flaring and, especially, anticurvature filing are important not only to gain a straight access for the apical preparation of the canal but also for safe preparation of the post space (7).

Curvatures not perceptible in the X-ray
Even if the cervical part of the canal is straight, a more apical curvature may limit the length of a post. The most dangerous curvatures are in the plane not perceptible on the X-ray picture. Only knowledge of the anatomy of the root prevents perforation during preparation of a post space, e.g. the palatal roots of upper bicuspids and molars.

Deviation of the prepared canal
Gates–Glidden drills as well as Peeso reamers and some specific drills for post systems have a non-cutting self-centering tip, which ensures that the preparation of the post space will not deviate from a guiding canal being enlarged concentrically. In the case of a root filled tooth, the center of the root filling is the guiding structure. When the root filling deviates from the original canal, the center of the root filling is no longer the center of the root. Enlarging a deviated canal preparation concentrically can cause a lateral perforation, depending on the amounts of deviation, enlargement and dentine bulk in that direction.

Use of end-cutting drills
Special care must be taken when using the end-cutting drills provided with many post systems. Even when driven by hand, they can easily deviate from the canal. Therefore, removal of the root filling and preparation of the canal space should be done using drills with a non-cutting tip prior to use of the drills for these post systems (8, 31).

Excessive length/diameter
When a post is longer than the straight portion of the canal, a perforation is likely to occur. With increasing diameter of the post, not only the fracture risk but also the risk of perforation increases significantly, therefore a post should always be as thin as possible, i.e. just thick enough to gain some guidance and retention within the canal.

Reinfection/bacterial leakage

For leakage in general, see Chapter 13.

Microleakage of cemented posts
A major aim of the root filling is to seal the canal tightly to prevent bacterial leakage from the oral environment to the periapical tissues. Preparing the canal for receiving a post removes a substantial amount of the root filling and may disturb the seal of the remaining filling.

The subsequent cementation of posts may again seal the canal and reduce the risk of infection (9, 49). Adhesive luting of posts leads to a further decrease of leakage (3). However, leakage may occur during post space preparation. Immediate post space preparation is less likely to cause leakage than after complete setting of the sealer (32) and a root filling without tight seal of the access cavity allows leakage of bacteria within a few weeks (5, 48), so the post space preparation and the subsequent luting of the post should be established immediately. Aseptic conditions are imperative during post space preparation and ideally a rubber dam should be used. If impossible, it must be substituted by adequate moisture control and the post space should be irrigated with antiseptic solutions such as sodium hypochlorite, chlorhexidine or alcohol.

Length of root fillings under posts: There is clinical evidence that leaving at least 3 mm of apical root filling under posts decreases the probability of occurrence of periapical lesions (23). *In vitro* studies have shown that a remaining apical root filling of 5 or 7 mm prevents leakage better than one of 3 mm (28, 32), therefore a residual root filling of 3 mm should be the absolute minimum.

Kinds of core build-ups

Core build-up without a post

If enough coronal tooth structure remains to yield retention to a core build-up, a post will not be necessary. The build-up will fill the access cavity, any substance loss caused by caries or other reasons and may increase the height of the abutment. It must be taken into account that in most cases the outward walls of the remaining tooth structure will be reduced in thickness or removed completely during abutment preparation and so will not contribute to the final build-up retention. The retention of the build-up must be achieved at the tooth structure that remains after the final preparation!

Modern dentine adhesives are able to retain composite fillings in cavities without any retentive form but they may be overrated in successfully bonding build-up and prosthodontic reconstruction alone. For build-ups, a mechanical retention in addition to dentine bonding should always be used to gain a maximum overall retention.

The possibilities to achieve mechanical retention are different between single- and multi-rooted teeth. The size of the pulp chamber (in width and depth) in multi-rooted teeth is of considerable advantage for achieving mechanical retention. Undercuts are a natural property of multi-rooted teeth, with divergent canals thus providing excellent mechanical retention.

Because forces acting on all teeth are different and depend on the degree of destruction, further mechanical retention may be necessary via grooves, parapulpal pins or posts. In anterior teeth the forces act in a more horizontal direction and their cross-sectional area is smaller than in posterior teeth, resulting in unfavorable lever-arm relations.

Whenever the remaining tooth structure and the pulpal space support sufficient retention for the build-up, a post will be dispensable and should be avoided

because the risks with the use of posts do not exceed the advantages in most cases.

Post and core systems

When a post is unavoidable there are different ways to establish it.

Prefabricated post/plastic core build-up

In contrast to a direct plastic build-up, an indirect one makes it necessary to remove undercuts, so that tooth structure valuable for strength and retention are removed. With a direct build-up the access cavity can be closed immediately after root filling. If this is done with a composite in combination with a suitable adhesive, the risk of bacterial leakage compared with a provisional closure is minimized. An adhesive build-up contributes more to the reinforcement of the tooth and minimizes the risk of fracture compared with a temporary material necessary during the period of manufacturing the laboratory-made post and core. These temporary materials do not bond to the tooth structure, they do not have the strength and it is necessary to remove them. Whenever a build-up with plastic material is possible it should be preferred (Core concept 12.2).

Cast post and core (direct/indirect technique)

To fabricate a cast post and core there are two different ways:

(1) The direct technique – an acrylic resin is used to form a core build-up directly in the mouth.

Core concept 12.2

The use of a prefabricated post in combination with a build-up in plastic material offers many advantages compared wtih a laboratory-made post:

(1) Saving of tooth structure:
 — undercuts can remain and serve for more retention.
(2) Immediate closure of the prepared canal.
(3) No need for a provisional restoration:
 — less danger of bacterial leakage
 — avoids higher fracture risk during provisional restoration
 — saves chairside time
 — saves cost.

In the case of a composite build-up, additional advantages are:

- Advanced esthetics
- Adhesive technique simply achievable
- Higher bond strength
- Decreased leakage.

(2) The indirect technique – making an impression and fabricating the post and core in the laboratory.

The resin used in the direct technique must be able to be burnt out completely during warming up in the casting procedure. It can be an autopolymerizing resin best used with a brush-on technique, applying alternately liquid and powder with a brush. A more convenient method is the use of a light-curing resin, owing to the individually determined working time and the absence of monomer vapors. Both resins can be prepared with the usual rotating instruments *in situ*. They can be used in combination either with a wrought precious alloy post, onto which the core part is cast, or with a burn-out acrylic post being lost in the cast procedure.

In the indirect technique there are also the two options of using a wrought precious alloy post to cast on or to cast the complete post and core from one metal. The mechanical properties of a wrought metal are superior to a cast one owing to the absence of voids and the more homogeneous structure being independent of the varying parameters of the casting procedure.

Indications for different kinds of core build-ups

The kind of build-up that is best suited for the individual situation depends on:

● The remaining tooth structure.
● The burden of the superstructure.

The ratio of these two factors influences not only the choice of build-up but also the prognosis of the long-term success.

In general, in all cases where sufficient retention can be gained without a post it should be avoided (Fig. 12.6). Whether a post and core should be of plastic material or a cast one is controversial. The plastic materials, especially composites, are usually preferred because their mechanical and adhesive properties have been improved.

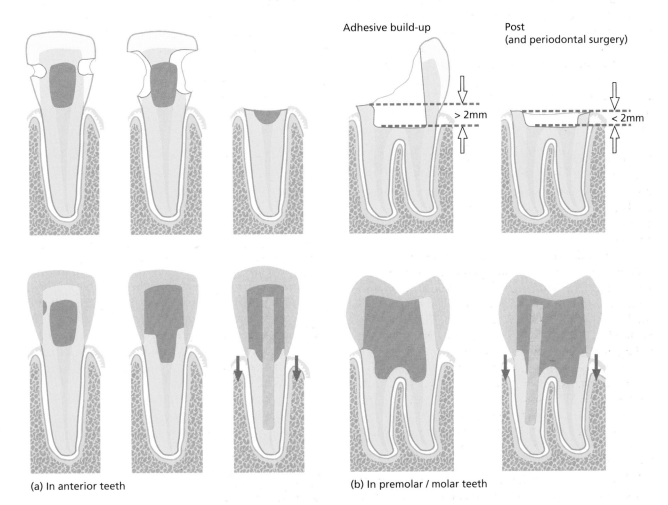

(a) In anterior teeth

(b) In premolar / molar teeth

Fig. 12.6 Indications for different kinds of build-ups in anterior teeth (a) and premolar / molar teeth (b).

Bonding techniques for strengthening tooth structure

When a tooth with an open apex needs endodontic therapy, both the endodontic treatment procedures and the final restoration are a challenge. Because the walls of the root are thin, it is much more susceptible to fracture (47) and therefore an effective reinforcement is a major concern for long-term success. An effective reinforcement can be achieved by filling the post-carrying part of the root with light-curing composite using a transparent light-conducting post. After removal of that post, a prefabricated metal post can be cemented (Fig. 12.7), gaining a higher overall fracture resistance than a custom-made cast post and core, which is adapted to a weakened canal wall (37). By using light-transmitting posts, a curing depth up to 11 mm can be achieved, depending on the diameter of the post (26).

The risk of fracture increases from the beginning of endodontic therapy, so effective protection is necessary between appointments during a longer lasting endodontic treatment aiming at apexification of thin-walled roots. The above-described technique can be used also before finishing the endodontic treatment, allowing access to the apical part of the canal. A strengthening effect of an internal composite reinforcement up to 3 mm apical to the cemento-enamel junction has been verified (19).

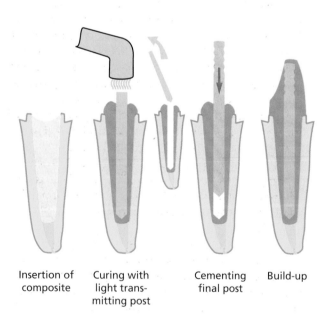

Insertion of composite   Curing with light trans-mitting post   Cementing final post   Build-up

Fig. 12.7   Clinical procedure for strengthening thin-walled root: insertion of composite; curing with light-transmitting post; cementing final post; build-up.

Core build-up materials

Amalgam

Amalgam has been widely used for a long time as a plastic core material. It offers good mechanical and handling properties and has shown its suitability for core build-ups used with posts, pins or other retentive features (17, 25, 30, 46). However, in the discussion about mercury toxicity, this material has gained a bad reputation in latter years and its use for that purpose has been restricted in some countries.

Composites

Composite is the material of choice for a plastic core build-up. In combination with dentine adhesives it offers the possibility of superior bond strength to the tooth structure over the entire surface, leading to higher retentive strength. Its mechanical properties make it suitable even for substitution of more than half of the coronal tooth structure. Depending on the kind and amount of fillers, its hardness can be determined similar to that of dentine, facilitating the final abutment preparation. Its modulus of elasticity should be equal to or higher than that of dentine, resulting in enhanced reinforcement. In anterior teeth it also has aesthetic advantages when used in combination with all-ceramic reconstructions.

Ceramics

Recently, high-performance ceramics were introduced as core build-up materials, especially in anterior teeth. They have not only esthetic advantages but also superior strength. Using a surface pretreatment that depends on the kind of ceramic, they are cemented adhesively to the tooth, gaining a stabilizing effect. The fabrication of a ceramic post–core build-up is comparable to that of a cast metal post and core, not only because it is also done in the laboratory but also because there is the option to use a ceramic pressed around a preformed ceramic post or to fabricate the post–core build-up in one material as glass-infiltrated alumina (20). As a third option, post and core can be separate parts bonded together during the insertion (22).

Cements

Even cements with the highest compressive strength – the metal-reinforced glass ionomer cements – are not suitable as a core build-up material. Compared with composite resins or amalgam in studies regarding frac-

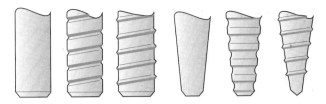

Fig. 12.8 Different types and shapes of posts.

ture resistance, composite resins and amalgam always performed much better.

Resin-modified glass ionomer cements and compomeres, respectively, achieve a fracture strength similar to that of composite, but they undergo a slow expansion under water sorption leading to cracks in overlaying ceramic crowns (40). Thus, they are likely also to exert stress to other restorations and tooth structure.

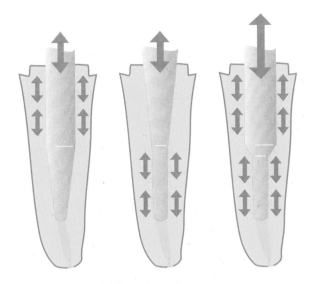

Fig. 12.9 Retention of different shapes of posts.

Post systems and materials

Post systems: cylindrical, tapered, screws

In general, prefabricated posts may be either cylindrical or conical in shape, or a combination of both. Their surface may be smooth, rough or equipped with retentive devices such as grooves or a tap (Fig. 12.8). The two basic shapes have advantages and disadvantages and the principle of gaining retention is different for both geometrical forms.

A smooth cylinder that fits exactly into its matching cylindrical hole has no retention by itself because there is no force perpendicular to the fitting surfaces pressing the cylinder's surface against the hole's wall. By cementing a cylindrical rod into the corresponding hole, a tensile force onto the rod is changed into a shear load onto the cementing agent. The retention depends on the shear bond strength between the luting agent and the two surfaces and the shear strength of that material. This method of force conduction is favorable with respect to the properties of the luting agents commonly used in dentistry.

Any cone-shaped rod fits exactly into its matching hole. Because of the oblique shape of this rod, vertical forces are transformed into radial forces acting on the hole's wall. The amount of this force pressing the rod's surface against the walls depends on the convergence angle. This force increases the friction because friction is a function of the force perpendicular to the interface. On the other hand, this force produces stress over the entire length in a radial direction where the root is most susceptible to longitudinal fracture. When the retention is lost in a conical post it is lost suddenly and completely,

in contrast to a parallel post where, after a first dislocation, there is still residual retention due to the parallel sites of the post.

A parallel post does not stress the root dentine at the walls of the post space but does not match the anatomical form of most of the roots. Thus, a parallel post of adequate diameter in the cervical area and of the same diameter in the apical area produces a potential point of fracture at the end of the post where the diameter of the root decreases, leaving a weak area in the remaining dentine wall. When the end of the post is not rounded or tapered, the sharp edge leads additionally to a peak in the stress of this area and the risk of perforations is high.

The shape of the post also has an influence on the insertion when a luting agent has to flow out of the prepared post hole. Although the space between a tapered post and its preparation diminishes continuously during insertion, a precisely fitting parallel post has a very small space for cement to escape from the very beginning of insertion. Thus, a parallel post must always have a venting groove for escape of the luting agent.

Each shape has distinct disadvantages of its own but by using suitable combinations (Fig. 12.9) these can be decreased. The most retentive one of these is a parallel post with a diameter decreasing in steps (right illustration in Fig. 12.9).

Surface structure, i.e. roughness, is of importance for both the post and the post's space. Different means are used to achieve sufficient surface roughness. Posts may be sandblasted, whereas the post's space may be roughened by mechanical means or chemically pretreated to gain micromechanical retention. Serrations of the post add significantly to retention.

Post materials

Metals

The most important mechanical property of a post material is Young's modulus for stiffness and tensile strength, resulting in fracture strength against bending forces. From that point of view stainless steel is superior to precious alloys and pure titanium. Under unfavorable conditions, which might be the case in the clinical situation, stainless steel is not resistant against corrosion. Corrosion may lead to loss of retention, structural weakening with subsequent post fracture or, most deleterious, to root fracture due to the expansion of the corrosion products. Stainless steel is therefore no longer licensed in Europe. Precious alloys showing no corrosion are somewhat weaker but still strong enough when used as a wrought post. They are the materials of choice for a cast post and core. Cobalt–chromium-based alloys are an economical alternative but they require troublesome work in the laboratory procedures.

The problems associated with the casting technology of titanium are due to the low specific weight and the high melting point, therefore it is necessary to check every cast object against porosities by X-rays but it cannot be excluded that microporosities still remain undetected to weaken a cast post and core. The mechanical properties of machined titanium alloy posts are superior compared with cast pure titanium individual post and cores (18).

Fiber-reinforced resins

Recently, epoxy-based carbon-fiber posts were marketed, followed by quartz and glass-fiber posts. They are luted adhesively and used in combination with a composite core material. *In vitro* studies have shown that the fracture resistance is lower compared with that of metal posts. But the mode of failure is fracture of the post or cervical root fracture, which is more favorable than the often much deeper root fractures of the metal posts. Furthermore, the fiber posts are easy to remove in the case of retreatment (27, 39).

Ceramics

In latter years new ceramics with high strength have come into clinical use as promising materials for full ceramic reconstructions: namely yttrium oxide partially stabilized zirconia and glass-infiltrated aluminium oxide ceramics (22). They offer high strength, the former produced as prefabricated posts and the latter used for custom-made post and core construction. Fabrication by cutting the shape out of a prefabricated block is also possible with these materials. Although a zirconia post is as strong as a titanium post and has a higher stiffness (1),

its use should be judged carefully. There are still no long-term clinical results and the removal of such a post if retreatment should become necessary might be impossible, or at least conducted with a very time consuming procedure, leading to excessive dentine loss and a high risk of lateral root perforations.

Preparation techniques for posts

Moment of post preparation

After finishing the endodontic treatment it is essential to take precautions so that the risk for bacterial leakage along the remaining root filling is avoided. The final restoration therefore should be established as soon as possible (5, 48). Another reason for an immediate preparation of the post space is so that the dentist is still familiar with the individual canal anatomy.

Heat

The safest method of removing the root filling material without leaving the canal is by hot instruments and they should be used always as a first step in achieving the post space preparation. A hot plugger is introduced into the canal, repeatedly softening and removing the gutta-percha until most of the length is cleared. The use of solvent agents to soften the gutta-percha is obsolete because their action cannot be limited and there is evidence of more leakage after their use (28).

Rotating instruments

The next step in preparing the post space is the use of rotating instruments. It is essential to begin with instruments equipped with a non-cutting tip. In contrast to Gates–Glidden drills, Peeso reamers ensure a straight preparation. The drills are used in ascending diameters with low speed to avoid excessive heat (36). Orifice openers can also be used. The size of the last file gives an orientation about the appropriate diameter for the post. As soon as the rotating instrument cuts into dentine over almost all of the circumference, the corresponding drill of the post system is used. These drills often have end-cutting tips so they must be used very carefully and only for the final preparation to avoid perforations. After completing the preparation, an X-ray should be performed with the post in place to ensure its proper positioning.

Length of posts

This is limited by the curvature of the root and the necessary root filling needed to prevent leakage. An absolute minimum of 3 mm of apical root filling should remain (23). The length of a cylindrical post may be limited owing to excessive weakening of the root at the apical end of the post.

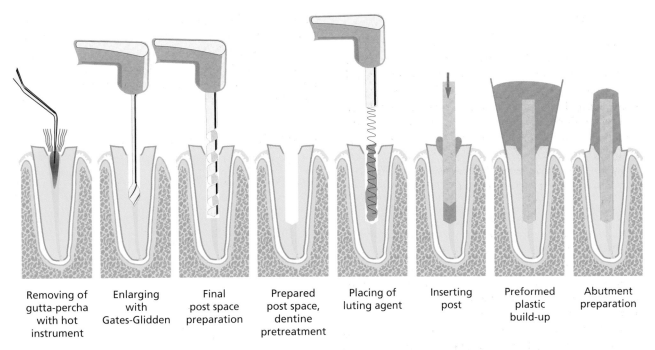

| Removing of gutta-percha with hot instrument | Enlarging with Gates-Glidden | Final post space preparation | Prepared post space, dentine pretreatment | Placing of luting agent | Inserting post | Preformed plastic build-up | Abutment preparation |

Fig. 12.10 Clinical procedure for preparing and inserting a post.

Cementing posts

The retention of a post depends more on factors such as shape, length and surface roughness than on the cementing agent. The cementing agent has to fill the gap between post and dentine wall and to transduce the forces between both. The classical cementing agent for fixed restorations is zinc phosphate cement. It is still the material of choice for metal posts in a standard situation because it is uncritical in handling and regarding dentine pretreatment. It is removable by ultrasonic instruments when retreatment is necessary. Resin cements are required for adhesive luting of ceramic or carbon-fiber posts. They require an adequate dentine pretreatment for removing or modifying the smear layer that is always present on mechanically treated dentine surfaces. On using dentine adhesives the manufacturer's instructions must be followed carefully. Of all resin cements, the most widely used and best proven contains active phosphate monomers. It has superior bond strength, especially towards metal. The curing has a distinct oxygen-prohibiting effect so that spreading on the mixing pad can prolong the working time.

In the cementing procedure it is essential to ensure dry conditions. The post space is rinsed with water and dried with paper points. Also, in the case of the use of zinc phosphate cement, removing the smear layer with ethylenediaminetetraaceticacid (EDTA) is recommended to clean the canal and enhance retention. The cement is mixed to a creamy consistency and applied with a lentulo spiral into the post preparation. The post is than seated carefully until it reaches the bottom of the preparation and left to harden undisturbed.

When using fast-setting resins the use of a lentulo spiral may be fateful because premature setting may hinder complete positioning of the post. When using these materials only the post is coated with the cement (21).

Prosthodontic reconstruction

Single tooth

The simplest case of prosthodontic reconstruction is the restoration of a single tooth. Often a prosthodontic reconstruction can be substituted by a composite filling (Fig. 12.11). When the composite is bonded to etched enamel and dentine by use of a suitable adhesive, the fracture resistance is increased considerably (11). As a temporary solution, an amalgam filling is also possible (Fig. 12.12). In the case of lost proximal ridges, a cuspal coverage should be established to reduce the risk of fracture (12, 13). Such an amalgam filling can last for some years and allow a proper observation period. Later on, the filling can remain as a core build-up and be prepared to receive the final cast restoration. This is also a cost benefit for the patient.

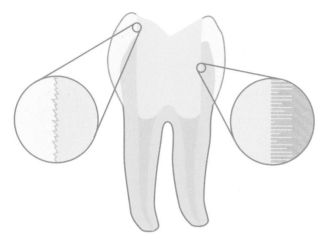

Fig. 12.11   Composite restoration.

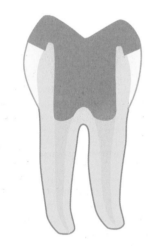

Fig. 12.12   Amalgam restoration.

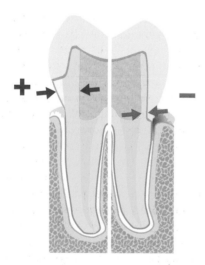

Fig. 12.13   Crown with different levels of preparation.

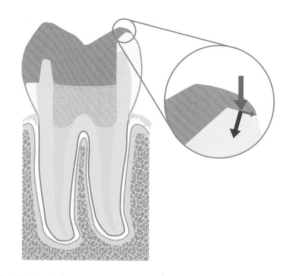

Fig. 12.14   Onlay.

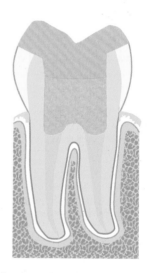

Fig. 12.15   Ceramic onlay.

When the crown preparation is carried out the margin of the preparation should end as high as possible to the occlusal in order not to weaken the cervical area, which is weakened from the inside during endodontic therapy (Fig. 12.13). For this reason a partial crown or an onlay (Fig. 12.14) with a maximum preservation of sound tooth structure is most desirable. In an onlay, even minimal embracing of a cusp ensures that occlusal forces cannot act in a horizontal direction (see detail in Fig. 12.14).

In the case of thin remaining walls of coronal tooth structure and esthetic demands, a full ceramic restoration (Fig. 12.15) offers the advantage of adhesive bonding throughout the entire surface (35) and can be made as a core build-up and crown restoration in one piece (Fig. 12.16), which is desirable in the case of substantial loss of tooth structure (6).

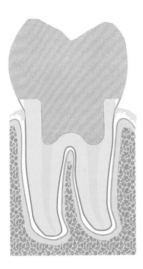

Fig. 12.16 Full ceramic 'endo-crown'.

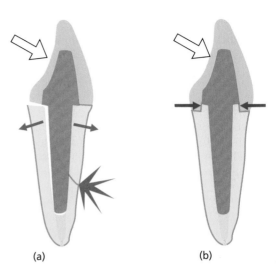

(a)   (b)

Fig. 12.17   (a) Risk of fracture without ferrule. (b) Effect of ferrule.

Preparation principles

Internal loss of tooth structure

The reduction of internal tooth structure takes place in several steps during the endodontic and restorative treatment:

- Access cavity
- Coronal flaring
- Preparing the root canal
- Preparing the post space (if needed)
- Removing undercuts, if a custom cast post and core will be established.

Although sufficient access and proper flaring are necessary for the success of endodontic treatment, every loss of dentine weakens the tooth (12). Thus, when a tooth serving or going to be used as an abutment needs endodontic treatment, the preservation of tooth structure must be considered during the endodontic procedure as well. When a tooth is already provided with a crown, it is highly recommended to remove the reconstruction before gaining access to the pulp chamber. This is done to achieve better orientation concerning two aspects: because the tooth has lost its natural shape, cervical or interradicular perforations are more likely to occur; and the amount of coronal dentine left is clearly visible. After endodontic treatment the decision for the kind of build-up is facilitated. Leaving the reconstruction in place makes the determination of the amount of coronal dentine impossible and allows only a blind estimation unless the reconstruction enables radiographic examination, as in the case of full ceramic crowns.

Ferrule design

Special care must be taken in the restoration of a tooth with a minimal amount of remaining coronal tooth

Key literature 12.3

In 1995 Libman and Nicholls (24) divided 25 extracted human central incisors into five groups and prepared them for complete cast crowns. Test teeth had cast dowel cores fabricated, with the ferrule height varying from 0.5 to 2.0 mm in 0.5-mm increments. The five control teeth did not have cast dowel cores. A 4.0-kg load was applied cyclically to each of the restored teeth at an angle of 135° to the long axis of each tooth at a rate of 72 cycles per minute. The load application point was predetermined by a waxing jig that was used to wax all crowns. An electrical resistance strain gauge was used to provide evidence of preliminary failure. Preliminary failure was defined here as the loss of the sealing cement layer between crown and tooth. The results of this study showed that the 0.5-mm and 1.0-mm ferrule lengths failed at a significantly lower number of cycles than the 1.5-mm and 2.0-mm ferrule lengths and control teeth.

structure, i.e. when the complete clinical crown is decayed and only the root remains. In this case a post will be necessary for sufficient retention. Generally, with decreasing root length the crown length will increase, resulting in an unfavorable ratio of leverage of crown versus root. Horizontal loads are supported and transferred by the post to the root, resulting in extreme tensile stress and thus increasing the risk of root fracture dramatically. A marginal preparation that embraces the root effectively participates in the transfer of horizontal forces onto the root and decreases the forces transferred by the post cervically on the opposite side (Fig. 12.17). Such an embracing collar is usually called a ferrule (Key literature 12.3). A prerequisite is the establishment of a ferrule of 1.5–2 mm (4, 14, 24, 41). If this is not possible, primarily a surgical crown lengthening procedure should be considered.

For prosthodontic reconstructions substituting lost teeth a higher burden onto the remaining abutment teeth must be considered.

References

1. Asmussen E, Peutzfeldt A, Heitmann T. Stiffness, elastic limit and strength of newer types of endodontic posts. *J. Dent.* 1999; 27: 275–8.

2. Ausiello P, De Gee AJ, Rengo S, Davidson CL. Fracture resistance of endodontically-treated premolars adhesively restored. *Am. J. Dent.* 1997; 10: 237–41.

3. Bachicha WS, DiFiore PM, Miller DA, Lautenschlager EP, Pashley DH. Microleakage of endodontically treated teeth restored with posts. *J. Endodont.* 1998; 24: 703–8.

4. Barkhordar RA, Radke RA, Abbasi J. Effect of metal collars on resistance of endodontically treated teeth to root fracture. *J. Prosthet. Dent.* 1989; 61: 676–8.

5. Barthel CR, Strobach A, Briedigkeit H, Göbel UB, Roulet JF. Leakage in roots coronally sealed with different temporary fillings. *J. Endodont.* 1999; 25: 731–4.

6. Bindl A, Mörmann WH. Clinical evaluation of adhesively placed Cerec endo-crowns after 2 years – preliminary results. *J. Adhes. Dent.* 1999; 1: 255–65.

7. DeCleen MJH. The relationship between the root canal filling and post space preparation. *Int. Endodont. J.* 1993; 26: 53–8.

8. Gegauff AG, Kerby RE, Rosenstiel SF. A comparative study of post preparation diameters and deviations using para-post and Gates Glidden drills. *J. Endodont.* 1988; 14: 377–80.

9. Gish SP, Drake DR, Walton RE, Wilcox LR. Coronal leakage: bacterial penetration through obturated canals following post preparation. *J. Am. Dent. Assoc.* 1994; 125: 1369–72.

10. Hansen EK. In vivo cusp fracture of endodontically treated premolars restored with MOD amalgam or MOD resin fillings. *Dent. Mater.* 1988; 4: 169–73.

11. Hansen EK, Asmussen E. In vivo fractures of endodontically treated posterior teeth restored with enamel-bonded resin. *Endodont. Dent. Traumatol.* 1990; 6: 218–25.

12. Hansen EK, Asmussen E. Cusp fracture of endodontically treated posterior teeth restored with amalgam. *Acta. Odontol. Scand.* 1993; 51: 73–7.
   1584 teeth with class II amalgam fillings after endodontic treatment done by 91 Danish dentists were analyzed. They were divided into subgroups treated before 1975 or after 1979. In the latter period the frequency and severity of fractures increased significantly. It is suggested that weakening of the cervical part of the root due to the introduction of Gates–Glidden burs and the use of expanding high-copper amalgam may be the most important reasons.

13. Hansen EK, Asmussen E, Christiansen NC. In vivo fractures of endodontically treated posterior teeth restored with amalgam. *Endodont. Dent. Traumatol.* 1990; 6: 49–55.

14. Huang TJG, Schilder H, Nathanson D. Effects of moisture content and endodontic treatment on some mechanical properties of human dentine. *J. Endodont.* 1992; 18: 209–15.

15. Hunter AJ, Feiglin B, Williams JF. Effects of post placement on endodontically treated teeth. *J. Prosthet. Dent.* 1989; 62: 166–72.

16. Isidor F, Brøndum K, Ravnholt G. The influence of post length and crown ferrule length on the resistance to cyclic loading of bovine teeth with prefabricated titanium posts. *Int. J. Prosthodont.* 1999; 12: 78–82.

17. Kane JJ, Burgess JO, Summitt JB. Fracture resistance of amalgam coronal-radicular restorations. *J. Prosthet. Dent.* 1990; 63: 607–13.

18. Kappert HF. Titan als Werkstoff für die zahnärztliche Prothetik und Implantologie [Titanium as a material for dental prosthetics and implants]. *Dtsch. Zahnärztl. Z.* 1994; 49: 573–83.

19. Katebzadeh N, Dalton BC, Trope M. Strengthening immature teeth during and after apexification. *J. Endodont.* 1998; 24: 256–9.

20. Kern M, Pleimes AW, Strub JR. Bruchfestigkeit metallischer und vollkeramischer Stiftkernaufbauten. [Fracture strengths of metallic and all-ceramic post-and-core restorations]. *Dtsch. Zahnärztl. Z.* 1995; 50: 451–3.

21. Kostka EC, Roulet J-F. Retention of posts luted with different materials after root filling with Eugenol containing sealer. *J. Dent. Res.* 1998; 77: 680.

22. Koutayas SO, Kern M. All-ceramic posts and cores: the state of the art. *Quintess. Int.* 1999; 30: 383–92.

23. Kvist T, Rydin E, Reit C. The relative frequency of periapical lesions in teeth with root canal-retained posts. *J. Endodont.* 1989; 15: 578–80.

24. Libman WJ, Nicholls JI. Load fatigue of teeth restored with cast posts and cores and complete crowns. *Int. J. Prosthodont.* 1995; 8: 155–61.

25. Lovdahl PE, Nicholls JI. Pin-retained amalgam cores vs. cast-gold dowel-cores. *J. Prosthet. Dent.* 1977; 38: 507–14.

26. Lui JL. Depth of composite polymerization within simulated root canals using light-transmitting posts. *Oper. Dent.* 1994; 19: 165–8.

27. Mannocci F, Ferrari M, Watson TF. Intermittent loading of teeth restored using quartz fiber, carbon-quartz fiber, and zirconium dioxide ceramic root canal posts. *J. Adhes. Dent.* 1999; 1: 153–8.

28. Mattison GD, Delivanis PD, Thacker RWJ, Hassell KJ. Effect of post preparation on the apical seal. *J. Prosthet. Dent.* 1984; 51: 785–9.

29. Mentink AGB, Creugers NHJ, Hoppenbrouwers PMM, Meeuwissen R. Qualitative assessment of stress distribution during insertion of endodontic posts in photoelastic material. *J. Dent.* 1998; 26: 125–31.

30. Oliveira FC, Denehy GE, Boyer DB. Fracture resistance of endodontically prepared teeth using various restorative materials. *J. Am. Dent. Assoc.* 1987; 115: 57–60.

31. Pilo R, Tamse A. Residual dentine thickness in mandibular premolars prepared with Gates Glidden and Para-Post drills. *J. Prosthet. Dent.* 2000; 83: 617–23.

32. Portell FR, Bernier WE, Lorton L, Peters DD. The effect of immediate versus delayed dowel space preparation on the integrity of the apical seal. *J. Endodont.* 1982; 8: 154–60.

33. Randow K, Glantz PO. On cantilever loading of vital and non-vital teeth. An experimental clinical study. *Acta. Odontol. Scand.* 1986; 44: 271–7.

34. Reeh ES, Douglas WH, Messer HH. Stiffness of endodontically-treated teeth related to restoration technique. *J. Dent. Res.* 1989; 68: 1540–44.

35. Roulet JF. Benefits and disadvantages of tooth-coloured alternatives to amalgam. *J. Dent.* 1997; 25: 459–73.

36. Saunders EM, Saunders WP. The heat generated on the external root surface during post space preparation. *Int. Endodont. J.* 1989; 22: 169–73.

37. Saupe WA, Gluskin AH, Radke RAJ. A comparative study of fracture resistance between morphologic dowel and cores and a resin-reinforced dowel system in the intraradicular restoration of structurally compromised roots. *Quintess. Int.* 1996; 27: 483–91.

38. Sedgley CM, Messer HH. Are endodontically treated teeth more brittle? *J. Endodont.* 1992; 18: 332–5.

39. Sidoli GE, King PA, Setchell DJ. An in vitro evaluation of a carbon fiber-based post and core system. *J. Prosthet. Dent.* 1997; 78: 5–9.

40. Sindel J, Frankenberger R, Krämer N, Petschelt A. Crack formation of all-ceramic crowns dependent on different core build-up and luting materials. *J. Dent.* 1999; 27: 175–81.

41. Sorensen JA, Engelman MJ. Ferrule design and fracture resistance of endodontically treated teeth. *J. Prosthet. Dent.* 1990; 63: 529–36.
    This study evaluated the fracture resistance of teeth provided with a cast post and core and crown with various ferrule designs and amounts of coronal tooth structure. One millimeter of coronal tooth structure above the shoulder preparation substantially increased the fracture resistance. A bevel of 1 mm at an angle of 60° at either the toothcore junction or the crown margin was ineffective. The thickness of axial tooth structure at the crown margin did not appreciably improve resistance to fracture.

42. Städtler P, Wimmershoff M, Shookoi H, Wernisch J. Kraftübertragung von vorgefertigten Wurzelkanalstiften. [The stress transmission of prefabricated root canal posts]. *Schweiz. Monatsschr. Zahnmed.* 1995; 105: 1418–24.

43. Standlee JP, Caputo AA, Collard EW, Pollack MH. Analysis of stress distributions by endodontic posts. *Oral Surg.* 1972; 33: 952–60.

44. Steele A, Johnson BR. In vitro fracture strength of endodontically treated premolars. *J. Endodont.* 1999; 25: 6–8.

45. Thorsteinsson TS, Yaman P, Craig RG. Stress analyses of four prefabricated posts. *J. Prosthet. Dent.* 1992; 67: 30–33.

46. Tjan AH, Dunn JR, Lee JK. Fracture resistance of amalgam and composite resin cores retained by various intradentinal retentive features. *Quintess. Int.* 1993; 24: 211–17.

47. Tjan AH, Whang SB. Resistance to root fracture of dowel channels with various thicknesses of buccal dentine walls. *J. Prosthet. Dent.* 1985; 53: 496–500.

48. Torabinejad M, Ung B, Kettering JD. In vitro bacterial penetration of coronally unsealed endodontically treated teeth. *J. Endodont.* 1990; 16: 566–9.

49. Wu MK, Pehlivan Y, Kontakiotis EG, Wesselink PR. Microleakage along apical root fillings and cemented posts. *J. Prosthet. Dent.* 1998; 79: 264–9.

Chapter 13
Apical and coronal leakage

William P. Saunders

Apical leakage

It was long considered that there was a link between the quality of the root canal obturation and failure. The leakage of tissue fluids apically around inadequate root fillings was cited as the most common cause of failure. The hollow tube theory (46) propounded that the stasis of fluid in the apical part of the root canal system, with subsequent degradation and the formation of toxic by-products, induced an inflammatory response in the periradicular tissues. An evaluation of failures in an extensive clinical study in the USA (22) suggested that over half could be attributed to a poor apical seal of the root filling. Several studies have shown that failure was correlated with voids present in the root filling in the apical part of the root canal system. Harty *et al.* (20), in a retrospective clinical study, showed that the prognosis for success in root canal treatment was poorer when there were voids apically in the root canal filling. Others attributed one of the major causes of failure to incomplete obturation of the root canal system (1, 39, 58).

Much of this correlation between obturation and failure was based upon an earlier *ex vivo* study (13). Extracted root-filled teeth were examined for quality of obturation using leakage with a radioisotope. Dow and Ingle (13) found that poorly obturated root canals allowed leakage of the isotope through the apical part of the root canal system. This study perpetuated the hollow-tube theory and was termed the percolation theory. The same principle was put forward; namely, that tissue fluids enter the root canal system in cases where there has been insufficient obturation. These fluids then break down and leak back out into the periradicular tissues to generate an inflammatory response. This process has also been termed apical leakage.

However, this would imply that all teeth that have undergone root canal preparation but have not been obturated would be likely to fail as a result of percolation. This is not the case and a number of cases have been reported where healing has occurred without the presence of a root canal filling (11, 27).

A number of subsequent studies have shown that sterile tissue fluid is unable to initiate and sustain an inflammatory reaction and it has now become well established that periradicular periodontitis is caused by micro-organisms or their by-products (4, 31, 54, 55, 60). The aim of root canal treatment is to reduce the microbial flora within the root canal system to allow the body's defenses to initiate and progress healing. It is a delicate balance between host response and infective load that affects healing. Cleaning and shaping the root canal system during root canal treatment removes necrotic and vital pulp tissue and reduces the number of micro-organisms. Further disinfection of the system is achieved using canal dressings that are antimicrobial. It is important that the root canal system is protected from ingress by micro-organisms when the root canal treatment is complete. Obturation with gutta-percha impedes this ingress by:

- Providing a physical barrier to the movement of micro-organisms and their by-products.
- Possessing inherent antimicrobial activity.

Unfortunately the commonly used materials for obturation of the root canal system do not provide a complete seal. Leakage does take place and this may be at such a level that the host response cannot cope and failure occurs.

Micro-organisms, their by-products and the products of tissue breakdown may leak through the apical delta of the root canal and generate an inflammatory response in the periradicular tissues. This also, rather confusingly, could be termed apical leakage. The leakage may be initiated by:

- Micro-organisms that remain in the root canal system after preparation has been completed. Indeed, it is probably impossible to remove all the micro-organisms and necrotic debris from the root canal system, especially from the apical delta, with currently available methods for root canal treatment.
- Subsequent ingress of micro-organisms from the oral cavity. The mouth is a limitless reservoir of micro-

organisms and any deficiencies in the coronal part of the tooth structure may allow invasion by micro-organisms themselves, their by-products or nutrients to sustain organisms already present in the root canal system or dentine. This ingress is known as coronal leakage and may eventually reach the apical tissues.

Coronal leakage

The oral cavity provides a constant source of micro-organisms, some species of which, if given the opportunity, will invade the root canal system of the root-filled tooth. Obturated root canals may be contaminated by micro-organisms in a number of ways:

- Delay in placing a definitive coronal restoration after root canal obturation. Various temporary cements have satisfactory sealing properties but all tend to dissolve slowly in the presence of saliva and the seal may be disrupted.
- Fracture of the coronal restoration or the tooth. Cracks within the coronal tooth structure or across a restoration may allow ingress of micro-organisms. These often occur without the knowledge of the patient and may be present for some time before treatment is undertaken.
- Through exposed dentinal tubules of a root where cementum is not present.
- Caries at the margin of the restoration. Caries progresses painlessly in root-filled teeth and it may be extensive before treatment is received.
- Preparation of post space during preparation of a post-retained restoration, especially when an indirect technique is used requiring the provision of a temporary post.

Marshall and Massler (32) first brought the concept of coronal leakage causing failure of root canal treatment to prominence. They used a radioactive tracer to examine the leakage around the coronal restoration. They speculated as to whether the overall seal of the root canal was changed if the coronal seal was broken. They also discussed the prognosis of root canal treatment if the quality of the obturation was poor but the coronal seal was good. It was shown that coronal leakage took place despite the presence of a coronal dressing. Allison et al. (2), when discussing the role of spreader penetration in the quality of the root canal obturation, also made reference to the effect that a poor coronal seal may have on clinical failure. In 1987, Swanson and Madison (56) revived the concept of coronal leakage as a cause of failure of root canal treatment. Madison and Wilcox (29) showed that if root canals were exposed to the oral envi-

Key literature 13.1

Ray and Trope (44) undertook a cross-sectional study of 1010 root-filled teeth. They examined full-mouth periapical radiographs that had been selected randomly. Only teeth that had been restored permanently were included, and teeth with post and core restorations were excluded. The technical quality of the root canal treatment and the coronal restoration were assessed as either good or poor. The periradicular tissues were also evaluated as to the presence or absence of inflammation.

The results showed that the overall rate of absence of signs in the periapical tissues was 61.07%. A good restoration resulted in significantly more cases of no inflammation compared with cases of good root canal therapy (80% versus 75.7%). Conversely, the presence of a poor restoration resulted in significantly more cases of inflammation periapically compared with poor root canal treatment (30.2% versus 48.6%). The combination of a good restoration and a good root canal treatment had a rate of absence of periradicular inflammation of 91.4%, whereas the combination of a poor restoration and a poor root canal treatment had a rate of absence of periradicular inflammation of 18.1%.

The conclusion from this study is that the technical quality of the coronal restoration was significant and perhaps of even more importance than the technical quality of the root canal treatment for health of the periradicular tissues.

ronment coronal leakage took place, which, in some cases, extended to the full length of the root.

Further studies have demonstrated the importance of coronal leakage in the failure of root canal treatment. Torabinejad et al. (59) examined the bacterial coronal leakage of single-rooted extracted root-filled teeth using two micro-organisms. They found that 50% of the teeth were contaminated along the whole length of the root filling after 19 or 42 days, depending on the organism. Interestingly, the motile organism *Proteus vulgaris* was slower to penetrate the root canal system than the non-motile *Staphylococcus epidermis*. Khayat et al. (26) determined the length of time required for the bacteria in natural saliva to penetrate root canals that had been obturated with either vertical or lateral condensed gutta-percha. All root canals were contaminated within 30 days whatever the obturation technique. The penetration of organisms in human saliva was also tested by Magura et al. (30). Salivary penetration was greater after 3 months than four earlier study periods. They considered this contamination to be significant clinically and suggested that root canal retreatment should be undertaken if obturated root canals were exposed to the oral environment for at least 3 months.

It has been recognized that the integrity of the coronal part of the root canal system is paramount for success (44). Ray and Trope's study (44) concluded that the quality of the coronal restoration was more important than the quality of the root canal treatment (Key literature 13.1). The same protocol for this study was applied by Tronstad *et al.* (61) but they found that although the coronal restoration was important for success the endodontic treatment quality was more significant. Ricucci *et al.* (45) had the opportunity to examine the periradicular status of teeth that had not been adequately restored for some time after root canal treatment. They concluded that a root canal system that was well obturated may prevent sufficient numbers of bacteria from penetrating to create a radiographically detectable apical periodontitis. Unfortunately this study was probably underpowered and in their discussion they stress that adequate protection of the coronal part of the root canal filling should be made to prevent leakage. Also in this study, the quality of the root canal treatments was good. This contrasts with the studies by Ray and Trope (44) and Tronstad *et al.* (61), where many of the root fillings were of poor quality.

There is therefore an important continuum between coronal leakage and apical leakage. Micro-organisms, toxins and nutrients enter the root canal system by coronal leakage, and, when they reach the apical part of the root canal, apical leakage into the periradicular tissues can ensue, creating a periradicular periodontitis. Saunders and Saunders (48) have reviewed the role of coronal leakage in the failure of root canal treatment.

Coronal leakage during root canal treatment

An access cavity to the root canal system provides a relatively easy way for microbial invasion to take place. It is essential that the microbial flora is kept to a minimum during root canal treatment. A rubber dam provides the most consistent way of protecting the root canal system from unnecessary contamination. Ideally it should be placed prior to gaining access to the pulp chamber. The crown of the tooth ideally should be disinfected using 30% H_2O_2 followed by 5% KI, but a 0.5% chlorhexidine solution is also beneficial. A temporary dressing should be leak-proof, certainly in the short-term. Studies *in vitro* have demonstrated that most of the materials available for temporary dressings, including cements and proprietary single-component setting pastes, are satisfactory in this respect, although the thickness of the material placed is a very important factor (19, 62). At least 3.5 mm should be placed to minimize the leakage risk (62). The results of these studies are somewhat conflicting, with one study showing that one material is leak-proof and another that the same material performed relatively poorly with considerable leakage.

A leakage study using a microbiological model showed that a light-cured single-paste material provided a better seal to *Streptococcus sanguis* than either Cavit or a fortified zinc oxide–eugenol cement (10). By contrast, another study using an electrochemical impedance technique showed that fortified zinc oxide–eugenol cement gave a better seal than either a light-cured resinous material or Cavit G (24). In a thorough *in vitro* study where seven commonly used temporary restorative materials were tested, only four materials did not exhibit leakage during the 8-week testing period. The fortified zinc oxide–eugenol cement and a polycarboxylate cement were the least effective in preventing leakage (3). If the temporary restoration is considered to be at risk from dislodgement, wear or subsequent leakage, then a two-tier dressing can be placed to give a double seal. The floor of the pulp chamber is covered with a small cotton pledget and the access cavity dressed with a zinc oxide–eugenol-based material covered by a glass polyalkenoate cement. The former has some bactericidal properties and the latter provides some chemical bonding to dentine and enamel, thereby reducing microleakage.

Coronal leakage after root canal treatment

The smear layer and coronal leakage

The interface between the gutta-percha root filling and the wall of the root canal is the weak link for leakage after root canal treatment and is one of the reasons why a sealer is recommended during obturation. However, despite the presence of sealer, it has been suggested that the sealer/canal wall interface is where most leakage takes place (21). When the root canal wall is instrumented mechanically, a layer of debris forms on the surface and extends into the dentinal tubules. This is known as the smear layer (34). This layer cannot be removed adequately with NaOCl or chlorhexidine irrigation fluids. Thus, unless specific efforts are made to remove this layer, most root-filled teeth will have a smear layer intact. The effect that the smear layer has on the prognosis of root canal treatment is unknown (8) but it may be broken down by bacterial toxins and acids (35, 36). This would then allow a pathway through which leakage could take place (41). The role of the smear layer was reviewed by Sen *et al.* in 1995 (52).

A number of studies have shown that coronal leakage may be reduced if the smear layer is removed, despite the method used for obturation (15, 57). Interestingly, if the smear layer is removed, some species of bacteria have more difficulty in adhering to the surface of the dentine (5). Conversely, the presence of the smear layer may actually prevent the penetration of dentine by micro-organisms (14, 28, 38). There is still controversy concerning the role of the smear layer in coronal leakage. If the smear layer is removed and the root filling leaks, subsequently micro-organisms may enter the dentinal tubules. The long-term effect that these micro-organisms may exert is unknown but it may be presumed that if nutrients leak into the tubules then the micro-organisms may multiply and move out into the root canal system. The use of chemically active sealers that bond to the wall of the root canal chemically may be an important way of preventing coronal leakage (43, 51).

Coronal leakage and molar teeth

It has been shown that coronal leakage is a significant problem in multi-rooted teeth (47). The presence of accessory canals in the floor of the pulp chamber may allow the spread of micro-organisms and their toxins into the furcation area (18, 53). The common practice of packing excess gutta-percha across the floor of the pulp chamber should be avoided because considerable leakage will take place (47). The use of amalgam, glass ionomer or cermet cement across the floor of the pulp chamber prevents this leakage (Clinical procedures 13.1 and 13.2). More recently it has been shown that a resin-modified glass ionomer provided a good barrier to coronal microbial leakage (7).

Post-retained restorations and coronal leakage

The removal of root filling to accommodate a post may compromise the seal of the obturation and allow leakage to occur more easily. The retention of 5 mm of well-condensed root filling apically is necessary whenever possible and great care should be taken when removing the existing root filling, especially if it has been present for some time. There is a tendency for the gutta-percha to be twisted or vibrated during removal and this may disrupt the seal (25). The post-space preparation can be undertaken immediately following obturation without deleterious effects on leakage (42), even with the core-carrier obturation methods (50). Clinically it seems that failure of root canal treatment in the presence of a post-retained restoration is a major problem (17, 49). The placement of an adequately cemented post provides as good a barrier to coronal leakage as an intact root filling (64).

Leakage studies

There have been many research studies carried out *in vitro* on leakage in endodontics. Wu and Wesselink (65) have critically reviewed these studies. A marker is usually employed, which may be a dye, radioisotope or bacteria. Root canal treatment is undertaken on extracted teeth and the root surfaces covered with an impervious substance, except for the apex or coronal openings, or both. The teeth are then placed in the

---

Clinical procedure 13.1   Protecting the root canals in molars from coronal leakage

(1) The root canals are obturated in the usual way (a).

(2) Excess gutta-percha and sealer are removed completely from the pulp chamber. The gutta-percha should be seared at the opening of each root canal with a hot instrument. The coronal gutta-percha should be condensed vertically into the root canal. The sealer is removed with a dental excavator and a pledget of cotton wool soaked in alcohol.

(3) The floor of the pulp chamber should be inspected carefully to ensure that the dentine surface is clean.

(4) The floor of the pulp chamber, together with the opening of the root canals, is covered with a layer of resin-modified glass ionomer (b).

(5) The tooth now can be restored with a core and extracoronal restoration.

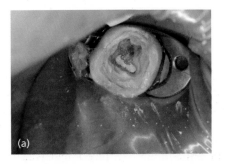

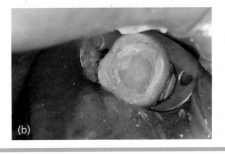

---

marker for varying times, are then split or rendered transparent and the depth of penetration by the tracer is measured. It was noted that there were marked inconsistencies in the results produced by various research workers; for example, aqueous solutions have been shown to penetrate further than isotopes (33). A qualitative volumetric method of measurement was considered to be a more accurate assessment of leakage. These include spectrophotometric measurements (12), an electrochemical method (23) and pressure methods using water to determine the volume of fluid movement (9, 63).

Microbiological models have been used *in vitro* in an attempt to match clinical conditions more closely (6, 16, 40, 63). In most cases, the filled root is sterilized and the

Clinical procedure 13.2

For the intact anterior tooth where only the access cavity has been cut in the crown:

(1) The root canals are obturated in the usual way.
(2) Excess gutta-percha and sealer are removed completely from the pulp chamber and 1–2 mm into the root canal itself.
(3) The root canal should be filled with a light-cured glass ionomer cement.
(4) A light-colored acid-etched composite resin restoration should then be placed in an effort to restore the strength of the crown, particularly at the cervical margin.

Not only will this technique increase the strength but the natural translucency of the enamel will not be as impaired as it would if gutta-percha were left in the entrance of the root canal because this can, particularly in the young tooth, be within the cervical one-third of the crown.

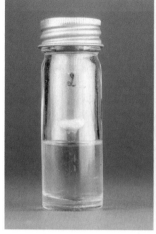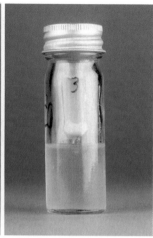

Fig. 13.1 Experimental set-up to demonstrate coronal leakage of bacteria through a root-filled tooth. The cloudy solution in the lower chamber (right) shows bacterial contamination.

coronal part is inoculated with a known microorganism. The time for the organisms to penetrate the root canal and enter an apical chamber, which contains a medium that changes colour when contaminated, is recorded (Fig. 13.1). Unfortunately most of these techniques are not quantitative, although efforts are being made to produce a quantitative method (37). The presence of the organism *Pseudomonas fluorescens* was detected using fluorimetry. The depth of penetration from the root apex toward the crown of the tooth was measured. Using this method Michailesco *et al.* (37) found no statistically significant differences in leakage results among lateral, vertical and thermomechanical condensation techniques.

Despite all the shortcomings of *in vitro* leakage tests, they provide a suitable initial screening of new materials and techniques for obturation. Further work is required *in vivo* to examine further the relationship between leakage of root fillings and periradicular tissue reactions.

Conclusions

The coronal leakage of micro-organisms, their by-products and nutrients from the oral cavity may be an important cause of failure of root canal treatment. All techniques used to obturate root canals leak over time, therefore there must be an important balance between the host response and the amount of contamination, notwithstanding the virulence of the organism. It may be that, for the most part, the host is able to cope with these low levels of infection. When the ingress reaches a certain level, an inflammatory response is triggered in the periradicular tissues with consequent bone resorption and resultant changes that are seen radiographically. This response is influenced by various factors concerning each individual. Therefore, it is very important to protect the root canal system from coronal leakage. This can be achieved by ensuring that:

(1) Microbial contamination is avoided during root canal treatment.
(2) The coronal aspect of the root filling is protected.
(3) A sound coronal restoration is placed immediately following root canal treatment.

References

1. Adenubi JO, Rule DC. Success rate of root fillings in young patients. *Br. Dent. J.* 1976; 141: 237–41.
2. Allison D, Weber C, Walton R. The influence of the method of canal preparation on the quality of apical and coronal obturation. *J. Endodont.* 1979; 5: 298–304.
3. Bobotis HG, Anderson RW, Pashley DH, Pantera EA Jr. A microleakage study of temporary restorative materials used in endodontics. *J. Endodont.* 1989; 15: 569–72.
4. Byström A, Sundqvist G. Bacteriologic evaluation of the efficacy of mechanical root canal instrumentation in endodontic therapy. *Scand. J. Dent. Res.* 1981; 8: 321–8.
5. Calas P, Rochd T, Druilhet P, Azais JM. *In vitro* adhesion of two strains of *Prevotella nigrescens* to the dentin of the root canal: the part played by different irrigation solutions. *J. Endodont.* 1998; 24: 112–15.
6. Chailertvanitkul P, Saunders WP, MacKenzie D, Weetman DA. An *in vitro* study of the coronal leakage of two root canal sealers using an obligate anaerobe microbial marker. *Int. Endodont. J.* 1996; 29: 249–55.
7. Chailertvanitkul P, Saunders WP, Saunders EM, MacKenzie D. An evaluation of microbial coronal leakage

in the restored pulp chamber of root canal treated multi-rooted teeth. *Int. Endodont. J.* 1997; 30: 318–22.

8. Czonstkowsky M, Wilson EG, Holstein FA. The smear layer in endodontics. *Dent. Clin. North Am.* 1990; 34: 13–25.

9. Derkson GD, Pashley DH, Derkson ME. Microleakage measurement of selected restorative materials: a new *in vitro* method. *J. Prosthet. Dent.* 1986; 56: 435–40.

10. Deveaux E, Hildelbert P, Neut C, Boniface B, Romond C. Bacterial microleakage of Cavit, IRM, and TERM. *Oral Surg.* 1992; 74: 634–43.

11. Donnelly JC. Resolution of a periapical radiolucency without root canal filling. *J. Endodont.* 1990; 16: 394–5.

12. Douglas WH, Zakariasen KL. Volumetric assessment of apical leakage utilizing a spectrophotometric dye recovery method (Abstract 512). *J. Dent. Res.* 1981; 60: 438.

13. Dow PR, Ingle JI. Isotope determination of root canal failure. *Oral Surg.* 1955; 8: 1100–104.

14. Drake DR, Wiemann AH, Rivera EM, Walton RE. Bacterial retention in canal walls *in vitro*: effect of smear layer. *J. Endodont.* 1994; 20: 78–82.

15. Gencoglu N, Samani S, Gunday M. Evaluation of sealing properties of Thermafil and Ultrafil techniques in the absence or presence of smear layer. *J. Endodont.* 1993; 19: 599–603.

16. Goldman LB, Goldman M, Kronman JH, Letourneau JM. Adaptation and porosity of poly-HEMA in a model system using two micro-organisms. *J. Endodont.* 1980; 6: 683–6.

17. Grieve AR, McAndrew R. A radiographic study of post-retained crowns in patients attending a dental hospital. *Br. Dent. J.* 1993; 174: 197–201.

18. Gutmann JL. Prevalence, location and patency of accessory canals in the furcation region of permanent molars. *J. Periodontol.* 1978; 49: 21–6.

19. Hansen SR, Montgomery S. Effect of restoration thickness on the sealing ability of TERM. *J. Endodont.* 1993; 19: 448–52.

20. Harty FJ, Parkins BJ, Wengraf AM. Success rate in root canal therapy: a retrospective study of conventional cases. *Br. Dent. J.* 1970; 128: 65–70.

21. Hovland EJ, Dumsha TC. Leakage evaluation *in vitro* of the root canal sealer cement Sealapex. *Int. Endodont. J.* 1985; 18: 179–82.

22. Ingle JI, Glick D. The Washington Study. In: *Endodontics* (1st edn) (Ingle JI, ed.). Philadelphia, PA: Lea & Febiger, 1965; 54–77.

23. Jacobson SM, Von Fraunhofer JA. The investigation of microleakage in root canal therapy. An electrochemical technique. *Oral Surg.* 1976; 42: 817–23.

24. Jacquot BM, Panighi MM, Steinmetz P, G'sell C. Evaluation of temporary restorations' microleakage by means of electrochemical impedance measurements. *J. Endodont.* 1996; 22: 586–9.

25. Jeffrey IWM, Saunders WP. An investigation into the bond strength between a root canal sealer and root-filling points. *Int. Endodont. J.* 1987; 20: 217–22.

26. Khayat A, Lee S-J, Torabinejad M. Human saliva penetration of coronally unsealed obturated root canals. *J. Endodont.* 1993; 19: 458–61.

27. Klevant FJH, Eggink JO. The effect of canal preparation on periapical disease. *Int. Endodont. J.* 1983; 16: 68–75.

28. Love RM. Adherence of *Streptococcus gordonii* to smeared and non-smeared dentine. *Int. Endodont. J.* 1996; 29: 108–12.

29. Madison S, Wilcox LR. An evaluation of coronal microleakage in endodontically treated teeth. Part 3. In vivo study. *J Endodont.* 1988; 14: 455–8.

30. Magura ME, Kafrawy AH, Brown CE, Newton CW. Human saliva coronal microleakage in obturated root canals: an *in vitro* study. *J. Endodont.* 1991; 17: 324–31.

31. Makkes PC, Thoden van Velzen SK, Wesselink PR, de Greeve PCM. Polyethylene tubes as a model for the root canal. *Oral Surg.* 1977; 44: 293–300.

32. Marshall FJ, Massler M. The sealing of pulpless teeth evaluated with radioisotopes. *J. Dent. Med.* 1961; 16: 172–84.

33. Matloff IR, Jensen JR, Singer L, Tabibi A. A comparison of methods used in root canal sealability studies. *Oral Surg.* 1982; 55: 402–7.

34. McComb D, Smith DC. A preliminary scanning electron microscopic study of root canals after endodontic procedures. *J. Endodont.* 1975; 1: 238–42.

35. Meryon SD, Brook AM. Penetration of dentine by three oral bacteria *in vitro* and their associated cytotoxicity. *Int. Endodont. J.* 1990; 23: 196–202.

36. Meryon SD, Jakeman KJ, Browne RM. Penetration *in vitro* of human and ferret dentine by three bacterial species in relation to their potential role in pulpal inflammation. *Int. Endodont. J.* 1986; 19: 213–20.

37. Michailesco PM, Valcarcel J, Grieve AR, Levallois B, Lerner D. Bacterial leakage in endodontics: an improved method for quantification. *J. Endodont.* 1996; 22: 535–9.

38. Michelich VJ, Schuster GS, Pashley DH. Bacterial penetration of human dentine *in vitro*. *J. Dent. Res.* 1980; 59: 1398–403.

39. Molven O, Halse A. Success rates for gutta-percha and Kloroperka N-O root fillings made by undergraduate students: radiographic findings after 10–17 years. *Int. Endodont. J.* 1988; 21: 243–50.

40. Mortensen DW, Boucher NE Jr, Ryge G. A method of testing for marginal leakage of dental restorations with bacteria. *J. Dent. Res.* 1965; 44: 58–63.

41. Pitt Ford TR, Roberts GJ. Tissue response to glass ionomer retrograde root fillings. *Int. Endodont. J.* 1990; 23: 233–8.

42. Portell FR, Bernier WE, Lorton L, Peters DD. The effect of immediate versus delayed dowel space preparation on the integrity of the apical seal. *J. Endodont.* 1982; 8: 154–60.

43. Ray H, Seltzer S. A new glass ionomer root canal sealer. *J. Endodont.* 1991; 17: 598–603.

44. Ray HA, Trope M. Periapical status of endodontically treated teeth in relation to the technical quality of the root filling and the coronal restoration. *Int. Endodont. J.* 1995; 28: 12–18.

45. Ricucci D, Gröndahl K, Bergenholtz G. Periapical status of root-filled teeth exposed to the oral environment by loss of restoration or caries. *Oral Surg.* 2000; 90: 354–9.

46. Rickert UG, Dixon CM. The controlling of root surgery. FDI 8me Congres Dentaire Internationale Paris. *C. Re. Gen. Sec.* 1931; IIIa: 15–22.

47. Saunders WP, Saunders EM. Assessment of leakage in the restored pulp chamber of endodontically treated multi-rooted teeth. *Int. Endodont. J.* 1990; 23: 28–33.

48. Saunders WP, Saunders EM. Coronal leakage as a cause of failure in root canal therapy: a review. *Endodont. Dent. Traumatol.* 1994; 10: 105–8.

49. Saunders WP, Saunders EM. Prevalence or periradicular periodontitis associated with crowned teeth in an adult Scottish sub-population. *Br. Dent. J.* 1998; 185: 137–40.

50. Saunders WP, Saunders EM, Gutmann JL, Gutmann ML. An assessment of the plastic Thermafil obturation technique. Part 3. The effect of post-space preparation on the apical seal. *Int. Endodont. J.* 1993; 26: 184–9.

51. Saunders WP, Saunders EM, Herd D, Stephens E. The use of glass ionomer as a root canal sealer – a pilot study. *Int. Endodont. J.* 1992; 25: 238–44.

52. Sen BH, Wesselink PR, Turkun M. The smear layer: a phenomenon in root canal therapy. *Int. Endodont. J.* 1995; 28: 141–8.

53. Sinai IH, Soltanoff W. The transmission of pathologic changes between the pulp and periodontal structures. *Oral Surg.* 1973; 36: 558–68.

54. Strindberg LZ. The dependence of the results of pulp therapy on certain factors. An analytical study based on radiographic and clinical follow-up examinations. *Acta Odontol. Scand.* 1956; 14 (Suppl. 21): 1–174.

55. Sundqvist G. Bacteriological studies of necrotic dental pulps. *Thesis.* Umea: Umeå University, 1976.

56. Swanson K, Madison S. An evaluation of coronal microleakage in endodontically treated teeth. Part 1. Time periods. *J. Endodont.* 1987; 13: 56–9.

57. Taylor JK, Jeansonne BG, Lemon RR. Coronal leakage: effects of smear layer, obturation technique, and sealer. *J. Endodont.* 1997; 23: 508–12.

58. Thoden van Velzen SK, Duivenvoorden HJ, Schuurs AHB. Probabilities of success and failure in endodontic treatment: a Bayesian approach. *Oral Surg.* 1981; 52: 85–90.

59. Torabinejad M, Ung B, Kettering JD. *In vitro* bacterial penetration of coronally unsealed endodontically treated teeth. *J. Endodont.* 1990; 16: 566–9.

60. Torneck CD. Reaction of rat connective tissue to polyethylene tube implants (part 1). *Oral Surg. Oral Med. Oral Pathol.* 1966; 21: 379–87.

61. Tronstad L, Asbjornsen K, Doving L, Pedersen I, Eriksen HM. Influence of coronal restorations on the periapical health of endodontically treated teeth. *Endodont. Dent. Traumatol.* 2000; 16: 218–21.

62. Webber RT, Del Rio CE, Brady JM, Segall RO. Sealing quality of a temporary filling material. *Oral Surg.* 1978; 46: 123–30.

63. Wu MK, De Gee AJ, Wesselink PR, Moorer WR. Fluid transport and bacterial penetration along root canal fillings. *Int. Endodont. J.* 1993; 26: 203–8.

64. Wu MK, Pehlivan Y, Kontakiotis EG, Wesselink PR. Microleakage along apical root fillings and cemented posts. *J. Prosthet. Dent.* 1998; 79: 264–9.

65. Wu MK, Wesselink PR. Endodontic leakage studies reconsidered. Part I. Methodology, application and relevance. *Int. Endodont. J.* 1993; 26: 37–43.

Chapter 14
Factors influencing endodontic retreatment

Claes Reit

The outcome of endodontic treatment

Essentially endodontic treatment is concerned with the removal of diseased or infected pulpal tissue, instrumentation and medication of the root canal system and, finally, the placement of a root filling. The ultimate objective is to protect the individual from a potentially painful and harmful infection and, at the same time, to preserve the affected tooth in the long term. The disease processes usually take place in body compartments hidden from direct inspection and therefore methods of evaluating the biological outcome of the treatment procedures are limited to observation of clinical symptoms, radiographic findings and histopathology of periapical biopsy specimens. Because clinical symptoms occur infrequently and periapical biopsies are difficult to obtain, the presence of pathological alterations is largely determined by radiographic diagnosis.

Evaluation of the outcome of endodontic therapy has a long tradition and numerous investigations based on radiographic examination have been published. A study with great impact on subsequent research was published by Strindberg in 1956 (62). Strindberg launched a system of criteria based on the absence or presence of radiographic rarefactions around the apex of the evaluated root. Basically Strindberg held that a periapical radiolucency diagnosed at the end of a predetermined healing period should be considered a sign of biological treatment 'failure'. Although Strindberg found that complete periapical healing sometimes did not occur until 10 years after treatment, he recommended a 4-year follow-up period as a cut-off before a final classification be made. The system provided a simple distinction between healthy and diseased roots and has been widely used as a tool to assess the general outcome of endodontic treatment but also to find factors that might influence postoperative healing (Fig. 14.1).

Investigations assessing the outcome of endodontic therapy often are designed as so-called follow-up studies. In these studies a cohort of patients are treated and followed clinically and radiographically for a certain period of time. Ideally such studies should be made prospectively and factors of interest randomized, but for ethical and practical reasons a retrospective (looking back in files and records) non-randomized approach more often has been used. However, this scientific strategy might bias the data produced and limit the confidence in conclusions made.

A substantial body of data have been collected from follow-up studies through the years. The accumulation of knowledge is impeded by the large variation among the investigations concerning factors such as case selection, sample size, treatment procedures, recall rate, length of observation period and radiographic interpretation. Regardless of the limitations, the studies clearly demonstrate that endodontic treatment can be a very reliable procedure. When teeth without apical periodontitis (irrespective of the pulp being vital or necrotic) are treated *lege artis*, a successful outcome might be expected in as many as 95% of cases. When treatment 'fails', i.e. periapical inflammation develops, it is most often caused by micro-organisms contaminating the root canal during treatment.

Compared with vital pulp cases, teeth with necrotic pulp and apical periodontitis are associated with less probability of treatment success. In such cases micro-organisms are present initially that, owing to the complexity of the root canal system, cannot be combated successfully. However, minute cleaning, medication and obturation of the canal will produce periapical healing in 80–85% of cases.

Factors influencing treatment outcome

Although endodontic treatment most often can be successful, some cases will fail and it is within the responsibility of the individual clinician to minimize this number. Therefore, knowledge of the various factors that will influence treatment outcome is of supreme importance. Such 'prognostic' factors might be found in the situation that precedes endodontic treatment (*preop-*

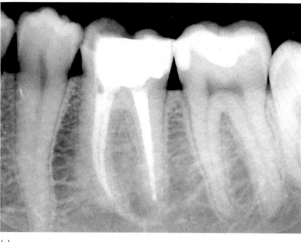 (a)

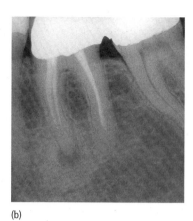 (b)

Fig. 14.1 Evaluation of treatment outcome according to Strindberg (62). (a) A 4-year follow-up of a first lower molar. The patient has no clinical symptoms and no signs of pathology are visible in the radiograph. The case is classified as a 'success'. (b) This tooth was treated 5 years ago for apical periodontitis. The periapical lesion has decreased but is still visible on the radiograph. The case is classified as a 'failure'.

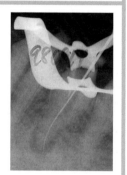

Core concept 14.1   Factors influencing treatment outcome

Preoperative factors

● Apical periodontitis

Operative factors

● Extent of canal preparation
● Quality of seal
● Procedural error

Postoperative factors

● Coronal leakage
● Post preparation

erative factors) or might be associated with the treatment *per se* (*operative* factors). Also, elements of the *postoperative* situation might exert influence on the long-term outcome (Core concept 14.1, Key literature 14.1).

Preoperative factors

In most studies general factors such as age, gender and health have not been demonstrated to influence significantly the treatment outcome. When local factors have been considered some investigators reported that certain teeth came out more favorable than others, but a systematic pattern among the studies and teeth has not been found. The only preoperative factor that con-

sistently has proven to influence significantly the treatment result is the diagnosis of apical periodontitis. Studies have reported 10–25% lower healing rate when radiographic signs of periapical disease are present compared with when they are not.

Operative factors

The apical extent of the root canal preparation is one of the major prognostic factors. The instrumentation ideally should be terminated at the constriction of the canal, which normally is located 1–2 mm from the root apex. Accordingly, Sjögren *et al.* (59) reported periapical health to be restored in 94% of teeth with apical periodontitis when the preparation, and root filling, ended within 0–2 mm of the radiographic apex. On the other hand, when preparations were made to a shorter distance from the apex, only 68% healed.

Overinstrumentation of the root canal should be avoided. When the instrument passes through the apical foramen it may induce displacement of infected dentine into the periapical tissues (Fig. 14.2). Within the dentine chips, micro-organisms are protected from the defense mechanisms of the host and may sustain inflammation and impair healing (69). More importantly, repeated overinstrumentation may enlarge the apical foramen and alter its original anatomy. Consequently, the root canal preparation will lose its apical resistance form, which often will result in overfill combined with an inadequate apical seal of the canal. Overfill of the root canal has been found to be associated with a decreased healing frequency in teeth with apical periodontitis. The

---

Key literature 14.1   Dependence of the results of pulp therapy on certain factors

In his influential thesis published in 1956, Strindberg (62) performed an analytical study of endodontic treatment results based on radiographic and clinical follow-up examinations. The case material consisted of 254 patients with 529 teeth and 775 roots treated by the author during a 6-year period. The root canals were instrumented by the use of Kerr files and Hedstroem files. Vital cases were mostly completed in two sessions. When a devitalizing agent was used (arsenic or paraformaldehyde paste) the treatment was extended to three appointments. The non-vital pulps were often treated in four or more sessions. The intracanal medicaments that were used varied considerably. Five percent chloramine solution was usually employed in vital cases. In non-vital cases rotation of the medicament (e.g. tricresol formalin, iodine preparations, oil of cloves, creosote) was preferred to prevent the bacteria from acquiring resistance to any one substance. The canals were filled with gutta-percha and either Alytit or an 8% solution of resin in chloroform as a binding agent. Although Strindberg's treatment methodology to a large extent must be regarded as obsolete, his scientific approach still is commendable.

Follow-ups were carried out over a period of 6 months to 10 years. The results of the therapy for a particular root were assessed at the radiographic examinations as a 'success' when the contours, width and structure of the periodontal margin were normal and the periodontal contours were widened mainly around the excess filling, and as a 'failure' when there was a decrease in the periradicular rarefaction, unchanged periradicular rarefaction and a new or an increase in the initial rarefaction.

After a follow-up period of 4 years, Strindberg found that 95% of cases without an initial rarefaction and 71% with an initial rarefaction could be classified as 'successes'. If the period was extended to include those observations that he had made beyond the 4-year point, the healing rate among the latter increased to 85%.

Strindberg's main idea was to study the impact of certain factors on periapical healing. He found that components such as *age, health status, number of interappointment dressings, treatment flare-up* and *root filling material* did not exert any significant influence on the therapeutic result. Among the statistically significant factors he reported *periradicular status, number of roots, canal preparation* and *type of root filling.* Healing was found less frequently among cases with an initial periapical radiolucency. Successful operations were carried out more often in three-rooted than in two-rooted teeth, which in turn displayed better results than single-rooted teeth. Where the apical part of the canal was mechanically widened only to a diameter corresponding to Hedstroem file no. 1, a higher proportion of success was obtained than when wider files were used. Negative influences were found if canals were prepared to or beyond the radiographic apex and if the root filling showed poor adaption to the root canal or was forced through the apical foramen.

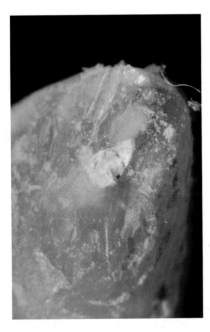

Fig. 14.2   The negative influence of overinstrumentation. A repeated instrumentation through the apical foramen will result in a 'tear-drop' anatomy and hinder a good-quality root-filling seal.

periapical reaction is probably not caused by the material *per se* (gutta-percha is well tolerated by the tissues) but rather by intracanal microbes. Numerous outcome studies have proven the significance of the quality of the root filling seal. An inadequate apical seal will allow tissue fluids to leak into the root canal and supply microorganisms with substrate, and also let bacterial products seep out into the periapical tissues. On the other hand, a defective coronal seal might provide the oral micro-organisms with an avenue for a postoperative infection of the root canal, resulting in a 'late' or sustained periapical inflammation.

If negative prognostic factors are accumulated, the chance of success will decrease substantially (15). For example, if an apical periodontitis case is overinstrumented and provided with a defective seal, the probability of healing will be very low. In an epidemiological study Bergenholtz *et al.* (6) found that 55% of overfilled roots with defective seals were associated with periapical radiolucencies. On the other hand, when root fillings ended within 2 mm of the apex and were assessed as adequate, only 12% demonstrated periapical radiolucencies.

Procedural errors such as perforations, broken instruments and ledge formations will not directly impede periapical healing. However, the prognosis of the treat-

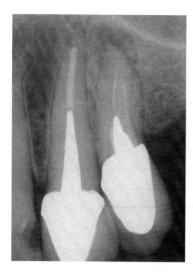

Fig. 14.3 Bacterial provocation of root-filling seal. In the first left upper premolar, an acute periapical lesion developed 1 year after placement of the post and crown. The root-filling seal is defective and microorganisms probably have entered the canals either via microleakage or during the restorative procedures.

ment is decreased if the complication obstructs the cleaning of an infected canal.

Postoperative factors

Data from recent studies indicate that the quality of the restoration of the tooth might exert an influence on the outcome of the endodontic treatment (46). Via defective margins, micro-organisms may enter and colonize a poorly sealed root canal (54) (Fig. 14.3). Furthermore, leaking saliva may dissolute the sealer and break the resistance against reinfection (57). However, provided that instrumentation and root fillings are carefully performed, the problem of coronal leakage may not be of great clinical importance (52).

The placement of a post in the root canal does not *per se* influence the outcome of endodontic treatment. However, the post preparation might break the root filling seal either by disturbing the adaptation of the material to the dentinal walls or by leaving too little gutta-percha remaining. Studies have shown that not less than 3 mm should remain in the apical part of the canal (29).

Prevalence of endodontic 'failures'

Assessment of the technical quality and the outcome of endodontic treatment at a population level has a long tradition in Scandinavian countries. Studies have reported a relatively high frequency of defective root fillings. It has been reported consistently that 25–35% of endodontically treated teeth are associated with periapical radiolucencies (6, 13, 17, 44). Similar findings during recent years have been reported from other areas of Europe and North America (9–11, 22, 33, 55, 56). The most frequently adopted study design, the cross-sectional survey, does not disclose the dynamics of the periapical reactions and therefore does not provide direct information on the frequency of 'failed' treatments. However, in a follow-up study Petersson *et al.* (42) found about equal numbers of healing and developing periapical radiolucencies in a population over a period of 11 years. Obviously there is a contradiction between what is possible with endodontic therapy (85–90% success) and what is actually obtained (60–70% success). It is an important task for the profession to try to close this gap.

At present the number of potential retreatment cases is huge; in Sweden (9 million inhabitants) it can be estimated to be about 2.5 million. However, the attitude to the clinical management of such cases has been found to vary substantially among clinicians (3, 21, 43, 48, 49, 60).

Variation in the management of periapical lesions in endodontically treated teeth

Variation in healthcare procedures was recognized early, at the beginning of the 20th century. In a classical study (2) of 1000 11-year-old schoolchildren in New York City it was found that 650 children had undergone tonsillectomy. The remaining 350 children were sent to a group of physicians. A total of 158 children were selected for tonsillectomy. Those rejected (182) were sent to another group of physicians and 88 of them were then suggested for tonsillectomy. After that, the remaining childen were examined by a third group of physicians, and then only 65 children remained for whom tonsillectomy had not been suggested. At that point the study was interrupted owing to a shortage of physicians to consult. This report inspired investigators to challenge the clinical consensus of a variety of medical (and dental) procedures. Troubled over the results of these studies, Eddy (14) concluded: 'Uncertainty creeps into medical practice through every pore. Whether a physician is defining a disease, making a diagnosis, selecting a procedure, observing outcomes, assessing probabilities, assigning preferences, or putting it all together, he is walking on a very slippery terrain. It is difficult for nonphysicians, and for many physicians, to appreciate how complex these tasks are, how poorly we understand them, and how easy it is for honest people to come to different conclusions.'

Key literature 14.2   Variation in management of endodontic 'failures'

Reit and Gröndahl (48) showed 35 dental officers from the Public Dental Health Organization in Sweden 33 endodontically treated teeth showing periapical radiolucencies of various sizes. The cases were presented with radiographs and the same clinical history: 'The actual patient, aged 45, is in good general health and presents with no clinical symptoms from his teeth or oral soft tissues. The present radiographs were taken at a routine examination. Root fillings are more than four years old. This is your first examination of the patient, who has no other dental problems and no further dental treatment is being considered.' For each case the clinicians made a choice among five options: no therapy indicated, wait 12 months, non-surgical retreatment, surgical retreatment or extraction.

In the figure each bar represents one case. In no case was the same option suggested unanimously by all examiners. In eight teeth all five options were suggested, and in 15 cases four of the alternatives. The number of teeth selected for therapy (surgical or non-surgical retreatment or extraction) had an interexaminer range of 7–26 teeth.

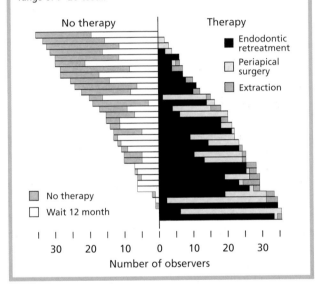

The large variation among clinicians when suggesting the treatment of endodontic cases was first demonstrated by Smith *et al.* (60). Several reports have confirmed that the mere diagnosis of a persistent periapical radiolucency in an endodontically treated tooth does not consistently result in suggestions for retreatment among clinicians (42, 43, 48, Key literature 14.2). For example, Reit and Gröndahl (49) found that only 39% of persistent periapical lesions diagnosed by practitioners were complemented by a retreatment decision.

Owing to their complexity, clinical decision problems have attracted interdisciplinary attention. In addition to interest from health professionals, philosophers, psychologists and economists have also contributed (12).

Two main areas of research and thinking can be identified: descriptive and prescriptive. Descriptive projects aim at mapping out and explaining how clinicians reason and make decisions. Prescriptive, or normative, projects, on the other hand, are concerned with how decisions should or ought to be made.

Clinical decision-making: descriptive projects

In studies of clinical reasoning several models have been suggested and used (12). Some investigators have focused on the artistic, or intuitive, aspects of clinical practice (45). In the tradition of 'judgement analysis', researchers have tried to reveal the pieces of information or 'cues' used at conscious or unconscious levels that influence a person's decision-making policy. This approach has been applied in several domains (8), including judgements of third molar removal (24). In a series of innovative investigations Kahneman *et al.* (23) explored a proposition that people most often rely on a small number of heuristic principles to make decisions.

Attempts have been made to explain the observed variation in the management of periapical lesions in endodontically treated teeth. Because several studies have demonstrated large interindividual variation in radiographic interpretation of the periapical area (see Chapter 2), it has been hypothesized that variation in retreatment decisions might be regarded as a function of diagnostic variation. However, studies of general practitioners have not supported this idea (49). The influence of components including risk assessment (50), clinical context (3, 60), cognitive factors (50) and overall dental treatment plans (43) has been explored. However, the complexity and multiplicity of factors present in each study have rendered interpretation of the results difficult. Kvist and Reit have proposed a model to explain endodontic retreatment behavior (27, 28, 51). In the 'Praxis Concept' (Advanced concept 14.1) it is suggested that dentists perceive periapical lesions of varying sizes as different stages on a continuous health scale, based on their radiographic appearance. Interindividual variation then could be regarded as the result of different cut-off points on the continuum for prescribing retreatment.

Endodontic retreatment decision-making: a normative approach

Probably the most highly developed normative decision-making model is the 'expected utility theory'

Advanced concept 14.1   The Praxis Concept

This theory hypothesizes that dentists conceive of periapical health and disease not as either/or situations but as states on a continuous scale. On this scale a major lesion represents a more serious condition than a smaller one. Variation between decision-makers then could be regarded as the result of the individual's selection of differing cut-off points on the scale for prescribing retreatment. Placement of the cut-off point is dependent on value but also is influenced by factors such as costs, quality of seal and accessibility to the root canal.

Personal values

- High costs   - Low costs
- Adequate seal   - Defective seal
- Difficult access   - Easy access

Retreatment   No retreatment

High degree of   Cut-off point   Perfect health
poor health

(Big periapical lesion)   (No periapical lesion)

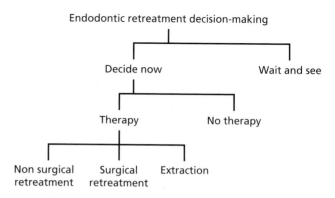

Fig. 14.4   The structure of the retreatment decision-making problem.

(EUT) (for a review, see Ref. 19). The philosophical foundation is to be found in classical utilitarianism, whereas its mathematical origins are even older. The advent of modern EUT is associated with the influential work of von Neumann and Morgenstern (40), which made some of the psychological assumptions of utilitarianism redundant. The theory was introduced to medicine by Ledley and Lusted (31) and, under the concept of 'clinical decision analysis', discussed in detail by Lusted (32) and Weinstein and Fineberg (68). Over the last 30 years clinical decision analysis has received increasing attention in medicine as well as dentistry (53).

Clinical decision analysis prescribes that the problem should be structured as a 'decision-tree', which logically displays the available actions and their possible consequences. Then the listed outcomes are assessed regarding probabilities and values ('utilities'). After this, the weighed sum (expected utility) of each strategy is computed and the action with the highest sum is chosen.

Reit and Gröndahl approached the management of periapical lesions in endodontically treated teeth from a decision analytical point of view. The problem was graphically structured (48) and later probabilities and utilities were produced and 'best' actions were calculated (47, 50). However, large parts of the critical information needed for calculations are very uncertain, therefore in the present context the decision-tree will be used only as a rational basis for clinical deliberations, with no explicit calculations being made.

The structure of the decision problem

The structure of the decision-making problem is logically and temporally displayed in Fig. 14.4. Before retreatment of a root filled tooth with apical periodontitis is actually allowed to start, there are basically three clinical questions that have to be answered and three choices that have to be made. When a periapical radiolucency is detected the clinician first has to question whether the corresponding lesion might be expected to heal or not. If there is a chance of healing, the case should be followed for an additional period of time. If it is thought that the patient will not benefit from further expectation, the second question will be raised: should the case be retreated or not? The choice is between accepting the situation as it is or trying to improve on it. This is the most difficult and complex of the choices that have to be made and no simple answers are available. If retreatment is favored there will be a question of which clinical procedure to use. Personal skills, knowledge of prognosis and cost-effectiveness estimations will influence this decision.

Choice 1: Decide now/wait and see

As mentioned above, endodontic treatment of teeth with apical periodontitis has good prognosis. The majority of the cases that will succeed show complete periapical healing within the first 2 years of root canal treatment. By extending the observation period, the healing frequency will increase and single cases have been reported not to heal until 10 years postoperatively (62). However, most investigators recommend the placement of a cut-off 4 years postoperatively, a time during which the healing curve flattens out. Thus, from a clinical point of view, a case initially treated for apical periodontitis might be observed for up to 4 years. If the lesion still persists, a decision has to be made between performing

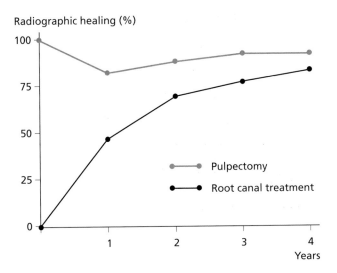

Fig. 14.5 Healing dynamics of the periapical tissues following treatment of vital and non-vital cases.

additional treatment or accepting the situation at hand (Fig. 14.5).

As a result of microbial contamination during intracanal treatment procedures, roots without preoperative signs of apical periodontitis may develop disease. Most such cases may be detected within 1 year of the original treatment (41). 'Late failures' most often are due to coronal leakage of microbes allowed to invade a defectively sealed root canal. Consequently, the diagnosis of a new periapical lesion in an endodontically treated root normally is regarded as a sign of root canal infection. Spontaneous healing is not expected to occur and therefore an extension of the observation period is not meaningful. Together with the patient, the clinician has to decide whether retreatment is indicated.

Occasionally transient apical radiolucencies develop around the apices of root filled teeth (62). Periapical inflammatory reactions with subsequent bone resorption might be elicited as responses to toxic components of antimicrobial medicaments and root filling materials. Toxicity usually decreases over time and inflammation resolves. Clinically this possibility should be considered if the radiolucency is associated with an overfill or is diagnosed within the first months of completed root canal treatment.

Choice 2: Therapy/no therapy

If a periapical lesion is not expected to heal, several factors have to be considered when choosing between retreating the root or not. For example, what is the probability that the detected periapical radiolucency represents disease? What are the general and local risks that have to be taken if the periapical disease is not treated? If retreatment is carried out, what are the risks of complications? What is the opinion of the patient, does he or she have any preferences? Are there any moral implications to be considered? (Core concept 14.2.)

To decide whether retreatment should be carried out or not is complex and each case can be the subject of contraproductive overdone deliberation. In the everyday situation it normally gives the best consequences if a few simple principles are followed (Core concept 14.3).

It is assumed that the best overall consequences are obtained if dentists' primary suggestions to patients are to perform endodontic retreatment. The persistent lesion is an expression of a root canal infection and people benefit from having their infections treated. For the medically uncompromised patient the general health hazard is probably low and therefore false-positive diagnoses should be avoided. There is no solid scientific evidence to distinguish among grades of periapical disease.

This first principle in Core concept 14.3 is quite dogmatic and leaves no room for deliberation. It implies that if retreatment is suggested and accepted no specific arguments are needed. However, if a persistent lesion is diagnosed and retreatment is not selected, then specific arguments have to be put forward. These are found in the second principle.

Respecting patient autonomy implies that the patient is fully informed regarding the situation but does not want retreatment. Attitudes to periapical disease vary among persons and subjectivity and personal values must be allowed to influence the decision-making process.

On an individual basis, potential risks associated with a retreatment procedure (e.g. root fracture following post removal, or nerve injury as a result of periapical surgery) might be judged to be too high. The objectively assessed risks (the probability of a certain event) should be weighed against the subjectively evaluated benefit of retreatment. When the patient's costs for retreatment are considered (treatment fee, drugs, loss of income, suffering), the cost/benefit ratio might be too low to be accepted.

Probability of disease

Biopsies obtained from periapical areas showing radiolucencies have demonstrated the presence of pathologically altered tissue (granulomas, cysts) in about 95% of investigated cases (7, 61). It has been demonstrated convincingly that these reactions are mainly caused by microbial irritants present either in the root canal (30, 34, 38, 64) or in the periapical tissue (63, 67).

Risks of untreated disease

The risks of leaving a root with chronic periapical disease untreated are not very well known. The infected root canal as a potential threat to systemic health is discussed in detail elsewhere in this book. The topic has been argued since Hunter in 1901 suggested that oral micro-organisms could disseminate throughout the system and cause disease in other body compartments. Currently the evidence base is very weak and a general risk assessment is still very much a subject of personal opinion (35).

From a local point of view Eriksen (16) estimated the incidence of possible exacerbations per year to be less than 5%. The composition of the intracanal microbial flora of the root filled tooth generally varies from that of the necrotic pulp. It is not known if this difference influences the risk.

Risks of retreatment procedures

Clinical procedures may injure the tooth or the surrounding tissues. In order to re-enter the root canal tooth substance, crowns or posts often must be removed, implying risks of weakening the tooth or of causing direct fractures. Surgical retreatment might, for example, lead to mandibular nerve injury or to a visible retraction of the marginal gingiva. These risks have to be presented to the patient, included in the decision-making and accepted before retreatment starts.

Personal preferences

Personal values will influence the decision-making process. As mentioned above, given identical information and similar diagnostic findings, patients (and doctors) will not choose the same clinical management of a certain disease. For example, some persons will be very eager to have a bacteria-caused periapical inflammation in a root filled tooth treated whereas others will be more reluctant.

The concept of value is multidimensional but it seems reasonable to suppose that there is a close connection between an individual's values and his or her value judgements. It has been suggested that one may apprehend values in acts of preferring (19, 40). This means that when faced with a choice, the values of an individual are reflected in his or her preference behaviour. To measure preferences, various rating scales or the so-called 'Standard Gamble' technique (Advanced concept 14.2) have been used (65, 66).

Reit and Kvist (51) transformed the Standard Gamble technique to suit an endodontic retreatment situation and investigated the subjective value of periapical health and disease among dental students as well as endodontic specialists (27). Substantial interindividual variations were registered in the evaluation of symptomless periapical lesions in root filled teeth. It was found that, at a subjective level, some persons will benefit much more from endodontic retreatment than others.

Ethical principles

Ethical reflection is a fundamental component of medical decision-making. The utilitarian idea that it is the consequences, and only the consequences, of an action that will determine its moral value has been a central thought in Western moral philosophy, but it is still a very controversial one. Traditionally, dentists and physicians have had a paternalistic approach to clinical practice. Today, however, patient autonomy is widely regarded as the primary ethical principle, emphasizing the importance of determining patient values. Besides respect for autonomy, the principles of beneficence (doing good to patients), non-maleficence (avoiding doing harm) and justice are often stressed in biomedical ethics (4).

Choice 3: Non-surgical/surgical retreatment

The root filled tooth can be retreated using either an orthograde or a retrograde approach to the canal. In the orthograde or *non-surgical retreatment* the tooth is re-entered through the crown, the root filling removed and the canal once again negotiated before it is reobturated (Fig. 14.6). The main objective of the non-surgical retreatment is to eradicate potential intracanal micro-organisms, thus allowing the periapical tissue to heal.

Advanced concept 14.2   The Standard Gamble

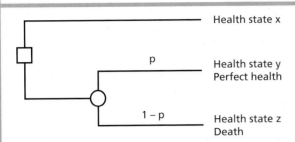

The subject is given a choice between two alternative courses of action. The options available are to continue living in the state of health described in a scenario (health state *x*) or to take a 'gamble'. The gamble most often is some type of treatment, e.g. surgery, that may lead to the restoration of health (health state *y*) but risks are involved and the patient might die (health state *z*). The probability (*p*) of attaining the best outcome of the gamble is systematically varied until the subject is indifferent between continuing to stay in health state *x* and taking the gamble. In this situation the value or 'utility' of the two alternative actions is the same. This means that the utility of health state *x* (U_x) equals the relative sum of the utilities of state *y* (U_y) and state *z* (U_z). The formal expression will be:

$$U_x = (p)(U_y) + (1 - p)(U_z)$$

If perfect health is given a utility of 1 and death is given a utility of 0, then $U_x = (p)(1) + (1 - p)(0)$, i.e. $U_x = p$.

An example will make it easier to understand the method. Imagine that you have become blind and have not been able to see for a couple of years. A new surgical method is very promising and is offered to you. The problem is that there is a risk that you might die as a result of the surgical procedure. In the Standard Gamble the chance of survival or risk of dying is varied to find the frequency when you are indifferent between staying blind or being treated. Using the formula above, a person who is indifferent when there is a 10% risk of dying values the state of being blind to 0.90 on a scale from 1 to 0. Another person will perhaps be indifferent when there is only a 1% risk of dying, resulting in a utility value of 0.99.

As an alternative to the orthograde approach, root canals might be retreated from a retrograde direction. A *surgical retreatment* will include removal of the periapical soft-tissue lesion, resection of the root tip and placement of a retrofill (Fig. 14.7). Using this methodology, complete eradication of an intracanal microflora must not be expected. Rather, if the retrofill is effective, remaining microbes will be entombed in the root canal and shut off from periapical communication.

Several factors must influence the choice between non-surgical and surgical retreatment of a case, and aspects of biological outcome, costs and risks have to be deliberated.

Data on the outcome of non-surgical retreatment are most often available as part of general follow-up studies (for a review, see Ref. 20). Reported success rates in these investigations vary between 56% and 88%. The issue has been addressed specifically only by a few authors. After 2 years of observation, Bergenholtz *et al.* (5) found, in a prospective study, complete resolution of apical radiolucencies in 48% of 234 retreated roots. Decreased size of the radiolucency was observed in a further 30%. After a follow-up period of 5 years, Sundqvist *et al.* (64) reported complete resolution in 74% of 54 retreated teeth. Information on the outcome of surgical retreatment is abundant. Many methods have been adopted and reported success rates vary between 30% and 90% (20). In a comprehensive review of the literature, Hepworth and Friedman (20) tried to estimate the success rate of retreatment by means of a weighted average calculation, reporting 59% and 66% for surgical and non-surgical approaches, respectively.

Outcome studies have focused almost exclusively on either surgical *or* non-surgical retreatment procedures. However, Allen (1), in a retrospective analysis of 633 cases where either of the two methods was used, found no difference. These observations were corroborated in a prospective, randomized investigation by Kvist and

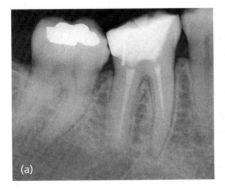
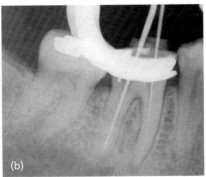
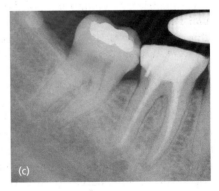

Fig. 14.6   Non-surgical endodontic retreatment. (a) The first lower molar was treated for pulpitis. (b) A periapical radiolucency developed 2 years postoperatively in the mesial root, signalling the presence of an intracanal infection. (c) The root canals were re-entered and subjected to antimicrobial procedures before they were refilled.

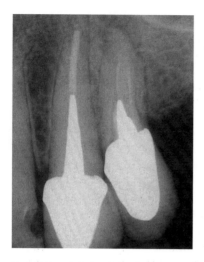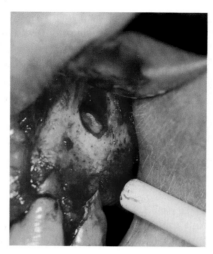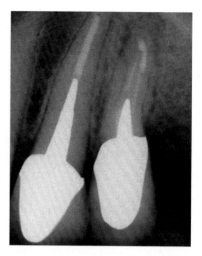

Fig. 14.7   Surgical endodontic retreatment. Following the placement of a post and crown, the second upper premolar developed periapical pathosis. The case was retreated surgically with removal of the soft-tissue lesion, apicoectomy, preparation of the apical portion of the canal with ultrasonic instruments and placement of a super EBA retrofill.

> ### Core concept 14.4   Case-related factors influencing retreatment choice
>
> - Etiology of the lesion
> - Access to the root canal
> - Monetary costs
> - Quality of original treatment
> - Position of the tooth
> - Personal skills

Reit (25, Key literature 14.3), who failed to show any systematic difference in the outcome of surgical and non-surgical endodontic retreatment.

Scientific data do not support the notion of a systematic difference in healing potential between surgical and non-surgical retreatment. However, whether the recent rapid development in technology (e.g. nickel–titanium instruments, rotary systems, surgical microscopes, ultrasonic retrotips, new retrofilling materials) will change this situation remains to be seen.

Because there seems to be no evidence for a systematic preference for one retreatment approach over the other, the choice has to be based on individual case-related factors (Core concept 14.4).

Etiology of the lesion

In the majority of endodontic 'failures' the periapical radiolucency is caused by an intracanal infection. However, in some cases the causative agent might be found in the periapical tissue, demanding a surgical retreatment approach. Bacteria such as *Actinomyces israelii* and *Propionibacterium propionicum* have been found to be able to prevail outside the root canal (18, 58).

Additional strains have been observed (63, 67) but the prevalence of extraradicular microbes in chronic apical periodontitis is controversial.

Periapical lesions in endodontically treated teeth may be associated with non-microbial agents such as foreign body reactions to root filling materials (37) and the development of cysts. Periapical cysts are classified as 'pocket' cysts and 'true' cysts. The pocket cyst has the epithelial-lined cavity open to the root canal and might be expected to heal after conventional endodontic treatment (36). The cavity of the true cyst is completely enclosed by epithelial lining, which might make the dynamics of the cyst independent of any intracanal treatment measures. Thus, traditionally it has been supposed that true cysts have to be enucleated surgically in order to heal.

Clinically it is very difficult to differentiate between cases with different etiology of the periapical reactions. No accurate tests are available but cysts are expected to be more prevalent among major lesions (39).

Access to the root canal

Endodontically treated teeth are often restored. In order to re-enter the root canal, crowns sometimes have to be perforated and posts removed. Such procedures will increase monetary costs and the risks for loosened crowns and root fractures. Therefore, the more complex the restoration, the more attractive the choice of surgical intervention.

Quality of original treatment

There is a strong correlation between the quality of the treatment (as reflected in the technical quality of the root filling) and the treatment outcome. In a canal with a defective seal (short, voids), non-surgical retreatment

Key literature 14.3   Surgical versus non-surgical retreatment procedures

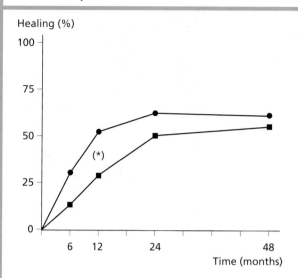

Kvist and Reit (25, 26) randomized 95 incisors and canines, classified as 'failures' according to the Strindberg (62) criteria, to surgical or non-surgical retreatment. Three randomization factors were considered: size of the periapical radiolucency, the apical position and the technical quality of the root filling. Clinical and radiographic follow-ups were made at 6, 12, 24 and 48 months postoperatively. To obtain identical radiographs at consecutive intervals, an impression was obtained of the patient's dental arch. The impression was attached to a modified Eggen device. The observers used a strict definition of periapical disease. Disputed cases were subject to joint evaluation.

At the 12-month follow-up a statistically significantly higher healing rate was found in favor of surgical (●) over non-surgical (■) retreatment (*). At the final 48-month examination no such difference between groups was registered. Four surgically retreated cases classified as healed did show a relapse of the apical radiolucency, or presented with clinical symptoms at later follow-up. In one non-surgically retreated tooth the periapical radiolucency did recur.

Significantly more patients reported discomfort (pain, swelling) after surgical retreatment than after non-surgical procedures. Analgesics significantly were consumed more often after surgery. Patients reported absence from work, mainly due to swelling and discoloration of the skin. Surgical retreatment tended to bring about greater indirect costs than non-surgical retreatment.

should be the first choice. Consequently, if the chances to improve the quality are small then surgical procedures should be considered.

Position of the tooth

Inaccessibility of the surgical site may be a contraindication for retrograde retreatment. The proximity of neurovascular bundles or the presence of thick alveolar bone might severely obstruct the possibility to cut, clean and seal the apical portion of the root.

Personal skills

Surgical and non-surgical retreatment procedures are often technically difficult and the results that can be achieved are highly dependent on the personal skills of the dentist. Therefore, complicated cases might benefit from being referred to a specialist or an experienced colleague.

Conclusion

Whether endodontic retreatment should be performed is a complex decision situation and many factors have to be considered. For the clinician it is important to appreciate the microbiology and pathology of the non-healing periapical lesion, as well as the technical potentials and limitations of retreatment. However, as important professional knowledge and skill might be it must be emphasized that the final decision is in the hand of the informed patient. The subjective meaning of the situation will vary among individuals. Remember that the patient is the expert on which symptoms are tolerable, which economic costs are acceptable and which risks are worth taking.

References

1. Allen RK, Newton CW, Beoen CE. A statistical analysis of surgical and nonsurgical retreatment cases. *J. Endodont.* 1989; 15: 261–6.
2. American Child Health Association. *Physical Defects: The Pathway to Correction.* American Child Health Association, 1934; 80–96.
3. Aryanpour S, van Niewenhuysen J-P, D'Hoore W. Endodontic retreatment decisions. *Int. Endodont. J.* 2000; 33: 208–18.
4. Beauchamp TL, Childress FF. *Principles of Biomedical Ethics.* New York: Oxford University Press, 1984.
5. Bergenholtz G, Lekholm U, Milthon R, Heden G, Ödesjö B, Engström B. Retreatment of endodontic fillings. *Scand. J. Dent. Res.* 1979; 87: 217–24.
6. Bergenholtz G, Malmcrona E, Milthon R. Röntgenologisk bedömning av rotfyllningens kvalitet ställd i relation till förekomst av periapikala destruktioner (Summary in English). *Tandläkartidningen* 1973; 65: 269–79.
7. Bhaskar SN. Periapical lesions, types, incidence, and clinical features. *Oral Surg.* 1966; 21: 657–71.
8. Brehmer B, Joyce CRB. *Human Judgement. The SJT View.* Amsterdam: Elsevier Science Publishers, 1988.
9. Buckley M, Spångberg LS. The prevalence and technical quality of endodontic treatment in an American subpopulation. *Oral Surg.* 1995; 79: 92–100.
10. De Cleen MJH, Schuurs AHB, Wesselink PR, Wu M-K. Periapical status and prevalence of endodontic treatment in an adult Dutch population. *Int. Endodont. J.* 1993; 26: 112–19.

11. De Moor RJG, Hommez GMG, De Boever JG, Delme KIM, Martens GEI. Periapical health related to the quality of root canal treatment in a Belgian population. *Int. Endodont. J.* 2000; 33: 113–20.

12. Dowie J, Elstein A. *Professional Judgement. A Reader in Clinical Decision Making.* Cambridge, UK: Cambridge University Press, 1988.

13. Eckerbom M, Andersson J-E, Magnusson T. A longitudinal study of changes in frequency and technical standard of endodontic treatment in a Swedish population. *Endodont. Dent. Traumatol.* 1989; 5: 27–31.

14. Eddy DM. Variations in physician practice: the role of uncertainty. *Health Aff.* 1984; 5: 74–89.

15. Engström B. Bacteriologic cultures in root canal therapy. *PhD Thesis.* Umeå, Sweden: University of Umeå, 1964.

16. Eriksen H. Epidemiology of apical periodontitis. In *Essential Endodontology* (Ørstavik D, Pitt Ford TR, eds). Oxford, UK: Blackwell Science, 1998.

17. Eriksen H, Bjertness E. Prevalence of apical periodontitis and results of endodontic treatment in middle-aged adults in Norway. *Endodont. Dent. Traumatol.* 1991; 7: 1–4.

18. Happonen RP. Periapical actinomycosis: a follow-up study of 16 surgically treated cases. *Endodont. Dent. Traumatol.* 1986; 2: 205–9.

19. Hargreaves Heap S, Hollis M, Lyons B, Sugden R, Weale A. *The Theory of Choice. A Critical Guide.* Oxford, UK: Blackwell, 1992.

20. Hepworth MJ, Friedman S. Treatment outcome of surgical and non-surgical management of endodontic failures. *J. Can. Dent. Assoc.* 1997; 63: 364–71.

21. Hülsmann M. Retreatment decision making by a group of general dental practitioners in Germany. *Int. Endodont. J.* 1994; 27: 125–32.

22. Imfeld TN. Prevalence and quality of endodontic treatment in an elderly urban population of Switzerland. *J. Endodont.* 1991; 17: 604–7.

23. Kahneman D, Slovic P, Tversky A. *Judgement under Uncertainty: Heuristics and Biases.* Cambridge, UK: Cambridge University Press, 1982.

24. Knutsson K, Brehmer B, Lysell L, Rohlin M. Judgement of removal of asymptomatic mandibular molars: influence of position, degree of impaction, and patient's age. *Acta Odontol. Scand.* 1996; 54: 348–54.

25. Kvist T, Reit C. Results of endodontic retreatment: A randomised clinical study comparing surgical and nonsurgical procedures. *J. Endodont.* 1999; 25; 814–17.

26. Kvist T, Reit C. Postoperative discomfort associated with surgical and nonsurgical endodontic retreatment. *Endodont. Dent. Traumatol.* 2000; 16: 71–4.

27. Kvist T, Reit C. The perceived benefit of endodontic retreatment. *Int. Endodont. J.* 2002; 35: 359–65.

28. Kvist T, Reit C, Esposito M, Mileman P, Bianchi S, Petersson K, Andersson C. Prescribing endodontic retreatment: towards a theory of dentist behaviour. *Int. Endodont. J.* 1994; 27: 285–90.

29. Kvist T, Rydin E, Reit C. The relative frequency of periapical lesions in teeth with root canal-retained posts. *J. Endodont.* 1989; 15: 578–80.

30. Langeland K, Block RM, Grossman LI. A histobacteriologic study of 35 periapical endodontic surgical specimens. *J. Endodont.* 1977; 3: 8–23.

31. Ledley RS, Lusted LB. Reasoning foundations of medical diagnosis. *Science* 1959; 130: 9–21.

32. Lusted LB. *Introduction to Medical Decision Making.* Springfield, IL: Charles C. Thomas, 1968.

33. Marques MD, Moreira B, Eriksen HM. Prevalence of apical periodontitis and results of endodontic treatment in an adult, Portuguese population. *Int. Endodont. J.* 1998; 31: 161–5.

34. Molander A, Reit C, Dahlén G, Kvist T. Microbiologic status of root filled teeth with apical periodontitis. *Int. Endodont. J.* 1998; 31: 1–7.

35. Murray CA, Saunders WP. Root canal treatment and general health. A review of the literature. *Int. Endodont. J.* 2000; 33: 1–18.

36. Nair PNR, Pajarola G, Schroeder HE. Types and incidence of human periapical lesions obtained with extracted teeth. *Oral Surg.* 1996; 81: 93–102.

37. Nair PNR, Sjögren U, Krey G, Sundqvist G. Therapy-resistant foreign body giant cell granuloma at the periapex of a root filled human tooth. *J. Endodont.* 1990; 16: 53–9.

38. Nair PNR, Sjögren U, Krey G, Kahnberg K-E, Sundqvist G. Intraradicular bacteria and fungi in root filled, asymptomatic human teeth with therapy-resistant periapical lesions: a long-term light and electron microscopic follow-up study. *J. Endodont.* 1990; 16: 41–9.

39. Natkin E, Oswald RJ, Carnes LI. The relationship of lesion size to diagnosis, incidence, and treatment of periapical cysts and granulomas. *Oral Surg.* 1984; 57: 82–94.

40. von Neumann J, Morgenstern O. *Theory of Games and Economic Behaviour.* Princeton, NJ: Princeton University Press, 1947.

41. Ørstavik D. Time-course and risk analyses of the development and healing of chronic apical periodontitis in man. *Int. Endodont.* 1996; 29: 150–55.

42. Petersson K, Håkansson R, Håkansson J, Olsson B, Wennberg A. Follow-up study of endodontic status in an adult Swedish population. *Endodont. Dent. Traumatol.* 1991; 7: 221–5.

43. Petersson K, Lewin B, Håkansson J, Olsson B, Wennberg A. Endodontic status and suggested treatment in a population requiring substantial dental care. *Endodont. Dent. Traumatol.* 1989; 5: 153–8.

44. Petersson K, Petersson A, Olsson B, Håkansson J, Wennberg A. Technical quality of root fillings in an adult Swedish population. *Endodont. Dent. Traumatol.* 1986; 2: 99–102.

45. Politser P. Decision analysis and clinical judgement. *Med. Decis. Making* 1981; 1: 361–89.

46. Ray HA, Trope M. Periapical status of endodontically treated teeth in relation to the technical quality of the root filling and the coronal restoration. *Int. Endodont. J.* 1995; 28: 12–18.

47. Reit C. Decision strategies in endodontics: on the design of a recall program. *Endodont. Dent. Traumatol.* 1987; 3: 233–9.

48. Reit C, Gröndahl H-G. Management of periapical lesions in endodontically treated teeth: a study on clinical decision making. *Swed. Dent. J.* 1984; 8: 1–7.

49. Reit C, Gröndahl H-G. Endodontic retreatment decision making among a group of general practitioners. *Scand. J. Dent. Res.* 1988; 96: 112–17.

50. Reit C, Gröndahl H-G, Engström B. Endodontic treatment decisions: a study of the clinical decision-making process. *Endodont. Dent. Traumatol.* 1985; 1: 102–7.

51. Reit C, Kvist T. Endodontic retreatment behaviour: the influence of disease concepts and personal values. *Int. Endodont. J.* 1998; 31: 358–63.

52. Ricucci D, Gröndahl K, Bergenholtz G. Periapical status of root filled teeth exposed to the oral environment by loss of restoration or caries. *Oral. Surg.* 2000; 90: 354–9.

53. Rohlin M, Mileman PA. Decision analysis in dentistry – the last 30 years. *J. Dent.* 2000; 28: 453–68.

54. Saunders WP, Saunders EM. Coronal leakage as a cause of failure in root canal therapy: a review. *Endodont. Dent. Traumatol.* 1994; 10: 105–8.

55. Saunders WP, Saunders EM, Sadio J, Cruickshank E. Technical standard of root canal treatment in an adult Scottish sub-population. *Br. Dent. J.* 1997; 182: 382–6.

56. Sidaravicius B, Aleksejuniene J, Eriksen HM. Endodontic treatment and prevalence of apical periodontitis in adult population of Vilnius, Lithuania. *Endodont. Dent. Traumatol.* 1999; 15: 210–15.

57. Siqueira JF Jr, Rocas IN, Lopes HP, Uzeda M. Coronal leakage of two root canal sealers containing calcium hydroxide after exposure to human saliva. *J. Endodont.* 1999; 25: 14–16.

58. Sjögren U, Happonen RP, Kahnberg K-E, Sundqvist G. Survival of *Arachnia propionica* in periapical tissue. *Int. Endodont. J.* 1988; 21: 277–82.

59. Sjögren U, Hägglund B, Sundqvist G, Wing K. Factors effecting the long-term results of endodontic treatment. *J Endodont.* 1990; 16: 31–7.

60. Smith J, Crisp J, Torney D. A survey: controversies in endodontic treatment and re-treatment. *J. Endodont.* 1981; 7: 477–83.

61. Spatafore CM, Griffin JA, Keyes GG, Wearden S, Skidmore AE. Periapical biopsy report: an analysis over a 10-year period. *J. Endodont.* 1990; 16: 239–41.

62. Strindberg LZ. The dependence of the results of pulp therapy on certain factors. *Acta Odontol. Scand.* 1956; 14(Suppl. 21).

63. Sunde PT, Olsen I, Lind PO, Tronstad L. Extraradicular infection: a methodological study. *Endodont. Dent. Traumatol.* 2000; 16: 84–90.

64. Sundqvist G, Figdor D, Persson S, Sjögren U. Microbiologic analysis of teeth with failed endodontic treatment and the outcome of conservative retreatment. *Oral Surg.* 1998; 85: 86–93.

65. Tengs TO, Wallace A. One thousand health-related quality-of-life estimates. *Med. Care* 2000; 38: 583–637.

66. Torrance GW. Measurements of health state utilities for economic appraisal. *J. Health Econ.* 1986; 5: 1–30.

67. Tronstad L, Barnett F, Riso K, Slots J. Extraradicular endodontic infections. *Endodont. Dent. Traumatol.* 1987; 3: 86–90.

68. Weinstein MC, Fineberg HV. *Clinical Decision Analysis.* Philadelphia, PA: W. B. Saunders, 1980.

69. Yusuf H. The significance of the presence of foreign material periapically as a cause of failure of root treatment. *Oral Surg.* 1982; 54: 566–74.

Part 5
CLINICAL METHODOLOGIES

Chapter 15
Radiographic examination

Ib Paul Sewerin

Introduction

Radiographic examination is essential before, during and after an endodontic procedure (Fig. 15.1). Radiographs may reveal information of significance for the assessment of the disease status of the tooth (e.g. root resorption processes) and the surrounding tissues (periapical inflammatory lesions). Radiographs also provide information about anatomy of importance to guide the clinician in his/her approach to the treatment procedures (Fig. 15.2a–d). The following observations are then critical:

(1) The number of root components and root canals.
(2) The possible presence of supernumerary roots and root canals.
(3) The length of the root components.
(4) The width of the root canals.
(5) Root deviations.
(6) Potential presence of obstacles.

During the treatment *per se* the operator is guided by radiographic examination, and after treatment the final result is controlled by radiography, immediately as well as after a period of observation (Fig. 15.3).

In addition, radiographs show how proximal roots are to anatomical structures such as the mandibular canal and the maxillary sinuses. A bony separation between root apices and the sinus may be absent (Fig. 15.2e). If precautions are not taken, the risk of perforating the sinus mucosa and forcing medicaments and root filling material into the sinus cavity is obvious. In the posterior parts of the mandible, a close relationship may exist between root apices and the mandibular canal, which implies a risk for damaging the mandibular nerve by overinstrumentation and overfilling (see further below).

Techniques in radiographic examination for endodontic purposes

Basic demands

In order to evaluate the health status of a tooth and its anatomy, depiction of the whole root complex, including the root apex/apices, the periodontal ligament space, the lamina dura and a surrounding 2 mm of bone, is mandatory. In the case of periapical bone loss, the whole periphery of the destruction should be exposed. For multi-rooted teeth and teeth that may present multi-rooted variations, angulated views are necessary to display each root component.

Imaging techniques

Conventional film radiography
Conventional radiography utilizing traditional x-ray machines, film and processing techniques is still the generally used method in dental practice. However, new alternative techniques have appeared and have been widely tested.

Digital radiography
In recent years digital radiography has progressed. Because the costs of digital radiography are still considerable, the method so far has gained only limited use. An outstanding advantage of this technique is that the radiograph is produced immediately or within a short period of 10–20 s. Digital imaging further offers the possibility of image enhancement, and it is also possible to make exact measurements directly from the computer image. However, no digital system yet has shown better results in determining canal length and file position or interpreting periapical lesions than conventional film imaging (11, 18, 23). In a study comparing diagnostic performance, using conventional D-speed and E-speed films and storage phosphor computed radiography, no significant differences were found (12). The digital

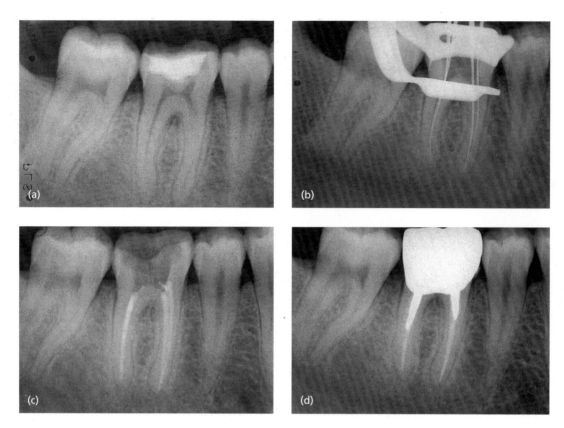

Fig. 15.1 Use of radiography during endodontic procedure: (a) diagnosis and treatment planning; (b) determination of working length; (c) control of root filling; (d) control of final treatment.

technique also includes subtraction programs, which means an improvement in identifying minor lesions and changes in radiographic density not visible by the naked eye. However, to be useful, identical projections are critical.

Other imaging techniques

Xeroradiographic images: produced by an electrostatic process, these were expected to facilitate visualization of early periapical lesions due to the edge enhancement of the technique, but this has not been the case (21).

Multimodal narrow-beam systems: producing sequential tomographic images, such systems have been shown to perform as well as conventional periapical radiography for detecting periapical bone lesions (20), but the equipment is expensive.

Microcomputed tomography (Fig. 15.4): this is a fascinating new methodology because it presents accurate, three-dimensional images of internal tooth morphology (5, 15). The method is complicated and time-consuming and until now has been used only for research purposes.

In conclusion, we are at the doorstep of the digital era in dental radiography and yet the new methods have not totally replaced conventional radiography in the daily practice of endodontics. Consequently, in the present chapter radiographic diagnosis and working procedures are based on conventional radiographic techniques. This chapter also is limited to radiography in relation to endodontic treatment of the adult patient.

Bisecting angle or paralleling technique?

Geometric considerations

Because exact measurements of root lengths are important for the proper instrumentation of root canal(s) in endodontic therapy, a radiographic technique resulting in minimum image magnification and minimum image distortion is crucial.

Before any treatment is started, an initial radiograph must be taken to serve as a preliminary guide for the procedures to be undertaken (Fig. 15.1a). Of the two classical techniques for obtaining periapical radiographs – the bisecting angle technique and the paralleling technique – the latter is recommended without reservations. The bisecting angle technique is maintained to secure

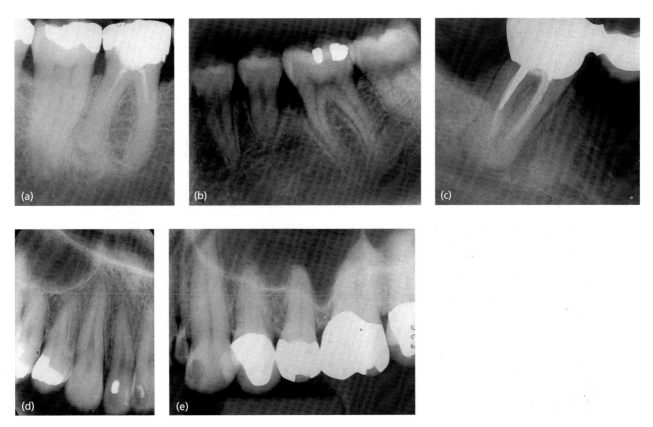

Fig. 15.2 Unpredictable radiographic findings of importance for endodontic treatment: (a) extraordinarily long roots of tooth 47 and hypercementosis of distal root component and angulation of mesial root component of tooth 46; (b) extraordinarily short roots of mandibular premolars; (c) likely inaccessible apical region due to root canal obturation and hypercementosis; (d) denticle in tooth 13 (courtesy of Dr G. Bergenholtz); (e) large maxillary sinus with recesses between roots of posterior maxillary teeth and a close relationship of roots to bony wall of sinus, representing a risk of intruding the maxillary sinus during instrumentation and root filling procedures.

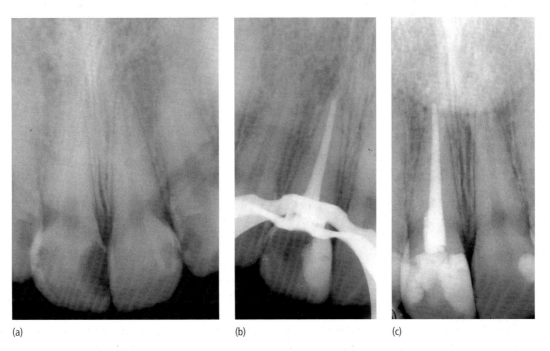

Fig. 15.3 Series of radiographs taken in conjunction with endodontic therapy of tooth 11: (a) initial radiograph showing a mesial, deep caries lesion prompting the treatment; (b) immediate postoperative radiograph demonstrating the dense root canal filling; (c) radiograph taken at a 2-year recall appointment showing normal periapical conditions and indicating a successful outcome (courtesy of Dr A. Gesi).

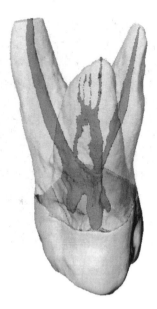

Fig. 15.4 Three-dimensional transparent reconstruction of the pulp chamber and the root canals in a permanent first upper molar (courtesy of Dr L. Bjørndal).

exact root lengths without magnification, but only in theory; for multi-rooted teeth with different distances between the root apices and the film, distortion always occurs (Fig. 15.5).

Forsberg and Halse (7) measured experimentally how the size of simulated periapical lesions was projected by the bisecting and the paralleling techniques. The bisecting technique often resulted in incorrect reproductions of the true lesion range, and reduction in size up to 50% was sometimes observed. It was concluded that the paralleling technique is far more accurate in imaging the extent of periapical lesions.

The paralleling technique is based upon the use of film-holding devices, among which a great number are available (Fig. 15.6a). For radiographs taken during the endodontic procedure certain problems exist, because these radiographs are taken under a rubber dam and often with instruments inserted into the root canal. Special film-holders allowing the presence of root canal instruments during exposure are available (Fig. 15.6b).

Working length determination

The ideal depth of instrumentation and thus the final position of the root filling must be determined with great accuracy. Two factors are in effect:

(1)   Any radiographic image will be magnified because there is a distance between the object (the tooth) and the film. The magnification varies with focus–object distance (a) and object–film distance

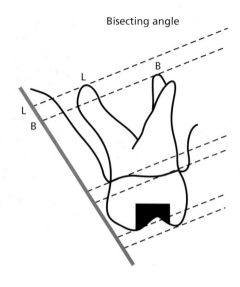

Bisecting angle

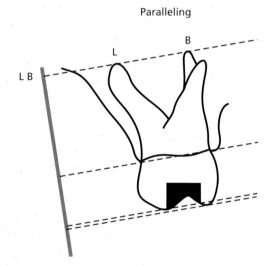

Paralleling

Fig. 15.5 Drawing demonstrating the principles of the bisecting angle and the paralleling techniques. In the bisecting angle technique the radiographic film is placed in close contact with the tooth crown. This position results in image distortion because the film plane and the longitudinal tooth axis form an angle. In the paralleling technique the film is positioned (using a film-holding device) parallel with the long axis of the tooth and thus minimizes distortion. L = lingual; B = buccal.

(b). To give two examples: if a is 150 mm (short cone technique) and b is 30 mm (typical maxillary incisor distance), the magnification will be 20%; if a is 300 mm (long cone technique) and b is 10 mm (typical mandibular molar distance), the magnification will be only 3%.

(2)   If the long axis of the tooth is angulated in relation to the film plane, elongation or shortening will appear on the radiograph. For multi-rooted teeth with facial and lingual roots, the problem is even

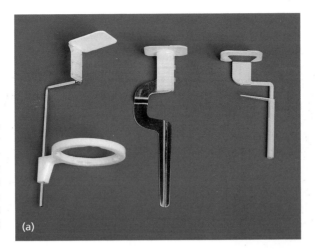
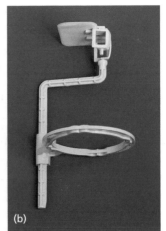

Fig. 15.6 Film-holders for use in endodontic radiography. (a) Devices for paralleling technique in initial radiograph: (right) XCP-holding device; (center) Eggen film-holder; (left) Hawe Super-Bite. (b) Device for working length determination with instrument in the root canal during radiographic exposure.

more complex because angulations of the buccal and lingual roots commonly differ in their relation to the main axis of the tooth.

It is nearly impossible to calculate the exact length of a root from a single radiograph, therefore working length determination by radiography is carried out in three steps:

(1) The initial radiograph, giving an overview of the root anatomy, provides a rough estimate of the root canal length. This radiograph should be taken with the paralleling technique to secure the least distortion possible.

(2) The radiograph serves as a guide for insertion of a root canal instrument to the approximated working length. The instrument must carry a stop, which is placed level with a reference point on the tooth surface (incisal edge or cusp tip).

(3) The true working length is decided from the subsequent radiograph, which will show the distance of the instrument tip to the radiographic apex. If the instrument ends more than 1 mm shorter or longer of what is considered to be an ideal length of instrumentation, then a new radiograph should be taken for an accurate estimate.

A simplified method allowing an immediate reading of the tooth length is to use a calibrated ruler (Fig. 15.7).

Note that bending of the film package may influence the apparent instrument and tooth length. Bending away from the apex will cause an elongation of the radiographic instrument ('trial file') length compared with the factual length (Fig. 15.8). Because film bending may be difficult to control in the mouth, the use of a stiff backing is desirable.

Another method for working length determination is the use of electronic devices (see Chapter 16).

Marinal

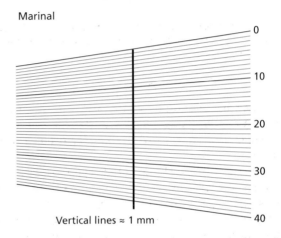

Vertical lines ≈ 1 mm

Fig. 15.7 Calibrated ruler for working length determination (Marinal®). A radiograph with an instrument of known length inserted is exposed. Any image magnification and/or distortion will be proportional for the instrument and the tooth, and the true (previous unknown) length of the tooth can be read directly.

Angulated views

Three-dimensional interpretation

A single radiograph only provides a two-dimensional perspective. Bone and dental structures then become superimposed and it is impossible to determine their position relative to each other, e.g. whether a structure is facial or lingual to another structure. In endodontics this applies to positions of roots and inserted instruments for working length determination. Taking two projections from different angles and a logical use of the principle of parallax enables the dentist to distinguish these positions.

The principle is based on the fact that the position of a structure close to the film remains more stable than a structure that is distant to the film when both structures are observed from viewing angles that are altered from the orthogonal projection. This is the essence of the 'Buccal object rule' and the popular 'SLOB rule' (Same Lingual, Opposite Buccal): it appears as if a 'lingual' structure (close to the film) 'moves' in the 'same' direc-tion as the tube, and a 'buccal' structure (distant to the film) moves in the 'opposite' direction, when the pro-jection angle is changed (Fig. 15.9).

Figure 15.10 shows two images of a maxillary first pre-molar from a full mouth survey: an orthogonal view (bitewing projection) shows one root filling and one post, whereas a mesial view (canine periapical projec-tion) reveals a buccal and a lingual root filling and, moreover, informs that the post is positioned in the lingual root component.

In producing angulated views for three-dimensional interpretation it is essential that the film is placed in exactly the same position for each exposure. The central x-ray beam should be angulated 20° mesially and dis-tally in relation to the orthogonal projection in the hori-zontal plane. It is of great help to use film-holders with a beam-guiding device (Fig. 15.6).

Extended use of full mouth surveys

In full mouth surveys, most teeth are depicted more than once and in different views. A comparison of these views often provides valuable information on root anatomies. Permanent mandibular incisors frequently contain two canals (6, 13). The faciolingual dimension of the canal is always clearly larger than in the mesiodistal dimension. A view strictly perpendicular to the facial surface pro-vides only limited information on the morphology of the pulp chamber and the root canals compared with angulated views. The routine canine projections often add valuable information about root canal anatomy

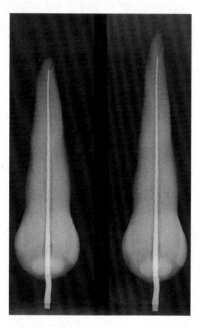

Fig. 15.8 Which is the true length of this canine? All exposure variables were the same, except that the film package was bent in the apical region in the right-hand image.

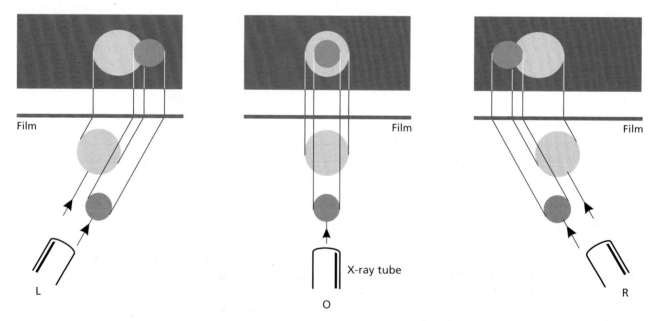

Fig. 15.9 The principle of parallax ('buccal object rule' or 'SLOB rule'). In an orthogonal view (O) the two structures (the large and the small ball) will appear superimposed on the film. The structure closest to the film (the large ball) is the most 'stable' when the two structures are viewed from the left (L) and from the right (R). The structure distant to the film (the small ball) will 'move' in the opposite direction as the x-rays focus.

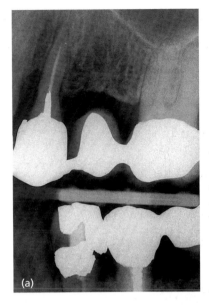
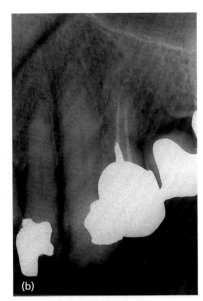

Fig. 15.10 (a) Orthogonal view in a bitewing radiograph reveals root filling and post in tooth 24. (b) Mesial view reveals two root fillings and the position of the post in the lingual canal.

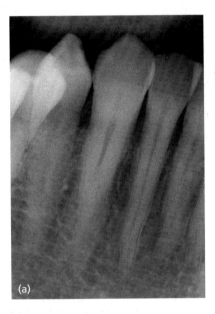
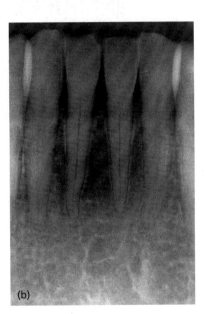

Fig. 15.11 Additional information obtained by combining different views from a full mouth survey: (a) mandibular canine projection; (b) incisor projection. Although teeth 42 and 41 show one canal in certain views, other views reveal divided canals in both. Also note the divided canal in the apical half of tooth 43.

of the incisors by depicting them in angulated views (Fig. 15.11).

Advantages and limitations of radiographs

By proper use of radiography, endodontic procedures are facilitated and the prospect for a successful result of the treatment is improved. However, the dentist should be cognisant of several limitations in the informative yield of the radiographs (Core concept 15.1; Case study 1).

Accessory canals, lateral branches and apical ramifications are most often so discrete that they cannot be expected to be visible in radiographs (19). Indeed, scanning electron microscopy (SEM) studies have revealed up to 16 apical foramina in permanent teeth and a variation of 0.2–0.38 mm in the distances between tips of the apices and the foraminal openings (10), but such ramifications are rarely identified unless they are filled by a contrasting medium, e.g. root filling material.

Radiographic diagnosis of sequelae to pulp necrosis

Expressions of periapical disease

Periapical pathoses nearly exclusively affect interior areas of the alveolar bone and are thus not accessible for

---

Core concept 15.1 Advantages of radiography and limitations in the interpretation of radiographs in endodontology

Advantages

Provides information regarding:

- Root morphology
  - stage of development (children and adolescents)
  - number of root components
  - number of root canals
  - diversions of root components.
- Previous endodontic treatment
  - length, density and adaptation of root filling.
- Periapical lesion
  - presence
  - extension
  - position
  - complications (e.g. cyst formation)
  - pathogenesis (e.g. parietal perforation).
- Root canal obstructions.
- Complications of endodontic treatment
  - fracture of instruments
  - root perforations
  - root fractures.
- Adjacent anatomical structure (e.g. mandibular canal, mental foramen, maxillary sinus).

Limitations

- The radiograph is two-dimensional, which means that:
  - structures may be obscured
  - overlapping structures cannot be separated
  - no conclusions can be drawn about the relationship between structures at different distances from the film.
- Radiography is a crude method of examination, and radiographically demonstrable bone lesions are always less extensive than the true lesions.
- The radiograph is a static image providing no information about the dynamics of disease processes.
- Diagnostic sensitivity and specificity are low.
- Intra- and interobserver variability are high.

---

direct visual inspection. Because clinical symptoms often are absent or scarce, imaging techniques such as radiography are therefore often the only means by which periapical lesions can be detected.

An osteolytic lesion will be visible only if there is loss of mineral to an extent that the difference of radiographic density is detectable by the naked eye. Several studies have pointed out that cortical bone lesions are easier to identify than lesions limited to the cancellous bone. This is due to the relatively higher loss of mineral lesions produced in cortical bone (4).

Any lesion starts as a discrete, hardly demonstrable radiolucency, which gradually may progress. In some cases the lesion becomes sharply demarcated, and in other cases it appears diffuse (Fig. 15.12). The latter is one explanation as to why there is wide inter- and intraobserver variability in the diagnosis of periapical lesions (8, 16, 21) (see also Chapter 14).

It is important to realize that the radiographic image tells us nothing about the age of a bony change or about its stage, e.g. whether it is progressing or healing or symptomatic (Fig. 15.13).

Apical periodontitis may produce various features in the radiograph suggesting that a lesion may be about to progress. Such indications include widening of the apical periodontal space and loss of lamina dura. However, these signs are also associated with teeth subjected to:

- Traumatic occlusion
- Ongoing orthodontic treatment (Fig. 15.14)
- A previous trauma.

Hence, the identification of a widened periodontal space or loss of lamina dura may or may not suggest that a root canal infection is ongoing (Fig. 15.15).

Periapical sclerosis
In certain cases of apical periodontitis a sclerosis may appear. The sclerotic zone may either surround the entire periapical radiolucency or occupy the whole lesion area (Fig. 15.16).

Differential diagnosis

Periapical radiolucencies may have causes other than an infected pulp necrosis and are therefore important to identify before a treatment decision is taken. Examples include:

- Anatomical structures
- Developmental and physiological phenomena
- Periapical scar tissue
- Traumatic injury
- Tumor
- Periapical lesion of periodontal origin
- Osteomyelitis
- Radicular cysts.

Distinguishing a fully formed radicular cyst from non-cystic lesions of apical periodontitis is another differential diagnostic issue that will be considered here.

Anatomical structures
Radiolucent anatomical structures may be projected over the apical area of teeth and simulate apical pathosis. This may be the case with mandibular premolars, where the mental foramen may project in the vicinity of

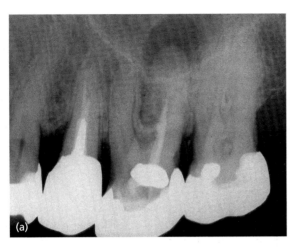

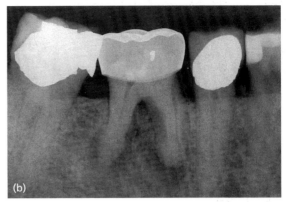

Fig. 15.12   Examples of radiographic distinctness of periapical lesions: (a) sharply demarcated lesion at palatinal root component of tooth 26; (b) diffusely demarcated lesion at mesial and distal root components of tooth 46, making it difficult to state the extent of the lesion.

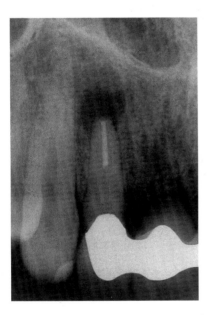

Fig. 15.13   The radiograph tells us nothing about the stage of a lesion (progressing, healing?). Essential for diagnosis of the periapical radiolucency of tooth 12 is information about previous findings (larger or smaller lesion?) and time of previous treatment. Actually, this tooth was surgically treated 2 months before the radiograph was taken ('empty' lumen may be a composite paste).

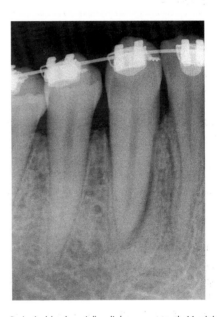

Fig. 15.14   Periapical (and mesial) radiolucency at tooth 44 originating from orthodontic treatment forces.

the root tip (Fig. 15.17). If the tooth through the radiolucency displays a clear periodontal ligament space around its circumference, it suggests representation of the mental foramen.

In the maxillary incisor region a pronounced incisive fossa as well as the incisive canal may be misinterpreted as a periapical lesion. Even the radiolucent zone on each side of the nasal septum, representing the air-filled nostrils, sometimes gives rise to questions on the possibility of periapical lesions associated with the maxillary central incisors (Fig. 15.18).

Developmental and physiological phenomena

One simple explanation of a periapical radiolucency may be that root formation has not terminated and the apical foramen is still open. In the primary dentition periapical radiolucencies are normal findings during stages of physiological resorption. Around retained primary teeth in adulthood with slowly progressing resorption, similar radiolucencies can be seen.

Periapical scar tissue

Surgical treatment of periapical lesions may sometimes result in the formation of scar tissue, leaving a permanent defect in the bone that is visible in the radiograph (Fig. 15.19). Typical findings indicative of scar tissue formation are, according to Molven *et al.* (14):

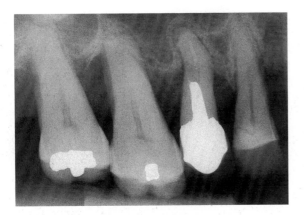

Fig. 15.15   Widened periodontal space at tooth 15.

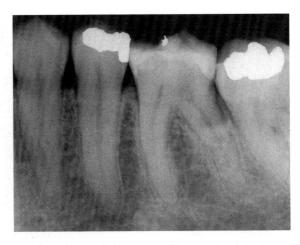

Fig. 15.17   Periapical radiolucency around the apex of tooth 35. Because the periodontal membrane space appears intact, it can be concluded that there is an overlapping of the mental foramen.

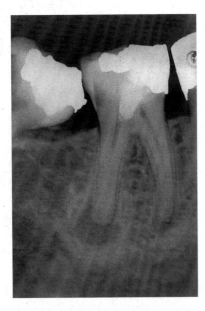

Fig. 15.16   Bone sclerosis bordering periapical lytic lesions at both roots of tooth 46.

- Reduction of the bony defect but persistence of a widened periodontal membrane.
- A pattern of irradiating fine bone trabeculae in contact with the root end.
- A solitary defect surrounded by compact bone but without root contact.

Traumatic injury

Typical results of acute physical traumas are luxation injuries (Fig. 15.20). Extrusive as well as lateral (facial) luxations will generate widened periapical spaces without pulp being necrotic or infected. The majority of dental injuries involve maxillary central incisors and may cause horizontal root fractures (3) (Fig. 15.21). Injured teeth should be followed radiographically to catch later development of lateral or periapical tissue changes (Fig. 15.22) and external root resorptions that may destroy the entire root structure.

Tumors

Radiographically one of the odontogenic tumors – the periapical cemental dysplasia – shows a close resemblance to a periapical lesion of infectious origin (Fig. 15.23). This tumor is easily distinguished from periapical inflammatory lesions because the pulp will appear vital and the tooth, in many cases, is intact and without any history of trauma. In later stages, the radiolucent area will be occupied by mineralizations that start in its central portion. Such lesions certainly do not require endodontic treatment.

Osteogenic sarcomas belong to the malignancies that may affect the jaws. If the origin of the tumor is adjacent to root structures, widening of the periodontal space and associated migration of neighboring teeth are typical signs. Although such a lesion is extremely rare, it should always be considered in cases when there is a periapical radiolucency on a tooth where the pulp is clearly vital (see Case study 2).

Metastases from malignant tumors elsewhere in the body may affect the jaws and also may be located in the periapical region of teeth. Radiographically they are characterized by indistinct borders. Often the compact bone is involved.

Periapical lesion of periodontal origin

A marginal periodontal destruction may reach and involve the periapical region. In most cases the route of infection is obvious, but sometimes a local marginal destruction may be obscure radiographically and the periapical lesion may be mistaken for a process of endodontic origin (Fig. 15.24).

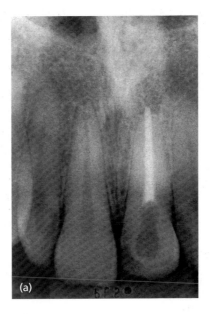

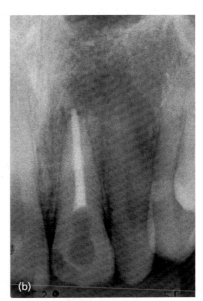

Fig. 15.18 (a) Questionable periapical lesion around the apex of endodontically treated tooth 21. (b) Distal view reveals that the 'lesion' is due to nostril radiolucency and nasal cartilage radiopacity.

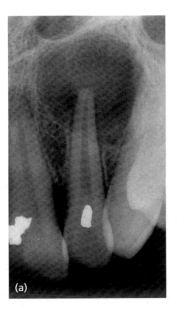

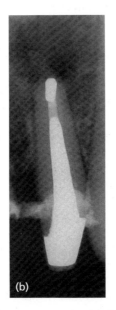

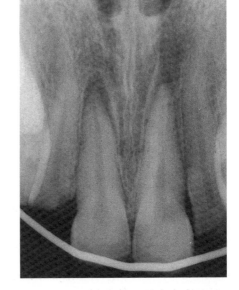

Fig. 15.19 (a) Preoperative radiograph showing cystic lesion at tooth 22. (b) Control radiograph 14 months after resection of root and retrograde root filling (amalgam), showing periapical bony scar around the apex of the tooth.

Fig. 15.20 Periapical radiolucencies of teeth 11 and 21 due to luxation following mechanical trauma.

In lesions of suspected combined endodontic and periodontal origin, pulp vitality may exclude the need for endodontic treatment, but in cases of non-vitality the two entities are often difficult to distinguish from each other.

Osteomyelitis
On very rare occasions endodontic infections may spread and involve large areas of surrounding bone and cause osteomyelitis (Chapter 9; Fig. 15.25). This condi-

tion is accompanied by severe pain and elevated body temperature. The radiographic image is characteristic and shows a linear pattern of radiolucent bone, leaving islands of normal bone, which later may become devitalized and transform to sequestrae.

Radicular cysts
A periapical inflammatory lesion eventually may transform to a radicular cyst (Chapter 9; Fig. 15.26). A sign indicating cystic transformation is a sclerotic zone bordering a distinct, fairly large radiolucent area. Cysts tend

to be larger than non-cystic lesions of apical periodontitis (granulomas), although there is a wide variation in the size of each. Only a few non-cystic lesions grow to a size exceeding $70\,mm^2$ (22), whereas cysts will expand continuously and finally may occupy a considerable portion of the jaw bone. However, a firm diagnosis is often not possible, especially when lesions are relatively small. From a treatment point of view the differential diagnosis is not important because both lesions are treated similarly by conventional endodontic therapy. Only if failing or if exudation through the root canal by cyst fluid prevents completion of endodontic therapy is surgical treatment indicated.

Information from radiographs essential to endodontic therapy

Producing radiographs of optimum image quality and interpreting them correctly serves an important basis for attaining high success rates of endodontic therapy.

Dental anatomy

Pulp cavity
On assessing a possible exposure of the pulp in carious teeth or the relation of the pulp to deep fillings, one has to understand two facts about the radiographic image:

(1)   The radiograph is two-dimensional and distances between two points will depend on the projection angle.
(2)   The radiographic image shows a burn-out effect.

This means that a pulp cavity with curved borders and tiny extensions of pulpal horns will not be depicted with clearly delineated margins. In general, the pulp cavity has a greater extension than is usually visualized by radiographs.

Root complex
In many cases the depiction of the root complex on a radiograph seems unsatisfactory but cannot be improved for anatomical reasons. Figure 15.27 shows an example of root apices of a maxillary first premolar that

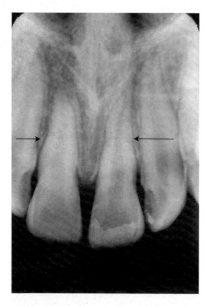

Fig. 15.21   Horizontal root fractures (arrows) following frontal injury (courtesy of Dr G. Bergenholtz).

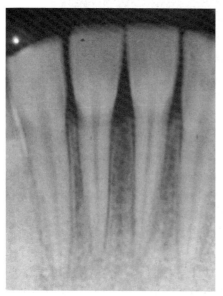
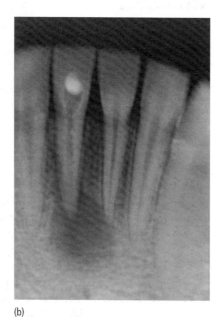

(a)   (b)

Fig. 15.22   (a) Radiograph of lower right incisor injured following a fall in the schoolyard. There are no visible pathological changes. (b) One year later a periradicular radiolucency was present and root canal treatment was initiated. Observe that the access opening is situated too far gingivally, which precludes access to a lingual canal (courtesy of Dr P. Hørsted-Bindslev).

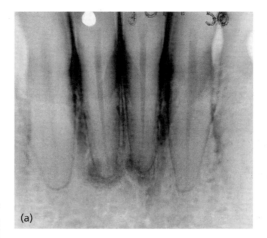

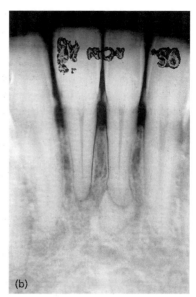

Fig. 15.23 (a) Periapical radiolucency around the apices of teeth 31 and 41 with vital pulp, diagnosed as periapical cemental dysplasia. (b) Later in the process, the radiolucency becomes filled by coalescent radiopacities of cementum (courtesy of Dr G. Bergenholtz).

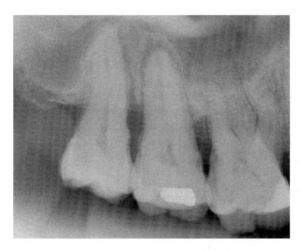

Fig. 15.24   Periapical radiolucency around the apex of tooth 16, presumably of periodontal origin.

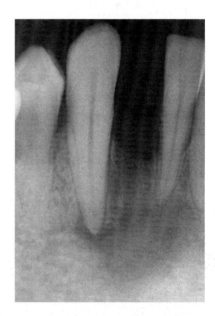

Fig. 15.25   Osteomyelitis in the apical area of tooth 43 in a 74-year-old man. Tooth 42 has been lost due to the infection. A widespread, diffusely demarcated radiolucency is seen.

are hardly distinguishable from the surrounding bone. Two factors determine how clearly visible and how distinct a root structure will be depicted in a radiograph:

(1) *The ratio between root volume and surrounding bone volume.* The thicker the root and the thinner the surrounding bone, the better the root will present itself, and vice versa. Gracile roots surrounded by thick and heavily mineralized bone may be camouflaged easily.

(2) *Root morphology and the direction of the central x-ray beam.* A flat lateral root surface depicted by x-rays parallel to its surface will appear with maximum definition compared with a rounded surface. An apex with a cut surface will appear more distinct than a pointed one.

Root canals

Information about root anatomy, i.e. number of roots, deviations, obstructions, root canal width, etc. (Fig. 15.2), which is essential for proper treatment planning, may be obtained in two ways: by tactile exploration during root canal instrumentation and by imaging methods, e.g. radiography. In general these two methods supplement each other and one cannot do without the other. Although it should be possible to identify all root canal orifices by direct visual examination, it is essential to employ radiographic examinations prior to initiation of therapy. Radiographs may reveal the number of roots and the expected number of canals as well as their courses and passages. Also, any aberrations from the normal pattern may be disclosed. For example, mandibular premolars and canines may present doublings of root complexes and supernumerary root canals (Fig. 15.28). Mandibular molars may also

exhibit supernumerary roots (*radix paramolaris* and *radix entomolaris*) with separate supernumerary root canals (Fig. 15.29). It should be noted that supernumerary roots may be camouflaged completely in ordinary, orthogonal projections.

Root curvatures

Deviations of root apices that are parallel to the film plane are normally clearly visualized, but deviations that are perpendicular to the film plane are hardly discernible. Therefore during endodontic treatment the clinician should anticipate that curvatures in such directions do occur and may pose a risk for causing a ledge or root perforation. If a trial file radiograph shows that the ideal working length is not reached, and if the operator feels an obstruction in the root canal, then a buccal or lingual curvature may be the cause (Fig. 15.30). In such cases an angulated view may reveal the existence of a curvature. Using the SLOB rule (see above), it is then possible to determine if the deviation is directed in a buccal or a lingual direction.

Root canal width

In order to carry out a successful endodontic treatment the root canal must be patent all the way to the apical region (Fig. 15.2). There may be a general narrowing of the canal, resulting in a (nearly) total obliteration, or there may be local obstructions due to mineralizations. On assessing these aberrations it should be borne in

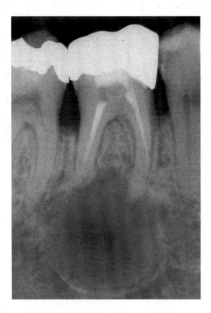

Fig. 15.26   Typical radicular cyst.

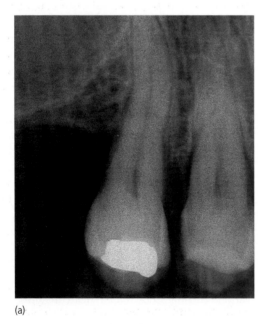

(a)

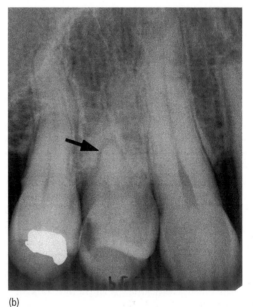

(b)

Fig. 15.27   Gracile root components of tooth 14, resulting in virtual radiographic invisibility: (a) premolar projection; (b) canine projection. Careful examination of original radiographs reveals two separated components of normal length. The structure marked with an arrow in (b), resembling a short root, represents the furcation between the root components.

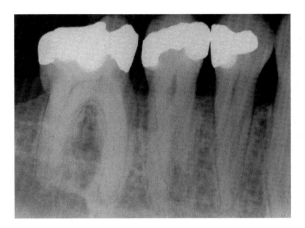

Fig. 15.28 Identification of the number of root canals. In tooth 46 two distinct canals are seen mesially, tooth 45 is a two-rooted variant with two separate canals and tooth 44 exhibits diversion of the apical half.

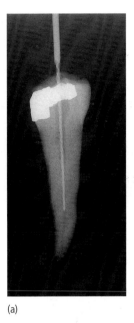 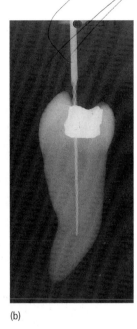

(a)   (b)

Fig. 15.30 (a) Facial view of a mandibular premolar with an instrument inserted showing a 'stop' 5 mm from apex. In a clinical situation the operator might try to force the instrument to a more apical level. (b) A mesial view tells us that the root has a buccal diversion. Efforts to force the instrument in a more apical direction would probably result in a lingual perforation of the root or an instrument fracture.

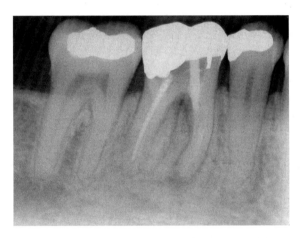

Fig. 15.29 A *radix entomolaris* located lingually in tooth 46. It has obviously not been identified during the endodontic treatment because it is not filled.

mind that the radiographic image of a root canal depends on:

- The morphology of the canal.
- Its extent in relation to the central x-ray beam.
- The ratio between hard-tissue volume and pulp canal volume.

This means that in certain cases, even if a canal seems totally obliterated, a root canal may be found and successfully treated.

Previous endodontic treatments

Root fillings and post materials
Root fillings may show apical or lateral voids and/or be either short or overfilled. Root filled teeth also may contain posts that are fabricated from various materials.

The most common core material for root fillings is gutta-percha, and a radiopaque root canal sealer is often added. Although these products have a virtually identical degree of radiopacity, it is somewhat below that of metal (Fig. 15.31).

In clinical practice, patients sometimes have root fillings with metallic cones as the core material (most often silver). Root fillings with silver cones and gutta-percha are easily distinguishable due to the radiopacity of the metal (Fig. 15.32).

The radiograph may also suggest the kind of post material being used. Identification of post material is of great significance for the assessment of whether post removal should be attempted or not in a retreatment effort. The radiopacity of post materials differs according to their atomic number (Z). Posts from gold ($Z = 79$) are highly radiopaque, whereas posts from carbon fibers ($Z = 6$) are radiolucent. Posts with radiopacities in-between these values are: palladium ($Z = 46$), zirconium ($Z = 40$), titanium ($Z = 22$) and silicium-inforced carbon ($Z(Si) = 14$) (Fig. 15.31).

Retrograde root fillings formerly were identified easily because amalgam was the most commonly used material. Today, retrograde root fillings are often made with various cements (e.g. glass ionomer cements, reinforced zinc oxide–eugenol cements, mineral trioxide).

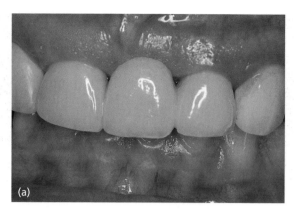
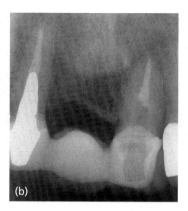

Fig. 15.31 Different root filling and post materials. (a) A 5-year-old porcelain metallic fused bridge from tooth 11 to tooth 22 (courtesy of Dr F. Isidor). (b) In tooth 11 there is a casted metallic post (possibly gold) and the remaining gutta-percha root filling. In tooth 22 the post is made from carbon fibers, which is radiolucent, and the canal appears empty except for the apical part, which is occupied by a gutta-percha filling (courtesy of Dr P. Hørsted-Bindslev).

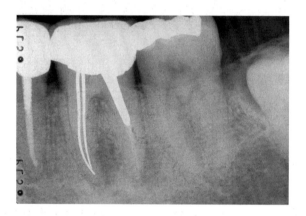

Fig. 15.32 Tooth 36 with two silver cone root fillings mesially and one gutta-percha root filling distally. Periapical radiolucencies are seen around both roots.

A retrograde filling also may be carried out with gutta-percha and a sealer (Chapter 20). There is a varying radiodensity of such materials, which makes them difficult to identify. A composite material introduced by Rud *et al.* (17) contains ytterbium trifluoride to produce (semi-)radiopacity (Fig. 15.33).

Treatment complications

Fracture of instruments
An undesirable complication to endodontic treatment is the separation of an instrument in the canal. The instrument is easily identified by radiography because of the radiopacity of the metal. In root filled teeth fractured instruments are more difficult to identify due to over-projection of the gutta-percha (Fig. 15.34).

Root fracture
Too violent handling during endodontic procedures may cause root fracture. More often, however, root fractures are seen as a late complication to endodontic treatment and post placement (Chapter 12). Fractures of this kind may be difficult to diagnose in an early stage, and they may not become evident until the fragments separate from each other and a periradicular radiolucency has appeared (Fig. 15.35).

Periapical extrusion of root filling material
Sealer as well as core material may be forced through the apical foramen in conjunction with the filling procedure (Fig. 15.36a–e). In many cases only minor initial symptoms follow, and root filling material may remain periapically for years without causing much irritation and may gradually disappear (Fig. 15.36a, b).

However, complications do occur. Figure 15.36c shows a case where a root filling has been forced into the maxillary sinus. Another serious complication is when root filling material is extruded periapically in the lower molar region or directly into the mandibular canal (Fig. 15.36d, e). Such a complication often causes either temporary or permanent paresthesia. The intracanalicular location is revealed by a horizontal extension of root filling material along the cranial border of the canal (Fig. 15.36e). Rapid surgical removal of the excess material may prevent long-term persistence of the paresthesia (9) (see Case study 3).

In the mandibular molar region, extrusion of root filling material through the thin lingual alveolar plate has been reported (1). Owing to the summarizing effect in radiography, a displacement of root filling material to the sublingual soft tissues may be mistaken for an intra-

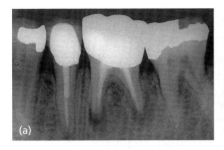
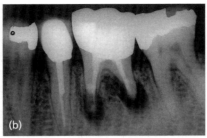
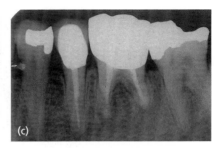

Fig. 15.33 Surgical treatment of periapical lesion on mesial and distal root components of tooth 36: (a) preoperative radiograph; (b) control radiograph after surgical procedure of retrograde root canal sealing with composite resin containing contrast medium; (c) healing after 1 year. (Courtesy Dr V. Rud.)

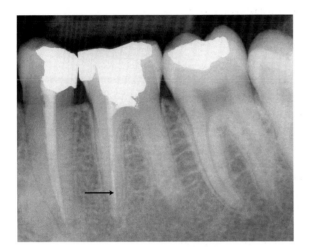

Fig. 15.34 Careful examination reveals a broken instrument in the mesial root component of tooth 36 (→). It may be situated in a non-filled root canal concealed by the root filling in the neighboring canal.

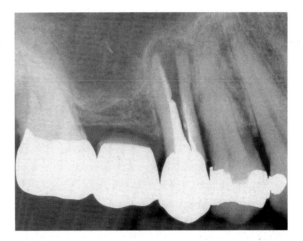

Fig. 15.35 Fracture of the root filled tooth 15, probably due to forces from the metallic post.

bony localization. A cross-sectional occlusal projection view will give the answer.

Iatrogenic root perforations

Instruments used for access opening or for canal preparation may be forced through the root canal wall and cause a perforation to the lateral surface of the root (Fig. 15.37). Also, perforations through the subpulpal wall may occur (for a review, see Ref. 2). In certain cases a false root canal may be created outside the root by the operator and, if unnoticed, a root filling may be placed in the periodontal space or in the surrounding bone rather than in the canal *per se* (see Case study 4).

Controls following completion of root filling

The immediate radiographic control of a completed root filling includes the same considerations as the initial demonstration of root anatomy. In order to depict all filled root canals without overlaps, angulated views are essential. Many root canals in single-rooted teeth

have faciolingual dimensions that are larger than the mesiodistal dimension. Often a circular cross-section of the canal is not obtained prior to root filling, with a risk of leaving narrow extensions of the root canal buccally and lingually unfilled. This indeed emphasizes the importance of angulated views. Figure 15.38a shows a central incisor with an apparently sufficient root filling. An angulated projection reveals severe torsion of the gutta-percha point (Fig. 15.38b).

Non-healing or emerging lesion

Because success cannot be guaranteed in endodontic treatment and because clinical symptoms are infrequently present in cases of periapical pathosis, radiographic control is essential. After completion of an endodontic treatment, a clinical and radiographic checkup should be scheduled within a 6–12-month period. If a tooth then is without clinical symptoms and is radiographically without a periapical radiolucency, the treatment is regarded as successful and need not be followed further. If a lesion persists or has appeared, the patient should be re-examined periodically until a decision about further treatment measures is taken (Chapter 14).

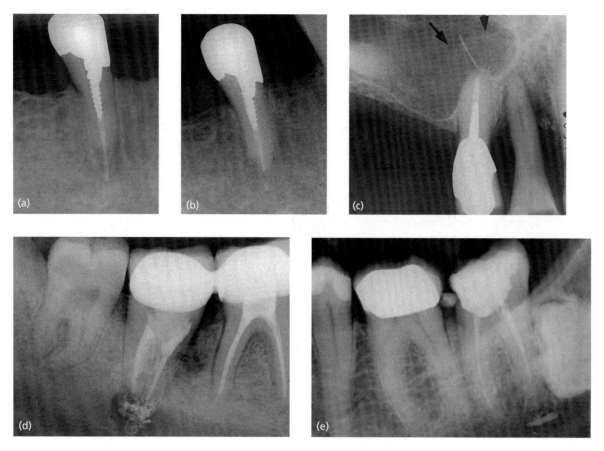

Fig. 15.36 (a) Surplus of root filling material periapically of tooth 45. No postoperative symptoms. (b) Resorption of some of the root filling material and normal periapical conditions 10 years later (courtesy of Dr P. Hørsted-Bindslev). (c) Root filling material forced into maxillary sinus, associated with irritative mucosal reaction (arrows). (d) Extrusion of root filling material through apical foramen and a close relation to mandibular canal. The patient suffered from paresthesia of the skin area innervated from the inferior alveolar nerve for months. (e) Root filling material forced into mandibular canal during endodontic treatment of tooth 37.

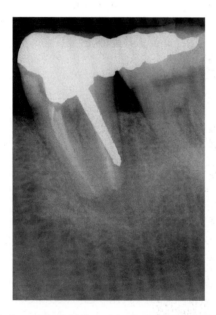

Fig. 15.37 Large periapical lesion originating from unsuccessful treatment of mesial canals and perforation of the distal root by a post.

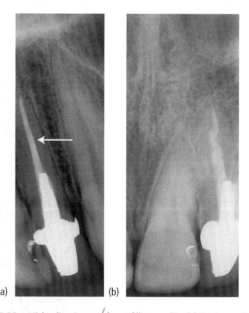

Fig. 15.38 Misleading image of root filling quality. (a) Canine projection of teeth 11 and 21. Varying radiopacity (→) may indicate curvature in root canal or a loose fit of the root filling. (b) An incisal projection reveals torsion of the gutta-percha point (courtesy of Dr P. Hørsted-Bindslev).

Case study 1

Root resorption due to apical periodontitis

A male patient felt discomfort and mild tenderness from tooth 26 for years. Apicectomy and retrograde root fillings of the buccal root components were performed. A control radiograph showed a well-delineated palatinal root component with a periodontal space of normal width (a). After a period of persisting symptoms the tooth was extracted. An extensive resorption of the palatal root component was found, indicating chronic periodontitis (b).

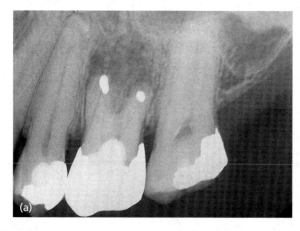

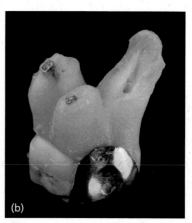

Case study 2

Differential diagnosis in periapical pathology

A 32-year-old healthy man was referred for an incidental radiographic finding of a widened periodontal membrane space around tooth 21. A pulp vitality test was positive. The tooth had changed its position and, furthermore, there was a hard swelling in the apical region of the facial alveolar bone. The findings are suggestive of a malignant disease and biopsy revealed an osteosarcoma.

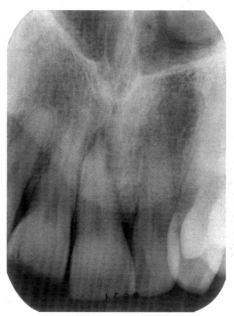

Case study 3

Root filling material intruding the mandibular canal

A 52-year-old woman had tooth 36 root filled. The patient soon felt pain and paresthesia developed in the mental region of the same side. The dentist removed the root filling but was unable to remove the material outside the apical foramen. A radiograph taken after removal of the root filling (a) showed sealer and 4 mm of gutta-percha in the periapical area, in close relation to or inside the mandibular canal.

The radiograph (b) was taken after surgical removal of the excess material and after new root filling. (Courtesy of Dr Jens Kølsen Petersen.)

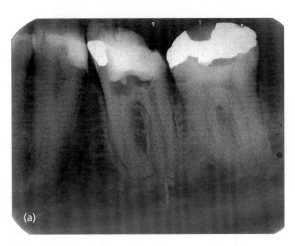 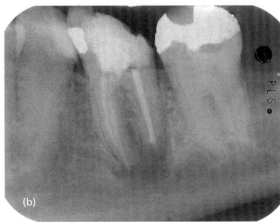

Case study 4

Value of angulated radiographic view

A 62-year-old female presented with symptoms from tooth 16. A radiograph was taken, which showed root fillings in the mesiofacial, distofacial and palatal canals and a metallic post in the palatal canal (a). An apical radiolucency is seen around the mesiofacial root component and it seems that a gutta-percha point is extending 3 mm through its apical foramen.

The angulated view below confirms the presence of root fillings and a post in the distofacial and palatal canals (b). However, it is demonstrated that the gutta-percha point, which was thought to belong to the mesiofacial canal, is located in the furcation.

A frontal tomogram confirms the diagnosis and shows that the gutta-percha point is intruded into the maxillary sinus and surrounded by a mucosal swelling (c).

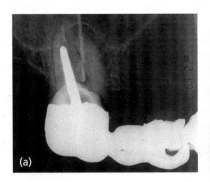 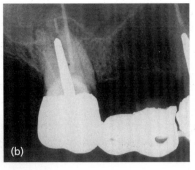 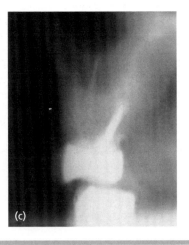

References

1. Alantar A, Tarragano H, Lefèvre B. Extrusion of endodontic filling material into the insertions of the mylohyoid muscle. *Oral Surg.* 1994; 78: 646–9.

2. Alhadainy HA. Root perforations. A review of literature. *Oral Surg.* 1994; 78: 368–74.

3. Andreasen JO, Andreasen FM. *Textbook and Color Atlas of the Traumatic Injuries to the Teeth.* Copenhagen: Munksgaard, 1994.

4. Bianchi SD, Roccuzzo M, Capello N, Libero A, Rendine S. Radiological visibility of small artificial periapical bone lesions. *Dentomaxillofac. Radiol.* 1991; 20: 35–9.
   The mean visibility index (MVI) of artificial periapical bone lesions was compared with six bone parameters: thickness of bone; thickness of the cortex; thickness of the spongiosa; density of the spongiosa; cortex/spongiosa ratio; and erosion of the cortex. The MVI was significantly associated with the erosion of the cortex and with the density of the spongiosa and the diameter of the lesion.

5. Bjørndal L, Carlsen O, Thuesen G, Darvann T, Kreiborg S. External and internal macromorphology in 3D-reconstructed maxillary molars using computerized X-ray microtomography. *Int. Endodont. J.* 1999; 32: 3–9.

6. Carlsen O. *Dental Morphology.* Copenhagen: Munksgaard, 1987.

7. Forsberg J, Halse A. Radiographic simulation of a periapical lesion comparing the paralleling and the bisecting-angle techniques. *Int. Endodont. J.* 1994; 27: 133–8.
   A simulated periapical 'lesion' was produced using an acrylic sphere (diameter 2.0 mm) covered with a radiopaque surface material. The 'lesion' was placed in close contact with the apical region of 60 extracted teeth and in continuation of the apical aperture. The teeth were radiographed at controlled angulations using bisecting angle and paralleling techniques. The investigation clearly indicated that the paralleling technique provides the most reliable information about the extent of a pathological process.

8. Green TL, Walton RE, Taylor JK, Merrell P. Radiographic and histologic periapical findings of root canal treated teeth in cadaver. *Oral Surg.* 1997; 83: 707–11.

9. Grötz KA, Al-Nawas B, Aguiar EG de, Schulz A, Wagner W. Treatment of injuries to the inferior alveolar nerve after endodontic procedures. *Clin. Oral Invest.* 1998; 2: 73–6.

10. Gutierrez JH, Aguayo P. Apical foraminal openings in human teeth. *Oral Surg.* 1995; 79: 769–77.

11. Hedrick RT, Dove SB, Peters DD, McDavid WD. Radiographic determination of canal length: direct digital radiography versus conventional radiography. *J. Endodont.* 1994; 20: 320–26.

12. Holtzmann DJ, Johnson WT, Southard TE, Khademi JA, Chang PJ, Rivera EM. Storage-phosphor computed radiography versus film radiography in the detection of pathologic periradicular bone loss in cadavers. *Oral Surg.* 1998; 86: 90–97.

13. Miyashita M, Kasahara E, Yasuda E, Yamamoto A, Sekizawa T. Root canal system of the mandibular incisor. *J. Endodont.* 1997; 23: 479–84.

14. Molven O, Halse A, Grung B. Incomplete healing (scar tissue) after periapical surgery – radiographic findings 8 to 12 years after treatment. *J. Endodont.* 1996; 22: 264–8.
    Twenty-four teeth treated by periapical surgery were observed for 8–12 years. Scar tissue healing at the 1-year control did not change for 22 teeth.

15. Nielsen RB, Alyassin AM, Peters DD, Carnes DL, Lancaster J. Microcomputed tomography: an advanced system for detailed endodontic research. *J. Endodont.* 1995; 21: 561–8.

16. Plonait D, Becker J, Barthel C. Können digitale Aufnahmeverfahren enorale Röntgenfilme bei der Diagnostik von Entzündungen im Kiefer ersetzen? *Dtsch. Zahnaerztl. Z.* 1997; 52: 745–8.

17. Rud J, Rud V, Munksgaard EC. Long-term evaluation of retrograde root filling with dentin-bonded resin composite. *J. Endodont.* 1996; 22: 90–93.

18. Sanderink GCH, Huiskens R, van der Stelt PF, Welander US, Stheeman SE. Image quality of direct digital intraoral x-ray sensors in assessing root canal length. The Radio VisioGraphy, Visualix/VIXA, Sens-A-Ray, and Flash Dent systems compared with Ektaspeed films. *Oral Surg.* 1994; 78: 125–32.

19. Scarfe WC, Fana CR, Farman AG. Radiographic detection of accessory/lateral canals: use of RadioVisioGraphy and Hypaque. *J. Endodont.* 1995; 21: 185–90.

20. Tammisalo T, Luostarinen T, Vähätalo K, Tammisalo EH. Comparison of periapical and detailed narrow-beam radiography for diagnosis of periapical bone lesions. *Dentomaxillofac. Radiol.* 1993; 22: 183–7.

21. White SC, Hollender L, Gratt BM. Comparison of xeroradiographs and film for detection of periapical lesions. *J. Dent. Res.* 1984; 63: 910–13.
    Histological diagnoses of periapical lesions on cadaver specimens were compared with radiographic diagnoses, scored by ten oral radiologists. In general, the observers detected about 70% of the cases with periapical disease, while simultaneously considering 10–15% of the normal surfaces to be abnormal.

22. White SC, Sapp JP, Seto BG, Mankovich NJ. Absence of radiometric differentiation between periapical cysts and granulomas. *Oral Surg.* 1994; 78: 650–54.
    The radiographic characteristics of 15 periapical cysts and 40 periapical granulomas were compared. Cysts were significantly larger than granulomas, but there was a wide variation in size of both types. There was no significant correlation between the density of a lesion and its size.

23. Yokota ET, Miles DA, Newton CW, Brown CE. Interpretation of periapical lesions using RadioVisioGraphy. *J. Endodont.* 1994; 20: 490–94.

Chapter 16
Root canal instrumentation

William P. Saunders and Elisabeth Saunders

Introduction

Root canal instrumentation involves the removal of soft and hard tissue, including pulp tissue, pulp stones and denticles and micro-organisms. It is important that diseased and infected tissue is removed as effectively as possible without damage to the patient, either in a general sense in relation to systemic health, or locally in relation to the periapical tissues and the tooth itself. Instrumentation also shapes the canal to accept a sound root filling effectively, thereby preventing the tooth from becoming a reservoir for microbial infection.

The complexity of the task

The root canal system of the tooth is nearly always complex, with each tooth displaying its own unique anatomy (Fig. 16.1).

Root canal curvature

Few root canals are straight, and even subtle curves introduce complexity into the instrumentation procedure. Straight root canals are found most frequently in maxillary central incisors, but curvature can occur in the roots of all tooth types. This curvature may be in a mesiodistal plane and is thus detected on periapical radiographic examination. Curves in a buccolingual plane are often not detected radiographically (Fig. 16.2). Instruments, especially those of relatively wide cross-sectional diameter and made from stiff metal, placed into a curved canal tend to remain straight within the root canal. This can lead to iatrogenic damage to the root canal system, which may compromise the success of the treatment. Not only the direction of the curve should be ascertained but also the degree of curvature and where the curvature starts on the root. A sharp curve starting in the apical one-third (Figs 16.3–16.5) will be more difficult to manage than a gentle curve beginning in the coronal one-third (Fig. 16.6).

Cross-sectional shape

A root canal with a round cross-section is easier to prepare than oval-shaped canals. A rotating instrument will cut a root canal with a round section uniformly, but instrumentation of a root canal with an oval cross-section inevitably precludes removal of tissue consistently from all the root canal wall. This means that it will not be as easy to clean an oval canal. Most often the narrowest dimension of the root canal lies in the mesiodistal plane, which is the one that is detected radiographically (Fig. 16.7) Some root canals, especially in specific ethnic groups, have extreme cross-sectional shapes, including the C-shaped canal. A ribbon-shaped canal is most often encountered in the distal root of mandibular molars (Fig. 16.8).

Number of root canals

The number of root canals contained within the root of a tooth forms a general pattern (Table 16.1). Of course, anomalies do occur and vigilance is necessary in interpreting radiographs; if in doubt, other radiographs should be taken at different angles mesiodistally to allow separation of canals on the processed image (see Chapter 15).

Mandibular incisors often have two root canals and two root canals are normally found in the maxillary first premolar. The mesiobuccal root canal of the maxillary first permanent molar often has two root canals. The minor mesiobuccal or mesiopalatal root canal (often termed MB2) may be difficult to find because it is often very narrow and the entrance is often covered by a lip of dentine (Fig. 16.9). This canal may have a separate apical foramen or may join the mesiobuccal canal as it extends apically. The mesial root of mandibular molars usually contains two root canals but these may not be discrete throughout their length and the presence of these fins and anastomoses makes instrumentation more difficult (Fig. 16.10).

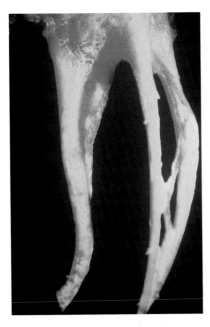

Fig. 16.1 Root canal morphology of mandibular molar showing complex anatomy.

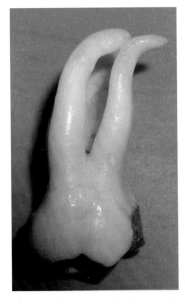

Fig. 16.3 Extracted maxillary left molar showing severe curvature of buccal roots in apical part of root. These would be very difficult to instrument without causing damage.

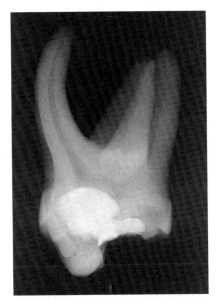

Fig. 16.2 Radiograph of extracted maxillary molar showing a mesiodistal projection. The buccal curvature of the palatal root is obvious.

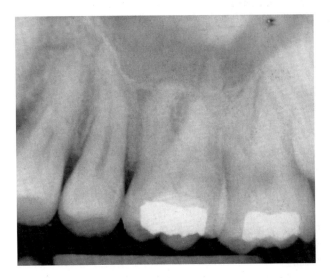

Fig. 16.4 Radiograph of maxillary first molar (tooth 26) showing curvature in apical portion of mesiobuccal root.

Root canal narrowing and obliteration

Dentine continues to be laid down throughout the life of the tooth with a vital pulp. Pulpal response to trauma and dental caries may cause reparative dentine to be deposited, with consequent narrowing and obliteration of part of the root canal system. This increased hard- tissue response usually begins in the coronal part of the root canal system and proceeds apically. It may take the form of pulp stones that are free within the root canal system or attached to the root canal wall. There may be generalized accumulation of hard tissue on the wall of the root canal, narrowing the lumen. In the pulp chamber of molars the hard tissue tends to form on the roof and the chamber becomes shortened vertically. Care must be taken in these cases, when gaining access to the

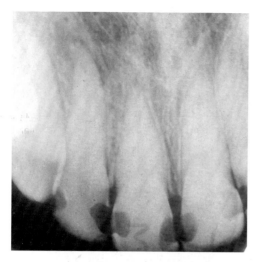

Fig. 16.5   Maxillary left lateral incisor tooth showing distal curvature of root canal in apical one-third. This curve probably extends palatally as well, which further complicates instrumentation.

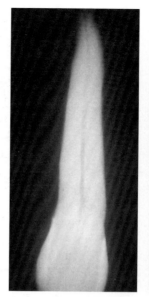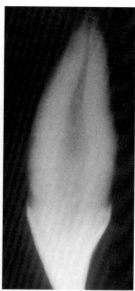

Fig. 16.7   Maxillary canine tooth: (left view) standard buccolingual radiographic projection; (right view) mesiodistal radiographic projection showing true size of root canal.

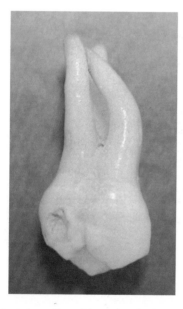

Fig. 16.6   Extracted maxillary right molar showing curvature of the mesiobuccal root. This curve, beginning about halfway down the root, will be relatively straightforward to instrument.

Apical configuration

The apical extent of instrumentation is very important. This should be at the junction of the pulpal tissue and the periodontal tissue and is located at the apical constriction (Fig. 16.13). In an immature tooth there may be no such constriction and great care must be taken to avoid overinstrumentation. Classic work carried out by Kuttler (17) demonstrated that the apical constriction lies 0.5–1 mm from the radiographic apex in most cases. However, in elderly patients extensive amounts of secondary cementum may be laid down, and the apical constriction will be situated coronally, up to approximately 3 mm from the radiographic apex. In addition, the main exit from the root canal is rarely positioned at the radiographic apex of the root.

Basic techniques

Access preparation

Access to the root canal system should allow its suitable cleaning and shaping without unnecessary damage or removal of too much coronal tooth tissue. Careful examination of an undistorted preoperative radiograph will allow some evaluation of the shape and number of root canals and the size of the pulp chamber. The presence of a radiopaque metal coronal restoration will prevent this evaluation and may complicate the initial access preparation of the root canal system. The decision to remove

root canal, to avoid damage to the floor of the pulp chamber (Fig. 16.11). In some cases the radiographic image of the tooth may indicate complete obliteration of the root canal. If a periradicular radiolucency is present, however, a patent canal often will be present (Fig. 16.12). The presence of coronal mineralization makes access to the root canal system much more difficult to achieve with the very real risk of perforation. General narrowing of root canals often makes them difficult to instrument.

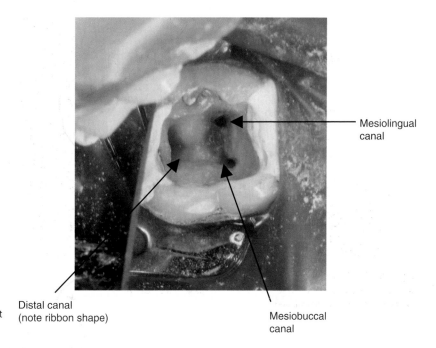

Mesiolingual canal

Distal canal (note ribbon shape)

Mesiobuccal canal

Fig. 16.8 The access cavity for a mandibular first molar.

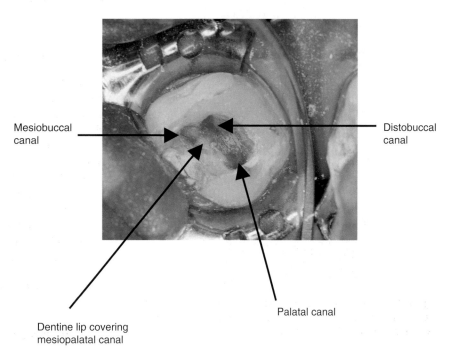

Mesiobuccal canal

Distobuccal canal

Dentine lip covering mesiopalatal canal

Palatal canal

Fig. 16.9 The access cavity for a maxillary first molar is triangular in shape with each of the main root canals at a corner of the triangle.

and eventually replace the coronal restoration is made easier if the marginal fit of the restoration is judged to be unsatisfactory or if there is obvious marginal leakage or dental caries. The removal of a metal restoration will allow better radiographic interpretation of the anatomy of the coronal part of the root canal system and will provide a better view of the access cavity by allowing more refracted light to enter the pulp chamber.

The access cavity should be prepared in such a way as to remove the entire roof of the pulp chamber and provide straight-line access to the root canals (Clinical procedure 16.1). Over the years a number of shapes and positions for access cavities have been recommended for each tooth in the dental arch (Fig. 16.14).

Initial penetration into the pulp chamber should be undertaken using a bur in a water-cooled high-speed

Table 16.1   Root canals in teeth of maxilla and mandible.

Maxilla

Central incisor	1 canal 100%
Lateral incisor	1 canal 100%
Canine	1 canal 100%
1st premolar	2 roots 57%
	Single root, 2 canals 16%
	Single root, 2 canals, 1 foramen 12%
	3 roots, 3 canals 6%
2nd premolar	1 canal 53%
	2 canals, 1 foramen 22%
	2 canals, 1 foramen 13%
	2 roots, 2 canals 11%
	3 roots, 3 canals 1%
1st molar	3 roots, 3 canals 38%
	4 canals 60%
	Mesiobuccal canal: 2 canals 60%
	2 foramina 20%
	1 foramen 80%
2nd molar	3 roots 60%
	1 mesiobuccal canal 70%
	2 mesiobuccal canals: 1 foramen 15%
	2 foramina 10%
	2 roots 25%
	1 root 10%

Mandible

Central incisor	1 canal 70%
Lateral incisor	1 canal 55%
	2 canals, 2 foramina: central 5%
	lateral 15%
	2 canals, 1 foramen: central 25%
	lateral 30%
Canine	1 canal 70%
	2 canals, 1 foramen 20%
	2 canals, 2 foramina 10%
1st premolar	1 canal, 1 foramen 74%
	Branching canal: 1 foramen 4%
	2 foramina 25%
2nd premolar	1 canal, 1 foramen 97%
	Branching canal: 1 foramen 12%
	2 foramina 3%
1st molar	2 mesial canals 60%, 1 foramen 40%
	1 distal canal 70%
	Distal canal: 2 canals, 1 foramen 35%
	2 canals, 2 foramina 10%
2nd molar	2 mesial canals 40%, 1 foramen 35%
	1 canal 25%
	1 distal canal 92%
	2 canals, 1 foramen 5%
	2 canals, 2 foramina 3%
	Can have a C-shaped distal canal

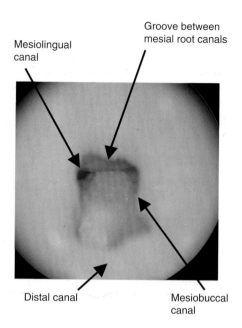

Fig. 16.10   The access cavity for a mandibular first molar, where the distal canal is obscured. Note the groove joining the mesial canals. This will contain pulp soft tissue.

Clinical procedure 16.1

Principles for preparation of the access cavity include:

● Complete removal of the roof of the pulp chamber to prevent retention of pulpal tissue under overhangs of dentine.
● Extension of the opening to include all root canals.
● Entrances of the root canals positioned at the periphery of the access cavity to ensure that instruments can be placed in the root canals easily without undue bending and stressing.
● Flaring the opening to allow proper visualization, especially if magnification is to be used.

---

handpiece. Special burs are available to penetrate metal restorations (Fig. 16.15a). It is important to reduce vibration and bur chatter to a minimum, especially in teeth with acute apical periodontitis. The basic outline of the cavity should be completed with these burs. Rubber dam placement may be delayed until the pulp chamber has been found, although the equipment should be ready for quick application. The decision on whether to place a rubber dam before or after access to the root canal system has been achieved depends on:

● The experience of the operator.
● The complexity of the root canal anatomy.
● The alignment of the tooth under treatment in relation to the adjacent teeth in the dental arch.

Directing the initial penetration of the pulp chamber over the widest root canal is less likely to result in iatrogenic damage to the floor of the pulp chamber. The anatomy of the floor of the pulp chamber is such that openings of the root canals usually can be traced by following the grooves in the floor. Subtle changes in color from a yellowish roof of the pulp chamber to a grayish floor also assist in finding root canal entrances (Fig. 16.16).

The use of ultrasonically powered instruments and magnification has revolutionized the controlled removal of tooth tissue when finding an opening into root canals. These instruments are used at low power settings and with a light touch. The tip of the instrument is cooled with a stream of air from the 3-in-1 syringe; water cannot be used because it interferes with vision. It is possible to pick small amounts of tooth structure away in a controlled manner. Often, openings to root canals have been partially covered by mineralized tissue. This must be removed with care to avoid perforation. Overhanging margins of the roof of the pulp chamber can be removed with a stainless steel fissure or tapered fissure bur, with a non-cutting tip, used in a slow-speed handpiece (Fig. 16.15b). This will avoid damage to the floor of the pulp chamber. Openings to the root canals can be investigated with a sharp-tipped endodontic explorer and denticles overhanging the root canal can be picked away. A long shank or swan-necked bur in a slow-speed handpiece that is rotating at no more than 1000 rpm should be used to find narrow root canals (Fig. 16.15b). Multiple radiographs at varying angles may be required to ensure that the relationship of the bur to the root canal is monitored. These should be taken after each millimetre progression of the bur. Again, the use of magnification helps to ensure that the bur is kept on track. Subtle changes in color and texture of the dentine should be looked for (Figs 16.8 and 16.9).

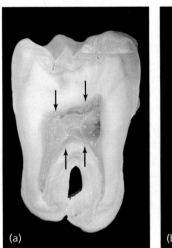 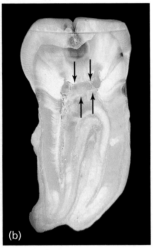

Fig. 16.11 (a) Large coronal pulp in a young molar (↑↓). (b) Hard-tissue apposition in the coronal pulp has narrowed the lumen, especially in the vertical dimension (↑↓). (Courtesy of Dr P. Hørsted-Bindslev.)

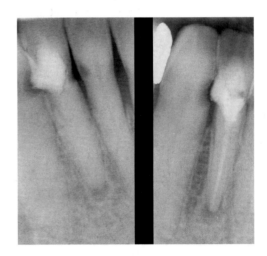

Fig. 16.12 Tooth 42 showing apparently calcified root canal in an elderly patient but endodontic treatment was feasible.

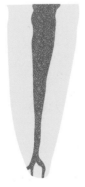 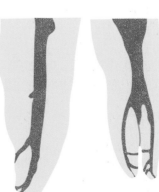 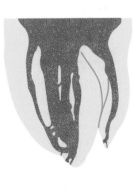

Fig. 16.13 Drawings depicting various configurations of apical constrictions and exit of canal at root surface.

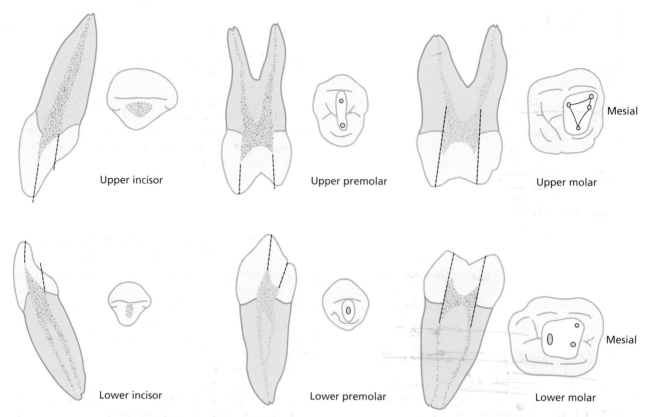

Fig. 16.14 Drawings showing typical access cavities to upper incisor, lower incisor, upper premolar, lower premolar and upper and lower molar.

Root canal instrumentation

Root canal instrumentation should enlarge the root canal system as a smooth taper from crown to apex, which includes the original canal, without causing damage to or needless weakening of the tooth (41) (Fig. 16.17).

Instruments and techniques have been developed to minimize iatrogenic damage. Of these, stripping and zipping canals are the most common.

Stripping

The root canal system does not always lie in the center of the root, and this eccentric placement means that uniform cutting of the canal wall will result in over-preparation of the inner wall, known as stripping. This is a particular problem on the distal surface of the coronal part of the mesial roots of mandibular molars (Fig. 16.18). Indiscriminate removal of tooth structure in this area may cause a strip perforation. To avoid such an occurrence, instrumentation must be carried out with regard to the anatomy of the tooth and overenlargement must be avoided; therefore a balance must be struck between removal of root canal wall to achieve a suitable shape and diameter to allow efficient delivery of irrigant and subsequent obturation. Using hand instruments in a rasping action or the injudicious use of Gates–Glidden burs increase the likelihood of stripping in the furcation region.

Zipping

Stainless-steel instruments placed into a curved root canal tend to straighten within the canal. This is because of the inherent rigidity of the metal. Flexibility of an instrument depends on a number of factors, including the material from which it is manufactured, the cross-sectional configuration and the diameter of the instrument. An instrument that is too stiff will cut more on the convex side of the curve than the concave side, thereby straightening the curve. This results in a phenomenon termed zipping (Fig. 16.19). The resultant hour-glass shape is very difficult to obturate and, if cutting is continued, perforation by the tip of the instrument may occur. It is to avoid these significant problems that modern root canal instruments have been developed.

Instruments

Alloys

The properties of root canal instruments are linked to alloy, taper, flute pattern and cross-sectional design.

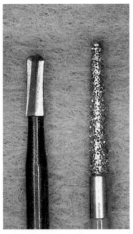

(a)

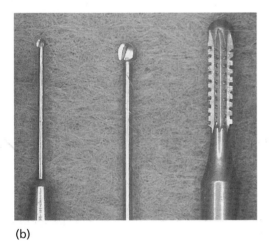

(b)

Fig. 16.15 (a) High-speed burs for initial access through the coronal restoration. (b) Burs used to locate entrances to root canals and modify the access cavity.

which means that it demonstrates an ability to return to some previously defined shape or size when subjected to an appropriate thermal procedure, approximately 125°C. The Ni–Ti instruments have about three times the elastic flexibility in bending and torsion compared with stainless-steel files. In the proportions used in endodontic instruments, Ni–Ti exhibits superelastic behavior that allows a return to the original shape when unloaded. The alloy undergoes a stress-induced martensitic transformation from a parent austenitic structure (Advanced concept 16.1). When the stress is released the material returns to austenite and its original shape.

These physical properties allow instruments made from Ni–Ti alloys to prepare severely curved root canals without permanent deformation. Nickel–titanium files cannot be made by twisting a tapered wire, as with many of the stainless-steel instruments, and are thus machined from a blank.

The major advantage of Ni–Ti is its ability to retain flexibility with increased taper. This has resulted in the development of groups of instruments that have a two- to six-fold greater taper than the ISO standardized 02 (Fig. 16.20). Hand Ni–Ti instruments are available, but these instruments are also manufactured for use in a constant-speed, high-torque handpiece running at between 150 and 350 rpm.

Nickel–titanium instruments are not immune from fracture and this may happen without any particular warning, although twisting or unwinding of the flutes may be observed. Like other root canal instruments, Ni–Ti instruments should not be overused and should be checked for distortion before each use (Fig. 16.21).

Titanium–aluminum
One manufacturer has produced an instrument that consists of an alloy containing 90% titanium and 5% aluminum by weight. This alloy does not have superelastic properties but is more flexible than conventional stainless steel. However, it has no advantages over flexible stainless steel in terms of cutting efficiency.

Modern root canal instruments are constructed of either stainless steel or nickel–titanium. Carbon steel instruments are also available but these are for one use only because they cannot be resterilized due to corrosion. This is uncommonly seen after sterilization of stainless-steel instruments and rarely occurs with nickel–titanium.

Newer alloys, including chrome–nickel steel and V-4 steel, provide good flexibility and produce better shaped root canal preparations than conventional instruments (4).

Nickel–titanium (Ni–Ti)
The introduction of nickel–titanium instruments has revolutionized root canal preparation. These alloys consist of approximately 55% nickel and 45% titanium by weight. Ni–Ti is known as a shape memory alloy,

Mesiobuccal canal

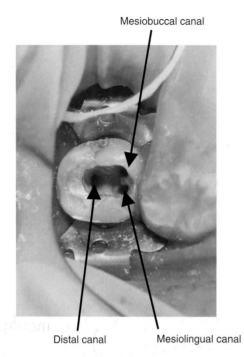

Distal canal   Mesiolingual canal

Fig. 16.16 The access cavity for a mandibular first molar is rectangular in shape, with each of the main root canals at the periphery of the rectangle. Note the grayish floor of the pulp chamber.

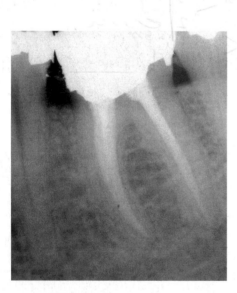

Fig. 16.17 Radiograph of completed root filling on mandibular first molar (tooth 36), showing good shaping of root canal with adequate taper and no iatrogenic damage.

Tip configuration

It was shown in the 1980s that the design of the tip of the instrument had an effect on cutting efficiency (26, 27). In these experiments the instruments used were of

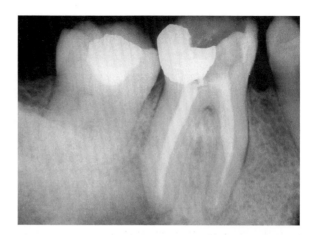

Fig. 16.18 Overenthusiastic use of mechanical instruments coronally in the mesial root of the mandibular molar has almost resulted in a strip perforation in the furcation.

a greater diameter at the tip compared with the canals, and thus a cutting tip was required for penetration. The triangular cross-sectional tip was better in narrow canals than those with a square cross-section. In addition, a pyramidal design was better than a conical shape. Another view was expressed that a cutting tip may cause damage during preparation of the apical part of the root canal. Luks in 1974 (19) suggested that the sharp tip of instruments made at that time should be removed with an emery board. Subsequently, Powell *et al.* (30, 31) demonstrated that the shape of root canal preparation with hand instruments using modified-tipped K files (safe-ended files) was superior to unmodified-tipped files. Sabala *et al.* (35) found that inexperienced students maintained the original canal curvature better with modified-tipped files compared with unmodified instruments. Many hand instruments now have a non-cutting tip (Fig. 16.22). Schafer *et al.* (41) compared simulated root canals prepared with a wide variety of hand instruments, including those manufactured from stainless steel and Ni–Ti. The best results were obtained with flexible instruments with non-cutting tips.

Instrument configuration

Root canal shaping may be carried out with hand-held or engine-driven instruments. These instruments now come in many configurations but are conventionally grouped according to ISO (International Organization for Standardization) and ANSI (American National Standards Institute) standards. The quality of instruments, sizing, physical properties and materials used for their manufacture come under these standards (see Core concept 16.1). The instruments can be separated further into groups, depending on the shape of the cutting part.

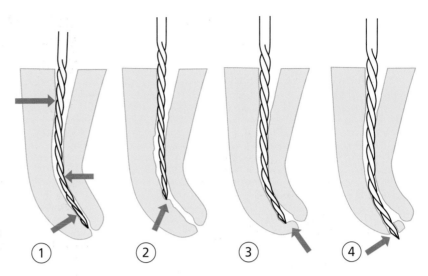

Fig. 16.19 The stiff instrument tends to straighten within the canal (1), causing ledge formation (2), zipping (3) or perforation (4).

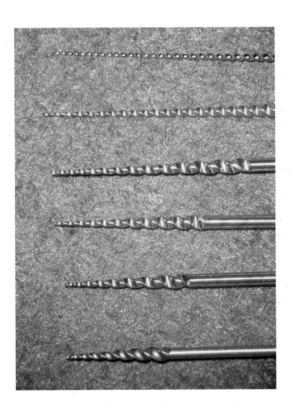

Fig. 16.20 Variably tapered instruments showing, in order from top, 02, 04, 06, 08, 10 and 12 tapers.

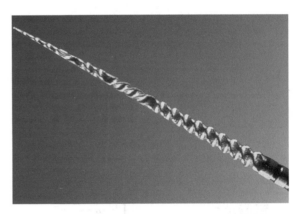

Fig. 16.21 Nickel–titanium instrument showing distortion of flutes.

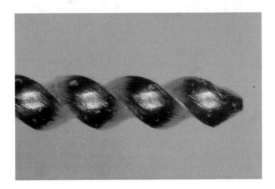

Fig. 16.22 Non-cutting tip of hand instrument.

Standardized instruments have cutting flutes 16 mm long and for each millimeter of file the diameter increases by 0.02 mm, so the final cutting part of the instrument (known as d2; see Fig. 16.23) is 0.32 mm wider than the first part of the cutting tip (known as d1). These files are thus known as 02 tapers.

These instruments are color coded and increase in diameter in set increments, the smallest diameter being 0.06 mm at d1 and increasing to 1.4 mm (Table 16.2). The length of the shaft of the instrument from the cutting tip to the handle may be 21, 25 or 31 mm. The longer instruments are useful when treating maxillary canines, which are over 25 mm long, and many molars can be treated with the 21-mm instruments.

Reamers

Reamers (Fig. 16.24) are made from stainless steel and may be square or triangular in cross-section. A tapered wire is twisted to create sharp cutting flutes that are present every 0.5–1 mm along the length of the instrument. Although the cross-sectional shape varies among manufacturers, the smaller sizes (nos 15–50) are usually square and the larger sizes triangular. The angle of the blades to the long axis of the reamer is about 10–30°, so these instruments are used in rotation where the flutes cut into and remove dentine from the wall of the root canal. The use of hand, stainless-steel ISO-sized reamers has declined in popularity because of their lack of flexibility (especially in large sizes), their inability to prepare canals with anything other than a round cross-section and their lack of cutting efficiency compared with other instruments.

Files

Files come in a number of configurations within the 02 taper standardization. The main generic types include: K files, flexible K files, Hedström files and S files.

K Files: manufactured in a similar manner to reamers except that the cutting spirals produced by twisting are much tighter. The cross-section can be triangular or square in shape. The angle of the cutting flutes to the long axis of the instrument is about 25–40° and hence they cut the wall of the root canal when used in rotation. K Files have a greater angular deflection than reamers and thus there is less risk of torsional fracture with these instruments compared with reamers (48).

Flexible K files (Fig. 16.25): essentially similar to K files except that the cross-sectional design is such that the instrument is able to flex more than the conventional K

Core concept 16.1

Standardization of cutting instruments includes:

- Diameter and taper of each instrument.
- Regimented increase in size.
- A numbering system based upon the diameter of the instrument at the cutting aspect of the tip.

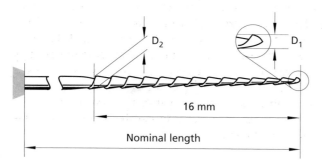

Fig. 16.23   Drawing showing a file with the distances marked d2–d3, etc.

Table 16.2   Coded sizes, diameter at d1 and color of standardized instruments.

Size	d1(mm)	Color
006	0.06	Orange
008	0.08	Grey
010	0.10	Purple
015	0.15	White
020	0.20	Yellow
025	0.25	Red
030	0.30	Blue
035	0.35	Green
040	0.40	Black
045	0.45	White
050	0.50	Yellow
055	0.55	Red
060	0.60	Blue
070	0.70	Green
080	0.80	Black
090	0.90	White
100	1.00	Yellow
110	1.10	Red
120	1.20	Blue
130	1.30	Green
140	1.40	Black

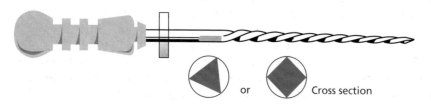

or   Cross section

Fig. 16.24   Reamer with 02 taper.

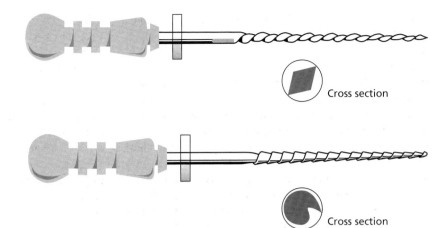

Fig. 16.25 Flexible K file with 02 taper.

Cross section

Fig. 16.26 Hedström file with 02 taper.

Cross section

file. They may be triangular in cross-section or a more elaborate rhomboid. In addition, they may be made from new stainless-steel alloys, titanium or nickel–titanium, which are more flexible. Most of the flexible K files are made by twisting a tapering blank. Some, however, are machined from a tapered blank. They cut the root canal wall if used in rotation or with a filing action. The angle between the cutting flutes and the long axis of these instruments varies between 23 and 30° at the tip and 45 and 50° at the end of the working part of the file. Schafer *et al.* (41) have shown that these flexible files are more efficient than conventional reamers and files in cutting dentine. However, there is now a distinct trend in contemporary endodontic practice toward the use of Ni–Ti instruments in preference to those manufactured from stainless steel.

Hedström files (Fig. 16.26): manufactured by machining a steel tapered blank that has a round cross-section. The machining produces a spirally tapered series of cones with cutting edges at the base of each cone. The angle between this cutting edge and the long axis of the instrument is about 60–65° and thus is designed for a filing motion. The instrument cuts only when being withdrawn from the root canal, and if rotated may break relatively easily because of the small core diameter. The cutting efficiency of Hedström files is greater than that of K files. Hedström files are used mainly for coronal flaring of root canals and to remove fractured instruments and gutta-percha in retreatment cases. Larger-sized Hedström files, being rigid, cause iatrogenic damage within the canal, including the formation of zips and elbows, when used in a filing motion (see below) (2, 4, 5).

S Files: in principle these are modified Hedström files. They are machined from a blank, have an 's'-shaped cross-section and are stiffer than Hedström files.

Movement of hand instruments during shaping of the root canal

Hand instruments may be used in a variety of ways to enlarge and shape the root canal system. The efficiency with which this shaping is done depends on the movement applied, the instrument type used and the material from which the instrument is made. Again, it is important to stress that the enlargement of the root canal must be achieved without iatrogenic damage.

Push–pull motion (Fig. 16.27)

A *push–pull* motion, especially when applied to Hedström files, will file dentine from the wall of the root canal. An amplitude of 1–2 mm is recommended but there are inherent difficulties with this method. These difficulties include grooving the root canal wall, unless a conscious effort is made to move the file circumferentially, and packing of debris ahead of the tip of the instrument, which may block the root canal. When K files were used with a filing motion, pronounced zips and elbows were created (1, 10). Because of the possibility of iatrogenic damage, rasping is not recommended for routine root canal preparation. However, it can be used in retreatment cases to aid the removal of gutta-percha root fillings.

Reaming (Fig. 16.27)

A reaming motion denotes a clockwise or anticlockwise rotation of the instrument in the canal. It is generally recommended to rotate the reamer a quarter-turn before removal to prevent the instrument from binding in the canal. Two techniques are described here.

Watch winding: a clockwise/anticlockwise rotation of the instrument through an arc of 30–60° while advancing into the root canal. This method is less aggressive than the quarter-turn and pull and should be used with

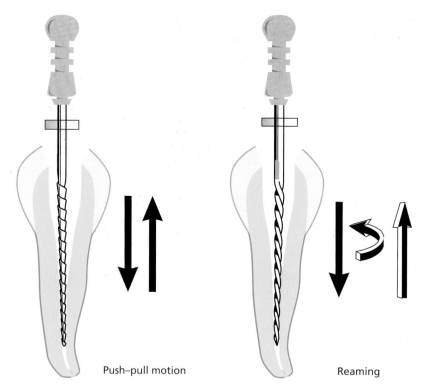

Push–pull motion   Reaming

Fig. 16.27 Drawing showing push–pull motion (left) and reaming (right).

light apical pressure. With precurved stainless-steel instruments (Fig. 16.28) this technique is extremely useful for initial negotiation of root canals, especially those that are severely curved or narrow. The apical part of the very curved root canal can be prepared using this motion.

The balanced force technique: devised by Roane *et al.* (34) and later endorsed by Charles and Charles (9) on the basis of a mathematical model. Although the mechanism as described by Roane *et al.* (34) has been challenged by Kyomen *et al.* (18), essentially the clinical result is the same.

This technique is essentially a reaming action using clockwise movement to insert the file and anticlockwise movement to remove dentine. The file is placed into the root canal until it binds against the wall. The file is then rotated through 60–90°. This creates threads within the dentine. The instrument is moved anticlockwise through 120–180° with apical pressure, which crushes and breaks off the dentine threads and enlarges the root canal.

A final clockwise rotation allows flutes to be loaded with debris and removed from the root canal (38). This technique has been shown to be efficient and less prone to cause iatrogenic damage (6, 45, 36, 37, 43). It appears to keep the instrument more centrally placed within the root canal and extrusion of debris apically is much reduced compared with other hand instrumentation techniques (3, 12, 25). The technique must be used with

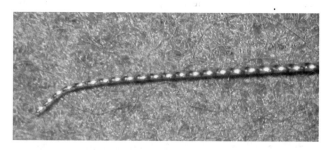

Fig. 16.28 Precurving of the tip of a fine instrument prior to negotiation of the root canal with a watch-winding movement.

straight instruments that are not precurved; modified-tipped instruments are recommended although non-modified-tipped instruments have been shown to produce satisfactory results (37). A technique of reverse balanced force instrumentation has been developed for use with variably tapered nickel–titanium files where the flutes of the instruments are machined in an opposite thread to normal files.

Specific features of root canal instruments

Cutting flutes

The configuration of the flutes of an instrument will affect its cutting ability. A flute with a positive rake angle planes the dentine surface whereas that with a negative rake angle scrapes the surface (Fig. 16.29). The greater

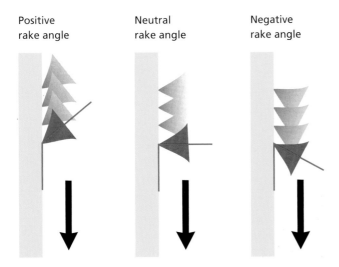

Positive rake angle   Neutral rake angle   Negative rake angle

Fig. 16.29 Rake angles.

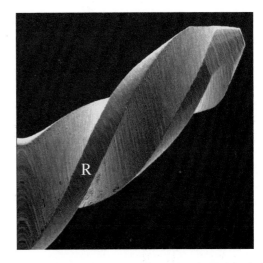

Fig. 16.30 Scanning electron microscope view of radial lands (R) on nickel–titanium instrument.

the positive rake angle, the more aggressive the cutting potential.

Cross-sectional configuration of files

The cross-sectional design of an instrument affects the number of cutting blades presented to the dentine and the flexibility of the instrument. The most commonly seen cross-sectional shapes are the square, triangular, round and rhomboid (Figs 16.24–16.26). More recently, U-shaped or radial land (Fig. 16.30), and more complex cross-sections based on the radial land, have been introduced. The U shape is basically triangular in shape but the points at each apex of the triangle have been flattened to give a flat planing surface. This U shape has been modified further to produce a complex fluting pattern in cross-section where the flute is shaped to allow more easy removal of debris from the cutting site but only two radial lands are present.

Rotary instruments

Not all root canal preparation is carried out using hand instruments and there is a trend for increased use of rotary instruments in all aspects of root canal preparation.

Gates–Glidden burs (Fig. 16.31) are, in effect, engine-driven reamers. Gates–Glidden burs come in various sizes from ISO 050 (size 1) to ISO 150 (size 6) and are available in 15- and 19-mm lengths. The tip of the instrument is elliptically shaped with short cutting flutes and a non-cutting tip. The instruments are designed so that if stressed they will fracture at the junction of the shank and the shaft. They are used to open root canals and flare the coronal straight part of the root canal but because they are relatively aggressive care must be taken to avoid overuse coronally, which may lead to strip perforation. Gates–Glidden burs should be used at no greater than 1500 rpm to ensure adequate control. They generate considerable swarf and should be used only when the root canal system is filled with irrigant fluid in order to avoid canal blockage. There is a tendency, especially at relatively high speed, for the bur to pull itself into the root canal and cause overcutting. This may lead to a poor final shape, often referred to as a 'coke bottle' shape.

Peeso reamers (Fig. 16.31) differ from the Gates–Glidden drill in having parallel-sided cutting flutes. They are available from ISO 070 (size 1) to ISO 170 (size 6), with and without non-cutting tips. Because they are less well controlled than Gates–Glidden drills, their use tends to be restricted to post space preparation.

Gates–Glidden burs and Peeso drills, although very popular, are being superseded by Ni–Ti rotary instruments specifically designed to give a better, more controlled shape coronally (Fig. 16.32a). Although engine-driven rotary instruments have been available for many years, the advent of Ni–Ti has seen exciting developments in the use of engine-driven instruments.

Basically there are two different designs of these instruments: a design with a cutting tip at the end of a long, slim and flexible shank (Fig. 16.32b); and a design resembling conventional hand instruments but with various tapers and cutting flute configurations different from hand files (Fig. 16.32c–e). Most of these instruments have a radial land design that prevents uncontrolled cutting into the canal wall. During rotation the land planes the wall of the root canal and the flutes direct the debris coronally away from the cutting surface. A recent introduction is a Ni–Ti rotary file with

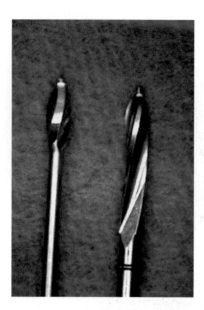

Fig. 16.31 Photograph of Gates–Glidden and Peeso reamer.

varying tapers along its length. This is claimed to be able to prepare severely curved canals without altering the natural shape or fracturing the instrument (Fig. 16.32f).

The most important feature of these Ni–Ti instruments is that the taper of the instrument can be increased to provide good shaping with consistent taper using fewer instruments. The rotary instruments are used in contra-angle handpieces running at a speed of 150–650 rpm. Some special motors and handpieces are manufactured with torque adjustment, which opens up the possibility of preventing deformation and separation of the instruments if they lock into the canal.

Despite the flexibility of Ni–Ti instruments, several studies have reported defects and breakage following the use of such instruments (7, 14, 32, 40, 50). Breakage has primarily occurred during the learning period because certain basic rules have not been followed (see Clinical procedure 16.2). The fractures have been divided into torsional and flexural fractures. Torsional fracture may be preceded by unwinding or reverse winding, which can be detected, whereas flexural fatigue fracture may occur without warning. It is therefore recommended to discard instruments after some time even though defects cannot be seen (see Clinical procedure 16.2).

Basic principles of root canal instrumentation

Step-down technique

The shape of the prepared root canal ideally should be a gradually increasing taper from the apical constriction to the coronal opening (42). Experience has shown that this is most predictably attained by the use of a step-down technique (Fig. 16.33).

With the step-down technique the coronal portion of the canal is prepared first. The apical region is then gradually approached with a range of instruments of smaller cross-sectional area, leaving behind a fully cleaned and tapered canal lumen. The working length is accurately measured when step-down instrumentation is within 2–3 mm of the apical constriction. In the step-back technique (Fig. 16.33), the working length is first established (see below) and then the apical part of the canal is cleaned and shaped, followed by preparation of the coronal parts with a sequence of larger instruments used in gradually increasing distances from the apical region.

Step-down is now regarded as the preparation technique of choice. It was originally described as the 'crown-down pressureless technique' (22) and underwent research scrutiny by Morgan and Montgomery (28). The advantages of this technique over step-back are outlined in Core concept 16.2.

In this technique the preparation is begun with Gates–Glidden drills or rotary Ni–Ti instruments and larger files in the coronal part of the root canal. Sequentially smaller files are then used until the apical constriction is reached. The balanced force technique should be used for hand instruments.

Most protocols for the use of Ni–Ti files in a rotating handpiece involve a crown-down approach. Before instrumentation is begun, it is helpful to increase the size

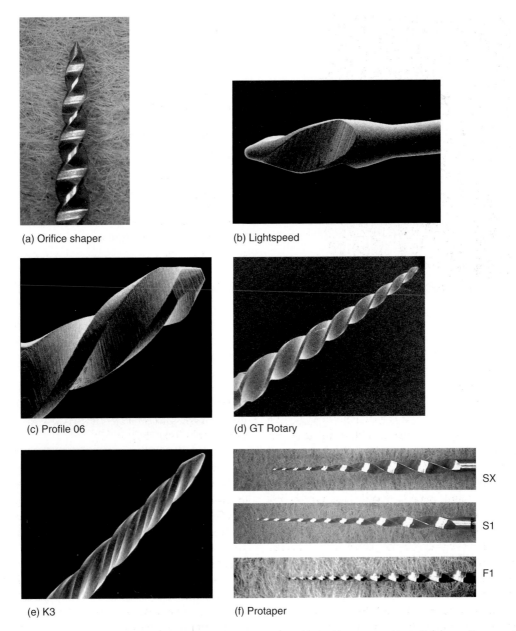

(a) Orifice shaper

(b) Lightspeed

(c) Profile 06

(d) GT Rotary

(e) K3

(f) Protaper

SX

S1

F1

Fig. 16.32 Nickel–titanium rotary instruments: (a) Orifice shaper; (b) Lightspeed; (c) Profile 06; (d) GT Rotary; (e) K3; (f) Protaper. (Courtesy of Dr P. Dummer and Dr S. Thompson.)

of the openings of the root canals with a rotating tapered instrument. This provides a guide path and allows easier entry to the root canal by all the other instruments. The root canal then should be investigated for patency. A small-sized hand file (08–15) with an 02 taper is precurved in its apical few millimeters, coated with a small quantity of lubricant or chelating paste (Fig. 16.34) and placed into the root canal with a stem-winding motion. It is advisable at this stage not to take this instrument to the full working length. The root canal then should be flared coronally, which will allow irrigant to be introduced more effectively into the root canal. A step-down

approach then can be adopted, using progressively smaller diameter instruments until the working length is within approximately 2 mm. The working length then is determined and apical preparation can be completed. The final refinement of the shape of the root canal then can be undertaken.

Methods to establish the working length

The apical extent for preparation of the root canal has been the subject of some controversy over the last few years. Preparation into the periradicular tissues beyond

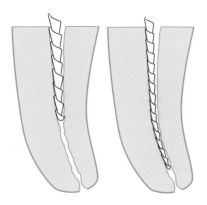
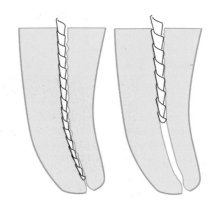

Step down
Dimensions of file decrease

Step back
Dimensions of file increase

Fig. 16.33 Drawing showing the principle of the step-down and step-back techniques.

Core concept 16.2

The step-down technique

- Provides less risk of extrusion of pulp debris, irrigant solution and dentine mud because there is less hydrostatic pressure generated in an apical direction.
- Reduces the risk of inoculation of endodontic pathogens into the periradicular tissues (15) because there is a marked tendency for the majority of microorganisms to be in the coronal part of the root canal system (44).
- Provides less likelihood for a change of the working length measurement during preparation.
- Facilitates adequate penetration of irrigant into the root canal system.
- Prevents binding of instruments except in the apical flutes, reduces the stress placed on the instrument and results in less risk of preparation errors such as zipping.

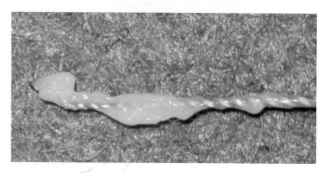

Fig. 16.34 The file should be coated with a lubricant prior to placement in the root canal.

laid down at the anatomical apex. Tactile detection of this constriction may be difficult clinically and impossible if there has been pathological root resorption apically.

The working length may be determined in a number of ways but whatever method is used it must be accurate, repeatable and carried out easily.

Measuring working length by radiography
Radiography is the most commonly used method. An undistorted periapical radiograph taken using a film-holder and a paralleling technique prior to treatment allows a good estimation of the tooth length to be made. A precurved instrument with a silicone stop on the shaft is placed into the root canal 1–2 mm short of the full working length. If preflaring of the root canal has been done prior to working length determination, then tactile sensation can be used to 'feel' for the apical constriction, although this takes some practice (46). In some cases there will be no proper tactile feedback, especially if the apical constriction has been destroyed, if there is immature development of the root end or if the root canal is

the root canal may cause an acute inflammatory reaction with postoperative pain and delayed healing. If there is subsequent overfilling, then there will be incomplete regeneration of the supporting periradicular tissues. Some authorities consider that the apical termination of the root filling should be at the cementodentinal junction (16). However, this anatomical landmark is impossible to detect radiographically. Therefore a better position is the smallest diameter of the root canal at the apex: the constriction or apical foramen (33). This may be regarded as the junction between the periodontal tissue and the pulpal tissue. Depending on the amount of secondary cementum that has been laid down at the apex, this position may be 0.5–3 mm from the radiographic apex (11, 13, 17). The distance tends to increase with the age of the patient as secondary cementum is narrow along most of its length. The root canal needs to be widened to a size of at least ISO 15 so that the apical part of the instrument may be seen clearly on a radiograph. The working length radiograph should be taken using a paralleling technique and a film-holder (see Chapter 15).

If the processed film shows the tip of the instrument to be more than 2 mm short of the radiographic apex and there is obvious root canal apically, then the stop should be readjusted and a further film exposed. If the radiograph shows the instrument to be long, then the stop should be adjusted accordingly and another radiograph taken. The working length should always be recorded in the patient's case notes together with the coronal reference point. Cusp tips are not very useful for this exercise and judicious flattening will help to provide a more positive landmark.

Measuring working length by electrical apex locators

Sunada (47) was the first to apply to endodontics the principle that the electrical resistance between the periodontal membrane and the oral mucosa was a constant value of 6.5 kΩ. This led to the introduction of the electrical apex locator (Fig. 16.35). One side of the electrical circuitry is connected to the root canal instrument and the other to a lip clip that connects with the oral mucosa. When the file is placed into the root canal and advanced to the apex to make contact with the periodontal tissues, the electrical contact is completed and visual and audible signals will be triggered. There are three types of apex locators: resistance type, impedance type and frequency-dependent type (23). Many of these locators, particularly the frequency-dependent types, are now so sophisticated that it is possible to obtain accurate readings even in the presence of fluids within the canal (Clinical procedure 16.3).

There is, however, a rather steep learning curve for the accurate use of an apex locator.

The accuracy of contemporary electrical apex locators is high (24), even up to 100%, with a tolerance level of 0.5 mm, in teeth with an apical foramen in the long axis of the tooth (29). However, it is still prudent to take a periapical radiograph with the working length file in place to confirm the position.

Paper points

A fine paper point placed into a dried canal and extended beyond the working length will absorb tissue fluid at the apex and, if withdrawn after just a few seconds in position, will allow measurement of the dry portion of the point and provide some indication of the working length.

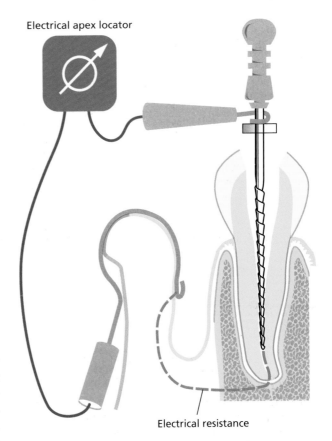

Electrical apex locator

Electrical resistance

Fig. 16.35 Drawing showing how the apex locator works.

Flare preparation

The coronal flare should be completed as soon as possible after confirmation that the root canal is patent and can be instrumented. An Ni–Ti engine-driven instrument of suitable taper is used in the coronal 3–5 mm of the root canal. This phase of preparation will allow irrigant and lubricant to be introduced more efficaciously into the root canal. Gates–Glidden drills can also be used judiciously in a step-down fashion in the coronal straight section of the root canal. Instruments of ISO sizes 110, 090 and 070 (Fig. 16.36) can be used but ISO 050 is not advised because there is a tendency for these smaller sized instruments to break too easily. The root canal system should be flooded with irrigant when using these instruments to avoid blockage of the root canal with debris. Root canal preparation then can be continued toward the apex using hand files of progressively smaller size. These should be used with a balanced force movement. Stainless steel (02 taper) or variably tapered Ni–Ti hand or rotary instruments can be used. The canal should be irrigated between each change of instrument and a small quantity of chelating

---

Clinical procedure 16.3   Electrical apex locators

(1)   Place lip clip, dampened with water, to provide sufficient electrical contact.

(2)   A root canal instrument attached to the second electrode is advanced until the apical foramen is reached. Contact must be made between instrument and canal wall at entrance and apex.

(3)   Move the instrument up and down 1–2 mm; the display will follow this movement.

(4)   A reading that is within the root canal but is obviously not at the apex may indicate the presence of a large lateral canal or a perforation. The reading also may be false if the instrument touches a metal restoration and, for some locators, if excessive moisture (especially sodium hypochlorite) is present within the pulp chamber.

(5)   Contact must be made between the instrument and the apical exit from the root canal. With an open or immature apex, this can be achieved by making a small but sharp curve at the tip of the file.

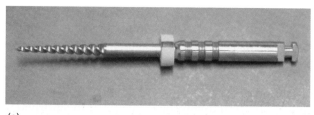

(a)

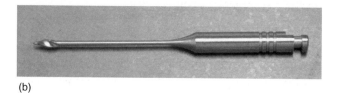

(b)

Fig. 16.36   (a) Rotary instrument with increased taper for coronal enlargement. (b) Gates–Glidden bur (ISO 090) for coronal enlargement.

lubricant picked up with each file prior to placement in the root canal.

Apical preparation

The amount of preparation carried out in the apical part of the root canal is the subject of considerable controversy. Some consider that it is unnecessary to widen the apical preparation because preflaring and patency filing will allow the irrigant to reach and be agitated in the apical part of the canal and therefore cleaning takes place. Others consider it necessary to remove infected dentine in the apical few millimeters of the root canal (49) and thus shaping should be carried out to at least a size ISO 30 file. Certainly the widening of the apical part of the root canal to a reasonable size after preparation of the coronal and middle sections allows easier placement of the needle for irrigation and also of the gutta-percha cone when cold lateral condensation is used for obturation.

Patency filing

Schilder (42) and Buchanan (8) stressed the need to avoid apical blockage by placing a small file through the apical constriction of the root canal, without enlargement. It is purported that this file stirs the apical debris back into the irrigation fluid, which is flushed subsequently from the root canal. The patency file also moves clean irrigating fluid into the apical portion of the root canal. This file should be used frequently but factors such as the movement of the file itself, the narrowness of the root canal and

the proximity to the apex all influence how often patency is used. The balanced force technique and the use of Ni–Ti rotary instruments tend to gather debris into the flutes of the instrument, thereby minimizing packing of debris toward the apex. It must be appreciated also that it is impossible to achieve patency of all the exits of the complex anatomy of the apical delta.

Finishing the root canal preparation

The presence of clean white dentine chips on the apical flutes of the master apical file, the presence of clean irrigating fluid and the presence of glassy smooth walls have all been used to indicate when canal preparation is complete. Each of these criteria is inaccurate and there has yet to be a reliable method devised. Certainly the wall of the root canal should be smooth with no ledge or interference. A spreader should be able to penetrate to within 2 mm from the apex. It should be possible to place the master apical file to the working length with only light apical pressure with the tip of the forefinger. It is impossible to tell how clean the root canal system is following instrumentation and it is of fundamental importance, therefore, that large volumes of a suitable irrigant are delivered to the root canal system during this process.

Irrigation

Irrigation of the root canal system is an essential and integral part of root canal preparation. It is the irrigant that actually does the cleaning of the system while the instrumentation shapes the root canal. The irrigant helps lubrication and flushes out debris generated during preparation. Sodium hypochlorite used in copious amounts not only is antimicrobial but also dissolves necrotic debris and is therefore more efficient than saline, sterile water or local anesthetic solution (see Chapter 11). Chlorhexidine also has a place as a root canal irrigant because it is antimicrobial and possesses substantivity, although it does not have the tissue-dissolving properties of sodium hypochlorite. At least 15 ml of fluid should be used to irrigate each root canal during mechanical instrumentation.

Removal of the smear layer

When the root canal is instrumented, organic and mineralized debris becomes impacted against the wall to form an amorphous layer known as the smear layer. This varies in thickness depending on the way the wall has been instrumented. Debris also extends into the dentinal tubules to form plugs of material. Various factors suggest that it should be removed prior to root filling (Fig. 16.37) (see further Chapter 11).

Technical aids

A number of technical aids have been introduced in endodontics to help provide more predictable instrumentation.

Surgical operating microscope

The use of the surgical operating microscope in root canal preparation (Fig. 16.38a) is now recognized as an invaluable tool. The ability to visualize the root canal system in fine detail gives the opportunity to clean and shape more efficiently. Microscopic examination of the floor of the pulp chamber (Fig. 16.38b) helps to identify the openings of the root canals, especially of additional root canals such as the mesiopalatal canal in the mesiobuccal root of the maxillary first molar (39). The use of the microscope, combined with the removal of coronal dentine with an ultrasonically powered pick, allows both conservative and accurate removal of tooth structure. Most operative procedures can be undertaken at ×6 to ×10 magnification and up to ×16 when experienced. The use of a high magnification of ×26 is useful for examination of the root canal system but it is difficult to operate at this level. The use of the operating microscope requires practice and it may take several months before full proficiency is reached.

Lasers

There has been considerable research into the use of lasers in root canal preparation, although to date these can be regarded only as experimental. Originally Nd:YAG and CO_2 lasers were investigated but with little

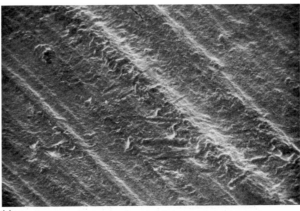

(a)

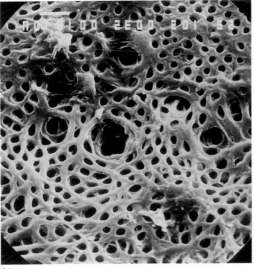

(b)

Fig. 16.37 (a) Smear layer on canal wall after mechanical instrumentation. (b) Root canal wall in middle one-third after removal of smear layer with citric acid and NaOCl. Open dentinal tubules are clearly seen.

improvement over conventional preparation techniques. Research continues using other types of lasers, including excimer lasers, with more promising results. It is hoped that lasers may be used to clean root canal systems and melt dentine to close dentinal tubules and seal the apical delta.

Ultrasonic instruments

Ultrasonic energy may be used to power K-type files. This energy is generated with either a magnetostrictive device or a piezoelectric crystal. The former generates considerable heat and requires a cooling unit for the handpiece. The energy generates a sinus waveform through the file with areas of maximum displacement (antinode) and areas of minimal displacement (node). The tip of the instrument is an antinode and, depending

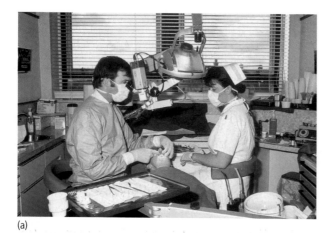

(a)

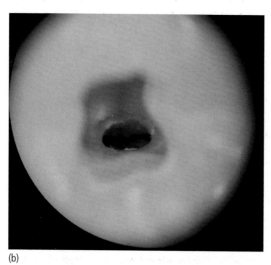

(b)

Fig. 16.38 (a) Operating microscope in use. (b) View of opening of distal root canal of mandibular molar as seen through the microscope (×16 original magnification).

on the power setting, produces an amplitude of up to 2 mm at a frequency of 30 kHz. The ultrasonic unit for endodontic use should be designed to accept sodium hypochlorite with no ill effects to the apparatus. The file is used with a constant stream of irrigant. The fluid may generate two phenomena: acoustic microstreaming and cavitation. The former occurs most often and results in eddy currents around the file, which develop hydrodynamic shear stresses that clean the wall of the root canal. Cavitation occurs as a result of pressure changes within the fluid. A cavity can form in the fluid and the following pressure change results in implosion, which can occur with a great force sufficient to clean the surface. Unfortunately the constraints of the instrument within a fine root canal prevent the consistent generation of these physical phenomena. However, the delivery of large amounts of irrigant aids debridement of the root canal

system. In addition, the activity of the instrument heats the irrigant, which, in the case of sodium hypochlorite, will improve its effects. The use of a small file with minimal contact to the root canal wall provides the best conditions for the use of ultrasonics. Care must be taken not to have the power setting too high, when the unconstrained tip of the instrument may fracture or cause damage to the wall of the root canal. As mentioned previously, ultrasonically powered instruments are used more frequently for removing coronal tooth tissue when finding root canals, and also to aid in the removal of fractured instruments and for root-end preparation in surgical endodontics.

Sonic instruments

Sonically powered instruments have a frequency of 1400–1500 Hz. This produces a single antinode at the tip of the instrument. On contact with the wall of the root canal the force is directed into the long axis of the file and cutting takes place. Special files are available for use with these units.

Non-instrumentation techniques for root canal preparation

An innovative technique for root canal treatment was introduced recently (20, 21). After access to the root canal system is gained, cleaning is achieved using NaOCl irrigation under alternating pressure fields generated by a vacuum pump and an electrically driven piston. Bubbles are formed in the irrigation fluid, which, with a subsequent increase in pressure, implode. This creates hydrodynamic turbulence that cleans the wall of the root canal, including the ramifications and fins. The pressure system operates below tissue pressure so there is little risk of extrusion of the irrigant into the periradicular tissues. The root canal system can be obturated using the same system. As yet, there is no published evidence of the clinical effectiveness of this technique.

Procedural errors during root canal preparation

There are several errors that may occur during root canal preparation.

Perforation

Perforation may occur at any time during the shaping of the root canal system but is more prevalent during the access and when undertaking apical shaping, especially in curved root canals. Sudden bleeding from the root canal system is indicative of a perforation. Injudicious use of large burs in the floor of the pulp chamber may

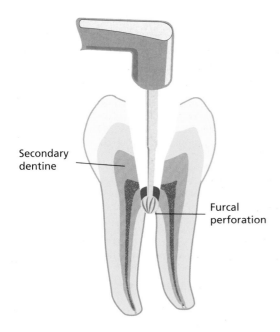

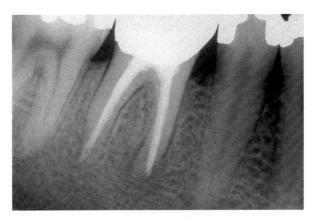

Fig. 16.40 Zipping of mesial root canal of mandibular right first molar (tooth 46). The stiff instruments have not followed the path of the canal and the apical part has not been instrumented and cleaned.

Fig. 16.39 Furcal perforation.

cause furcal perforation, which is difficult to repair (Fig. 16.39). Even the use of ultrasonically powered picks may cause this type of perforation. If there has been no loss of furcal bone it is best to repair the perforation immediately (Clinical procedure 16.4).

Ledging

A ledge results from repeated preparation or the insertion of a relatively large inflexible instrument to a particular level in the root canal, which is usually at the beginning of the curve (Figs 16.40 and 16.41). The ledge makes subsequent preparation apically very difficult or impossible. To attempt to bypass a ledge, a severe curve is placed in the apical 2 mm of a fine stainless-steel instrument and this is passed down the root canal with a stem-winding motion. The use of a lubricant such as EDTA paste is helpful. If the ledge can be bypassed then gentle filing may remove the ledge.

Fractured instruments

Instruments may fracture as a result of misuse or overuse (Fig. 16.42a). Instruments should be checked carefully to ensure that the cutting flutes are not damaged, and rotary instruments must be used at speeds and in a manner recommended by the manufacturers. The introduction of the operating microscope and ultrasonically powered picks allows dentine to be removed precisely so that in many cases fractured instruments may be freed and subsequently removed

---

> ### Clinical procedure 16.4 Treatment of a perforation in the floor of the pulp chamber during access preparation
>
> In a case with a necrotic pulp, a perforation is usually obvious because there is some bleeding. In the vital case, the pulp chamber should be irrigated gently with sterile saline or sodium hypochlorite solution, dried, and the floor of the pulp chamber examined carefully to establish where the perforation site is situated. If possible, the perforation should be repaired immediately. The bleeding is stopped with pressure using a sterile damp cotton-wool pledget applied for several minutes. Mineral trioxide aggregate is then mixed and placed over the perforation. It should be gently plugged into the defect. This material then can be covered with a resin-modified glass ionomer to protect the site, or a damp cotton-wool pledget can be placed in the pulp chamber. The tooth is then closed with a temporary dressing. The mineral trioxide aggregate takes about 4 h to set, so should be hard if the tooth is re-entered after 24 h. If there is extensive bone loss in the furcation it may be necessary to use a matrix to prevent the mineral trioxide aggregate from being pushed into the periradicular tissues. Matrices used include collagen and calcium sulfate.

(Fig. 16.42b). Unfortunately the canal is often overprepared during this procedure. If an instrument fractures during root canal treatment, the patient must be informed and the case notes suitably annotated. (For further reading, see Chapter 19.)

Conclusion

Root canal instrumentation is a difficult technical procedure that must be undertaken with diligence and skill.

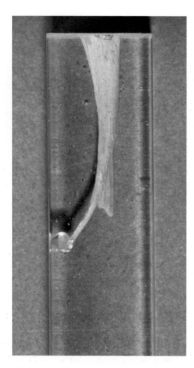

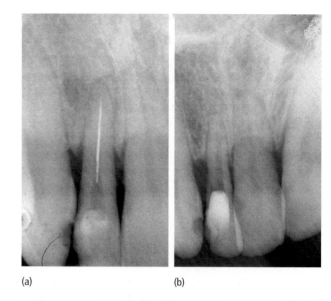

(a)   (b)

Fig. 16.42   (a) Fractured file in tooth 22. (b) This was removed using ultrasonic energy, resulting in overenlargement of the root canal.

Fig. 16.41   A simulated curved root canal in a plastic block shows severe ledging as a result of overinstrumentation with a rotary instrument. Preparation of the root canal apical to this damage is difficult.

It is important to get the root canal system as clean as possible and with a resultant shape that makes obturation with gutta-percha relatively straightforward. This biomechanical preparation should be done without causing iatrogenic damage to the tooth.

References

1.   Alodeh MHA, Dummer PMH. A comparison of the ability of K files and Hedström files to shape simulated root canals in resin blocks. *Int. Endodont. J.* 1989; 22: 226–35.

2.   Alodeh MHA, Doller PM, Dummer PMH. Shaping of simulated root canals in resin blocks using the step-back technique with K-files manipulated in a simple in/out filing motion. *Int. Endodont. J.* 1989; 22: 107–11.

3.   al-Omari MA, Dummer PM. Canal blockage and debris extrusion with eight preparation techniques. *J. Endodont.* 1995; 21: 154–8.

4.   al-Omari MA, Dummer PM, Newcombe RG. Comparison of six files to prepare simulated root canals. 1. *Int. Endodont. J.* 1992; 25: 57–66.
     A total of 300 simulated root canals of various angles and positions of curvature in clear resin blocks were prepared by hand using six file types. Each file type was used with a linear filing motion and an anticurvature stepback technique. Overall, preparation with Hedström files was significantly quicker than with any other file, whereas preparation with K files and K-Flex files took significantly longer. Fracture and deformation of instruments occurred substantially less often with Flex-R and Hedström files, but significantly more often with Unifiles. Loss of working distance occurred with all file types, but was significantly greater in canals prepared with K files. Unifiles and Hedström files were responsible for significantly more weight loss than the other files, whereas K files produced significantly less weight loss. Canals with rough undulating walls were created most often by Hedström files and Unifiles. Overall, under the conditions of this study, Flexofiles, Flex-R files and Hedström files appeared to be substantially more effective than K files, K-Flex files and Unifiles.

5.   al-Omari MA, Dummer PM, Newcombe RG, Doller R. Comparison of six files to prepare simulated root canals. 2. *Int. Endodont. J.* 1992; 25: 67–81.

6.   Backman CA, Oswald RJ, Pitts DL. A radiographic comparison of two root canal instrumentation techniques. *J. Endodont.* 1992; 18: 19–24.

7.   Barbakow F, Lutz F. The 'Lightspeed' preparation technique evaluated by Swiss clinicians after attending continuing education courses. *Int. Endodont. J.* 1997; 30: 46–50.

8.   Buchanan LS. Management of the curved root canal. *J. Calif. Dent. Assoc.* 1989; 17: 18–25.

9.   Charles TJ, Charles JE. The 'balanced force' concept of instrumentation of curved canals revisited. *Int. Endodont. J.* 1998; 31: 166–72.

10. Cimis GM, Boyer TJ, Pelleu GB. Effect of three file types on the apical preparations of moderately curved root canals. *J. Endodont.* 1988; 14: 441–4.

11. Dummer PMH, McGinn JH, Rees DG. The position and topography of the apical constriction and apical foramen. *Int. Endodont. J.* 1984; 17: 192–8.

12. Fairbourn DR, McWalter GM, Montgomery S. The effect of four preparation techniques on the amount of apically extruded debris. *J. Endodont.* 1987; 13: 102–8.

13. Green D. A stereomicroscopic study of the root apices of 400 maxillary and mandibular anterior teeth. *Oral Surg.* 1960; 13: 728–33.

14. Haikel Y, Serfaty R, Bateman G, Senger B, Allemann C. Dynamic and cyclic fatigue of engine-driven rotary nickel–titanium endodontic instruments. *J. Endodont.* 1999; 25: 434–40.

15. Hession RW. Endodontic morphology. III Canal preparation. *Oral Surg.* 1977; 44: 775–85.

16. Ingle JI, Bakland LK, Peters DL, Buchanan LS, Mullaney TP. *Endodontic Cavity Preparation in Endodontics* (4th edn) (Ingle JI, Bakland LK, eds) Baltimore: Lea & Febiger, 1994, 198.

17. Kuttler Y. Microscopic investigation of root apices. *J. Am. Dent. Assoc.* 1955; 50: 544–52.

18. Kyomen SM, Caputo AA, White SN. Critical analysis of the balanced force technique in endodontics. *J. Endodont.* 1994; 20: 332–7.

19. Luks S. *Luks Practical Endodontics.* Philadelphia, PA: JB Lippincott, 1974.

20. Lussi A, Nussbacher U, Grosrey J. A novel noninstrumented technique for cleansing the root canal system. *J. Endodont.* 1993; 19: 549–53.
    The aim of this study was to examine a non-instrumental technique for root canal preparation. A device that was able to develop controlled cavitation in the root canal was compared with a filing step-back technique using 3% NaOCl as an irrigant. Teeth in the three test groups were prepared with the new machine using 1, 2 or 3% NaOCl. The treatment time ranged from 16 to 32 min in the hand group and from 10 to 15 min in the machine groups. The teeth were then prepared for histological examination. The apical one-third of curved canals was significantly cleaner when using the machine and 3% NaOCl than with hand instrumentation.

21. Lussi A, Messerli L, Hotz P, Grosrey J. A new noninstrumental technique for cleaning and filling root canals. *Int. Endodont. J.* 1995; 28: 1–6.

22. Marshall FJ, Pappin J. *A Crown Down Pressureless Preparation Root Canal Enlargement Technique: Technique Manual.* Portland, Oregon: Oregon Health Sciences University, 1980.

23. McDonald NJ. The electronic determination of working length. *Dent. Clini. North Am.* 1992; 36: 293–307.
    This is a review paper that describes the development and the advantages and disadvantages of the various types and clinical use of apex locators.

24. McDonald NJ, Hovland EJ. An evaluation of the apex locator Endocater. *J. Endodont.* 1990; 16: 5–8.

25. McKendry DJ. Comparison of balanced forces, endosonic and step-back filing instrumentation techniques: quantification of extruded apical debris. *J. Endodont.* 1990; 16: 24–7.

26. Miserendino LJ, Moser JB, Heuer MA, Osetek EM. Cutting efficiency of endodontic instruments. Part II: Analysis of tip design. *J. Endodont.* 1986; 12: 8–12.

27. Miserendino LJ, Moser JB, Heuer MA, Osetek EM. Cutting efficiency of endodontic instruments. Part 1: A quantitative comparison of the tip and fluted regions. *J. Endodont.* 1985; 11: 435–41.

28. Morgan LF, Montgomery S. An evaluation of the crown-down pressureless technique. *J. Endodont.* 1984; 10: 491–8.

29. Pagavino G, Pace R, Baccetti T. A SEM study of *in vivo* accuracy of the Root ZX electronic apex locator. *J. Endodont.* 1998; 24: 438–41.

30. Powell SE, Simon JHS, Maze BB. A comparison of the effect of modified and nonmodified instrument tips on apical canal configuration. *J. Endodont.* 1986; 12: 293–300.

31. Powell SE, Wong PD, Simon JH. A comparison of the effect of modified and nonmodified instrument tips on apical canal configuration. Part II. *J. Endodont.* 1988; 14: 224–8.

32. Pruett JP, Clement DJ, Carnes DL. Cyclic fatigue testing of nickel-titanium endodontic instruments *J. Endodont.* 1997; 23: 77–85.

33. Ricucci D. Apical limit of root canal instrumentation and obturation. Part 1. Literature review. *Int. Endodont. J.* 1998; 31: 384–93.

34. Roane JB, Sabala CL, Duncanson MG Jr. The balanced force concept for instrumentation of curved canals. *J. Endodont.* 1985; 11: 203–11.

35. Sabala CL, Roane JB, Southard LZ. Instrumentation of curved canals using a modified tipped instrument: a comparison study. *J. Endodont.* 1988; 14: 59–64.

36. Saunders WP, Saunders EM. Effect of non cutting tipped instruments on the quality of root canal preparation using a modified double-flared technique. *J. Endodont.* 1992; 18: 32–6.

37. Saunders WP, Saunders EM. Comparison of three instruments in the preparation of the curved root canal using the modified double-flared technique. *J. Endodont.* 1994; 20: 440–4.

38. Saunders EM, Saunders WP. The challenge of preparing the curved root canal in today's root treatment cases. *Dent. Update* 1997; 24: 241–7.

39. Saunders WP, Saunders EM. Conventional endodontics and the operating microscope. *Dent. Clin. North Am.* 1997; 41: 415–28.
    This is a review of the use of the operating microscope in non-surgical root canal treatment. Included are clinical tips to improve efficiency with this treatment aid.

40. Sattapan B, Nervo GJ, Palamara JE, Messer HH. Defects in rotary nickel–titanium files after clinical use. *J. Endodont.* 2000; 26: 161–5.

41. Schafer E, Tepel J, Hoppe W. Properties of endodontic hand instruments used in rotary motion. Part 2. Instrumentation of curved canals. *J. Endodont.* 1995; 21: 493–7.

42. Schilder H. Cleaning and shaping the root canal. *Dent. Clin. North Am.* 1974; 18: 269–96.

43. Short JA, Morgan LA, Baumgartner JC. A comparison of canal centering ability of four instrumentation techniques. *J. Endodont.* 1997; 23: 503–7.

44. Shovelton DS. The presence and distribution of microorganisms within non-vital teeth. *Br. Dent. J.* 1964; 117: 101–7.

45. Southard DW, Oswald RJ, Natkin E. Instrumentation of curved molar root canals with the Roane technique. *J. Endodont.* 1987; 13: 479–89.

46. Stabholz A, Rotstein I, Torabinejad M. Effect of preflaring on tactile detection of the apical constriction. *J. Endodont.* 1995; 21: 92–4.

   The efficacy of tactile detection of the apical constriction in flared and nonflared root canals. In the nonflared group a size 15 or 20 K-file was used to detect the apical constriction, whilst in the second group the coronal portion of the root canal was preflared prior to testing the apical constriction. After placing a size 15 or 20 file in each root canal, a radiograph was taken, and the distance between the tip of the file and the radiographic apex was measured. The location of the file tip was classified into three categories: (a) within 1 mm short of the radiographic apex; (b) underextended, more than 1 mm short of the radiographic apex; and (c) overextended beyond the radiographic apex. In the non-flared group, 32.3% of the root canals were classified in category a, as compared with 75.0% in the preflared group. Over 26% of the root canals in the unflared group and approximately 4% of the canals in the preflared group were included in category b. Files inserted in preflared root canals had a significantly lower incidence of overextension than those placed in nonflared canals (21% versus 41%). The ability to determine the apical constriction by tactile sensation was significantly increased when the canals were preflared (P < 0.0001).

47. Sunada I. New method for measuring the length of the root canal. *J. Dent. Res.* 1962; 41: 375–8.

48. Tepel J, Schafer E, Hoppe W. Properties of endodontic hand instruments used in rotary motion. Part 3. Resistance to bending and fracture. *J. Endodont.* 1997; 23: 141–5.

49. Wu M-K, Wesselink PR. Efficacy of three techniques in cleaning the apical portion of curved root canals. *Oral Surg.* 1995; 79: 492–6.

   This study examined the cleaning of mesiobuccal canals of human mandibular molars with an average curvature of 25° using step-back, crown-down pressureless or balanced force techniques with 2% NaOCl as an irrigant. The cleaning efficacy of these techniques was evaluated by counting the remaining surface debris under a stereomicroscope with a calibrated eyepiece micrometer. The results indicated that the apical portion of the canal was less clean than the middle and coronal portions regardless of the technique performed, and that the balanced force technique produced a cleaner apical portion of the canal than did the other techniques studied. They were able to enlarge the apical stop to size 40–60 using the balanced force technique without recognizable transportation. They considered that enlargement to size 25 1 mm from the apex and to size 35 3 mm from the apex may be insufficient to clean the apical part of the root canal system.

50. Yared GM, Bou Dagher FE, Machtou P. Cyclic fatigue of ProFile rotary instruments after clinical use. *Int. Endodont. J.* 2000; 33: 204–7.

Chapter 17
Root canal filling materials

Gottfried Schmalz

Introduction

Purpose

It has been well established that bacteria play the primary role in the etiology and pathogenesis of apical periodontitis, therefore the fully instrumented root canal has to be provided with a tight and long-lasting obturation in order to prevent bacteria (and antigens) from spreading from (or through) the canal system to the periapical area. Thus, a root canal filling material should prevent infection/reinfection as a cause of inflammation. Together with an acceptable level of biocompatibility (inert material) this shall provide the basis for promoting healing of the periodontal ligament or for maintaining its health.

In addition to this traditional concept of the purpose of a root canal filling material, recently ideas have been promoted that a root canal filling material also should be able to actively stimulate regeneration of the periodontal connective tissue attachment apparatus, especially after a sometimes aggressive treatment procedure or after apical pathosis. Relevant materials may be osteoconductive (serve as a scaffold for the ingrowth of precursor osteoblasts) or osteoinductive (inducing new bone formation by differentiation of pluripotent local connective tissue cells into bone-forming cells).

Classification

Root canal filling materials may be divided into three types:

- Cones
- Sealers
- Combinations of the two.

Cones are prefabricated root canal filling materials of a given size and shape (taper). Sealers are pastes and cements that are mixed and hardened by a chemical setting reaction after a given amount of time. This time varies between the various preparations, from minutes up to days. Owing to several reasons outlined later, combinations of cones and sealers are currently recommended. Still less commonly used are thermoplastic materials (gutta-percha preparations), which are heated for better adaptation to the root canal wall, or are melted, injected into the root canal in a liquid state and then hardened by cooling. Again, these materials are normally recommended to be used together with a sealer.

Limitations

As will be shown in this chapter, all materials recommended for root canal filling have advantages and disadvantages and there is no material/method available so far that fulfills all requirements, therefore clinicians are well advised to observe carefully the new developments and the relevant scientific literature. It also should be kept in mind that clinical properties of root canal filling materials depend substantially upon the treatment technique: e.g. the amount of sealer used may determine the tissue reactions and the amount of leakage for some materials due to factors such as shrinkage during setting, the formation of pores or enhanced solubility (40). Therefore, the selection and the use of a root canal filling material must be part of a conclusive treatment concept. Finally, there is no magic material by which the tedious work of correct diagnosis and chemomechanical preparation of the root canal system can be circumvented.

Selection

Root canal filling materials should be selected on the basis of a critical evaluation of the presented evidence (preferably reports in scientific journals) in relation to the requirements, which will be mentioned below. Sometimes, however, contradicting results are reported for the same material. This may be due to the special circumstances of both the test method involved and the preparation of the specimens (tested freshly after mixing or in a set state). Thus, the clinician should ask for a set of tests preferably performed in a comparative (i.e. controlled) way, testing the new product against one or more currently accepted preparations. Selection of a suitable root canal filling material is a challenge for the clinician regarding both his/her level of updated information and his/her ability for critical assessment of the presented information.

Requirements

Root canal filling materials may be considered as implants and thus should fulfill the requirements of such a device concerning technical, biological and handling properties (Core concept 17.1).

Technical properties

Technical properties are mainly related to sealing aspects, taking into account that the success of a root canal filling significantly depends upon the prevention of infection/reinfection of the apical and lateral peri-

odontal ligament and the adjacent bone. In cases of material extrusion beyond the apex, which is associated with elevated rates of clinical failure (63), resorption of the material would be desirable. However, this is in contradiction to the required insolubility, therefore utmost care must be exerted to avoid overfilling.

Biological properties

Biological properties are related to preventing systemic and local tissue irritation for both the patient and the dental personnel and to stimulating regeneration of the apical region. The risk (frequency and severity of adverse effects) for general health impairment as a consequence of the use of root canal filling materials is generally low. Single cases of allergic reactions of patients and medical personnel have been reported. More dramatic are local effects, especially in the context of overfilling beyond the apex and eventually into the mandibular canal (see below).

There are also some inherent contradictions between the requirements for a root canal filling material that have to be weighed against each other, e.g. antibacterial properties versus local toxicity. Bacteria in the root canal should be removed by chemomechanical debridement. However, the complex anatomy of the root canal system makes debridement difficult, especially in the apical delta region. Furthermore, bacteria have been demonstrated to invade dentinal tubules up to 1 mm and thus they may not be removed totally by chemomechanical debridement. Therefore, thorough cleaning, shaping and irrigation with disinfectants may not result in a completely sterile root canal system. Owing to the fact that microleakage cannot be prevented by any material/method available today, percolation followed by bacterial penetration and growth may occur. Antimicrobial activity of root canal sealers should compensate for these imperfections, although this is not supported by direct scientific evidence.

On the other hand, it was consistently demonstrated that sealers with high antimicrobial activity, such as formaldehyde-releasing ZnOE (zinc oxide–eugenol), are also toxic. Furthermore, sealers that release substances may, at the same time, disintegrate. Therefore, antibacterial properties of a root canal filling material based on the release of antibacterial substances from the sealer should not compromise its physical properties (such as stability and sealability) or biological properties. Some materials (e.g. epoxy resin sealers) are antimicrobially active only during the setting period, which is an interesting approach. For a short period residual bacteria may be killed (toxicity is accepted); in the long run, the material is not toxic, leaving time for the surrounding tissues to heal.

Core concept 17.1   Requirements for an ideal root canal filling material

Technical

- No shrinkage.
- No solubility in tissue fluids, undisturbed setting in the presence of moisture.
- Good adhesion/adaptation to dentine or combining materials (cones, sealers).
- No pores and water absorption.
- No tooth discoloration.

Biological

- No general health problems or allergies for patients and dental personnel.
- No irritation of local tissues.
- Sterile.
- Antimicrobial – no enhanced bacterial growth.
- Stimulation of the periapical healing process.

Handling

- Radiopaque: ISO 6876 (62) requires > 3 mm aluminum (dentine has 0.6–0.7) (radiopacity of dental materials is measured as mm aluminum equivalent).
- Setting in an adequate time, allowing sufficient time for obturation and x-ray control.
- Easy to apply and easy to remove (e.g. for post placement or revision) using solvents, heat or mechanical instrumentation.

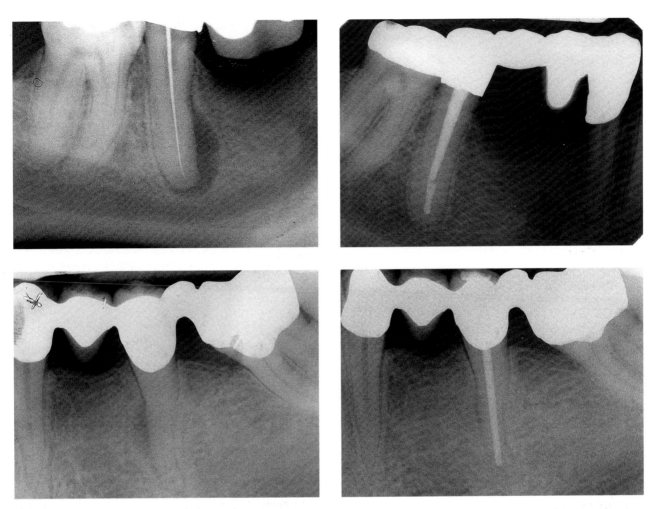

Fig. 17.1   Lateral and apical regeneration of an osteolytic process after shaping and cleaning the root canal and filling with cones and a sealer of temporary toxicity (gutta-percha with an epoxy resin sealer).

Apical healing has been observed after elimination of bacteria and a radiographically tight sealing of the root canal system (Fig. 17.1). *Active* stimulation of apical regeneration is – so far – based on the release of calcium hydroxide from the root canal filling material. However, again it should be required that such a release of active substances from a root canal filling material does not interfere with the stability of the material and does not increase leakage.

Handling properties

Handling properties shall facilitate the actual use of the material and the control of the technique/treatment result. The length of the root canal filling is of utmost importance for the clinical success of a root canal filling and a sufficient radiopacity is needed for x-ray control. Setting conditions must be adjusted to the special situation of the root canal filling techniques and relevant

requirements may be different for regular root canal fillings (slow setting allowing for condensation and eventual correction after x-ray control) and retrograde fillings (fast setting for better moisture control during the operation).

The ideal root canal filling material has not been developed yet. Compromises have to be made between the different requirements in relation to the special clinical situation. New formulations, however, should be checked *critically* against this list of requirements (Core concept 17.1).

Biocompatibility

An acceptable level of biocompatibility is an essential requirement for a suitable root canal filling material. According to EU regulations (Medical Device Directive 93/42 EEC) valid within the EU and in Switzerland,

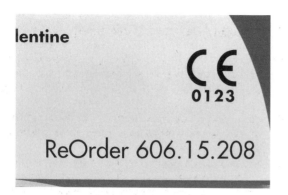

Fig. 17.2 The CE sign on the package shows that the material has passed a risk assessment procedure; note the number that identifies the supervising body ('Notified Body').

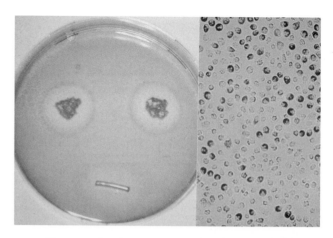

Fig. 17.3 Cytotoxicity test with a polyketone root canal sealer: zone of decolorization around the test specimen (left) indicates moderate toxicity; the partial loss of dye (neutral red) from the cells (right) indicates moderate cell damage.

Iceland, Liechtenstein and, Norway, root canal filling materials have to successfully pass a clinical risk assessment procedure before they are allowed to be marketed. The CE sign on the package (Fig. 17.2) shows that the material is in conformity with the essential requirements of this directive: namely safety, efficacy and quality. Although for this process the term 'clinical risk assessment' is being used, it should be noted that a new root canal filling material does not necessarily have to pass any clinical testing if the manufacturer assumes from preclinical and other data (e.g. so-called 'historic' data from similar/identical materials that are on the market already and/or have been tested in the past) that the material is both safe and effective. The dentist should therefore ask the manufacturer for clinical data (see below), because he/she is finally responsible for the selection of the material in the single patient situation and the patient relies on his/her independent expertise (57). The timespan for which a root canal filling material shall be *in situ* (years) should be reflected in the timespan of clinical tests. There are so far no official regulations concerning recommended periods for a clinical test in root canal filling materials. In analogy to filling materials, a time of 1 year for excluding catastrophic failures and a timespan of 3–5 years for the final testing may be advisable. Products without a CE mark must not be used in those countries where the aforementioned EU Directive in effective.

Root canal filling materials come into close and prolonged contact with living tissues of patients (e.g. bone, connective tissue, the sinus maxillaris, the N. alveolaris inferior) and of dental personnel (e.g. skin of hands). Possible adverse reactions are of systemic toxic, allergenic (immunological) or local toxic nature. Accordingly, a large number of different test methods have been designed to test the different aspects of the biocompatibility of root canal filling materials. Relevant methods have been included in international standards (ISO

10993 or ISO 7405) (57). Normally, *in vitro* cytotoxicity tests are performed first using different cell cultures (e.g. periodontal ligament fibroblasts or osteoblasts) for measuring local toxic effects (Fig. 17.3). Cytotoxicity is regarded as a measure of the basic material property to damage cells and thus cause inflammation (56). Furthermore, cytotoxicity may impair the local defense by causing damage to essential cells of the immune system (11). A possible influence of a material on the genetic information apparatus of cells is tested in genotoxicity/mutation assays, e.g. using cells or bacteria. Antimicrobial properties, being of special interest for root canal filling materials, can be tested *in vitro*, exposing different bacterial strains to the materials and measuring the growth pattern. Relevant bacteria comprise those present in the oral environment, especially in infected root canals (mainly Gram-negative anaerobic rods). Recently, there has been increasing interest in yeast (mainly *Candida albicans*) infection in cases of apical periodontitis.

The clinical relevance of these *in vitro* test methods is limited, because they do not take the complex clinical situation of the apical region of a tooth into account. Data from such tests provide basic information on the material and can be used to explain certain clinical reactions, e.g. in relation to extrusion of root canal material over the apex. They are by themselves not sufficient to show the biocompatibility of a material (56).

In vivo biocompatibility test methods are mainly performed on laboratory animals. Relevant tests involve the implantation of a material into the subcutaneous/muscle tissues of rats, mice or rabbits (Fig. 17.4). These tests are mainly designed to test the local toxic potential. Of special interest are endodontic usage tests (e.g. in dogs and monkeys), in which the material is applied as

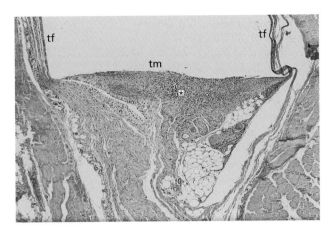

Fig. 17.4 Tissue reaction 14 days after subcutaneous implantation (rat) of a set polyketone root canal sealer filled into a Teflon tube: accumulation of inflammatory cells (mainly polymorphonuclear neutrophilic granulocytes) at the contact area (*) with the test material indicates moderate toxicity; no tissue reaction at the contact area with the Teflon tube. tm = test material, tf = Teflon tube (negative control and material carrier).

---

used later with the patient, i.e. for filling root canals. With such an approach special issues such as apical repair (e.g. new cement formation) or the formation of hard tissue after treatment of teeth with open apices (root-end closure) can be studied, because this requires the interaction of different specialized cell types that so far cannot be simulated in *in vitro* tests or in implantation studies. Although endodontic usage tests are closer to the clinical situation than *in vitro* tests, again they have disadvantages, e.g. results of endodontic usage tests depend strongly on the treatment method and there are indications that these tests do not provide a sensitive discrimination among endodontic materials of widely different chemical composition (50).

The allergic potential of dental materials is tested preclinically mainly on guinea pigs, which provides a rough estimate. Patients who show clinical symptoms of an allergic reaction toward a dental material may be subjected to special allergy tests, which apply a series of materials on the skin (e.g. patch test). Positive patch test results together with corresponding clinical symptoms (e.g. swelling, redness, itching) are indicative of a material-related allergy. For allergy testing and for avoiding relevant allergenic products in the sensitized patient, the composition of the material to be used must be known.

None of the test models described so far for assessing the biological properties of root canal filling materials can be said to be identical to the clinical situation under which the material is used, therefore clinical trials are essential. These clinical trials (including x-rays) are conducted with the prime target organ, the human tooth.

> ### Core concept 17.2 Factors influencing leakage
>
> (1) *Root canal anatomy and preparation.* Oval and keyhole-shaped profiles of the root canals and unsuitable cleaning and shaping impede the correct application of the root canal filling material.
> (2) *Access cavity.* Bacteria may penetrate an obturated root canal within a few days/weeks if the access cavity is not sufficiently sealed (coronal leakage).
> (3) *Smear layer.* Removal using citric acid (10–50%) or EDTA (ethylenediaminetetraacetic acid) (17%) may influence leakage, although results are unequivocal. The effect depends apparently upon the sealer used.
> (4) *Hemostasis/dryness of the root canal.* The wall of the root canal must be clean and dry for a tight adaptation of the sealer to the wall.
> (5) *Root canal filling material.* Stability, adhesion to dentine and lack of pores.
> (6) *Sealer thickness and obturation technique.* Thick layers of root canal sealers (e.g. a ZnOE sealer or a calcium hydroxide sealer) showed more leakage than a thin one (40), which may be due to the fact that most sealers contain pores or dissolve faster in thick layers. A thin layer of root canal sealer is therefore generally recommended.

However, they are unsatisfactory because they do not allow for histological evaluation and a substantial amount of calcium must be lost (>30%) before it can be detected in standard x-rays. This demonstrates that the biocompatibility of a new material cannot be evaluated by one test alone, but a set of tests is necessary to cover the different aspects of biocompatibility.

Leakage/sealing

It is generally believed that the main cause for failure of endodontic treatment is the lack of seal of the root canal filling (apical and coronal leakage), facilitating bacterial growth. Many studies (about 25% of the current endodontic literature) are devoted to leakage and sealability. Leakage mainly occurs between the root canal filling and the root canal wall, although there are some reports showing leakage between sealer (ZnOE or glass ionomer cement) and gutta-percha and throughout the sealer. Leakage is influenced by the root canal filling material itself and by a number of other factors (Core concept 17.2).

Results reported in the literature on leakage depend greatly upon the test methods used. Test methods most often used are performed *in vitro* and include dye penetration, additionally with pressure, centrifugation or vacuum. Other authors used bacterial penetration or fluid transport (73). The clinical relevance of these *in vitro* studies is questionable and contradictory results have been reported for the same material using different methods (6), therefore these tests are – at most – valid in a comparative manner whereby a new material is compared with a clinically established one. *In vivo* usage tests (e.g. on experimental animals) reveal more relevant results but are more difficult to perform and more uncontrollable variables (e.g. application technique) are included. Again, a set of different test methods is necessary to evaluate the leakage properties of a new root canal filling material. Leakage data reported in the literature for root canal filling materials therefore should be regarded with caution because, as with data for other properties (e.g. biological), they are only mosaic stones that need other properties to determine the clinical usefulness of the new material.

Gutta-percha cones

Gutta-percha is the most common cone material used for root canal filling. Silver was used in the past but has been abandoned because of the mediocre sealing qualities, even when used together with sealers, and because of high corrosion leading to tooth discoloration and local tissue reactions (Fig. 17.5). Titanium cones are available and have good biocompatibility, but they show low radiopacity and poor adaptation to the root canal wall in cases of a non-circular cross-section of the shaped root canal. This requires a comparatively high amount of sealer and therefore aggravates the seal of the filling. In narrow and curved canals, where the application of

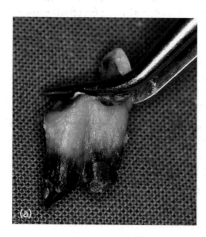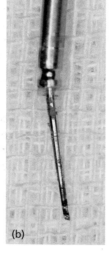

Fig. 17.5 (a) Discoloration of a root after root canal filling with a silver cone. (b) Removed silver cone showing signs of severe corrosion.

gutta-percha points is difficult, these cones may be considered.

Gutta-percha cones are the material of choice for filling the major part of the canal volume. The clinician should carefully select materials with exact dimensions and a composition that is not tissue irritating. Gutta-percha cones (even standardized ones) do not as such fit optimal to the shaped root canal and therefore must be compacted and used together with sealers; the less sealer necessary, the better.

Composition

Gutta-percha is a natural product that consists of the purified coagulated exudate of mazer wood trees (*Isonandra percha*) from the Malay archipelago or from South America. It is a high-molecular-weight polymer based on the isoprene monomer. Two forms of gutta-percha are relevant for dental products: the α- and the β-form. The β-form is used in most gutta-percha cones (less brittle than the α-form) but the α-form is used for injectable products because of its better flow characteristics.

The composition of gutta-percha cones (Table 17.1) varies considerably between different manufacturers. This and the fact that gutta-percha is a natural product (with varying molecular weight) may be the reasons for different properties being reported for different brands. Formerly, cadmium (Cd)-based dyes were added to provide a yellow color, which should facilitate removal (if necessary; e.g. for revision). Modern gutta-percha preparations use other colorants and do not contain any *intentionally* added Cd compounds (zinc oxide may contain low levels of Cd impurities). Some gutta-percha preparations contain calcium hydroxide or chlorhexidine, with the aim of enhancing their antibacterial activity (temporary root canal dressing) and stimulating apical healing. Clinical experience is limited so far.

Gutta-percha cones are supplied by the manufacturers in different sizes (length, diameter, taper; Table 17.2). Standardized cones frequently are used and the idea of having a cone that corresponds closely to the shape and the dimensions of the prepared root canal is striking.

Table 17.1 Typical composition of gutta-percha cones.

Components	Composition (%)
Zinc oxide	66
Metal sulfates (radiopacity)	11
Gutta-percha	20
Additives like colophony (rosin, mainly composed of diterpene resin), pigments or trace metals	3

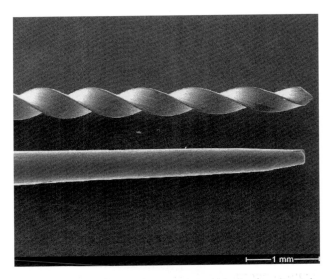

Fig. 17.6 Scanning electron microscope picture of the tip of a gutta-percha cone and the corresponding root canal file; note the discrepancies in shape.

Table 17.2 Dimensions of gutta-percha cones.

Type of cone	Size
Standardized cones	Corresponds in diameter and taper (2%) to root canal shaping instruments according to ISO 6877. The sizes of the gutta-percha cones range from ISO 10 to ISO 140 (Fig. 17.8)
Accessory cones	Larger taper, descriptive size, may be used for lateral compaction
Greater taper cones	Cones with a 4% or 6% (and up to 12%) taper used together with special engine-driven root canal shaping instruments (see Chapter 16)
Compaction cones	Taper corresponds to the taper of finger-spreaders

However, there are discrepancies between the shapes of the cones and the shaping instruments (Fig. 17.6), and the actual dimensions of the gutta-percha cones show considerable variation. Therefore, it is advisable to check the dimensions of each cone by a suitable gauge prior to use (Fig. 17.7). Some manufacturers offer gutta-percha cones with a color coding according to the ISO system for the different sizes (ISO 10–ISO 140) (Fig. 17.8) and/or with a millimeter scale to control the length of insertion. Cones with a 4% or 6% (and up to 12%) taper are offered in sizes using the ISO numbering system (i.e. 10–140); however not only the taper but also the (apical) diameters may be different from the standardized cones. Depending on the shaping system, the taper of gutta-percha cones may be constant over the 16 mm length of the cone or it may be limited to the apical part of the cone.

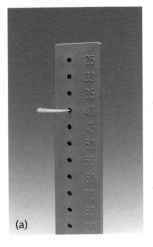
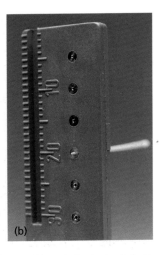

Fig. 17.7 (a) Gauge for controlling the size of the actual gutta-percha cone. (b) The actual cone is too thin, because it reaches out of the gauge.

Gutta-percha may be used *per se* (i.e. cold) in combination with a sealer. Owing to the thermoplastic properties, gutta-percha may be used also in a heated state, which allows closer adaptation to the canal walls (Fig. 17.9). The products consist of a plastic core (carrier) coated by α-phase gutta-percha for improved flow characteristics and to reduce shrinkage after cooling. Gutta-percha also may be liquefied at a temperature of 70°C (Ultrafil) or 160/200°C (Obtura II) and injected directly into the root canal.

Technical properties/leakage

Gutta-percha cones are flexible (elastic) at room temperature, become plastic at about 60°C and are volume-constant under mouth conditions. Heating leads to expansion (and cooling to contraction), a fact that reduces the sealing quality of warm or liquid gutta-percha application (when used without a sealer). Gutta-percha is soluble in organic solvents such as eucalyptus oil.

Gutta-percha *per se* does not adhere to the canal walls, regardless of the obturation technique applied, resulting in marked leakage. Therefore, gutta-percha (used cold and heated) is generally recommended to be used together with a sealer. For an optimal seal the sealer layer generally should be as thin as possible, therefore the skill of the operator plays an important part in the success of the treatment by correctly compacting gutta-percha, whereas it is apparently of minor importance which method of compaction is applied.

Biological properties

No systemic–toxic reactions toward gutta-percha have been reported in the literature. Concerning the Cd

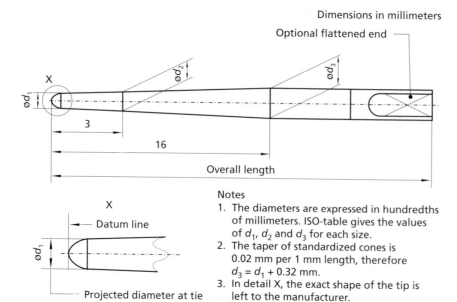

Dimensions in millimeters

Optional flattened end

Notes
1. The diameters are expressed in hundredths of millimeters. ISO-table gives the values of d_1, d_2 and d_3 for each size.
2. The taper of standardized cones is 0.02 mm per 1 mm length, therefore $d_3 = d_1 + 0.32$ mm.
3. In detail X, the exact shape of the tip is left to the manufacturer.

Fig. 17.8 Scheme for the dimensions of a standardized gutta-percha cone according to ISO 6877; $d_1 \times 100 =$ size designation of gutta-percha cone (ISO 10–ISO 140).

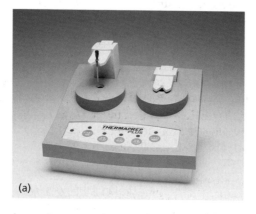

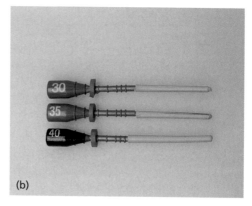

Fig. 17.9 Oven for warming gutta-percha cones (a) and the corresponding cones (b).

content of 'older' gutta-percha (produced up to the 1980s; information from manufacturers), no systemic reaction is to be expected owing to the small masses involved and the low solubility. Allergic reactions towards gutta-percha are extremely rare. One case was reported of a suspected allergic reaction during a root canal treatment with a patient who was sensitized to natural latex. No latex gloves were worn during treatment, but pain, swelling of lips and diffuse urticaria developed after treatment. After 4 weeks the gutta-percha cone was removed and the symptoms abated. The allergy was attributed by the authors to the fact that pure gutta-percha and natural latex are fabricated from natural substances derived from trees of the same botanical family (10). No further cases have been reported. Cones made from synthetic gutta-percha are available.

In several cell culture studies, gutta-percha proved to be non-cytotoxic or only a little cytotoxic, depending on the product (Fig. 17.10). Generally, gutta-percha is well tolerated by animal tissues (e.g. rat and mice connective tissue), inducing the formation of a collagenous capsule with no/almost no inflammation (Fig. 17.11). Interestingly, it was found that *in vitro* and *in vivo* some gutta-percha preparations were more toxic than others (27, 55). After subcutaneous implantation of large particles in guinea pigs only mild reactions occurred, whereas small gutta-percha particles (50–100 μm) caused an accumulation of macrophages and giant cells (typical of a foreign body reaction), which may impair apical healing (64). This shows that gutta-percha is by no means a homogeneous group of materials, and that the tissue reaction also depends upon the particle size.

The elevated temperatures involved in the application of injectable liquefied gutta-percha or of heat-mediated condensation/compaction techniques have been the motive for several investigations into the involved risk

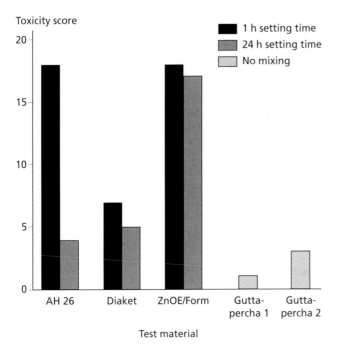

Toxicity score

■ 1 h setting time
■ 24 h setting time
□ No mixing

Test material

Fig. 17.10 Cytotoxicity of different root canal filling materials; human cells were exposed to eluates of the materials and the effect upon cell growth was measured; high scores indicate strong cytotoxicity. For sealers, effects of freshly mixed materials and set materials were measured; for gutta-percha, two brands were tested. ZnOE/Form = formaldehyde-containing ZnOE sealer (55).

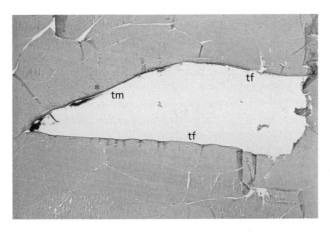

Fig. 17.11 Tissue reaction 7 days after intramuscular implantation of gutta-percha: no inflammatory cells can be observed at the contact area with the test material (*), which indicates good biocompatibility. tm = test material, tf = Teflon tube (negative control and material carrier).

Table 17.3 Temperature measurements for liquefied gutta-percha.

Technique	Intracanal temperature (°C)	Tooth surface temperature rise (°C)
Ultrafil	70	
Obtura II	Max. 61	Max. 8.9
Warm vertical condensation	45–80	3–7
Thermomechanical compaction	55–100	14–35

which reflects the cooling process during application (70).

However, the main target tissue (the periodontal ligament) is separated from the heated gutta-percha by dentine, which, owing to its low thermal conductivity, acts as a thermal isolator. Its effectiveness depends on the dentine thickness, therefore temperature measurements at the surface of the root are clinically more relevant. It is generally accepted that a temperature rise of approximately 10°C above normal body temperature is critical if maintained over 1 min; over 5 min more consistent bone damage will occur (20). Again, the highest temperatures were measured on the root surface with the thermomechanical compaction technique, with differences depending on the rotational speed of the compacting instrument. After stopping compaction, heat is dissipated in 15–30 s for a less than 10°C elevation (53).

The reaction of the target tissues (periodontal ligament) after injection of heated gutta-percha into the root canals of a dog showed no evidence of inflammation. In the case of overfilling, an acute inflammatory reaction was observed briefly after insertion and a chronic/ foreign body reaction was found in long-term experiments (41). The classical warm vertical condensation or the warm lateral condensation did not cause any heat-related periodontal damage in monkeys and miniature pigs at the coronal, middle or apical segments of the root. Contrary to these data, thermomechanical compaction of gutta-percha with a sealer caused tissue damage (see Key literature 17.1).

In conclusion, for melted injectable gutta-percha, no tissue damage is expected due to rapid cooling during application and isolation of the dentine layer. If this layer is not present, e.g. after overfilling, a tissue reaction may occur. No such risks exist for the classical warm condensation technique, with the use of heated instruments or with the prewarming of gutta-percha cones. The use of sealers further reduces temperature rises. However, with the thermomechanical compaction technique most elevated temperatures on the root surfaces were recorded, as well as tissue damage with cementum resorption and ankylosis.

for adverse clinical effects. Intracanal temperatures have been measured, the highest being for the thermomechanical condensation technique (see Chapter 18) (Table 17.3). Interestingly, for liquefied gutta-percha (Obtura II), which is heated to more than 160°C, the intracanal temperature shows a maximum of only 61°C,

Key literature 17.1

Saunders (54) studied histologically the effect of thermomechanical compaction (10,000 revolutions per minute) of gutta-percha with a calcium hydroxide sealer upon the cementum of ferret teeth. Twenty days after root filling, 20% of the experimental teeth showed signs of surface resorption of cementum in the central section of the root with no signs of inflammation. After 40 days, 28% showed resorption and, of these, 22% exhibited ankylosis of alveolar bone to cementum. Controls with lateral condensation showed no resorption or ankylosis. The authors conclude that heat generation by this method is sufficient to stimulate surface resorption and ankylosis in the longer term.

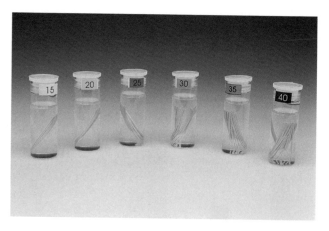

Fig. 17.12 Gutta-percha cones delivered ('germ-free') in an aqueous solution of ethanol and hexetidine.

Antimicrobial properties

It was reported that gutta-percha revealed some antimicrobial properties, the active substance being ZnO from which zinc ions (Zn^{2+}) are mobilized by hydrolysis. Other authors found some brands of gutta-percha active against anaerobically cultivated isolates from root canals. The occurrence and the size of the detected zones varied with the bacteria used for testing and the brand of the gutta-percha cone (69).

Handling properties

Gutta-percha cones are usually supplied by the manufacturer in a non-sterile way. Storage in commonly used disinfectants may have a negative influence on the mechanical properties of the cones and should be avoided, unless evidence is presented that the cones are not damaged. Rather, an effective surface disinfection (e.g. with 5.25% NaOCl) immediately prior to use is advisable; the cones afterwards should be rinsed in 70% alcohol to prevent NaOCl crystals forming on the gutta-percha cone. Recently, gutta-percha cones that are 'free of living germs' (declaration of the manufacturer) have been marketed (Fig. 17.12). Gutta-percha cones should be stored cool and dark in order to prevent enhanced hardening and brittleness due to further crystallization and/or oxidation. A technical problem with the use of heated gutta-percha is the higher frequency of extrusion of root canal sealer.

Gutta-percha can be removed mechanically owing to its comparatively soft consistency, for example, by conventional hand file or by rotary instruments (see Chapter 19). Chloroform is not recommended due to its possible carcinogenicity. Gutta-percha preparations using a plastic carrier can be removed using organic solvents, e.g. eucalyptus oil. The carrier can be bypassed by endodontic instruments. The radiopacity of gutta-percha was measured to be between 6.14 and 8.8 mm Al (62) and this is considered to be sufficient.

Sealers

Sealers are used to fill voids and minor discrepancies of fit between the gutta-percha cones and the root canal wall. Without a cone, leakage increases significantly, probably owing to the fact that sealers may shrink during setting, pores may develop and the solubility of the sealers is enhanced when used in thick layers; the net effect is volume dependent, which is the main reason for using no more sealer than is absolutely necessary. Therefore, the use of sealers without any cone, as was recommended in the past, is today obsolete. An ISO standard for dental root canal sealing materials (ISO 6876) is being published and it describes mainly technical and radiopacity requirements for such materials.

Sealers comprise a heterogeneous group of materials with different compositions (Core concept 17.3). Sealers commonly used will be discussed in more detail in the following paragraphs. In former times, gutta-percha dissolved in chloroform was commonly used as a sealer. However, sealing qualities are regarded as being poor owing to shrinkage toward the center of the material mass after chloroform evaporation. Furthermore, the use of chloroform is discouraged because of its inherent health problems (e.g. carcinogenicity).

Composite resins/dentine bonding agents were tested as root canal sealers in a few studies. They are reported to achieve a good seal, with penetration of the resin into the dentinal tubules, although there are apparently difficulties in applying the material to the apical one-third of the canal (42). Removal of the set resin is difficult and thus problems occur when a re-entry is needed.

Recently, calcium phosphate cements (CPCs) have been described as root canal sealers. They consist of tetracalcium phosphate and either dicalcium phosphate dihydrate or anhydrous dicalcium phosphate mixed with a 1M solution of sodium phosphate dibasic heptahydrate. Reports on the sealing properties are still unequivocal, apparently being dependent upon the actual formulation. Biological reactions are favorable: after implantation no or only mild inflammatory reactions occurred. After correct application and even after deliberately overfilling root canals, the CPC caused no or only minimal alterations. There was even a potential for promoting cementum-like hard-tissue deposition (76).

Silicone as a basis for root canal sealers was introduced in 1984. The first product was based on a condensation polymerizing silicone ('C-Silicone') and, after subcutaneous implantation in rats, this material was initially mildly irritating and in the long run virtually non-toxic (28). In comparison with calcium hydroxide and ZnOE sealers it proved to be the material that was the least tissue irritating. Recently, a root canal sealer with an additional polymerizing silicone ('A-Silicone') became available (Fig. 17.13). A-Silicones, used as impression materials, are known to be more dimensionally stable than C-Silicones, which release ethanol during polymerization. In different *in vitro* studies this sealer was used together with the thermoplastic technique and the lateral condensation technique and proved to provide, in most cases, better sealing properties than calcium hydroxide- or epoxy-based sealers (18). A-Silicones (as impression material) tested non-toxic both *in vitro* and after implantation into experimental animals (58). Yet, so far, no reports are available on the long-term clinical behavior of silicone root canal sealers.

Zinc oxide–eugenol sealers

Zinc oxide–eugenol (ZnOE) sealers have been used for many years and ample clinical experience exists with these materials. However, sealing ability and biological properties are, in general, inferior compared with other

---

> ### Core concept 17.3 Classification of root canal sealers
>
> Sealers commonly used are based on:
>
> - Zinc oxide and eugenol (ZnOE)
> - Polyketone
> - Epoxy resin
> - Glass ionomer cement
> - Calcium hydroxide.
>
> Sealers under investigation/recently marketed are based on:
>
> - Composite resins/dentine bonding agents
> - Calcium phosphate cements
> - Silicones.

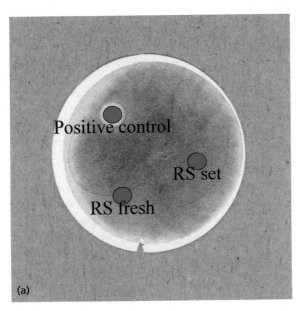
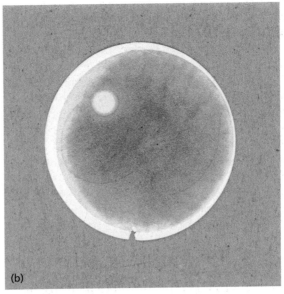

Fig. 17.13 (a) Cell culture toxicity test on L929 mouse fibroblasts of an 'A-Silicone' root canal sealer. The cells are growing beneath the filter (circular grey area). A positive control (5% phenol), the freshly prepared sealer and the set sealer are placed on top of the filter in three different rings. (b) The cells beneath fresh and set material are not damaged, whereas all cells beneath the control are dead. (Courtesy of Dr D. Ørstavik.) RS = root sealer.

root canal sealers. Because of its tendency for disintegration it is still recommended as root canal filling material for deciduous teeth. However, it has not been shown that disintegration of the material occurs parallel to tooth resorption. Formaldehyde-releasing ZnOE root canal sealers should not be used anymore because of their inherent toxicity potential. The European Society of Endodontology discourages the use of these materials (23).

Composition

These sealers comprise a fairly large group of different preparations. Additionally to the standard composition of ZnOE sealers (Grossman sealer, Table 17.4) some preparations further contain thymol or thymol iodide for increasing the antimicrobial effects. Also, hydroxyapatite or calcium hydroxide has been added for improving apical healing. In some sealers eugenol is partially or totally replaced by oil of cloves, Peru balsam or eucalyptol. Oil of cloves is a natural product that contains 60–80% eugenol. The ZnOE sealers may contain colophony (a rosin, mainly diterpene resin acids) to give body, to impart adhesiveness to the sealer and to reduce the solubility/disintegration of the sealer.

Modified ZnOE preparations are composed of: 60% zinc oxide, 34% alumina and 6% natural resin (powder); or 62.5% ortho-ethoxy benzoic acid and 37.5% eugenol (liquid). Another frequently used cement contains 80% ZnO and 20% PMMA (polymethylmethacrylate) in the powder, and the liquid is eugenol. These materials are preferably used for temporary fillings of the access cavity and for root-end fillings. Some ZnOE-based sealers contain paraformaldehyde (e.g. 7% of the powder), with the claim of long-term disinfection by the release of formaldehyde.

The ZnOE preparations harden in a humid environment by forming a ZnOE chelate compound. The mix sets within 24h but the speed can be regulated by the addition of resins, calcium phosphates or zinc acetate. The setting reaction is reversible, releasing eugenol and zinc ions under hydrolytic conditions.

Table 17.4 Typical composition of a ZnOE sealer.

Powder	Liquid
Zinc oxide (42%)	
Staybelite resin (27%)	Eugenol
Bismuth subcarbonate (15%)	(4-allyl-2-methoxyphenol)
Barium sulfate (15%)	
Sodium borate, anhydrous (1%)	

Technical properties/leakage

Several studies showed *apical* leakage around ZnOE sealers that increased with storage time (measured up to 2 years), in thick layers more than in thin layers (40). Sealing properties of ZnOE sealers were inferior in comparison to other sealers (epoxy resin or calcium hydroxide sealers) but better than those of glass ionomer cements. Adhesion of ZnOE sealers to gutta-percha cones is sufficient. Also, *coronal* leakage was greater for a ZnOE sealer (when used with a lateral condensation technique) than for a calcium hydroxide sealer, probably due to the relatively high solubility of the ZnOE sealer (5). Acid end-products of Gram-negative bacteria penetrated a seemingly well-obturated canal within 12 weeks. These acid end-products are able to induce inflammation, e.g. by stimulation of interleukin-1β (a protein that belongs to the group of cytokines and plays an essential role in immune/inflammatory reactions) secretion of cells (15). Modified ZnOE cements appear to have better sealing qualities (see root-end filling).

A ZnOE preparation releasing formaldehyde partially dissolved in contact with vital pulp tissue, and particles of the sealer were dislocated at varying distances from the contact site up to the periapical ligament (36). Removal of the smear layer (17% EDTA) improved (coronal) sealing and in EDTA-pretreated canals different ZnOE sealers showed homogeneous penetration into the root dentine tubules, up to 600μm deep.

From these data it can be concluded that the sealing properties of ZnOE sealers in general are somewhat inferior to most other available materials. Removal of the smear layer improves the seal.

Biological properties

Eugenol, a phenol derivative, has attracted prime interest from a biological point of view. Systemic toxicity was evaluated to be low and eugenol is an accepted nutrition additive. However, eugenol is a known contact allergen, as well as colophony and Peru balsam. Eugenol and its derivatives are used in fragrances, and allergies toward fragrances may be related to eugenol. Cases of allergic reactions toward ZnOE-containing temporary filling materials have been reported (33), but apparently not for root canal sealers. In some cases, dental personnel reported contact dermatitis toward eugenol-containing materials (38). Formaldehyde, which is released from certain ZnOE sealers, is a known allergen. A female patient, a few hours after the application of a high formaldehyde-containing root canal paste, reported urticaria of the lower jaw that rapidly cleared with oral corticosteroids. In the skin test, the patient reacted positive toward the formaldehyde-containing liquid of the root canal paste (19).

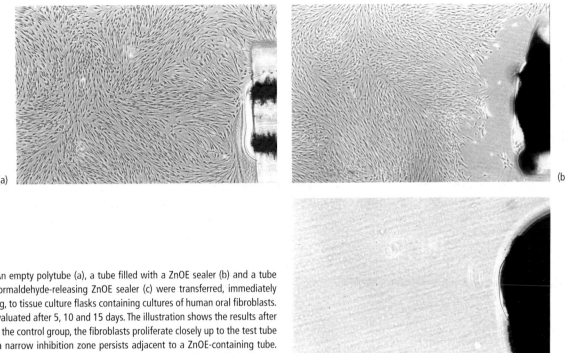

Fig. 17.14 An empty polytube (a), a tube filled with a ZnOE sealer (b) and a tube filled with a formaldehyde-releasing ZnOE sealer (c) were transferred, immediately after obturating, to tissue culture flasks containing cultures of human oral fibroblasts. Toxicity was evaluated after 5, 10 and 15 days. The illustration shows the results after 15 days. In (a), the control group, the fibroblasts proliferate closely up to the test tube (right). In (b) a narrow inhibition zone persists adjacent to a ZnOE-containing tube. In (c), where the tube contained a formaldehyde-releasing sealer, no vital cells are seen (3). (Courtesy of Dr P. Hørsted-Bindslev.)

Eugenol is cytotoxic and the same has been shown frequently for ZnOE with different cell culture systems, especially after mixing but also in a set state. Even higher cytotoxicity was observed with formaldehyde-containing ZnOE sealers, which were classified as highly/extremely cytotoxic (Fig. 17.14) (3) and reveal strong cytotoxic effects (Fig. 17.10) even after several elutions of the hardened specimens (27). A ZnOE sealer without paraformaldehyde tested non-mutagenic. Mutagenicity of formaldehyde, with paraformaldehyde being one of its sources, has been demonstrated.

Some components of ZnOE sealers have neurotoxic effects. Eugenol inhibited nerve conductance *in vitro* in experiments with different nerve tissues. Furthermore, eugenol has both local and general anesthetic effects. Taking into consideration the concentrations involved, a possible neurotoxic effect of eugenol may be reversible *in vivo* (12). On the contrary, formaldehyde irreversibly suppressed nerve conduction in concentrations that may be reached in patients with formaldehyde-containing root canal sealers owing to the high solubility of formaldehyde in water (12). The concentration in root canal sealers and in formocresol pastes is much higher (2–19%) than that needed for *in vitro* destruction of nerve and muscle excitability. Accordingly, a ZnOE sealer in direct contact with the nerve caused complete but reversible inhibition of the nerve conductance, whereas formaldehyde-containing root canal sealers completely

and irreversibly inhibited the nerve conductance (13). The results with the formaldehyde-containing sealers suggest permanent damage of the nerve *in vivo*.

In addition to the observed allergic reactions, ZnOE root canal sealers may influence the immune system. *In vitro* investigations (11) showed both stimulatory (low concentrations) and inhibitory (higher concentrations) effects of extracts of ZnOE sealers on immune-competent cells, with and without formaldehyde. The stimulatory effect may indicate that these materials evoke or accentuate an inflammatory reaction in the apical region *in vivo* (11). After intramuscular injections of a mixture of pulp tissue with a formaldehyde-releasing root canal filling material, a marked immune response (lymphocyte proliferation and elevated antibody titers) was observed with this material (8).

A ZnOE sealer consistently has shown an initial inflammatory effect on the periapical tissues after obturation of ferret root canals, whereas only three out of ten showed inflammation after root filling with a calcium hydroxide formulation (34). A paraformaldehyde-containing ZnOE sealer produced extensive inflammation and tissue necrosis after intramuscular implantation (Fig. 17.15) and when used in root canals of dogs' teeth. Such a sealer significantly impaired apical tissue repair. Severe reactions occurred after overfilling (35, Key literature 17.2). When used as a root canal sealer in human teeth, a formaldehyde-releasing ZnOE sealer

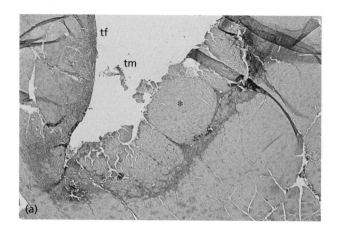 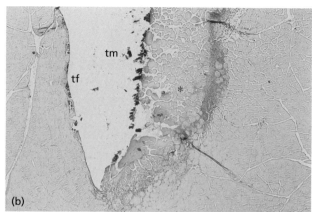

Fig. 17.15 Tissue reaction 7 days after intramuscular implantation of a formaldehyde-releasing ZnOE sealer: extended area of inflammatory cells and necrotic tissue at the contact area with the test material (*) indicates strong toxicity for the material after mixing (a) and after 7 days of setting (b). tm = test material, tf = Teflon tube (negative control and material carrier).

> **Key literature 17.2**
>
> Hong *et al.* (35) performed experiments on the incisors of monkeys. They deliberately overfilled the root canals (thus simulating a worst-case situation) with two ZnOE sealers, one releasing for-maldehyde and, the other not. The tissue reaction was evaluated histologically. The formaldehyde-releasing ZnOE sealer caused severe periapical inflammation even after 6 months; the formaldehyde-free sealer evoked milder alterations. Under the same experimental conditions a calcium phosphate sealer (experimental material) produced only minimal tissue reactions and even new bone was formed. Based on their results the authors recommend materials that alter periapical tissues as little as possible, to prevent severe and chronic tissue reactions after inadvertently overfilling the root canal.

evoked a strong inflammatory reaction of the contacting pulp tissue 6 months after placement, and in corresponding animal experiments particles from this sealer were scattered in the adjacent tissue and surrounded by foreign body cells (multinuclear giant cells, macrophages) (36). From these data it can be concluded that ZnOE sealers have a moderate local toxicity that is strongly enhanced by the addition of paraformaldehyde. There are reports indicating favourable clinical results using sealers containing formaldehyde. However, as mentioned, clinical outcome depends on many variables and is by itself no proof of acceptable biological properties.

Zinc oxide–eugenol sealers with paraformaldehyde were reported to induce aspergillosis of the sinus maxillaris if the material is overfilled into the sinus. A typical x-ray shows a homogeneously clouded antrum with one or more round-to-oval radiodense objects (Fig. 17.16). Clinical symptoms are inconclusive: most patients report intermittent pain and tenderness of the cheek. Other patients have no clinical symptoms and aspergillosis may be detected incidentally at an x-ray examination (7).

Antimicrobial properties: These could be demonstrated even 7 days after mixing on a variety of micro-organisms, including *Enterococcus faecalis* suspensions and anaerobic bacteria. This effect was stronger than the effect produced with calcium hydroxide products but less than an effect from an epoxy resin sealer (Fig. 17.17). Apparently, eugenol is the main antimicrobial agent. Ørstavik (48), in an experimental model of contaminated dentinal tubules, has shown that a ZnOE sealer in the pulp chamber disinfected the dental tubules to a depth of 250 μm (Fig. 17.18). Formaldehyde-releasing ZnOE sealers show extensive antimicrobial properties (Fig. 17.17).

Handling properties

Zinc oxide–eugenol-based sealers are easy to handle. They can be mixed to a smooth paste, which allows enough time for obturation and control (x-ray) before setting. Removal can be performed with organic solvents. The radiopacity of different ZnOE sealers was 5.16–7.97 mm Al (62) and thus can be regarded as sufficient.

Polyketone sealer

The polyketone sealer has good mechanical and sealing properties and no effects on general health are to be expected. On the other hand, the relatively short period for setting may be a problem, especially when compli-

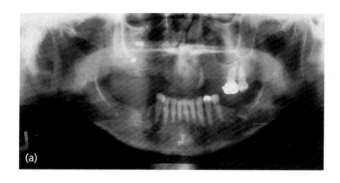
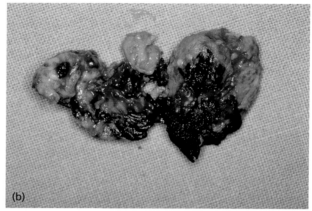

Fig. 17.16   X-ray of a maxillary sinus with suspected aspergillosis from an overfilled root canal in the right sinus: round to oval radiodense objects in the right sinus indicate aspergillosis; the responsible tooth was extracted (a) and the tissue was removed from the sinus (b). (Courtesy of Dr Härle.)

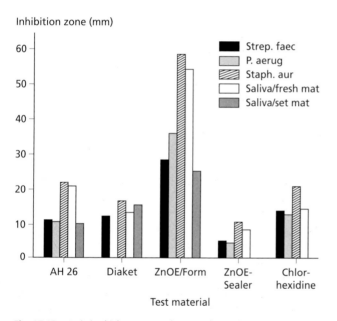

Fig. 17.17   Antimicrobial properties: distance of growth inhibition zone for several root canal sealers and different bacterial strains. Large zones indicate extensive antimicrobial properties; ZnOE/Form = formaldehyde-containing ZnOE sealer (47).

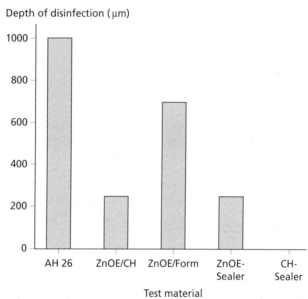

Fig. 17.18   Antimicrobial properties: depth of dentine at which bacteria (*Enterococcus faecalis*) were killed by the root canal sealers; ZnOE/Form = formaldehyde-containing ZnOE sealer; ZnOE/CH = calcium hydroxide-containing ZnOE sealer (48).

cated compaction techniques are used and teeth with more than one root canal are to be treated. However, this may be advantageous in a root-end filling situation. The material is only moderately toxic and apparently does not actively stimulate the healing of apical tissues.

Composition

There has been one commonly used polyketone-based root canal sealer on the market since 1952 (Table 17.5). During setting, a chelate between the ketone and zinc is formed.

Table 17.5   Composition of a polyketone sealer.

Powder	Liquid
Zinc oxide (97%)	Propionylacetophenone (76%)
Bismuth phosphate (3%)	Copolymers of vinyls (23.3%)
	Dichlorophen (0.5%)
	Triethanolamine (0.2%)

Technical properties/leakage

The polyketone-based sealer proved to have acceptable technical properties (sufficient strength, low shrinkage and good adhesion to dentine). Leakage studies showed that this material had lower microleakage scores than the other tested sealers (ZnOE sealers and a glass ionomer cement).

Biological properties

There are no reports available indicating any systemic–toxic effect or allergic reactions. Cell culture experiments for local toxic effects consistently showed cytotoxic reactions that were less pronounced than those reported with paraformaldehyde-containing ZnOE sealers and that decreased after setting (Fig. 17.10). The material was shown to be non-mutagenic in a commonly used bacterial mutation test (59). The sealer showed partial inhibition of nerve conductance *in vitro*, which was partially reversible (13).

When mixed to sealer consistency, the polyketone sealer was shown to cause chronic inflammation after intraosseous implantation and in subcutaneous tissue. The reactions resolved totally or partially with increasing postoperative observation periods. A thicker consistency showed better biocompatibility with bone. A mild inflammatory reaction occurred when used (and overfilled) in rat molars (46). It was resorbed slowly with a tendency toward fibrous encapsulation. In a comparative study the polyketone sealer showed marked antibacterial properties (4). Antimicrobial activity was dependent upon the bacterial strain used for testing (Fig. 17.17) and was generally less distinct than with epoxy sealers.

Handling properties

The sealer hardens rather rapidly (approximately 6 min is stipulated by the manufacturer), which may create a problem with complex lateral condensation methods and when more than one canal needs to be filled. The short setting time, however, is an advantage when the sealer is used for a root-end filling. Radiopacity is sufficient (4.4 mm Al). The sealer is very difficult to remove and thus must be used together with gutta-percha cones.

Epoxy resin sealers

Epoxy resin sealers have comparatively good mechanical and sealing properties. No effects on general health are expected and allergic reactions are apparently rare. Antimicrobial properties are good, especially in a freshly mixed state. Cytotoxicity is moderate to low (set state). Mutagenicity is mainly observed shortly after mixing and no unacceptable risk is expected for the patient.

Table 17.6 Composition of epoxy sealer.

Powder	Liquid
Bismuth (III) oxide (60%)	Bisphenol-A-diglycidylether (BADGE)
Hexamethylene tetraamine (25%)	
Silver (10%)	
Titanium dioxide (5%)	

For a follow-up product adamantane amine, *N,N′*-dibenzoyl-5-oxanonane-diamine-1,9-TCD-diamine is used as a catalyst

For dental personnel, a 'No Touch Technique' is recommended.

Composition (Table 17.6)

The original preparation (AH26), although still on the market in some countries, has been replaced by a follow-up product (AHPlus, Topseal).

Because the silver in AH26 may lead to tooth discoloration due to the formation of black silver sulfides, preparations are available without silver, and bismuth oxide is added for radiopacity. A newly developed preparation (AHPlus) is also based on an epoxy resin (BADGE) but contains a different catalyst.

The setting reaction of AH26 lasts about 1–2 days (at body temperature) and is a polymerization process during which formaldehyde is released, but the concentration is more than 300-fold less than that of a formaldehyde-releasing ZnOE formulation (66). The AHPlus is set after about 8 h. There are indications that AHPlus does not release formaldehyde.

Technical properties/leakage

The epoxy-based sealer showed good mechanical properties as well as excellent adhesion/adaptation to dentine. After initial volumetric expansion, the sealer showed some shrinkage when tested at longer intervals. In general, *in vitro* and *in vivo* studies with the material showed better sealing properties than with any other sealer tested, although it was far from perfect because an increasing storage time (up to 2 years) decreases the sealing quality (40). The use of third-generation dentine bonding agents improved significantly the seal of AH26 to destine via lateral condensation (44). However, there is very little experience with this combination, especially concerning the tissue reaction toward potentially (cyto)toxic dentine bonding agents. Studies on the sealing properties of AHPlus compared with AH26 show inconsistent results. If the smear layer is removed from the root canal walls, AH26 is able to flow into the orifices of the dentinal tubuli (Fig. 17.19), which is the reason for the comparatively good adhesion of AH26 to

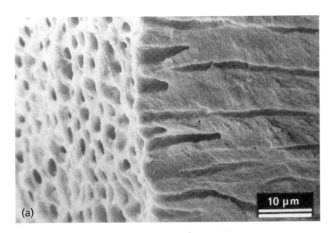 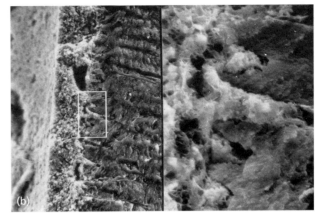

Fig. 17.19 (a) Scanning electron micrograph of root canal dentine after smear layer removal with citric acid. (b) AH26 used as a sealer on a smear-layer-free dentine surface: the sealer enters the dentinal tubuli. (Courtesy of Dr A. Petschelt.)

dentine. Alcohol residues in the canal may impair adhesion of AHPlus to the canal walls.

Biological properties

Epoxy resins are biologically active molecules but no reports are available in the literature on systemic–toxic reactions caused by epoxy-based sealers. One case of allergic reaction toward AH26 was reported after root canal filling, characterized by erythema of the face and the neck and a positive skin test (Fig. 17.20) (37). Positive reactions to AH26 have also been observed in the guinea pig maximization test (32).

The cytotoxicity of AH26 is related to the setting reaction: freshly mixed, the material is cytotoxic, but after setting it is not toxic or only slightly toxic (Fig. 17.10) (55). Cytotoxicity was related to the initial release of formaldehyde during setting. *In vitro* AH26 showed some inhibition of the nerve conductance, which was partially reversible (13).

In both *in vitro* and *in vivo* experiments AH26 was mutagenic (21, 30, 49), especially in a freshly mixed state (59, 61). The cause for the mutagenic reaction may be formaldehyde formed during the setting reaction or the epoxy monomer (BADGE). The AHPlus (which also contains BADGE) was also shown to be mutagenic, but only immediately after mixing (60). In contrast to studies with AH26, an almost tenfold higher amount of AHPlus is needed to elicit similar mutagenic effects and no mutagenicity was observed 24h after mixing (43, 60). The mutagenicity data are difficult to interpret. After exposure to an enzyme mix containing esterases, BADGE is further hydrolyzed to a compound that is no longer mutagenic (59). Because the set material in most studies was non-mutagenic, we conclude that it can be used in the patient situation but care should be taken for the dental personnel, who may come into frequent contact

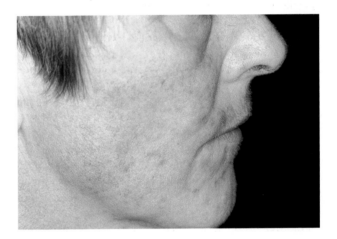

Fig. 17.20 Allergic reaction toward an epoxy resin sealer. A couple of hours following root filling of tooth 46 the patient developed swelling and erythema of the right side of the face and neck. Redness of the oral mucosa around tooth 46 was experienced and the tooth became tender to percussion. The symptoms subsided after a couple of days. The root filling was removed and the canals were later obturated without complications using gutta-percha points and ZnOE cement. Before obturation a strong positive patch test reaction to bisphenol-A-ethyldimetacrylate (BISEMA), bisphenol-A-glycidyldimetacrylate (BISGMA) and epoxyacrylate was demonstrated. The patient recalled that almost similar symptoms had arisen 6 months previously when another tooth was root filled. However, the previous reactions were not as serious. (Courtesy of Dr P. Hørsted-Bindslev.)

with the unpolymerized material. Therefore, a 'No Touch Technique' is recommended.

After subcutaneous, intramuscular or intraosseous implantation into different small laboratory animals, the epoxy sealers proved to be toxic initially but the reaction resolved partially or even totally with prolonged postoperative observation periods (Fig. 17.21). As was observed with cytotoxicity, the toxic reaction *in vivo* was

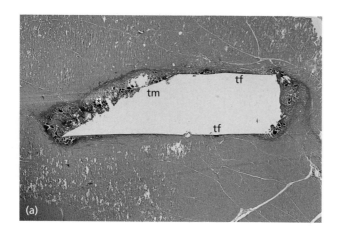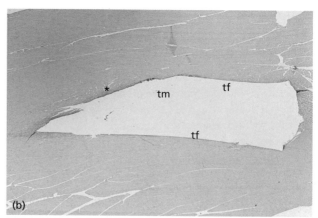

Fig. 17.21 Tissue reaction 7 days after intramuscular implantation of AH26: an accumulation of inflammatory cells (mainly polymorphonuclear neutrophilic granulocytes) at the contact area between the test material and the tissue (*) indicates moderate toxicity of the material directly after mixing (a); the tissue in contact with the set material shows no inflammatory cells (*) and is therefore virtually non-toxic (b). tm = test material, tf = Teflon tube (negative control and material carrier).

related to the setting reaction: immediately after mixing, implanted samples caused a severe reaction, but after 7 days of setting before implantation no toxic reaction occurred. In rat molars after overfilling an inflammatory reaction was observed. Overfilled AH26 was solubilized and phagocytized.

Antimicrobial properties: These have been demonstrated consistently for AH26 (Fig. 17.17). As was shown with the local toxicity, the antimicrobial effect decreased with increasing setting time. Compared with ZnOE, calcium hydroxide and glass ionomer cement sealers on the model of infected root dentine AH26 showed the strongest antimicrobial effect (Fig. 17.18) (31), probably due to the initial release of formaldehyde (66).

Handling properties

Epoxy-based sealers have been used for more than 40 years worldwide and their handling properties are usually considered to be good. Radiopacity is sufficient (6.66 mm Al). However, the materials set to a hard mass that, in a clinically relevant time, is virtually non-soluble even for organic solvents. Therefore, this material must be used together with gutta-percha cones.

Glass ionomer cement (GIC) sealer

The main problems of the glass ionomer cement (GIC) sealer are related to leakage, which again may be due to moisture sensitivity during setting. The formation of pores may be another problem. On the other hand, these materials offer the possibility to strengthen the root due to chemical binding to dentine, therefore further test results and/or material improvements should be monitored.

Composition

More than 10 years ago a GIC (Ketac-Endo) was introduced as a root canal sealer. This material basically contains ground silicates (calcium–sodium–fluor–phosphor silicate) in the powder and polyacrylic acid, malenic acid or tartaric acid in the liquid. The setting reaction, which is sensitive to both moisture and desiccation, starts as dissolution of the particle surfaces followed by an acid–base reaction by which the metal ions from the powder (first calcium and later aluminum) 'replace' the protons of the carboxylate groups and form a non-soluble matrix into which the remnants of the particles are embedded.

Technical properties/leakage

The good adaptation and chemical adhesion to the dentine provided the rationale for using GICs as root canal sealers. In contrast to all other sealers, a single cone technique was described with the idea of strengthening the root canal with a thick layer of GIC. Gutta-percha was recommended only for better re-entry. The GICs have shown good mechanical properties in other applications but the presence of pores reduces the sealing quality considerably.

In vitro leakage studies revealed contradicting results: some authors conclude that, in general, Ketac-Endo showed greater dye penetration than other sealers such as ZnOE and AH26, and that there was no significant difference between the lateral condensation and the single cone technique for Ketac-Endo. On the other hand, no difference in apical dye penetration between Ketac-Endo and AH26 was reported and an even better seal was formed when used as a thin layer (74). These differences may be due to problems of the test method (the GIC sealer seems to absorb the dye) or to the sensitivity of the setting process of GICs with respect to moisture. No bacterial penetration was observed after 60 days when Ketac-Endo was used with a one-cone technique. As was observed with other sealers, leakage increased with increasing storage time (2-year observation period) (40).

Biological properties

Glass ionomer cements have been used for more than 25 years in different applications in dentistry, but there are no reports available in the corresponding literature about systemic–toxic or allergic reactions. Cell culture experiments with GICs consistently show some cytotoxicity of the freshly mixed material. After setting, no or only minimal cytotoxicity occurred. However, for optimal setting the correct water balance is necessary: either too much or too little moisture leads to insufficient setting combined with enhanced solubility and cytotoxicity. This may be a problem in a root canal with an open apex and with the sealer in direct contact with the living tissue. After subcutaneous implantation in rats a mild inflammation was observed after 5 days with the GIC, which further diminished with time (120 days), compared with a ZnOE sealer that produced a stronger inflammation even after 120 days (39). A GIC root canal sealer was non-mutagenic in a commonly used bacterial test system (21).

Antimicrobial properties: The antimicrobial properties of a GIC sealer compared with other sealers (ZnOE sealers, calcium hydroxide sealer) on anaerobic bacteria were somewhere between the ZnOE sealers (strong activity) and the calcium hydroxide preparations (weak activity) (1). On bovine dentine models with infected root dentine, the GIC showed the lowest activity in comparison with a ZnOE sealer, a calcium hydroxide sealer and an epoxy sealer (31). Antimicrobial activities of GICs may be due to the initially low pH and the fluoride release.

Handling properties

Basically, handling of these materials seems uncomplicated. However, the working time in the mouth is limited to 7 min. This may cause some problems if the material is used with the lateral condensation technique on teeth with several root canals. It should also be kept in mind that the mixed material should not be stored much longer than 7 min outside the capsule, because the water evaporates and the paste tends to thicken. The mixed material can be kept inside the capsule for about 40 min. The radiopacity of the materials is sufficient. The material cannot be removed from the canal under clinical conditions once it has set and thus must be used with gutta-percha cones.

Table 17.7 Main components of a calcium hydroxide sealer.

Base paste	Catalyst paste
Calcium hydroxide (32%)	Disalicylates (36%)
Colophony (32%)	Bismuth carbonate (18%)
Silicon dioxide (8%)	Silicon dioxide (15%)
Calcium oxide (6%)	Colophony (5%)
Zinc oxide (6%)	Tricalcium phosphate (5%)
Others (16%)	Others (21%)

Calcium hydroxide (CH) sealers

Calcium hydroxide sealers have inferior technical properties compared with polyketone or epoxy resin preparations. Leakage studies show inconsistent results, with a tendency for less sealing quality compared with other sealers. From a biological point of view, calcium hydroxide sealers are very favorable materials and they exhibit – at least in a freshly mixed state – considerable antimicrobial activity. Furthermore, they belong to the few materials that apparently stimulate apical healing and hard-tissue formation (root-end closure). Further research with these materials should be monitored carefully.

Composition

These sealers were introduced in an attempt to stimulate periapical healing with bone repair through the release of calcium hydroxide (Table 17.7). The setting reaction is based on the salicylate compounds. One ZnOE sealer contains calcium hydroxide as an addition to the powder. This material, however, should be considered more as a ZnOE sealer because most effects (e.g. cytotoxicity) are related to this group of sealers. Some authors recommend the use of calcium oxide, which after contact with fluids is partially transformed into calcium hydroxide. It is reported to have the same properties as calcium hydroxide but with the potential of better intratubular penetration and removal of unmineralized extracellular matrix.

Calcium hydroxide sealers release OH^- and Ca^{2+} ions. The amount varies between different brands, but the clinical significance of this difference is not known. Release of these ions is markedly higher when suspensions are used. Calcium hydroxide sealers evoked an increase of pH when placed in distilled water (48 h after setting) of 9.14 and 8.6; under the same conditions, pure calcium hydroxide paste increased the pH to 12.5. When calcium hydroxide sealers are used together with lateral condensation of gutta-percha, the outer dentine surface does not become alkaline, in contrast to the use of calcium hydroxide suspensions. The authors conclude that after setting of calcium hydroxide sealers no OH$^-$ ions are available anymore for diffusion through dentine (22).

Technical properties/leakage

Mechanical properties of calcium hydroxide sealers are inferior compared with polyketone-, epoxy- or GIC-based sealers. The desired release of OH$^-$ ions may be associated with degradation of the sealer, enhancing leakage. Degradation of salicylate-based materials is known from their application as pulp capping agents. Studies clearly indicate significant volumetric expansion, disintegration and high solubility of a calcium hydroxide sealer following long-term observations. Apparently, some calcium hydroxide sealers dissolve at a relatively high rate, especially when used in a thick layer (75). The bond to dentine is weak (71).

Some *in vitro* studies showing less leakage for a calcium hydroxide sealer than for an epoxy sealer and a ZnOE sealer could not be confirmed *in vivo*. In vitro leakage studies with the commonly used dye methylene blue are problematic because calcium hydroxide decolorizes methylene blue. Coronal leakage for bacteria after up to 90 days of exposure proved to be less for a calcium hydroxide sealer than for a ZnOE sealer, when used with the lateral condensation technique (14). After 2 years of storage, leakage of a calcium hydroxide sealer increased (40). The removal of the smear layer has no effect on coronal leakage of a calcium hydroxide sealer when applied together with the lateral condensation technique.

Biological properties

There are no reports available in the literature about systemic–toxic or allergic effects on calcium hydroxide sealers. Their cytotoxicity was generally low (compared with other commonly used sealers) when tested in different cell culture systems (27). In a more complex cell culture system capable of demonstrating both cytotoxicity and the influence on immunocompetent cells, a calcium hydroxide sealer was nearly innocuous (11). A salicylate-based calcium hydroxide sealer was non-mutagenic in an *in vitro* bacterial test system (21). However, both a calcium hydroxide sealer and a calcium hydroxide-containing ZnOE sealer induced *in vitro* a fast and complete inhibition of nerve conductance when in direct contact with the nerve. After 30 min of contact, the nerve conduction was irreversibly blocked by both materials (9).

After implantation in rats and guinea pigs, calcium hydroxide sealers initially caused a severe reaction that diminished after several months and was finally lower than with a ZnOE sealer. In root canals of ferrets (34), all teeth with the ZnOE material showed an inflammatory reaction at their apices, whereas only three out of ten showed this effect with the calcium hydroxide-formulation. Furthermore, a calcium hydroxide sealer evoked the most extensive apical hard-tissue formation; a pure calcium hydroxide preparation induced less hard tissue and gutta-percha had the least effect (65).

Antimicrobial properties: for calcium hydroxide sealers these properties have been shown in several *in vitro* experiments, and the activity may even increase with time due to partial disintegration of the sealer. The mechanism of this antimicrobial activity was related to the high pH; the buffer capacity of body fluid will reduce the effect with time. However, it was also consistently demonstrated that ZnOE sealers exhibited a stronger antimicrobial effect than calcium hydroxide products regardless of the micro-organisms tested (1). In accordance with these studies, the calcium hydroxide sealer did not disinfect the dentinal tubules infected with *Enterococcus faecalis* after 4 h (Fig. 17.18) (48). This is in line with the observation that Enterococci, which are frequently isolated from persistent root canal infections, were found to be resistant to calcium hydroxide.

Root-end closure

A 'root-end closure' is the induction of calcified tissue formation to obturate the dental apical foramen; it was first reported in 1960. In several experiments with monkeys, osteocementum/cementoid substances at and around the open root apices were developed after the application of a calcium hydroxide suspension for 3 and 6 months. Clinical success rates are in the range of 74–100% (Fig. 17.22).

The mechanism of inducing hard-tissue formation by calcium hydroxide preparations is not yet elucidated. It is apparently related to the high pH and the released calcium ions from the material, which promote a state of alkalinity of the adjacent tissues – a condition that arrests root resorption and favors repair, due to an inhibition of osteoclastic activities. It has been postulated further that Ca^{2+} acts on the process of cell differentiation and on macrophage activation and that acids produced by osteoclasts are neutralized and calcium phosphate complexes are formed. It was suggested that activation of ATP, which accelerates bone and dentine mineralization, and the induction of TGF-β (transforming growth factor β), which represents a group of signaling molecules, play a central role in biomineralization. A further factor is the profound antimicrobial activity of calcium hydroxide sealers (68).

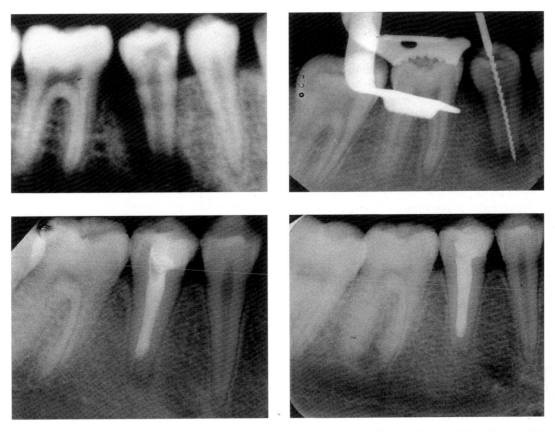

Fig. 17.22 Root-end closure of a lower premolar after treatment with a calcium hydroxide suspension for 6 months (lower left image). For the final root canal filling (lower right image) an epoxy sealer with gutta-percha was used. (Courtesy of Dr B. Thonemann.)

Handling properties

Handling properties of calcium hydroxide sealers are adequate; the radiopacity is regarded as sufficient. The material can be removed with common rotary instruments from the root canal.

Materials for retrograde fillings (root-end fillings) and replantation

These materials are used to create an apical seal and to permit regeneration of the periodontal ligament apparatus. Contrary to conventional root canal filling therapy, these materials are used in a surgical environment characterized by early moisture access and a bony defect.

A number of different materials have been used for root-end fillings, such as gutta-percha, composite resins, glass ionomers, amalgams, modified ZnOE cements and a polyketone sealer. Potentially applicable are mineral trioxide aggregates (MTAs) and calcium phosphate cements. Preformed titanium inlays in combination with

standard ultrasonic preparation were recommended (cemented with a modified ZnOE cement), as well as ceramic inserts. Amalgam used to be very popular, but the potential to release metallic components into the surrounding tissue has made amalgam a controversial material in this context.

The classical material for root-end filling – amalgam – has been gradually abandoned. Modified ZnOE cements, a polyketone sealer (thick consistency) used with or without metallic/ceramic inserts or a light-cured GIC were successfully used instead. However, reports on cementum deposition are unequivocal. A resin composite has shown promising results in the hands of a single group and MTAs apparently have the potential to stimulate further apical healing and thus may – after further clinical experience is gained – replace other materials for this purpose.

Composition

Modified ZnOE cements have been described above (see ZnOE sealers). A composite resin recommended for retrofills was based on bisphenol-A-glycidyldimetacrylate/triethyleneglycoldimetacrylate (BISGMA/TEGDMA, 1:1), containing silver or (more recently) ytterbium trifluoride for radiopacity. It is used together with a dentine bonding system (52). Mineral trioxide aggregates comprise a mixture of tricalcium silicate, tricalcium aluminate, tricalcium oxide and silicate oxide. Hydration of the powder results in a colloidal gel that solidifies to a hard structure in less than 4h.

Technical properties/leakage

The good mechanical properties of amalgams were the reason for their widespread use in the past. Data reported on the marginal seal of amalgams are, however, controversial. A polyketone sealer and a GIC sealer were reported to produce a better seal than various amalgams. Good sealing ability of a light-cured GIC was reported, probably due to the fast setting and little moisture sensitivity. Modified ZnOE cements have also been shown to produce a good seal, as well as a composite resin. Mineral trioxide aggregate produced a better seal than amalgam, being the most effective root-end-filling material against bacterial penetration in comparison with amalgam and two modified ZnOE sealers (25).

Biological properties

The group of materials used for root-end filling is rather heterogeneous. Especially for composite resins and amalgams, much literature is available on real or claimed systemic–toxic effects. The same is true for allergies. The reader is referred to corresponding text books. However, in general, there is no contraindication for the use of any of the mentioned materials due to systemic–toxic or allergenic effects. In the single patient situation, materials must not be used that contain a substance to which the patient is sensitized.

Cell culture experiments for local toxic effects show consistently that all setting materials used for root-end filling are cytotoxic initially after mixing. In the set state, cytotoxicity decreases to different levels characteristic of each material. Mineral trioxide aggregate, a fairly new root-end filling material, is less cytotoxic than amalgam, ZnOE or epoxy sealers (51). Implantation studies are available for all root-end filling materials, because they are used for other applications (e.g. filling technique). In parallel with cell culture experiments, the local toxic reaction decreases with increased aging of the material. The same is basically true for antimicrobial properties. For details, see the paragraphs on the specific materials above.

Of special clinical relevance are usage tests. Poor sealing properties, measured in animal experimentation

---

> **Key literature 17.3**
>
> In a study in dogs by Harrison et al. (29), root canals were obturated with a ZnOE material (IRM) or amalgam and then the root ends were resected. Orthograde fillings with gutta-percha/ZnOE sealer were used as controls. The test materials evoked no inhibition of osseous wound healing and cementum was present in contact with all materials after a 45-day observation period. However, Chong et al. (16) modified this test method: after artificial infection of root canals *before* the root resection and application of the root-end filling, amalgam in experiments up to 8 weeks caused persistent inflammation in the apical area. Better results were observed with a ZnOE material and a light-cured GIC. It was concluded that the poor sealing properties of amalgam were the main reasons for the negative test result and that in a corresponding clinical situation a ZnOE material or a light-cured GIC is recommended.

(Key literature 17.3), are in line with the poor clinical long-term prognosis of amalgam root-end fillings, as was reported by some authors (26).

A polyketone sealer with and without tricalcium phosphate (TCP) showed in dogs after 60 days a preosteoid/cementoid-like matrix in direct and intimate approximation to the root-end filling material (72). A dentine-bonded resin composite (Gluma-Retroplast) used in monkeys for root-end fillings without intentionally infected canals evoked cementum coverage, indicating optimal tissue tolerance. However, if the root canal was infected, less favorable results were observed. The resin material hardly entered the apical cavity and thus provided only a superficial seal (2).

Root-end fillings with MTA in monkey and dog teeth showed cementum coverage over the filling, whereas amalgam produced inflammation and no cementum layer on the material. Mineral trioxide aggregate stimulates cytokine release from bone cells with the potential of actively promoting hard-tissue formation (67).

Clinical data indicated inferior clinical success rates when amalgam was used compared with other materials (26). Further disadvantages are the potential of staining of the mucosa, scattering of particles during placement and corrosion. For modified ZnOE cements, good clinical results are reported over a period of up to 14 years (17). For composite resins only a few clinical studies are published, but a clinical success rate of about 90% was reported recently (52).

Handling properties

Owing to the special surgical environment mentioned above, good handling properties are important. Whereas ZnOE (and amalgam) harden in a moist environment, conventional GIC is susceptible to moisture and desiccation. Light-cured products may have certain advantages in this respect because of fast setting. It had been reported also that it is not easy to apply dentine bonding agents and a resin devoid of voids into a rather small apical cavity. Root-end filling materials should have a radiopacity greater than that of root canal filling materials.

Mandibular nerve injuries

These injuries after root canal filling therapy occur rather seldom in daily practice but they are dramatic in each single case. At least four different pathogenic mechanisms have been proposed:

- Instrumentation beyond the apex and mechanical severance.
- Combined effect of regional analgesia and mechanical nerve damage.
- Degeneration of the nerve due to the mechanical compression caused by filling the materials in the nerve canal.
- Toxicity/neurotoxicity of the root canal filling material.

Irreversible sensory nerve damage may involve frequent paresthesia, which constitutes altered sensation of pain, touch or temperature. Symptoms are the sensation of warmth, cold, burning, aching, prickling, tingling, pins and needles, numbness, itching and formication (feels as if ants are crawling on the skin) (45). In the endodontic literature most cases have resulted from overfill of paraformaldehyde-containing sealers in the vicinity of the inferior alveolar nerves. Long-term paresthesia of up to 13 years has been described. A survey of the literature in the year 1988 (12) has shown that more than 40 cases of root canal cements associated with paresthesia of the inferior alveolar nerve have been reported in the past two decades. Most of these patients have been treated with materials that contain (para)formaldehyde. The reaction of ZnOE sealers with the addition of formaldehyde was irreversible unless surgical treatment was performed. This is in line with data from *in vitro* experiments on different nerve tissues described above, which have shown an irreversible effect on nerve conductance from formaldehyde-releasing root canal sealers. Thus, there are indications that the material and especially the release of formaldehyde may play a major role in these injuries (12).

There are also case reports on paresthesia after overfill of AH26, which was attributed to the short-term release of formaldehyde during setting. A 4-month paresthesia was reported to be eugenol-induced. Another case caused by ZnOE was reversible. Six cases of paresthesia after overfill of gutta-percha/chloropercha were reported and the symptoms resolved after a maximum of 3 months (45).

Single cases were reported for other root canal filling materials/techniques. Melted gutta-percha (thermomechanical compaction used with a CH-based sealer) was extruded into the mandibular canal causing severe nerve injury with persistent local paresthesia (numbness and intermittent bouts of 'pins and needles' in the lip and chin). A few days later the area of paresthesia was replaced by anesthesia. After surgical removal from the periapical area and from the nerve canal, anesthesia was replaced by paresthesia. The authors assume that the reason for this adverse reaction was the elevated temperature by which the gutta-percha was extruded out of the root canal (24).

It can be concluded that with most of the currently used root canal filling materials detrimental effects on local nerve tissues were observed when the root canals were dramatically overfilled and the local nerve fibers were involved. However, most cases are described in connection with formaldehyde-releasing sealers with long lasting/irreversible damage to the nerve tissues. The clinician should be aware of this situation and be familiar with preventive measures when choosing the root canal filling material. These are:

- *Appropriate treatment technique*: to reduce the risk that the filling material is displaced beyond the apex and into the vicinity of the nerve.
- *Appropriate material selection*: use root canal filling materials with the least possible (neuro)toxic effects.

References

1. Abdulkader A, Duguid R, Saunders EM. The antimicrobial activity of endodontic sealers to anaerobic bacteria. *Int. Endodont. J.* 1996; 29: 280–83.
2. Andreasen JO, Munksgaard EC, Fredebo L, Rud J. Periodontal tissue regeneration including cementogenesis adjacent to dentin-bonded retrograde composite fillings in humans. *J. Endodont.* 1993; 19: 151–3.
3. Arenholt-Bindslev D, Hørsted-Bindslev P. A simple model for evaluating relative toxicity of root filling materials in cultures of human oral fibroblasts. *Endodont. Dent. Traumatol.* 1989; 5: 219–26.
4. Barkhorder RA. Evaluation of antimicrobial activity *in vitro* of ten root canal sealers on *Streptococcus sanguis* and *Streptococcus mutans*. *Oral Surg.* 1989; 68: 770–72.
5. Barnett F, Trope M, Rooney J, Tronstad L. In vivo sealing ability of calcium hydroxide-containing root canal sealers. *Endodont. Dent. Traumatol.* 1989; 5: 23–6.

6. Barthel CR, Moshonov J, Shuping G, Orstavik D. Bacterial leakage versus dye leakage in obturated root canals. *Int. Endodont. J.* 1999; 32: 370–75.

7. Beck-Mannagetta J. Zinc and aspergillus. *Oral Surg.* 1996; 81: 138–40.

8. Block RM, Sheats JB, Lewis RD, Fawley J. Cell-mediated immune response to dog pulp tissue altered by N2 paste within the root canal. *Oral Surg.* 1978; 45: 131–42.

9. Boiesen J, Brodin P. Neurotoxic effect of two root canal sealers with calcium hydroxide on rat phrenic nerve in vitro. *Endodont. Dent. Traumatol.* 1991; 7: 242–5.

10. Boxer MB, Grammer LC, Orfan N. Gutta-percha allergy in a health care worker with latex allergy. *J. Allergy Clin. Immunol.* 1994; 93: 943–4.

11. Bratel J, Jontell M, Dahlgren U, Bergenholtz G. Effects of root canal sealers on immunocompetent cells *in vitro* and *in vivo*. *Int. Endodont. J.* 1998; 31: 178–88.

12. Brodin P. Neurotoxic and analgesic effects of root canal cements and pulp-protectiong dental materials. *Endodont. Dent. Traumatol.* 1988; 4: 1–11.

13. Brodin P, Roed A, Aars H, Orstavik D. Neurotoxic effects of root canal filling materials on rat phrenic nerve *in vitro*. *J. Dent. Res.* 1982; 61: 1020–3.

14. Chailertvanitkul P, Saunders WP, MacKenzie D. Coronal leakage in teeth root filled with gutta-percha and two different sealers after long-term storage. *Endodont. Dent. Traumatol.* 1997; 13: 82–7.

15. Chailertvanitkul P, Saunders WP, MacKenzie D, Weetman DA. An in vitro study of the coronal leakage of two root canal sealers using an obligate anaerobe microbial marker. *Int. Endodont. J.* 1996; 29: 249–55.

16. Chong BS, Pitt Ford TR, Kariyawasam SP. Tissue response to potential root-end filling materials in infected root canals. *Int. Endodont. J.* 1997; 30: 102–14.

17. Dorn SO, Gartner AH. Retrograde filling materials: a retrospective success-failure study of amalgam, EBA, and IRM. *J. Endodont.* 1990; 16: 391–3.

18. Ebert J, Loeffler T, Zels H, Petschelt A. Sealing ability of Rockoseal®-automix under different conditions. *J. Dent. Res.* 1999; 78: 320.

19. El-Sayed F, Seite-Bellezza D, Sans B, Bayle-Lebey P, Marguery MC, Bazex J. Contact urticaria from formaldehyde in a root canal dental paste. *Contact Dermatitis* 1995; 33: 353.

20. Eriksson AR, Albrektson T. Temperature threshold levels for heat-induced bone tissue injury: a vital-microscopic study in the rabbit. *J. Prosthet. Dent.* 1983; 50: 101–7.

21. Ersev H, Schmalz G, Bayirli G, Schweikl H. Cytotoxic and mutagenic potencies of various root canal filling materials in eukaryotic and prokaryotic cells in vitro. *J. Endodont.* 1999; 25: 359–63.

22. Esberard RM, Carnes DL Jr, del Rio CE. Changes in pH at the dentin surface in roots obturated with calcium hydroxide pastes. *J. Endodont.* 1996; 22: 402–5.

23. European Society of Endodontology. Consensus report of the European Society of Endodontology on quality guidelines for endodontic treatment. *Int. Endodont. J.* 1994; 27: 115–24.

24. Fanibunda K, Whitworth J, Steele JG. The management of thermomechanically compacted gutta percha extrusion in the inferior dental canal. *Br. Dent. J.* 1998; 184: 330–32.

25. Fischer EJ, Arens DE, Miller CH. Bacterial leakage of mineral trioxide aggregate as compared with zinc-free amalgam, intermediate restorative material, and Super-EBA as a root-end filling material. *J. Endodont.* 1998; 24: 176–9.

26. Frank AL, Glick DH, Patterson SS, Weine FS. Long-term evaluation of surgically placed amalgam fillings. *J. Endodont.* 1992; 18: 391–8.

27. Geurtsen W, Leyhausen G. Biological aspects of root canal filling materials – histocompatibility, cytotoxicity, and mutagenicity. *Clin. Oral. Invest.* 1997; 1: 5–11.

28. Gorduysus MO, Etikan I, Gokoz A. Histopathological evaluation of the tissue reactions to Endo-Fill root canal sealant and filling material in rats. *J. Endodont.* 1998; 24: 194–6.

29. Harrison JW, Johnson SA. Excisional wound healing following the use of IRM as a root-end filling material. *J. Endodont.* 1997; 23: 19–27.

30. Heil J, Reifferscheid G, Waldmann P, Leyhausen G, Geurtsen W. Genotoxicity of dental materials. *Mutat. Res.* 1996; 368: 181–94.

31. Heling I, Chandler NP. The antimicrobial effect within dentinal tubules of four root canal sealers. *J. Endodont.* 1996; 22: 257–9.

32. Hensten-Pettersen A, Orstavik D, Wennberg A. Allergenic potential of root canal sealers. *Endodont. Dent. Traumatol.* 1985; 1: 61–5.

33. Hensten-Pettersen A, Jacobsen N. Perceived side effects of biomaterials in prosthetic dentistry. *J. Prosthet. Dent.* 1991; 65: 138–44.

34. Holland GR. A histological comparison of periapical inflammatory and neural responses to two endodontic sealers in the ferret. *Arch. Oral Biol.* 1994; 39: 539–44.

35. Hong YC, Wang JT, Hong CY, Brown WE, Chow LC. The periapical tissue reactions to a calcium phosphate cement in the teeth of monkeys. *J. Biomed. Mater. Res.* 1991; 25: 485–98.

36. Hørsted P, Hansen JC, Langeland K. Studies on N2 cement in man and monkey – cement lead content, lead blood level, and histologic findings. *J. Endodont.* 1982; 8: 341–50.

37. Hørsted P, Söholm B. Overfölsomhed overfor rodfyldningsmaterialet AH26. *Tandlaegebladet* 1976; 80: 194–7.

38. Kanerva L, Estlander T, Jolanki R. Dental nurse's occupational allergic contact dermatitis from eugenol used as a restorative dental material with polymethylmethacrylate. *Contact Dermatitis* 1998; 38: 339–40.

39. Kolokuris I, Beltes P, Economides N, Vlemmas I. Experimental study of the biocompatibility of a new glass-ionomer root canal sealer (Ketac-Endo). *J. Endodont.* 1996; 22: 395–8.

40. Kontakiotis EG, Wu MK, Wesselink PR. Effect of sealer thickness on long-term sealing ability: a 2-year follow-up study. *Int. Endodont. J.* 1997; 30: 307–12.

41. Langeland K, Liao K, Costa N, Pascon EA. Efficacy of Obtura and Ultrafil root filling devices. *J. Endodont.* 1987; 13: 135.

42. Leonard JE, Gutmann JL, Guo IY. Apical and coronal seal of roots obturated with a dentine bonding agent and resin. *Int. Endodont. J.* 1996; 29: 76–83.

43. Leyhausen G, Heil J, Reifferscheid G, Waldmann P, Geurtsen W. Genotoxicity and cytotoxicity of the epoxy resin-based root canal sealer AH plus. *J. Endodont.* 1999; 25: 109–13.

44. Mannocci F, Ferrari M. Apical seal of roots obturated with laterally condensed gutta-percha, epoxy resin cement, and dentine bonding agent. *J. Endodont.* 1998; 24: 41–4.

45. Morse DR. Endodontic-related inferior alveolar nerve and mental foramen paresthesia. *Compend. Contin. Educ. Dent.* 1997; 18: 963–78.

46. Muruzabal M, Erausquin J. Response of periapical tissues in the rat molar to root canal fillings with Diaket and AH-26. *Oral Surg.* 1966; 21: 786–804.

47. Ørstavik D. Antibacterial properties of root canal sealers, cements and pastes. *Int. Endodont. J.* 1981; 14: 125–33.

48. Ørstavik D. Antibacterial properties of endodontic materials. *Int. Endodont. J.* 1988; 21: 161–9.

49. Ørstavik D, Hongslo JK. Mutagenicity of endodontic sealers. *Biomaterials* 1985; 6: 129–32.

50. Ørstavik D, Mjor IA. Usage test of four endodontic sealers in *Macaca fascicularis* monkeys. *Oral Surg.* 1992; 73: 337–44.

51. Osorio RM, Hefti A, Vertucci FJ, Shawley AL. Cytotoxicity of endodontic materials. *J. Endodont.* 1998; 24: 91–6.

52. Rud J, Rud V, Munksgaard EC. Periapical healing of mandibular molars after root-end sealing with dentine-bonded composite. *J. Endodont.* 2001; 34: 285–92.

53. Saunders EM. *In vivo* findings associated with heat generation during thermomechanical compaction of gutta-percha. Part I. Temperature levels at the external surface of the root. *Int. Endodont. J.* 1990; 23: 263–7.

54. Saunders EM. *In vivo* findings associated with heat generation during thermomechanical compaction of gutta-percha. Part II. Histological response to temperature elevation on the external surface of the root. *Int. Endodont. J.* 1990; 23: 268–74.

55. Schmalz G. *Die Gewebeverträglichkeit zahnärztlicher Materialien – Möglichkeiten einer standardisierten Prüfung in der Zellkultur.* Stuttgart, Georg Thieme Verlag, 1981.

56. Schmalz G. Use of cell cultures for toxicity testing of dental materials – advantages and limitations. *J. Dent.* 1994; 22 (Suppl. 2): S6–11.

57. Schmalz G. Biological evaluation of medical devices: a review of EU regulations, with emphasis on in vitro screening for biocompatibility. *ATLA* 1995; 23: 469–73.

58. Schmalz G, Merkle D. Die lokale toxische Wirkung von Abdruckmaterialien. *Zahnärztl Prax.* 1985; 36: 6–13.

59. Schweikl H, Schmalz G. Evaluation of the mutagenic potential of root canal sealers using the salmonella/microsome assay. *J. Mater. Sci. Mater. Med.* 1991; 2: 181–5.

60. Schweikl H, Schmalz G, Federlin M. Mutagenicity of the root canal sealer AHPlus in the Ames test. *Clin. Oral Invest.* 1998; 2: 125–9.

61. Schweikl H, Schmalz G, Stimmelmayr H, Bey B. Mutagenicity of AH26 in an in vitro mammalian cell mutation assay. *J. Endodont.* 1995; 21: 407–10.

62. Shah PM, Chong BS, Sidhu SK, Ford TR. Radiopacity of potential root-end filling materials. *Oral Surg.* 1996; 81: 476–9.

63. Sjögren U, Hägglund B, Sundqvist G, Wing K. Factors affecting the long-term results of endodontic treatment. *J. Endodont.* 1990; 16: 498–504.

64. Sjögren U, Sundqvist G, Nair PN. Tissue reaction to gutta-percha particles of various sizes when implanted subcutaneously in guinea pigs. *Eur. J. Oral. Sci.* 1995; 103: 313–21.

65. Sonat B, Dalat D, Günhan O. Periapical tissue reaction to root fillings with Sealapex. *Int. Endodont. J.* 1990; 23: 46–52.

66. Spångberg LS, Barbosa SV, Lavigne GD. AH26 releases formaldehyde. *J. Endodont.* 1993; 19: 596–8.

67. Torabinejad M, Pitt Ford TR, McKendry DJ, Abedi HR, Miller DA, Kariyawasam SP. Histologic assessment of mineral trioxide aggregate as a root-end filling in monkeys. *J. Endodont.* 1997; 23: 225–8.

68. Tronstad L, Andreasen JO, Hasselgren G, Kristerson L, Riis J. pH changes in dental tissues after root canal filling with calcium hydroxide. *J. Endodont.* 1980; 7: 17–21.

69. Weiger R, Manncke B, Löst C. Antibakterielle Wirkung von Guttaperchastiften auf verschiedene, endodontopathogene Mikroorganismen. *Dtsch. Zahnärztl. Z.* 1993; 48: 658–60.

70. Weller RN, Koch KA. *In vitro* radicular temperatures produced by injectable thermoplasticized gutta-percha. *Int. Endodont. J.* 1995; 28: 86–90.

71. Wennberg A, Orstavik D. Adhesion of root canal sealers to bovine dentine and gutta-percha. *Int. Endodont. J.* 1990; 23: 13–19.

72. Williams SS, Gutmann JL. Periradicular healing in response to Diaket root-end filling material with and without tricalcium phosphate. *Int. Endodont. J.* 1996; 29: 84–92.

73. Wu MK, Wesselink PR. Endodontic leakage studies reconsidered: Part I. Methodology, application, and relevancy. *Int. Endodont. J.* 1993; 26: 37–43.

74. Wu MK, De Gee AJ, Wesselink PR. Leakage of four root canal sealers of different thickness. *Int. Endodont. J.* 1994; 27: 304–8.

75. Wu MK, Wesselink PR, Boersma J. A 1-year follow-up study on leakage of four root canal sealers at different thicknesses. *Int. Endodont. J.* 1995; 28: 185–9.

76. Yoshikawa M, Hayami S, Tsuji I, Toda T. Histopathological study of a newly developed root canal sealer containing tetracalcium-dicalcium phosphates and 1.0% chondroitin sulfate. *J. Endodont.* 1997; 23: 162–6.

Chapter 18
Root filling techniques

Paul Wesselink

Introduction

Filling the instrumented root canal is the final step in the fulfilment of an endodontic treatment. Regardless of whether the treatment was undertaken to remove a vital pulp (pulpectomy), a necrotic and/or infected pulp (root canal therapy) or a previous root canal filling (retreatment), the prime objective of the root filling is to prevent microbial organisms from entering, growing and multiplying in the empty space that resulted from the instrumentation procedure (Fig. 18.1). Root filling also serves as a wound dressing against which healthy periapical tissue can be laid down.

Specific objectives

After a pulpectomy a wound surface remains that will not heal with epithelium as it does with wounds in other body sites. Such a wound is therefore vulnerable to infection. Wound infection may be induced inadvertently in conjunction with the treatment procedure, e.g. from improper rubber dam isolation or by bringing chips of carious dentine to the apical region of the root canal. It may also follow leakage of bacterial organisms from the oral environment after completion of the filling where it incompletely seals the canal space. The latter is known as coronal leakage (see Chapter 13). Therefore, a hermetic and permanent seal of the wound surface is essential to allow proper healing after pulpectomy and to prevent bacterial organisms from later accessing the periapical tissue if, for any reason, the coronal restoration breaks down. Core concept 18.1 summarizes the overall functions of root fillings.

In the treatment of a tooth with an infected, non-vital pulp (i.e. root canal therapy), instrumentation and irrigation with a disinfecting solution will not always eliminate the microbial organisms. If such a root canal is left unfilled or improperly filled, residual organisms may continue to grow and multiply (Chapter 11). It needs to be recognized that microbial organisms require both space and nutritional elements for growth (Chapter 8), therefore in root canal therapy the root filling has two additional objectives:

(1) To prevent nutritional elements from accessing the pulpal space along any entrance to the root canal space, including apical foramina, accessory canals and the oral access cavity.
(2) To eliminate space for further growth of microorganisms that may have survived the biomechanical preparation.

Most often it is sufficient to block the portal of exit to the periapical tissue. However, lateral or accessory canals may also allow egress of bacterial elements to the periodontium, therefore it is essential that the entire length of the instrumented canal becomes completely filled. This means that all portals of exit to the periodontal tissue should be sealed and it is from this aspect that the quality of root fillings in general is assessed (see below).

Selecting a root canal filling material

A variety of factors determine the choice of a root canal filling material. Although a primary requirement is to allow a complete fill of the instrumented root canal(s), it should also be biologically compatible because it will often be in direct contact with vital tissue. In other words, except for a variety of technical and physical demands, a root filling material should also satisfy the requirements that are requested from implant materials (Chapter 17).

The most critical technical and physical requirements of a root filling material are:

- *Ability to adapt to the shape of the canal.* After cleaning and shaping, root canals may still harbor various irregularities that can allow space for bacterial growth. It has been shown that in many situations it is impossible to create a round and smooth root canal without removing so much of the inner root canal wall that the root structure is weakened. Therefore,

Core concept 18.1

The overall function of a root filling is to occupy the instrumented root canal space to allow proper healing of the periapical tissue. Specifically it attempts:

(1) To prevent leakage of bacterial organisms, bacterial elements and nutritional elements from the oral environment to the root canal (coronal leakage).

(2) To hold back any surviving bacteria in dentinal tubules and uninstrumented parts of the root canal space.

(3) To prevent release of bacterial elements in the other direction, i.e. from the root canal to the apical environment (apical leakage).

(4) To prevent leakage of nutritional factors from the periapical tissue to the canal space.

1. Stops coronal leakage
2. Entombs surviving bacteria
3. Stops influx of periapical tissue fluid and release of bacterial elements

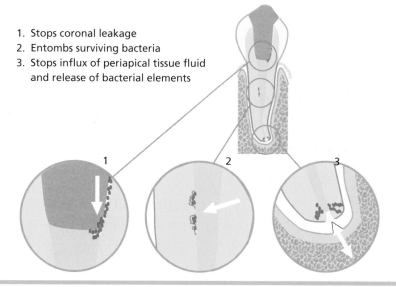

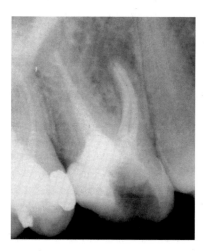

Fig. 18.1   Radiograph depicts an optimal root filling of a mesiobuccal root of an upper molar where two canals have been filled within the confines of the root. (Courtesy of Dr Gunnar Bergenholtz.)

to provide a tight seal, a root canal filling material should be able to fill these irregularities.

- *Length control.* A root canal filling material should allow a technique that keeps the entire material within the canal space. Extrusion of material to the periapical tissue compartment is undesirable because it may cause both cytotoxic and neurotoxic irritation (27, 34, 4). It may also produce a foreign body reaction (34). Furthermore, clinical outcome studies indicate that extrusion and overextension of root filling material negatively influence the healing of the periapical tissue (10, 30).

- *Safety.* The material and the technique used for its application should be safe for the patient. The demand for biocompatibility has already been stated (see also Chapter 17), but the technique should not pose risks for root fracture, require overzealous instrumentation or cause damage to the periodontal ligament by, for example, detrimental temperature increases or extrusion of material.

- *Insoluble.* Because of the risk for coronal leakage and the fact that root filling material may be exposed to percolation of tissue fluid at the apical foramen, it is important that it is not affected by moisture. Therefore, after setting, a root filling material should be insoluble in both saliva and tissue fluid.

- *Removable.* A root filling may not be performed perfectly at the first attempt or may turn out to be defective at a follow-up. The outcome of a treatment may also be such that one can suspect ongoing root canal infection. In these instances, retreatment and refill-

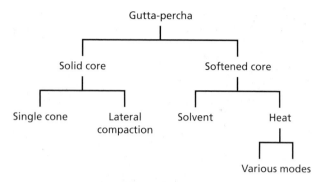

Gutta-percha

Solid core   Softened core

Single cone   Lateral compaction   Solvent   Heat

Various modes

Fig. 18.2 Outline of techniques to fill root canals with gutta-percha.

ing of the root canal may be necessary (Chapter 19). Therefore the material used should be removable by simple means without involving the risk of damaging the root structure or the periapical tissue.

- *Radiopaque.* In order to judge whether the root canal has been sufficiently filled, a most important requirement is that the root filling is discernible in a radiograph, i.e. it should be radiopaque.

Hardly any root filling material tested so far has been able to satisfy all these demands, yet a formulation based on gutta-percha as one of the principal ingredients has stood the test of time and has been widely used since the end of the 19th century. It is still the material of choice in most countries. By pressure or by softening with heat or organic solvent, gutta-percha is suitable for application in instrumented root canals using a variety of techniques. Combined with a sealing agent, the material can be adapted to the shape of root canals and serve as a reasonably insoluble and non-porous core of filling. At the same time, it is fairly easy to remove if necessary. Gutta-percha formulations also satisfy biological demands (Chapter 17) and, because of the universal use of gutta-percha-based formulations in endodontics, only techniques that are based on this material will be considered in the present chapter.

Root filling techniques for gutta-percha

There are various methods for delivering and packing gutta-percha in root canals and they can be divided into solid core and softened core techniques (Fig. 18.2). Solid core techniques imply that unsoftened gutta-percha cones are fitted to the instrumented canal(s) (Fig. 18.3a) and cemented to the canal walls with a root canal sealer. Techniques exist whereby either a single cone or multiple cones are placed in the root canal space (Fig. 18.4). In softened core techniques gutta-percha is plasticized either prior to or after insertion in the root canal by

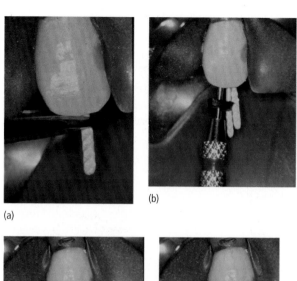

(a)   (b)

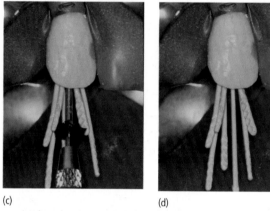

(c)   (d)

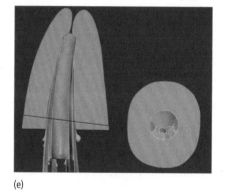

(e)

Fig. 18.3 Outline of the lateral compaction technique. Master cone fit (a), lateral compaction with spreader following addition of one accessory cone (b), continued lateral compaction (c) and further addition of accessory cones (d). Root filling is complete when it is not possible to place another accessory cone further than 2 mm into the root canal (e). In (e) the transverse red line indicates where the cross-sectional view to the right is taken.

solvent or heat. Also, these techniques often make use of a sealing agent to supplement the filling.

Gutta-percha cones

For solid core techniques, gutta-percha cones of different lengths, sizes and shapes may be employed. In

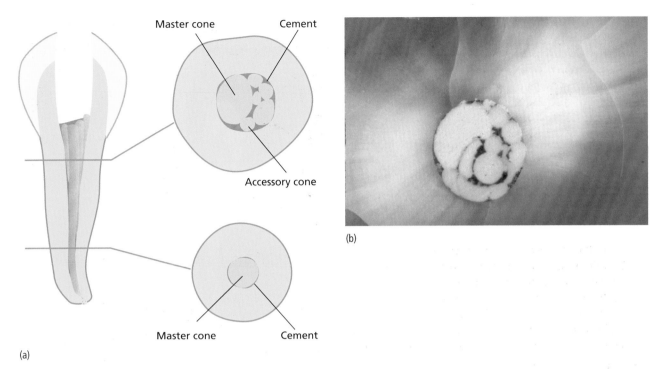

Master cone   Cement

Accessory cone

(b)

Master cone   Cement

(a)

Fig. 18.4 (a) Sketch showing a cross-sectional cut through a root canal filled with a master cone and multiple accessory cones. (b) The cross-sectional cut shows a true filling where the sealer (black material) unites the cones and fills out space laterally to the root canal wall.

general, cones are round and have a tapered form so they gradually increase in size from the tip. So-called 'standardized' cones were designed to match the size and taper of the root canal instruments used to shape the canal at its apical end. In early days these cones had a rather small taper of 2%, corresponding to the ISO standard root canal instruments (see Chapter 16). Nowadays there are cones standardized to fit canals prepared with differently tapered instruments. Hence, there are cones with 4% and 6% tapers (see Chapter 17). Also available are 'conventional' cones, which are not standardized and classified as fine, medium and large.

Root canal sealers

Unsoftened gutta-percha does not adhere to dentine and softened gutta-percha may shrink after cooling as a result of being heated or from evaporation of the solvent used, thus leaving gaps between the material and the root dentine (47). Naturally such defects may allow either coronal or apical leakage, or both, to cause or maintain apical periodontitis. It is, therefore, considered necessary to use a cement or sealer that forms a tight connection between the gutta-percha and the root dentine. In general, it is believed that this layer should be as thin as possible because, upon setting, sealers may shrink and dissolve in a moist environment (7, 18).

The above-mentioned consideration has led to the development of gutta-percha techniques that aim to create a filling consisting of a well-adapted mass of gutta-percha with a thin layer of root canal sealer between the gutta-percha and the root dentine. In this respect, consideration is similar to that with cast restorations, where well-fitting margins are created to leave as little cement as possible between the metal and the tooth structure.

As a general trait, but to a varying extent, root canal sealers in the initial setting phase are cytotoxic and bacteriotoxic and thereafter most sealers become substantially less bioactive (27, 41). Thus, as little contact as possible with the apical pulp tissue or periapical tissue is desirable and, in particular, overfilling of sealer material should be avoided. Several reasons for this view can be claimed:

(1) Except for being initially cytotoxic, all root canal sealers may potentially elicit allergic reactions (13), although animal and clinical observations indicate that sensitization via the root canal occurs rarely. It is occasionally reported (19, 11).

(2) Root canal cements in contact with nerve tissue, e.g. when inadvertently extruded into the mandibular canal, may cause anesthesia and long-lasting paresthesia as well as painful events (4, 25, 36).

(3) Although sealer material may be dissolved and resorbed by vital tissue over time, components of sealer material may be found in the periapical tissue many years after filling, where it causes ongoing phagocytic reactions (23, 30). Root filling material also may be found in several peripheral organs (9).

Currently used root canal sealers may be divided into four groups:

- Zinc oxide–eugenol based.
- Resin based.
- Dentine-adhesive materials.
- Materials to which medicaments have been added.

The benefits, uses and problems of each are discussed below and summarized in Core concept 18.2. For a more detailed description of these materials, the reader is referred to Chapter 17.

Zinc oxide–eugenol-based sealer

Once zinc oxide–eugenol materials set, they form a weak porous product and are decomposed in tissue fluids (43, 40, 23). Nevertheless, these materials are regarded to be clinically satisfactory (26). Practically all zinc oxide–eugenol sealers are cytotoxic and the response may be more long lasting compared with most other sealers (27, 30). Potential for sensitization exists (13, 11). Zinc oxide–eugenol cements are commercially available as Hermetic, Tubliseal, Procosol and Kerr pulp canal sealers, and form the basis of many medicament-containing sealers.

Resin-based sealers

Well-known resin-based materials are AH26 and AHPlus (De Trey Dentsply) and Diaket (Espe). Both AH26 and AHPlus consist of an expoxy resin. They are thin fluid materials that set slowly in 34 h (23, 7). The long setting time may sometimes be an advantage because it gives sufficient time to correct deficiencies in the root canal filling that were noticed at the postoperative radiographic check. Diaket is a mixture of vinylpolymerizates that sets in about 7 min, which makes it less suitable in techniques that require some waiting time (23).

These resin-based sealers elicit an initial severe inflammatory reaction that subsides after some weeks and thereafter seems well tolerated by the periapical tissues (26, 27). The sealer AH26 has been shown to have both a strong allergenic and a mutagenic potential (13, 24). The clinical implications of these findings, however, are unclear but contact allergy to this material has been reported (14).

Core concept 18.2   Properties of different sealers

Zinc oxide–eugenol-based sealers

- Reasonable seal
- Dissolve in fluids
- Long-lasting cytotoxicity
- Sensibilization

Resin-based sealers

- Good seal
- Initial cytoxicity
- Once set, biocompatible
- Allergenic

Gutta-percha-based sealers

- Moderate seal
- Initial cytotoxicity
- Shrinkage
- Plasticize gutta-percha

Dentine-adhesive sealers

- Good seal
- Set very quickly
- Good biocompatibility
- Difficult to remove

Formaldehyde-containing sealers

- Zinc oxide–eugenol based
- Severe long-lasting cytotoxicity
- Sensibilization

Calcium-hydroxide-containing sealers

- Release calcium hydroxide, which may result in disintegration
- Once set and integrity is maintained, no calcium hydroxide leaches out and no effect can be expected
- Initial antibacterial effect
- Risk of dissolution over time

Dentine-adhesive materials

Adhesive cements have been tested as a root canal filling material in an attempt to improve the sealing quality of sealers. Cyanoacrylate, calcium phosphate, polycarboxylate and glass ionomer cements have all been used. Of these, only glass ionomer cements have been widely marketed (Ketac-Endo, Endion). Although *in vitro* and in long-term studies favorable results were obtained, the materials have never gained great popularity, probably because they set too quickly (4 min) (18). Although quite biocompatible, glass ionomers are difficult to remove for retreatment.

Materials to which medicaments have been added

These materials may be divided into two groups:

(1) Materials based on the inclusion of strong disinfectants and/or antiphlogistic agents to suppress possible postoperative pain.
(2) Materials based on calcium hydroxide.

In the first group the added disinfectant is paraformaldehyde and the anti-inflammatory component is often a corticosteriod. Examples of brands in this category of sealers are Endomethasone, N2, Spad and Rocanal. If deposited in the periapical tissue, these filling materials may give rise to severe inflammatory reactions and thus do not satisfy the requirement for biocompatibility (29, 22). Paraformaldehyde also causes allergic reactions (8).

Calcium hydroxide is known to stimulate the formation of hard tissue at the foramen and therefore has been incorporated as an active component in several root canal sealers. The most popular commercial calcium-hydroxide-based cements are calciobiotic root canal sealer (CRCS, a zinc oxide–eugenol-based sealer), Sealapex (a polymeric resin-based sealer) and Apexit (a colophonium-based salicylate resin).

In vitro leakage studies have shown their sealing ability to be similar to the zinc oxide–eugenol cements or, in the long run, slightly less favorable (18). The latter observation supports the concern that during long-term exposure to tissue fluid calcium hydroxide may leach out of the cement, which may result in a loss of root filling integrity (48, 38).

Root filling techniques employing gutta-percha and sealer

These can be divided into solid core and softened core techniques (Core concept 18.3).

Solid core techniques

Whether a single-cone or multiple-cone technique (lateral compaction; Fig. 18.2), the most important step in solid core methods is to select and fit a cone (point) of gutta-percha to the apical 3–4 mm of the canal. This cone is often referred to as the *master cone*. Cones come in various tapered shapes and it is critical that the fitting procedure is given considerable attention, because the

---

Core concept 18.3   Root filling techniques

Solid core techniques

Single cone

- Simple
- Quick
- Good length control
- Round standard preparation required

Lateral compaction

- Good length control
- Not one compact mass of gutta-percha
- Time-consuming technique
- Supposed risk of root fracture

Softened core techniques

Warm lateral compaction

- Moderate length control
- Time-consuming technique
- Heat may damage periodontium

Warm vertical compaction

- Poor length control
- Sealer extrusion
- Heat may damage periodontium

Injection-molded gutta-percha

- Quick technique
- Poor length control
- Heat may damage periodontium

Thermomechanical compaction

- Quick technique
- Poor length control
- Heat may damage periodontium
- Instrument fracture risk

Core carrier

- Quick technique
- Sealer extrusion
- Gutta-percha may be stripped off carrier in curvature
- Difficult to remove for retreatment
- In combination with posts, inconvenient technique

Chloroform-resin

- Quick technique
- Potential health hazard effects on dental personnel over long time use

cone should fit tightly to the apical portion of the root canal.

Single cone

The single-cone technique consists of matching a cone to the prepared canal. For this technique a type of preparation (Chapter 16) is advocated so that the size of the cone and the shape of the preparation are closely matched. When a gutta-percha cone fits the apical portion of the canal snugly, it is cemented in place with a root canal cement.

Although the technique is simple, it has several disadvantages and cannot be considered as one that seals canals completely. After preparation, root canals are seldom round throughout their length, except possibly for the apical 2 or 3 mm. Therefore, the single-cone technique, at best, only seals this portion. *In vitro* research has shown that the single-cone technique permitted significantly more dye penetration than other techniques (1, 3) (see also Advanced concept 18.1).

Lateral compaction

In lateral compaction techniques additional secondary points are inserted and compacted laterally around the master cone to reduce the thickness of the sealer layer (Figs 18.3 and 18.4). In this technique, after cementing the master cone in position, specially designed spreaders – long, tapered, pointed instruments – are placed in the canal as far apically as possible and the master cone is laterally compacted against the wall. Next, the spreader is removed and the first auxillary point forced fully to place. The canal is filled in this way until it is not possible to place another accessory cone further than 2–3 mm into the root canal. Excess gutta-percha is then removed with a heated instrument at the canal orifice and final compaction is completed by vertical pressure with a plugger or condensor – an instrument with a flat apical tip.

The advantage of the lateral compaction technique in comparison with the single-cone technique is that it reduces the amount of sealer left in the canal. Because the relation between the but end of the cones and the reference point of the preparation can be monitored during the filling procedure, the length control of the filling is quite good and usually no filling material is extruded beyond the foramen. The seal in comparison with other techniques is good (44).

The disadvantage of the lateral compaction method is that the root filling does not consist of a homogeneous mass of material but rather of a large number of individual points tightly pressed together and joined by a frictional grip of cementing substance (Fig. 18.4b). In spite of this criticism the technique has been used for many years with considerable success and appeared clinically to be an improvement over the single-cone technique (15, 32).

Softened gutta-percha techniques

In an attempt to overcome the deficiencies of the cold lateral compaction technique, heat and solvents have been applied to render gutta-percha plastic. Gutta-percha is then compacted to create a homogeneous root canal filling of greater density throughout the canal than solid-core techniques can provide.

In recent years several modes of utilizing heat have been developed to soften gutta-percha. In principle, heat softening can be carried out inside the root canal or outside: the latter in the form of injecting preheated gutta-percha and the former by applying heat after insertion of unsoftened cones. These techniques will now be described in some detail.

Techniques employing heat inside the canal

Warm lateral compaction: this technique evolved as a compromise between lateral compaction of cold gutta-percha and the vertical compaction of warm gutta-percha (see below). The technique is similar to lateral compaction of cold gutta-percha but here a heated spreader is initially advanced into the mass of gutta-percha cones placed in the canal (Fig. 18.5). Following its removal a cold spreader is inserted, and the space thus obtained is filled up with accessory cones. The process is repeated until the canal is completely filled. Originally, it was advised to insert a heated spreader after every accessory cone. In practice, usually after

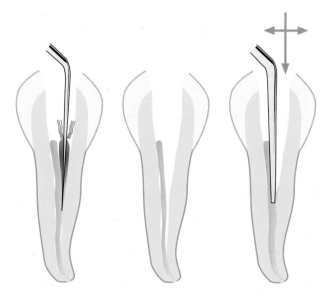

Fig. 18.5 Demonstration of gutta-percha compaction with hot instrument.

Advanced concept 18.1 Leakage tests

Randomized, controlled, clinical studies that compare the efficacy of various root filling materials and techniques as to their ability to promote a successful outcome of endodontic therapy are lacking. Therefore, to select the material and method, results of *in vitro* leakage tests are often claimed. Although having limited clinical value *per se*, together with biocompatibility testing (Chapter 17) they contribute information of importance for the choice. A common denominator for these methods, which are described below, is that extracted teeth are employed that have been instrumented and filled with the materials and techniques to be tested.

Dye penetration

After filling, either the coronal portion or the root tip is exposed to a dye that will penetrate any voids in and around the root filling. After the dye exposure, either transverse or longitudinal sections of the roots are cut at different levels, or the teeth are demineralized and made clear by chemicals. The length of dye penetration along the root filling is a measure of leakage around the filling.

An advantage of this technique is that it is a relatively simple and inexpensive way to acquire preliminary evaluation of the sealing quality of a root filling. A disadvantage is that it does not provide a quantitative evaluation because it gives no information about the volume of leakage and the size of the void. Entrapped air in the voids, furthermore, may hinder penetration of dye into the void, giving an underestimation of its length (46). Also, the method leads to destruction of the specimens studied, making an evaluation of the same root filling at several time periods impossible. Some filling materials may discolor the dye, resulting in an underestimation of the leakage.

Microbial penetration

A coronal and an apical reservoir are attached to the tooth containing the root filling. The coronal reservoir is filled with a bacterial suspension and the apical container is given culture medium. If bacteria or microorganisms pass along the root filling, it will reach the apical reservoir and result in growth turbidity of the medium (37, 46). An advantage of this technique is that bacterial leakage is measured, which may seem more relevant biologically than small dye particle leakage. The disadvantage is that in order to prevent contamination this system requires considerable attention. It is not quantitative because even one bacterium will result in growth. Whether a bacterium passes along a filling in 10 or 20

days does not really give an indication about the difference in quality of these fillings. Only complete voids from crown to apex can be detected.

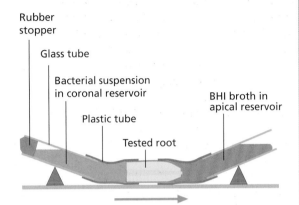

Fluid transport

At both ends, tubes filled with water are attached. At one end the water is applied under pressure. At the other end, a fine glass capillary tube is attached that contains a small air bubble to measure the fluid transport, if any, as indicated by movement of the air bubble. The method is a simple and inexpensive model. It gives quantitative data and allows the leakage pattern to be followed over time, because the specimen is not destroyed during the evaluation process (45). The disadvantage is that it only detects voids that run from crown to apex, with dead-end tract or cul-de-sac voids not being detected.

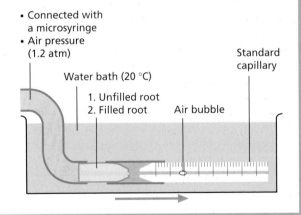

every three to four accessory cones the gutta-percha mass is heated and the compaction is continued. There are devices in which the spreader is heated electrically in a few seconds and thereafter quickly cools down again (e.g. Touch 'n Heat, EIE/Analytic).

The advantage of warm lateral compaction is that it leads to a homogeneous mass that, *in vitro*, permitted significantly less leakage than cold lateral compaction (17). A distinct disadvantage is that the softening of the

gutta-percha may lead to overextension of root filling material.

Warm vertical compaction: the objective is to obliterate the canal with a filling material softened by heat and packed with sufficient vertical pressure to force it to flow into the root canal system, including accessory and lateral canals. A non-standardized master cone is selected and adjusted so that it is loose in the coronal and the middle third, fits to the apical terminus of the preparation and is snug in its apical extent. The canal is lightly coated with sealer. The cone is plasticized with a hot instrument. Next, the soft gutta-percha is compacted with a cold plugger in an apical and lateral direction.

Recently, a new instrument, System B Heat Source, was introduced to simplify the down-pack of gutta-percha. This technique has been described as the *continuous wave technique* (21). The advantage of this system is that the tip of the instrument acts as a heat carrier and cold plugger at the same time. The tip of the plugger of this instrument maintains a temperature of 200°C throughout the down-pack procedure, permitting a smooth continuous progression of the plugger to a depth just shy of the apical terminus. The coronal portion of the canal is back-filled with small segments of warmed gutta-percha, injectable gutta-percha or an additional cone is compacted with the System B.

The advantage of the warm vertical compaction technique is that it results in a well-adapted homogeneous mass of gutta-percha to the canal wall that requires a minimum of sealer. The disadvantage is that the technique almost consistently leads to extrusion of filling material.

Techniques employing heat outside the canal

Injection technique: gutta-percha is thermoplastically molded and ejected out of a needle into the canal. For this technique there are two versions. The Obtura system (Fig. 18.6a) uses a pressure syringe in which the gutta-percha is warmed to 200°C and expressed into the canal through a needle as fine as 25 gauge (0.5 mm diameter). The gutta-percha leaves the needle at approximately 70°C.

Pluggers are prefitted to ensure that they match the middle portion of the canal while not contacting the dentine wall. A little root canal cement is wiped along the canal wall and gutta-percha is passively injected into the root canal. In 5–10 s the softened gutta-percha will fill the apical segment and begin to lift the needle out of the root. During this lifting by the softened, flowing mass, the middle and the coronal portions of the canal are continuously filled until the needle reaches the canal orifice. Compaction of the material follows to adapt the gutta-percha to the canal walls.

Because of concern over the high temperature generated, a thermoplasticized low-temperature (70°C) gutta-percha was developed along with a slightly different delivery system, Hygienic Ultrafil (Fig. 18.6b), where the canule with gutta-percha is heated in a specially designed heating device. The injection technique is used as the sole technique to fill the canal but is also frequently applied for the so-called back-pack phase of vertical compaction once the apical fill has been properly compacted.

Advantages of the injection technique are similar to those of warm vertical compaction. It also appears to be very useful in wide canals with an apical stop (Fig. 18.7a) and in cases of internal resorption (Fig. 18.7b).

The disadvantage is that here it may be even more difficult to control the level of the root filling, with a possible under- or overfill ensuing. Shrinkage of the gutta-percha during cooling may result in voids, which may make it necessary to use continuous compaction with pluggers during cooling. For this reason a segmental filling technique where small portions are injected and compacted with pluggers has been advocated.

Thermomechanical compaction: gutta-percha is plasticized by frictional heat and inserted by means of a compactor that forces the material apically. The compactor is an engine operated instrument resembling a Hedström file, but with the blades directed toward the blunt-tipped end, and operates on the principle of the reverse turning

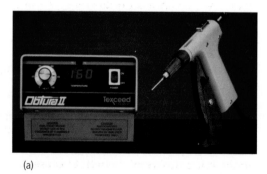
(a)

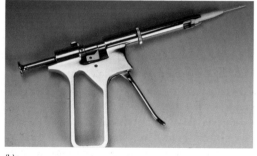
(b)

Fig. 18.6 Two commonly used devices to provide thermoplasticized gutta-percha for injection: (a) the Obtura system; (b) the Hygienic Ultrafil system.

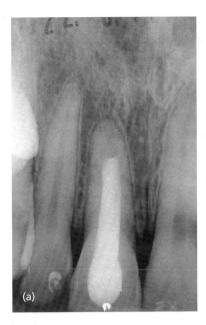
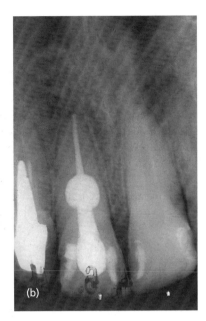

Fig. 18.7   (a) Filled root canal of traumatized incisor. (b) Internal resorption.

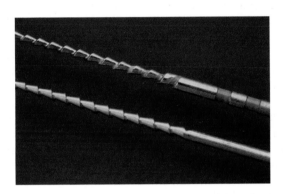

Fig. 18.8   Profiles of a compactor (top) and a Hedström file (bottom).

screw (Fig. 18.8). The technique with which this method gives best results is different from the original one suggested, where only one cone slightly larger than the master apical file and a compactor of the same size as the master apical file was used. To improve the reliability of the technique, thermomechanical compaction has been used following lateral compaction of the apical part of the canal, resulting in a reduction of dye penetration *in vitro* (35).

The advantage is that it is a very fast technique leading to a compact mass of gutta-percha that, in wide canals, resulted in less leakage than lateral compaction (16). The disadvantage is that the technique requires a lot of practice to get consistent results. In inexperienced hands, instrument fracture, extensive extrusion or poorly compacted fillings may occur. If the instrument is used by accident, when rotating clockwise it may perforate the foramen and fracture, leaving part of the instrument in the periapex.

Core carrier technique: a metal or resin core coated with gutta-percha is used (Thermafil, Soft core) (Fig. 18.9). After root canal preparation the correct size of the cone is selected and heated in a special oven for 45 s. After heating, the cone is pushed with pressure into the canal that is coated with sealer. Next, the coronal part is removed from the core that remains in the canal and the gutta-percha is then compacted in the canal orifice with a hand plugger.

The advantage of the technique is that, once the cone is properly heated in the oven, with this system the canal can be well obturated in all its dimensions within a short time. So far, this system has been evaluated only *in vitro* and it seems reasonable to assume that at least in straight canals the technique is about as good as lateral compaction of gutta-percha (2).

The disadvantage of the system is that, especially in curved canals, there is the risk of the gutta-percha being stripped off and apically only the metal or resin core being cemented (12). In almost all studies it appeared that, just as with most of the other warm gutta-percha techniques, sealer is extruded beyond the apical foramen (2).

Warm gutta-percha techniques – concluding remarks

Although it is known that dentine is a good insulator, concern exists as to whether the high temperatures that may develop in the canal during the application of warm gutta-percha and heating devices are transferred to the outer surface of the root to cause damage to the periodontal ligament. *In vitro* the temperature rise at the root surface may be as high as 15–30°C (21), leading to

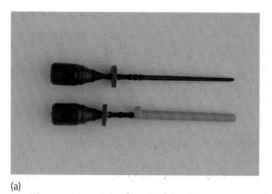

(a)

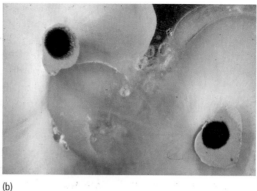

(b)

Fig. 18.9 The principle for the core carrier technique: (a) uncoated and gutta-percha coated cores; (b) a cross-sectional cut of two filled canals with the core material in the middle.

periodontal tissue injury. In experimental animals root resorption and ankylosis have been observed with these techniques (31).

The warm gutta-percha techniques have much to commend them and undoubtedly the resultant root filling appears to be homogeneous and, from radiographs, seems to fill the root canal space well. Yet there is no evidence to show that these techniques result in higher clinical success than for instance cold lateral compaction. So far, *in vitro* studies have not answered the question as to which of these techniques results in the least leakage (44).

Techniques employing solvent

Chloroform-resin technique: based on softening the master gutta-percha cone in chloroform for a few seconds prior to insertion. The master cone then should be cut approximately 2 mm short of the working length and is moved to length by a slight pumping movement. As a sealing agent in the canal, 6% resin in chloroform is used. This technique is not commonly practised, primarily owing to the alleged risk for shrinkage of the root filling after evaporation of the softening agent and the potential carcinogenecity of chloroform (Chapter 17).

Procedures prior to root canal filling

Smear layer removal

The instrumented dentine surface of the root canal interior is covered with a debris layer that sticks to its underlying structure and consists of (pre)dentine, pulpal remnants and, in previously infected root canals, microbial elements. By its presence it may jeopardize a proper seal of the root canal space.

Studies indicate that removal of the smear layer reduces leakage of fluid and bacterial elements along the root filling. Thus, it is not unreasonable to see the smear layer as a weak link, which should be removed to allow better adherence of the root filling to the root canal wall (33). To remove the smear layer, irrigation with EDTA (15%) followed by a sodium hypochlorite flush seems to be effective (33).

Drying canal

It is critical that, prior to root filling, the canal is completely evacuated of irrigation solution to allow good adaptation of the filling material. This is accomplished easiest by aspiration with a syringe, followed by drying with one or two paper points to the full working length. It may be necessary to measure up the paper points so that they are not extruded into the apical tissue, where they may cause bleeding or where fragments may be left to cause a foreign body reaction. The last point should not show signs of fluid present after its removal (28). It is important to note that if tips continue to be wet by bleeding or exudation, root filling should be postponed and the canal dressed temporarily (see Chapter 11). To eliminate moisture 90% alcohol is often used but the efficacy of this extra procedure has been questioned (42).

Sealer placement

Because a thin layer of sealer between the gutta-percha and canal wall is preferred, it seems desirable to coat the complete canal wall with sealer prior to applying the core material. Generally, it is recommended that a file be used that is one size smaller than the last instrument used for enlargement and set just short of the working length. A small amount is gathered on the blades of the instrument, which is carried up by rapidly 'twirling' the handle counter-clockwise. The procedure is repeated until the canal appears to be coated liberally with cement. The point itself is 'buttered' in cement and slowly passed into the root canal, allowing time for the cement to flow back in a coronal direction.

Assessing root filling quality

After the root filling procedure the quality of the fill should be checked radiographically with regard to the extent the instrumented canal was filled. An acceptable fill should reach the working length, as indicated by the trial file, and completely fill the canal space over its entire length (Core concept 18.4). Proper assessment is often difficult in an orthogonal view, therefore an angulated view is often essential (Fig. 18.1), not least to be able to observe the quality of fills in two- and multi-rooted teeth. If the root filling does not fill the canal properly, i.e. if there is a short fill or if the fill displays obvious voids, the filling should be adjusted (see Core concept 18.4). Often, complete removal and reinsertion of a new filling is the best strategy in such cases rather than adjustment by compaction. An overextended filling normally cannot be corrected owing to the diffuse spreading of sealer material.

Core concept 18.4   Assessment of root filling quality

(1)   Optimal outcome of root filling after pulpectomy. From the radiograph it can be seen that the length of the filling is to an appropriate working length (a) and it appears to densely fill the canal space in its entirety (b).

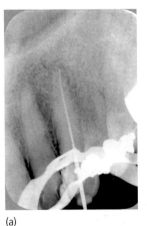 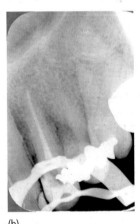

(a)   (b)

(2)   Too short a fill of an upper canine (retreatment case).

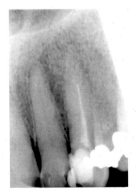

(3)   Obvious lateral spaces to the root canal walls (retreatment case).

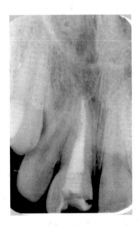

(4)   Overextended root filling on both the mesial and distal canals but it appears to fill out the canal space properly. No retreatment because of the limited potential to remove the excess root filling material.

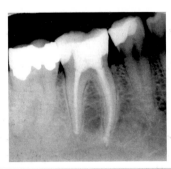

Filling of the pulp chamber and coronal restoration

Because of the potential presence of accessory canals near the floor of the pulp chamber of multi-rooted teeth and the fact that exposure of the root canal filling to saliva and bacteria seriously deteriorates the quality of the seal, application of a well-sealing, colored dentine-adhering cement is recommended (20, 37, 5). In the case of retreatment, to be able to locate the canal again this material should have a color distinct from dentine but not to the extent that it discolors the crown of the tooth.

Considering the negative effect of the oral fluids on the quality of the root canal filling, it is not surprising that the quality of the coronal restoration may also influence the outcome of endodontic treatment, particularly if the root canal is not perfectly sealed. It is recommended that a good coronal restoration be placed immediately after root canal filling. Therefore, the root filling material should be removed at or just apical from the canal orifice, and in single-root teeth just apical to the cemento-enamel junction, because all root canal cements stain dentine to cause tooth discoloration (39). In cases where a cast restoration is indicated, a core material is placed. This procedure is deleted if a post and core are indicated shortly after filling the canal. In that case, space for a post may be created right after filling the root canal, leaving at least 3–4 mm of gutta-percha in the canal (6).

Conclusions and recommendations

Insufficient research has been carried out to determine which technique under certain given conditions (root canal anatomy, apical constriction, preparation shape) is the most appropriate (44). However, there are indications that the risk for leakage of bacteria and bacterial elements is larger when the single-cone technique is used than with the use of other techniques (1, 3). Therefore, the clinician is advised to make him or herself confident with one or two of the techniques described. It needs to be recognized that no root filling technique can make up for an improper root canal preparation.

References

1. Beatty RG. The effect of standard or serial preparation on single cone obturations. *Int. Endodont. J.* 1987; 20: 276–81.
2. Becker TA, Donnelly JC. Thermafil obturation: a literature review. *Gen. Dent.* 1997; 45: 46–50.
3. Beer VR, Gängler P, Beer M. In-vitro Untersuchungen unterschiedlicher Wurzelkanalfülltechniken und -materialien. *Zahn-. Mund-. Kieferheilk.* 1986; 74: 800–806.
4. Brodin P, Roed A, Aars H, Ørstavik D. Neurotoxic effect of root filling materials. *J. Dent. Res.* 1982; 61: 1020–23.
5. Chailertvanitkul P, Saunders WP, Saunders EM, *et al.* An evaluation of microbial coronal leakage in the restored pulp chamber of root canal treated multirooted teeth. *Int. Endodont. J.* 1997; 30: 318–22.
6. De Cleen MJH. The relationship between the root canal filling and post space preparation. *Int. Endodont. J.* 1993; 26: 53–8.
7. De Gee AJ, Wu M-K, Wesselink PR. Sealing properties of Ketac-Endo glass ionomer cement and AH26 root canal sealers. *Int. Endodont. J.* 1994; 27: 239–44.
8. Fehr B, Huwyler T, Wütrich B. Formaldehyd- und Paraformaldehyd-allergie. *Schweiz. Monatsschr. Zahnmed.* 1992; 102: 94–6.
9. Feiglin B, Reade PC. The distribution of (^{14}C)leucine and ^{85}SR labeled microspheres from rat incisor root canals. *Oral. Surg.* 1979; 47: 277–81.
10. Friedman S. Treatment outcome and prognosis of endodontic therapy. In *Essential Endodontology* (Ørstavik D, Pitt Ford TR, eds). Oxford: Blackwell Science, 1998; 367–91.
11. Grade AC. Eugenol in Wurzelkanalzementen als mögliche Ursache für eine Urtikaria. *Endodontie* 1995; 2: 121–5.
12. Gutmann JL, Saunders WP, Saunders EP, *et al.* An assessment of the plastic Thermafil obturation technique. Part 2. Material adaptation and sealability. *Int. Endodont. J.* 1993; 26: 179–83.
13. Hensten-Pettersen A, Ørstavik D, Wennberg A. Allergenic potential of root canal sealers. *Endodont. Dent. Traumatol.* 1985; 1: 61–5.
14. Hørsted P, Søholm B. Overfølsomhed overfor rodfyllnings materialet AH26. *Tandlaegebladet* 1976; 80: 194–8.
15. Kerekes K, Tronstad L. Long-term results of endodontic treatment performed with a standardized technique. *J. Endodont.* 1979; 5: 83–90.
16. Kersten HW, Fransman R, Thoden van Velzen SK. Thermomechanical compaction II. A comparison with lateral condensation in curved canals. *Int. Endodont. J.* 1986; 19: 134–40.
17. Kersten HW. Evaluation of three thermoplasticized gutta-percha filling techniques using a leakage model in vitro. *Int. Endodont. J.* 1988; 21: 353–60.
18. Kontakiotis EG, Wu M-K, Wesselink PR. Effect of sealer thickness on long-term sealing ability: a 2-year follow-up study. *Int. Endodont. J.* 1997; 30: 307–12.
19. Longwill DG, Marshall FJ, Creamer RH. Reactivity of human lymphocytes to pulp antigens. *J. Endodont.* 1982; 8: 27–32.
20. Madison S, Wilcox LR. An evaluation of coronal microleakage in endodontically treated teeth. Part III. In vivo study. *J. Endodont.* 1988; 14: 455–8.
21. McCullagh JJ, Setchell DJ, Gulabivala K, *et al.* A comparison of the infrared thermographic analysis of temperature rise on the root surface during the continuous wave of condensation. *Int. Endodont. J.* 2000; 33: 326–32.
22. Negm MM. Biologic evaluation of SPAD II. A clinical comparison of Traitement SPAD with the conventional

root canal filling technique. *Oral. Surg.* 1987; 63: 487–93.

23. Ørstavik D. Weight loss of endodontic sealers, cements and pastes in water. *Scand. J. Dent. Res.* 1983; 91: 316–19.

24. Ørstavik D, Hongslo JK. Mutagenicity of endodontic sealers. *Biomaterials* 1985; 6: 129–32.

25. Ørstavik D, Brodin P, Aas E. Paraesthesia following endodontic treatment: survey of the literature and report of a case. *Int. Endodont. J.* 1983; 16: 167–72.

26. Ørstavik D, Kerekes K, Eriksen HM. Clinical performance of three endodontic sealers. *Endodont. Dent. Traumatol.* 1987; 3: 178–86.

27. Ørstavik D, Mjör IA. Histopathology and X-ray microanalysis of the subcutaneous tissue response to endodontic sealers. *J. Endodont.* 1988; 14: 13–23.

28. Petschelt A. Das Trocknen des Wurzelkanals. *Dtsch. Zahnärztl. Z.* 1990; 45: 222–6.

29. Pitt Ford TR. Tissue reactions to two root canal sealers containing formaldehyde. *Oral. Surg.* 1985; 60: 661–4.

30. Ricucci D, Langeland K. Apical limit of root canal instrumentation and obturation. Part II. *Int. Endodont. J.* 1998; 31: 394–409.

31. Saunders EM. In vivo findings associated with heat generation during thermo-mechanical compaction of gutta-percha. Part II. Histological response to temperature elevation on the external surface of the root. *Int. Endodont. J.* 1990; 23: 258–64.

32. Seltzer S, Bender IB, Turkenkopf S. Factors affecting successful repair after root canal therapy. *J. Am. Dent. Assoc.* 1963; 67: 651–62.

33. Sen BH, Türkün M, Wesselink PR. The smear layer: a phenomenon in root canal therapy. *Int. Endodont. J.* 1995; 28: 141–8.

34. Sjögren U, Sundqvist G, Nair PR. Tissue reaction to gutta-percha particles of various sizes when implanted subcutaneously in guinea pigs. *Eur. J. Oral. Sci.* 1995; 103: 313–21.

35. Tagger M, Tamse A, Katz A, *et al.* Evaluation of the apical seal produced by a hybrid root canal filling method, combining lateral condensation and thermatic compaction. *J. Endodont.* 1984; 10: 299–303.

36. Teeuwen R. Schädigung des Nervus alveolaris inferior durch überfülltes Wurzelkanalfüll-material. *Endodontie* 1999; 8: 323–36.

37. Torabinejad M, Ung B, Kettering JD. In vitro bacterial penetration of coronally unsealed endodontically treated teeth. *J. Endodont.* 1990; 16: 566–9.

38. Tronstad L, Barnett F, Flax M. Solubility and biocompatibility of calcium hydroxide-containing root canal sealers. *Endodont. Dent. Traumatol.* 1998; 4: 152–9.

39. Van der Burgt, Plasschaert AJM. Bleaching of tooth discoloration caused by endodontic sealers. *J. Endodont.* 1986; 12: 231–4.

40. Von Fraunhofer JA, Branstetter J. The physical properties of four endodontic sealers and cements. *J. Endodont.* 1982; 8: 126–30.

41. Weiss EI, Shallav M, Fuss Z. Assessment of antibacterial activity of endodontic sealers by a direct contact test. *Endodont. Dent. Traumatol.* 1996; 12: 179–84.

42. Wilcox LR, Wiemann AH. Effect of a final alcohol rinse on sealer coverage obturated root canals. *J. Endodont.* 1995; 1: 256–8.

43. Wilson AD, Clinton DJ, Miller RP. Zinc oxide-eugenol cements. IV. Microstructure and hydrolysis. *J. Dent. Res.* 1973; 52: 253–60.

44. Wu M-K, Wesselink PR. Endodontic leakage studies reconsidered. Part I. Methodology, application and relevance. *Int. Endodont. J.* 1993; 26: 37–43.

45. Wu M-K, De Gee AJ, Wesselink PR, Moorer WR. Fluid transport and bacterial penetration along root canal fillings. *Int. Endodont. J.* 1993; 26: 203–8.

46. Wu M-K, De Gee AJ, Wesselink PR. Fluid transport and dye penetration along root canal fillings. *Int. Endodont. J.* 1994; 27: 233–8.

47. Wu M-K, Fan B, Wesselink PR. Diminished leakage along root canal fillings filled with gutta-percha without sealer over time: a laboratory study. *Int. Endodont. J.* 2000; 33: 121–5.

48. Zmener O, Guglielmotti MB, Cabrini RL. Biocompatibility of two calcium hydroxide-based endodontic sealers. A quantitative study in the subcutaneous connective tissue of the rat. *J. Endodont.* 1988; 14: 229–35.

Chapter 19
Non-surgical retreatment

Pierre Machtou and Claes Reit

Introduction

Endodontic treatment is not always successful and peri-radicular inflammatory lesions might persist or develop postoperatively. Such 'failures' are most often caused by micro-organisms that have either survived the conventional treatment procedures or invaded the root canal system at later stages via coronal leakage. In order to combat the infection, the root canal has to be renegotiated using either an orthograde (non-surgical retreatment) or a retrograde (surgical retreatment) route of entry. It is the aim of the present chapter to review specifically the non-surgical retreatment procedures.

In terms of objectives there are no differences between the primary treatment of the infected root canal system and a retreatment, i.e. micro-organisms should be eliminated and the space hermetically sealed with a biocompatible filling material. However, retreatment cases often are technically complicated and require high skills by the dentist. Because endodontically treated teeth are frequently prosthodontically restored, canals regularly have to be re-entered through crowns. The canals might be obstructed by posts, insoluble filling materials or separated instruments. Furthermore, during the previous treatment a variety of procedural errors such as canal blockage, ledging, apical transportation and root perforation may have occurred.

Indications

Clinical outcome studies have failed to show any systematic difference between a surgical and non-surgical approach to retreatment (1, 17). Consequently the selection of retreatment procedures primarily has to be based on case-specific factors such as the technical quality of the root filling and the personal valuation of risks and monetary costs.

The typical indication for non-surgical retreatment is a case classified as a 'failure' in which the canals are poorly sealed. As soon as it is possible to improve on the quality of the previous instrumentation and obturation, the non-surgical approach should be considered as the primary choice. However, an orthograde route may be contraindicated subjectively if the patient regards the costs or risks of the procedures to be unacceptably high. The monetary costs will increase if crowns, bridges and posts have to be removed and later replaced. In certain situations access openings through the crowns of abutment teeth and removal of posts might increase the risk of bridges loosening and roots fracturing.

Non-surgical retreatment might be indicated also for preventive reasons. In conjunction with the placement of new crowns or posts, the root filling seal inevitably will be challenged by oral micro-organisms. A poor fill might not resist such provocation and thus allow micro-organisms to invade the root canal, therefore the replacement of defective root fillings always should be considered when new prosthodontic restorations are to be conducted.

Core concept box 19.1 summarizes the critical steps in non-surgical retreatment, and these are discussed in more detail below.

Access to the root canal

Because defect restorations might allow oral micro-organisms to invade the root canal system, amalgam and composite fillings frequently have to be removed completely prior to retreatment. Sometimes crowns and bridges have to be disassembled. Dismantling enables the clinician to assess the actual axis of the tooth and the remaining coronal structure, excavate recurrent or hidden caries and look for cracks, missed or additional canals. The decision to retain a restoration may be taken only when the latter is well fitting and fulfills esthetic, functional and periodontal requirements, and if the access preparation will not seriously damage it. In the case of an access cavity via a metallic restoration, care should be taken to make the occlusal outline wide enough at the start to allow for controlled manipulation

Clinical procedure 19.1   Crown removal technique

(1) With a transmetal bur, a slot is made on the buccal aspect of the crown to reach the tooth structure, starting at the gingival margin and stopping in the middle of the occlusal surface.

(2) An ultrasonic insert is then worked to disaggregate the cement bond and help the placement of an elevator to force apart the crown and then dislodge it. The procedure is safe, expedient and, if needed, the crown can be relined to be reused as a temporary one. For bridges, the abutments are separated and individually removed.

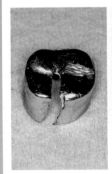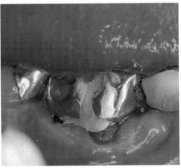

Advanced concept 19.1   Alternative crown removal techniques

(1) The Metalift Crown Removal System is recommended to gently remove individual crowns because the procedure is simple and highly efficient with minimal damage to the prosthetic crown (a tiny hole is created on the occlusal surface) and tooth structure. A self-tapping instrument threads the metal on the occlusal surface, pushes against the dentine, breaks the cement layer and results in a loosening and lifting of the restoration.

(2) The Coronaflex forceps may be used when maintenance of the crown integrity is mandatory. The forceps are placed at the margins of the crown. Then the Coronaflex handpiece is positioned against the forceps arch to ensure an axial pulling direction, and several impulses are delivered to lift off the crown.

(3) To remove permanently or temporarily cemented bridges without any damage, the parachute technique should always be used in conjunction with air-driven pneumatic crown removers such as the Kavo Coronaflex or the Easy Pneumatic Crown and Bridge Remover from Dentco. The technique allows the removal of bridges in an axial pulling direction. The parachute technique uses metallic wires placed through two or more embrasures of the bridge in order to create loops acting as a rest for a metal rod. Via a curved insert, the pneumatic handpiece delivers a lot of energy in an axial pulling direction that breaks the cement bond.

19.1). The latter techniques are too aggressive and dangerous for the tooth structure. They are unpleasant and painful for the patient and a crown or tooth fracture may often ensue.

Removing cores and posts

Composite and amalgam cores are easily removed with a high-speed handpiece bur. When a post is present, care must be taken not to damage the protruding head in the pulp chamber. In the case of a composite core, the difference in color between the metallic post and the filling material acts as a guide and makes the procedure easy. Amalgam cores should be drilled in a concentric fashion, starting from the outline of the cavity and moving closer and closer to the post. In both cases, with good illumination and magnification an ultrasonic tip placed in a piezoelectric ultrasonic unit is well suited to remove residual pieces of restorative material around the post and on the pulp chamber floor.

To remove a cast post and core in one piece from a single-rooted supporting tooth, the 'parachute' technique works well. First the metallic core has to be pierced right through with a transmetal bur. A metallic wire is then passed through the hole and tied with a knot to create a

of the endodontic instruments without interfering or scraping the cavity walls. Metal chips may be shaved off the walls and forced into the canal to create irreversible blockage, especially in mandibular teeth. Owing to their own weight, the shavings will not stay in suspension in the irrigating solution.

Removing crowns and bridges

Disassembling implies the use of a transmetal bur (Clinical procedure 19.1) to cut off the crown while preserving at best the underlying tooth structure, instead of using 'tapping off' techniques with crown-removers in order to break the luting cement (Advanced concept

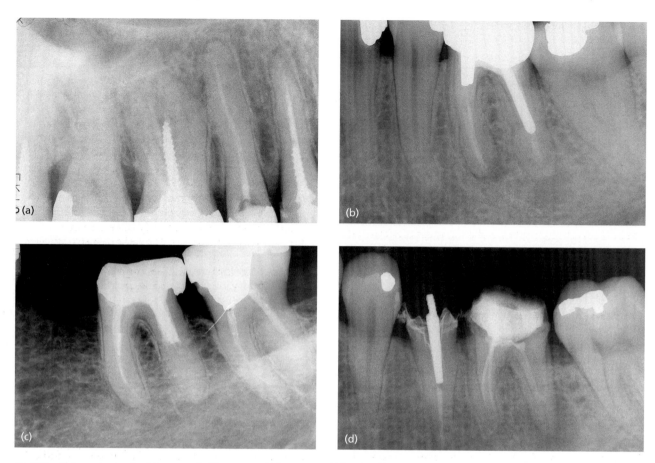

Fig 19.1   Radiographs showing (a) screwposts, (b) cast posts, (c) Para post and (d) carbon-fiber post (distal canal in first molar).

loop, acting as a rest for the Coronaflex or the Pneumatic Crown Remover (see Advanced concept 19.1).

Depending upon the number of posts present, cast cores should be separated into two or more pieces with transmetal burs to isolate each post. Utmost care is needed when reaching the pulp chamber floor, especially in the case of a very hard core such as those fabricated of NiCr. In many instances, the huge amount of vibration delivered during the drilling of the core, coupled with the use of ultrasonics, is sufficient to loosen the post.

When considering post removal it is essential to make a careful assessment of the root anatomy and the type, length and width of the post (Fig. 19.1). *Screw posts* or *threaded posts* usually should be unscrewed after sufficient ultrasonic vibration with a piezoelectric unit. A 10-min session of ultrasonics is considered to be the minimum amount of time needed to expect efficacy.

Passive conical or *parallel posts* along with *cast posts* are good indications for using a post removal system. Either the Gonon (Chige, USA) or its refined clone the Ruddle Post Removal System (Analytic Endodontics) may be used. Both devices are safe, efficient and predictable. Their use is similar and based on the principle of a

corkscrew: one force is applied on the tooth structure, providing the fulcrum, while the pulling force is placed on the post (21).

When a post is broken deep inside the canal, the Masserann kit (Micro Mega, France) should be the preferred post-removal device because it is more conservative for the root structure. Alternately, the post may be troughed with one of the suborifice ultrasonic tips in a dry operating field. While grooving around the post, the ultrasonic energy will vibrate the post and loosen it. Providing coaxial light and magnification, the advent of the surgical microscope (7) has made these procedures easier and allows them to be conducted in a controlled manner.

After post removal, some residual luting cement may have been left in the canal beyond the apical tip of the post. This can be removed easily with the use of a suborifice tip or an ultrasonic file.

Access to the apical area

Before attempting to reach the apical portion of the canal, the obturating material that obstructs the space

has to be removed. In order to avoid the risk of definitive canal blockage or pushing and extruding debris into
the periapical tissues, a pronounced crown-down instrumentation procedure should be used. As a complicating
factor, root canal instruments might have fractured and
been left in the canal; in a retreatment situation they
have to be removed or at least passed.

Removing gutta-percha

Gutta-percha is quite easy to remove but an organic
solvent is often a necessary adjunct, especially in the
case of densely filled or curved canals. Chloroform is
the best solvent for gutta-percha but great concern exists
as to its potential carcinogenicity and mutagenicity.
However, McDonald and Vire (22) reported that there
were no negative health effects to the dentist or assistant and air vapor levels were well below mandated
maximum levels when chloroform was used in common
endodontic treatment procedures. The report concluded
that with careful and controlled use chloroform can be a
useful adjunct in the practice of dentistry. Several alternatives to chloroform have been suggested, such as
eucalyptol, methyl chloroform, halothane and rectified
white turpentine, but all solvents are toxic and, whenever possible, retreatment should be carried out without
using solvents (2).

When gutta-percha-filled canals demonstrate some
degree of taper, a rotary nickel–titanium instrument is
used at 1200 rpm. This will generate sufficient heat to
soften the gutta-percha, which is evacuated in a coronal
direction owing to the flute design of the instrument (5).

When a canal is small and curved it is safer to use
chloroform to avoid creating a ledge or a perforation.
The coronal portion of gutta-percha is removed with
either a hot heat carrier or plugger or by using an appropriate sized Gates–Glidden drill or an orifice shaper (or
similar) at 1200 rpm. Using a glass syringe, two or three
drops of chloroform are introduced into the newly
created reservoir inside the root canal. The softened
gutta-percha then can be removed with Hedström files
in an apical direction.

The 'wicking technique' – flushing the canal with
solvent followed by drying it with paper points – helps
to remove any residual gutta-percha and sealer and
gives the irrigation solution access to the canal walls
during subsequent cleaning and shaping procedures
(28). (See Advanced concept 19.2.)

Removal of sealers, cements and pastes

It is critical that any residual sealer is eliminated from
the canal walls because bacteria may be harbored in the
interface (39). Moreover, successful removal will allow

> ### Advanced concept 19.2   Removing Thermafil plastic carriers
>
> The Thermafil obturators were introduced about 10 years ago. First
> marketed with metallic carriers, they were later modified and plastic
> replaced the metal. Currently, the obturators are available with a
> special grooved plastic carrier designed to make retreatment easier.
>
> Plastic carriers are easily removed initially using first a 0.04
> tapered rotary file placed at the groove location and rotated at 1200
> rpm with light pressure. The frictional heat melts the gutta-percha,
> which allows the instrument to advance apically. When resistance
> to progression is felt, switch to a 0.06 tapered rotary file and work
> it at 300 rpm. Owing to the greater taper, the instrument will bind
> between the plastic carrier and the dentine and exert an extracting
> force. As a last resort, an H-file used in conjunction with chloroform
> will engage the softened plastic carrier and lift it out (14). Once the
> carrier is removed, the wicking technique must be used to eliminate
> any residual gutta-percha before reinstrumentation.

irrigation of the contaminated walls during the canal
reinstrumentation (10). This step in the retreatment procedure is difficult and is often overlooked.

In paste-filled teeth, generally some paste is present in
the pulp chamber. During the access cavity preparation,
the clinician has to clean out the pulp chamber floor with
an ultrasonic tip and the amount of time taken indicates
the type of paste that has been used. Most of the time it
is a zinc oxide–eugenol paste that is removed easily. To
dissolve the paste inside the root canals, a solvent must
be used (Clinical procedure 19.2). Tetrachloroethylene
(Endosolv E, Septodont, France) is recommended but
xylene, orange solvent, eucalyptol or eugenol are also
efficient. A zinc oxide–eugenol paste that is easily dissolved with these solvents is N2.

For several pastes (epoxy resins, bakelites, glass
ionomers, zinc phosphates) no efficient solvents are
available (8). Currently, the best method is to use a
piezoelectric ultrasonic unit with either an ultrasonic tip
or an easy-to-fit file system. If the procedure can be monitored permanently under the surgical microscope, it can
be more predictable. Of course, only straight parts of
root canals can be managed in this way, but fortunately
the densest portion of the paste is usually the coronal
one and the apical portion is often not set.

Removing silver cones

Silver cones were introduced in endodontics by Jasper
(15) 70 years ago to simplify the obturation of curved
and narrow canals. Their widespread use has led to
numerous endodontic failures. Often canals with silver
cones are underprepared and, with a defective seal,

Clinical procedure 19.2   Removing soluble pastes

(1) The four-wall access cavity is flooded with the solvent and an explorer firmly probes the canal orifice, brings the solvent in contact with the paste and starts the first penetration.

(2) Select a 21-mm Hedström file whose size is adapted to the canal width. The H-file has a sharp tip and aggressive flutes on pulling, so the filling material can be removed laterally as the instrument penetrates into the paste. The material is removed in a coronal-apical direction, using smaller files as the apical portion of the canal is reached. Irrigate copiously with NaOCl to flush out debris and renew the solvent.

(3) It must be anticipated that a ledge is present at the terminus of the previous obturation. Therefore, if an obstruction or blockage is felt, the penetration should be stopped, a radiograph taken and specific measures implemented (see later).

coronal and apical leakage will bring about metallic corrosion. Today, silver cones are considered outdated but are still in use.

Various techniques have been described to retrieve silver cones (20) (Clinical procedure 19.3), but their removal depends mainly on two factors: being able to grab them; and the canal morphology, i.e. whether it is possible to bypass them with a K-file (33).

Removing broken instruments

It is not uncommon to find broken instruments left inside the root canal system. An instrument usually fractures when an overaggressive manipulation has tightly locked its tip in the root dentine. One should realize that the broken instrument itself is not a direct cause of treatment failure but rather an indirect one, because it may have prevented cleaning, shaping and filling of the apical portion of the root canal. Therefore, the therapeutic goal is either to retrieve the fractured instrument or to bypass it in order to get access to the uncleaned portion of the canal (Core concept 19.2 and Clinical procedures 19.4 and 19.5).

New technological advances such as surgical microscopes, powerful piezo-electric ultrasonic units and refined ultrasonic instruments have significantly increased the possibilities to retrieve separated instruments. As a rule, any broken instrument even partially located in the straight portion of the canal that can be visualized in the microscope should be removed. However, if the fragment is close to the foramen or protrudes beyond it, surgical endodontics is indicated.

Clinical procedure 19.3   Removing silver cones

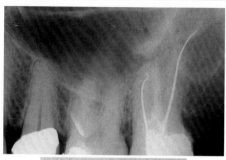

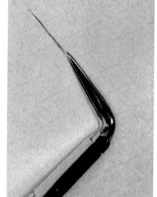

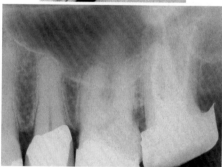

(1) A preoperative radiograph gives information about length and fitting of the cone, and whether the coronal head is protruding into the pulp chamber. If there is a crown, a second radiograph must be taken after crown removal.

(2) The restorative material is carefully eliminated from the pulp chamber with an ultrasonic tip, being careful not to damage the fragile silver cone end. At this stage, no attempt should be made to pull out the cone, unless it is very loose.

(3) Flood the access cavity with Endosolv E and try to bypass the cone with a no. 08 or 10 K-file to dissolve and break up the sealer around the cone. Then enlarge this pathway to allow the placement of a no. 15 K-file.

(4) Work a no. 15 or larger ultrasonic file alongside the cone with a short amplitude and in-and-out movements under copious water irrigation to float out the cone. If unsuccessful, then:

(5) Grasp the coronal end of the cone with a modified Steiglitz forceps, whose beaks have been made thinner, and use the tooth structure as a fulcrum to pull out the cone. If resistance is felt, indirect ultrasonics is applied on the beaks of the pliers close to the cone, to help dislodge it.

Core concept 19.2   Clinical strategies in canals with fractured instruments

(1)   Try to remove the fragment.

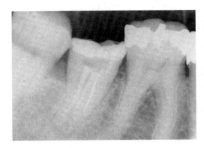 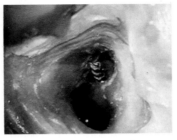 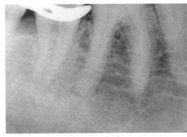

(2)   If removal is not successful, attempt to bypass the instrument and incorporate it in the subsequent root filling.

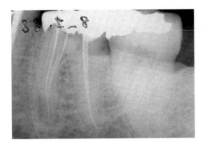 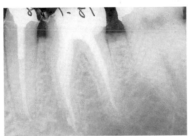 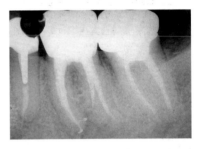

(3)   If the instrument cannot be bypassed, clean the canal up to the fragment and seal the space. Observe the case for a period of time before apical surgery is conducted.

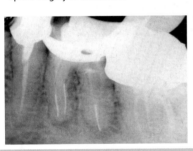 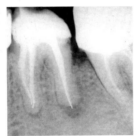 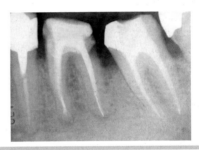

Instrumentation of the root canal

Reshaping the root canal

Reshaping the root canal system may be done by hand or by rotary instrumentation. In any case, the crown-down and patency concepts should be used to allow passive apical progression of the endodontic instruments working in a progressively deeper intracanal reservoir of sodium hypochlorite. The constant use of the patency file will move the irrigating solution into the restricted apical area to clean it. The apical preparation is done last, keeping in mind that a sufficiently deep shape should be produced to enable copious renewal of irrigation during final flushing and to pack the canal three-dimensionally. If NiTi rotary instrumentation is

elected, a smooth path guide to the canal terminus must be obtained beforehand for safe shaping of the root canal.

One should be aware that the requested reshaping of an already instrumented canal might create an overenlargement of the root canal space (40), therefore the danger zones of the root anatomy should have been assessed thoroughly before starting the retreatment. Avoiding canal deviation during reinstrumentation should be a permanent concern (27).

Apical obstructions

When canals have been underfilled, obstructive calcifications might be found in the apical unfilled portion. After coronal pre-enlargement and relocation of the

Clinical procedure 19.4   Removing stainless-steel instruments

(1) If the fragment can be bypassed, use the technique described for floating out silver cones. If unsuccessful, do not insist and proceed to cleaning and shaping. Often, the fragment is eliminated during these procedures, but if not it will be entombed in the filling material.

(2) If the instrument cannot be bypassed, get a straight radicular access to it. This is done using a sequence of K-files from no. 10 to no. 35, followed by an ascending sequence of Gates–Glidden drills from no. 1 to no. 5, paying attention not to damage the root structure. In curved canals, this step provides a relocation of the canal orifice.

(3) At this stage the instrument can be seen in the microscope. Depending upon the depth of its location in the canal, select an appropriate ultrasonic suborifice tip to make a trench around it. Under vision control and with a permanent light stream of air given by the Stropko syringe, rotate the tip anti-clockwise against the coronal end of the fragment to vibrate it, unwind it and then lift it out.

Clinical procedure 19.5   Removing fractured rotary NiTi instruments

Nickel–titanium alloys are brittle, so using ultrasonics may break the instrument. Radicular access is gained as described earlier, and a staging platform is created to gain better lateral access around the fragment (28). This is done with a no. 1 or 2 modified Gates–Glidden drill, whose working head has been sectioned with a bur at the maximum cross-sectional diameter. Then a 1.8-cc syringe with a blunt needle slightly larger than the instrument is selected. After the canal has been dried with pure alcohol and the Stropko, 1 cc of Core-Paste (Den-Mat) is loaded in the syringe and a small excess of material is extruded from the needle. The needle is removed from the syringe and wiped clean. The loaded needle is placed over the fractured instrument and the material is allowed to set for 5 min. The instrument is removed with a counter-clockwise twist.

Clinical procedure 19.6   Bypassing a ledge

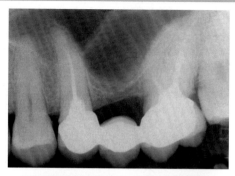

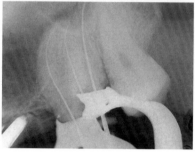

(1) Flood the canal with RC Prep or a similar product such as File-Eze (Ultradent, USA) or Glyde (Dentsply-Maillefer).

(2) Select a no. 10 SS K-file, place a sharp 1-mm curvature at the tip and orient the directional stop toward the file tip.

(3) Insert the file in the canal with the tip directed toward the canal curvature.

(4) Pick gently with very short strokes, searching for a catch. This procedure will move the irrigant and help to disintegrate the dentine mud. If unsuccessful, rebend the file tip and repeat the same procedure while slightly reorienting the tip.

(5) When a catch is felt, slightly wiggle the file back and forth while maintaining a light apical pressure.

(6) When the block is bypassed, move the file in an up-and-down motion to smooth the ledge. After obtaining a good glide path, copious irrigation with sodium hypochlorite should replace the lubricating gel.

canal orifice with Gates–Glidden drills, the coronal portion of the canal is copiously rinsed with sodium hypochlorite and then thoroughly dried with paper points and the Stropko syringe. At this stage, and if possible, the intracanal anatomy should be inspected carefully under the microscope to get information about the obstruction. Then, a small-size precurved K-file in association with a lubricating gel is worked with a slight pecking motion to try to find a catch. As long as a catch is felt at the tip of the K-file, apical progression should be continued and checked periodically with a radiograph until the canal terminus is reached.

Ledges

Often a ledge has been formed at the end of the previous obturation of the canal. Most of the time a ledge is the result of an inadequate angle of access to the root canal and goes hand in hand with canal blockage. Pre-flaring the coronal portion of the canal with K-files and relocating the canal orifice with Gates–Glidden drills are preliminary steps to bypassing a ledge (Clinical procedure 19.6) and recovering patency.

If the ledge is located in the apical portion of the canal, the fitting of the gutta-percha cone may be frustrating and repeatedly unsuccessful. Once the canal has been

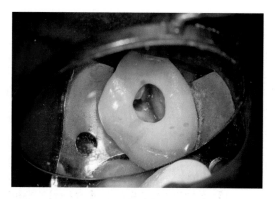
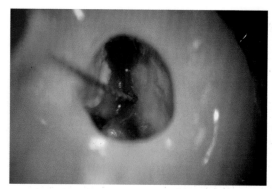
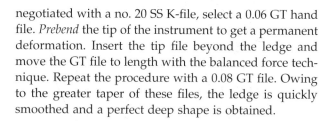
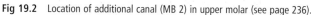

Fig 19.2 Location of additional canal (MB 2) in upper molar (see page 236).

negotiated with a no. 20 SS K-file, select a 0.06 GT hand file. *Prebend* the tip of the instrument to get a permanent deformation. Insert the tip file beyond the ledge and move the GT file to length with the balanced force technique. Repeat the procedure with a 0.08 GT file. Owing to the greater taper of these files, the ledge is quickly smoothed and a perfect deep shape is obtained.

Missed canals

Sometimes missed canals can be seen overtly in well-angulated radiographs but often they must just be suspected, e.g. when a tooth is reacting to thermal stimuli or is sore after an apparently adequate treatment (36).

After the main canals have been completely cleaned and shaped, the pulp chamber floor should be examined thoroughly. At this stage in the treatment this area is well cleaned by the irrigating solution. A careful inspection of the floor anatomy is made under high magnification and with good illumination. Shifts in dentine color and anatomic grooves may lead to the orifice of an additional canal (Fig. 19.2). An ultrasonic tip might be used on the pulpal floor to uncover hidden orifices and calcified canals.

Perforation repair

Furcal or root perforations might happen during root canal therapy, post space preparation or as a result of the extension of an internal resorptive defect. According to Ruddle (28), the four dimensions of a perforation that have to be analysed are its *level*, *location*, *size* and the *time* that has elapsed since its occurrence.

At a coronal level the inflammatory process that evolves as a response to the perforation might communicate with the gingival pocket and establish a periodontal defect. It is therefore favorable to seal the perforation site at an early stage before any major bone resorption has taken place. A wide perforation will be

---

> ### Clinical procedure 19.7   Perforation repair: the internal matrix technique
>
> (1) After cleaning the perforation walls with 0.5% NaOCl, the working length is established using an apex locator and several paper points. The consistently wet portion of the paper point indicates the level of the perforation.
>
> (2) Small pieces of Collacote are cut and sequentially packed with a prefitted plugger through the perforation site and into the bony lesion until a solid barrier is established at the borderline of the root defect.
>
> (3) The perforation site is copiously rinsed with 2.5% NaOCl and then dried. Finally, the defect is covered with a restorative material such as Super EBA, a glass ionomer or a composite.

more difficult to seal than a small one. The sites are mostly elliptical because an instrument usually perforates the canal wall at an oblique angle. Non-surgical repair is less affected by the location of the perforation than a surgical approach to treatment, which can be impossible in certain areas of the root.

Through the years numerous techniques and materials to repair perforations have been described. In this chapter two techniques are described (see Clinical procedures 19.7 and 19.8): the one-visit internal matrix technique using absorbable bovine collagen (Collacote, Calcitek, USA) (18); and the two-visit technique using mineral trioxide aggregate (MTA, Pro Root Dentsply-Maillefer)(37).

Antimicrobial treatment

Microbiota of the root filled tooth

Compared with the microbiota of non-treated pulps, little is known about the flora associated with failed root

---

Clinical procedure 19.8   Perforation repair: the MTA technique

First visit

(1) After cleaning the perforation site with 0.5% NaOCl, the working length is established using an apex locator and several paper points. The consistently wet portion of the paper points indicates the level of the perforation.

(2) The MTA is mixed with distilled water to a thick cement consistency, carried to the perforation defect with a Messing gun and gently packed with a plugger. It is then smoothed and a wet cotton pellet is placed against the MTA because the material needs moisture to set. The access cavity is temporarily filled with Cavit and the patient is dismissed.

Second visit: 48 h later

(1) After removal of the Cavit and the cotton pellet, the MTA hardness is probed with a sharp explorer. If found to be hard:

(2) The definitive obturation is made with the same restorative materials as used with the matrix technique.

Core concept 19.3   Features of the microbiota of the 'failed' root canal

- Few strains (1 or 2)
- Gram-positive micro-organisms predominate
- Dominance of facultatives over anaerobes
- *E. faecalis* frequently found

Clinical procedure 19.9   Standardized antimicrobial retreatment strategy

(1) Remove smear layer with citric acid or EDTA.

(2) Fill the root canal with 5% iodine potassium iodide or Churchill's solution for 10–15 min. Churchill's solution consists of iodine (16.5 g), potassium iodide (3.5 g), distilled water (20 g) and 90% ethanol (60 g).

(3) Prepare a mix of calcium hydroxide paste and the iodine compound used. Fill up the canal by means of a Lentulo spiral.

(4) Make a recall appointment 1–2 weeks later. Repeat steps (1) and (2) and obturate the canal.

It must be observed that sampling of root filled canals is fraught with difficulties. Initially it has to be preceded by removal of the sealing material. This physical activity might influence the anaerobes more negatively because they are generally more vulnerable. Yet, the composition of the described flora is as would be expected, i.e. more robust and treatment-resistant micro-organisms may remain after completed root canal therapy. The intracanal antimicrobial treatment acts as a selection procedure, favoring a certain type of microbiota either resistant to applied antimicrobial measures or able to survive in such a restrained nutritional habitat.

Antimicrobial retreatment strategies

When treating the non-vital pulp, calcium hydroxide often is recommended as the routine interappointment dressing. Few organisms will survive when directly exposed to calcium hydroxide, but several factors may impair its antimicrobial potency in the root canal. Complex anatomy will make it difficult to pack satisfactorily the whole canal system with paste (31). Also, calcium hydroxide lacks the potential to reach microbes colonizing the dentinal tubules (25). Furthermore, some species such as enterococci (6, 29) and yeasts (38) may resist high pH levels and thus show low sensitivity to calcium hydroxide. Therefore, in a retreatment situation other medicaments are likely to have greater potential.

A *standardized retreatment strategy* (Clinical procedure 19.9) must include measures to combat a potential *E. faecalis* infection. It has been observed that enterococci are sensitive to iodine compounds. Safavi *et al.* (29) infected dentinal tubules of human teeth with *E. faecium* and treated the canals with 2% iodine potassium iodide (IPI). A 10-min period of medicament–dentine contact was sufficient to prevent growth. The presence of a smear layer on the canal walls may delay the intratubule

canal treatments. In canals where major portions have been left unnegotiated, it is reasonable to assume that the flora are similar to those of the necrotic pulp (34). Consequently, in such cases the procedures recommended for primary treatment should be applied also in retreatment. However, when canals have been instrumented in their main parts a strikingly different composition of the recovered microflora has been found (9, 23, 24, 26, 34).

Instead of polymicrobial microbiota, often only one or two strains are detected in failed cases. The micro-organisms are predominantly Gram-positive with a slight dominance of facultative over obligate anaerobes (Core concept 19.3). *Enterococcus faecalis* is rarely found in primary samples of the necrotic pulp but has been recovered frequently in obturated canals. Among culture-positive teeth, *E. faecalis* was found in 24% by Engström (9), in 47% by Molander *et al.* (23) and in 71% by Peciuliene *et al.* (26). Attention also has been attracted to such species as actinomyces (12, 32, 35), candida (30, 38) and enteric rods (11, 16, 19).

antibacterial activity of a medicament (25), therefore in a clinical situation the application of IPI should be preceded by a smear-layer-removal procedure. Owing to its vaporization, IPI has a long-distance bactericidal effect. However, its duration in the root canal has been shown to be very short (9, 24) and therefore should not be left as an interappointment dressing. Instead, IPI in a mix with calcium hydroxide paste has been proposed (23).

There are several reasons (microbial and non-microbial) why an endodontic treatment fails and a standardized retreatment protocol will not consider these various reasons. As an alternative, *individualized monitoring* of retreatment cases might be designed based on intracanal microbiological sampling (Advanced concept 19.3).

Preventive retreatment

Intracanal micro-organisms have been recovered in root filled teeth *without* apical periodontitis (9, 23). However, the lack of a visible periapical radiolucency does not necessarily imply the absence of periapical pathosis. Attention must be paid to the possibility of periapical healing, although microbes survive in the root canal. Consequently, when a canal is retreated on a preventive indication, the case should be regarded as potentially infected. Also, patency filing through the foramen should be avoided. As long as there is no pathway to the

periapex, a periapical tissue response will not develop. If an avenue is opened up, nutritional supply will increase and an inflammatory reaction may be induced. Supportive clinical data have been presented showing that the development of periapical radiolucencies *after* retreatment is significantly associated with over-instrumentation and overfilling of the root canal (3). Bergenholtz et al. (4) diagnosed postoperative periapical radiolucencies in 3% of cases where the root fillings ended short of the apex, and in 18% when canals were overfilled.

Prognosis

Data on the outcome of non-surgical retreatment are most often available as part of general endodontic follow-up studies (for a review, see Ref. 13). Reported success rates in these investigations vary between 56% and 88%. The issue has been addressed specifically only by a few authors. After 2 years of observation, Bergenholtz et al. (3) found, in a prospective study, complete resolution of apical radiolucencies in 48% of 234 retreated roots. Decreased size of the radiolucency was observed in a further 30%. After a follow-up period of 5 years, Sundqvist et al. (34) reported complete healing in 74% of 54 retreated teeth. In this study microbiological samples were obtained at the time of root filling and only in two of six 'positive' cases did healing take place (33%). Three of the 'failed' canals did contain E. faecalis and in one canal A. israelii was detected. The samples were 'negative' in 44 cases and 35 of these showed radiographic signs of healing (80%).

Based on the available data, the prognosis of retreatment seems not to be as good as that of initial treatment. However, three out of four cases retreated non-surgically might be expected to heal. When retreatment is conducted for preventive reasons, and procedures are kept within the canal, failures might be anticipated in very few cases.

References

1. Allen RK, Newton CW, Brown CE. A statistical analysis of surgical and non surgical retreatment cases. *J. Endodont.* 1989; 15: 261–6.
2. Barbosa SV, Burkhard DH, Spangberg LSV. Cytotoxic effects of gutta-percha solvents. *J. Endodont.* 1994; 20: 6–8.
3. Bergenholtz G, Lekholm U, Milthon R, Heden G, Ödesjö B, Engström B. Retreatment of endodontic fillings. *Scand. J. Dent. Res.* 1979; 87: 217–23.
4. Bergenholtz G, Lekholm U, Milthon R, Engström B. Influence of apical overinstrumentation and overfilling on re-treated root canals. *J. Endodont.* 1979; 5: 310–14.

5. Bramante CM, Betti LV. Efficacy of Quantec rotary instruments for gutta-percha removal. *Int. Endodont. J.* 2000; 33: 463–7.

6. Byström A, Claesson R, Sundqvist G. The antibacterial effect of camphorated paramonochlorophenol, camphorated phenol and calcium hydroxide in the treatment of infected root canals. *Endodont. Dent. Traumatol.* 1985; 1: 170–5.

7. Carr GB. Microscopes in endodontics. *J. Calif. Dent. Assoc.* 1992; 20: 55–61.

8. Cohen AG. The efficiency of different solvents used in the retreatment of paste-filled root canals. *Master Thesis*, Boston University, 1986.

9. Engström B. The significance of enterococci in root canal treatment. *Odontol. Revy* 1964; 15: 87–106.

10. Friedman S. Treatment outcome and prognosis of endodontic therapy. In *Essential Endodontology* (Ørstavik D, Pitt-Ford T, eds). London: Blackwell Science.

11. Haapasalo M, Ranta H, Ranta K. Facultative Gram-negative enteric rods in persistent periapical infections. *Acta Odontol. Scand.* 1983; 41: 19–22.

12. Happonen R-P. Periapical actinomycosis: a follow-up study of 16 surgically treated cases. *Endodont. Dent. Traumatol.* 1986; 2: 205–9.

13. Hepworth MJ, Friedman S. Treatment outcome of surgical and nonsurgical management of endodontic failures. *J. Can. Dent. Assoc.* 1997; 63: 364–71.

14. Ibarrola JL, Knowles KI, Ludlow MO. Retrievability of Thermafil plastic cores using organic solvents. *J. Endodont.* 1993; 19: 417–19.

15. Jasper EA. Root canal therapy in modern dentistry. *Dent. Cosmos* 1933; 75: 823–9.

16. Kaufman A, Henig EF. The microbiologic approach in endodontics. *Oral Surg.* 1976; 42: 810–16.

17. Kvist T, Reit C. Results of endodontic retreatment: a randomized clinical study comparing surgical and nonsurgical procedures. *J. Endodont.* 1999; 25: 814–17.

18. Lemon RR. Non surgical repair of perforation defects. Internal matrix concept. *Dent. Clin. N. Am.* 1992; 36: 439–57.

19. Little JA. *Klebsiella pneumoniae* in endodontic therapy. *Oral Surg.* 1975; 40: 278–81.

20. Lovdahl PE, Gutmann JL. Problems in nonsurgical root canal retreatment. In *Problem Solving in Endodontics* (2nd edn) (Gutmann JL, Dumsha TC, Lovdahl PE, Hovland EJ, eds). St Louis: Mosby-Year Book, 1992.

21. Machtou P, Cohen A, Sarfati P. Post removal prior to retreatment. *J. Endodont.* 1989; 15: 552–4.

22. McDonald MN, Vire DE. Chloroform in the endodontic operatory. *J. Endodont.* 1992; 18: 301–3.

23. Molander A, Reit C, Dahlén G, Kvist T. Microbiological status of root filled teeth with apical periodontitis. *Int. Endodont. J.* 1998; 31: 1–7.

24. Möller ÅJR. Microbiological examination of root canals and periapical tissues of human teeth. *Odontol. Tidskr.* 1966; 74.

25. Ørstavik D, Haapasalo M. Disinfection by endodontic irrigants and dressings of experimentally infected dentinal tubules. *Endodont. Dent. Traumatol.* 1990; 6: 142–9.

26. Peciuliene V, Reynaud AH, Balciuniene I, Haapasalo M. Isolation of yeasts and enteric bacteria in root filled teeth with chronic apical periodontitis. *Int. Endodont. J.* 2001; 34: 429–34.

27. Peters O, Barbakow F. Apical transportation revisited or 'Where did the file go?' *Int. Endodont. J.* 1999; 32: 131–7.

28. Ruddle CJ. Nonsurgical endodontic retreatment. *J. Calif. Dent. Assoc.* 1997; 25: 769–99.

29. Safavi E, Spångberg L, Langeland K. Root canal dentinal tubule disinfection. *J. Endodont.* 1990; 16: 207–10.

30. Se BH, Piskin B, Demirci D. Observation of bacteria and fungi in infected root canals and dentinal tubules by SEM. *Endodont. Dent. Traumatol.* 1995; 11: 6–9.

31. Sigurdsson A, Stancill R, Madison S. Intracanal placement of Ca(OH)$_2$: a comparison of techniques. *J. Endodont.* 1992; 18: 367–70.

32. Sjögren U, Happonen R-P, Kahnberg K-E, Sundqvist G. Survival of *Arachnia propionica* in periapical tissue. *Int. Endodont. J.* 1988; 21: 277–82.

33. Stabholtz A, Friedman S, Tamse A. Endodontic failures and re-treatment. In *Pathways of the Pulp* (6th edn) (Cohen S, Burns RC, eds). St Louis: Mosby Company, 1994.

34. Sundqvist G, Figdor D, Persson S. Microbiologic findings of teeth with failed endodontic treatment and the outcome of conservative re-treatment. *Oral Surg.* 1998; 85: 86–93.

35. Sundqvist G, Reuterving C-O. Isolation of *Actinomyces israelii* from periapical lesion. *J. Endodont.* 1980; 6: 602–6.

36. Tidwell E, Witherspoon DE, Gutmann JL, Vreeland DL, Sweet PM. Thermal sensitivity of endodontically treated teeth. *Int. Endodont. J.* 1999; 32: 138–45.

37. Torabinejad M, Chivian N. Clinical applications of Mineral Trioxide Aggregate. *J. Endodont.* 1999; 25: 197–205.

38. Waltimo TMT, Sirén EK, Ørstavik D, Haapasalo MPP. Susceptibility of oral *Candida* species to calcium hydroxide in vitro. *Int. Endodont. J.* 1999; 32: 94–8.

39. Wilcox LR, Krell KV, Madison S, Rittman B. Endodontic retreatment: evaluation of gutta-percha and sealer removal and canal reinstrumentation. *J. Endodont.* 1987; 13: 453–7.

40. Wilcox LR, Swift ML. Endodontic retreatment in small and large curved canals. *J. Endodont.* 1991; 17: 313–15.

Chapter 20
Surgical retreatment

Peter Velvart

Introduction

Micro-organisms lodging in root filled canals may cause endodontic treatment failures. In order to eradicate the microbes in such cases, the root canal system has to be renegotiated and retreated. If the canals are poorly filled and fairly easy to access, an orthograde route of re-entry generally is recommended (Chapter 19). However, in many cases non-surgical retreatment may not be feasible from technical as well as financial aspects. Furthermore, failures might be caused by factors located outside the root canal, such as micro-organisms colonizing the periapical tissues, cysts and foreign-body reactions (Chapter 9). In such cases a surgical approach to retreatment may be considered (Fig. 20.1).

Although extensively debated over the years, there is little evidence to suggest that cysts are unable to heal following conventional endodontic therapy. But Nair (45) has drawn attention to the fact that some radicular cyst cavities do not have a direct connection with the root canal space. These so-called true radicular cysts are thought to be autonomous processes and are therefore not likely to respond to conventional therapy. From a clinical point of view, however, there are no means by which the existence of such a pathological condition can be determined. Consequently, all radiolucent lesions associated with non-vital pulps, whether cyst or not, should be seen as treatable by conventional means and be subjected to surgery only if healing cannot be attained. In surgical endodontic retreatment the procedural objectives are to expose the root tip and the periapical tissues by means of raising a mucoperiostal flap and, if necessary, cutting through the cortical bone. The treatment aims to combat a potential intracanal infection (usually the root tip is cut and the apical part of the canal is instrumented and sealed). Core concept 20.1 summarizes the typical indications for surgical retreatment.

General outline of the procedure (Core concept 20.2)

Following local anesthesia (step 1) a mucoperiostal flap is raised (step 2). If the periapical tissue response has not perforated the cortical bone plate, bone has to be removed (step 3) to provide access to the root tip. The soft-tissue lesion is then curetted (step 4) and the root tip is cut (step 5). Usually a root end preparation is made (step 6) and a filling (retrofill) is placed (step 7). The surgical procedure is finished with meticulous cleaning of the wound area and repositioning and suturing of the flap (step 8).

Local anesthesia

Proper pain control is required to perform the surgical procedure and to achieve optimal postsurgical comfort. Two kinds of medicaments are used: anesthetics and analgesics.

Choice of anesthetic agent
Anesthetic agents are most effective in a non-ionized form within a pH range near 7.4. In this state the drug can easily penetrate the nerve membranes and displace the calcium ions at the membrane receptor sites. The sodium channels are then blocked and upon nerve stimulation the membrane will remain in a polarized state. In acutely inflamed tissue the pH is lowered. In such an environment the anesthetic may remain in ionized form. The result can be lesser penetration of the drug, leading to inadequate anesthesia. This is one possible explanation as to the deficient pain control sometimes experienced when operating on acutely inflamed tissue. Endodontic surgeries should therefore not be performed in such instances, if possible. There are several anesthetics suitable for surgical pain control. Because allergic reactions to anesthetic drugs occur mainly to ester-based agents (such as procaine) (24), anesthetics

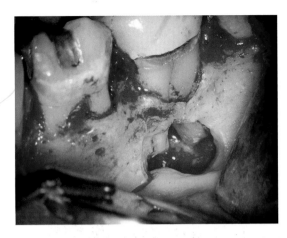

Fig. 20.1 Clinical photograph showing access to the root tips of a lower second molar in an endodontic surgical procedure, where retrograde instrumentation and root filling were carried out. (Courtesy of Dr G. Bergenholtz.)

based on amide groups are preferred. Good and profound anesthesia can generally be obtained with Articain, Lidocain and Bupivacain.

Vasoconstrictors

A vasoconstrictor is added to local anesthetics to reduce the blood flow at the injection site. This serves two important purposes:

(1) To retain the agent longer in the tissue, thereby extending the time for the anesthetic effect.
(2) To enhance hemostasis.

The reduced blood flow will also decrease absorption of the anesthetic and minimize systemic toxic effects.

The most widely used vasoconstrictor is epinephrine. This sympathomimetic agent causes vasoconstriction by stimulating specific membrane-bound receptors on the vascular smooth-muscle cells. The pharmacological action of epinephrine depends largely on the type of receptors present in the tissue. There are two types of adrenergic receptors: alpha vasoconstrictive and beta vasodilating receptors. Similar to mucosal and gingival tissues, alpha-adrenergic receptors predominate in the apical periodontium. Thus, upon its penetration to these tissue sites, the effect of epinephrine will be contraction of blood vessels. In skeletal muscles, on the other hand, vessels are controlled by beta-adrenergic vasodilating receptors (41). This means that injection of epinephrine to muscle tissue will result in increased blood flow and cause the opposite of the desired hemostatic effect (5). For this reason, the anesthetic should be administered to mucosal tissue only and close to the bone in the area in focus for the operation.

Concentrations of vasoconstrictor among anesthetic solutions vary between 1:50 000 and 1:200 000. The higher the concentration, the better the hemostatic effect.

Most widely used is the concentration 1:100 000–200 000. Although this concentration is adequate for non-surgical needs (31), it will not produce sufficient hemostasis for surgical procedures. For this purpose, at least 1:80 000 or rather 1:50 000 is recommended. It has been found that the use of 1:50 000 epinephrine results in good visualization of the surgical site, reduced surgery time and decreased postoperative bleedings and blood loss (5). High concentrations of epinephrine may cause an undesirable increased heart rate, cardiac contractility and peripheral vascular resistance. These systemic effects can be reduced by using several measures (see Core concept 20.3).

It should be realized that sufficient hemostasis can be achieved only if the anesthetic has reached the tissue. Therefore, on inferior alveolar nerve blocks the anesthetic must be administered also to the surgical site to obtain adequate hemostasis, even though blood flow peripheral to such nerve blocks becomes reduced (29).

Flap raising

The success of any surgical procedure depends largely upon the extent to which adequate access can be obtained. Endodontic surgery first requires exposure of the bone overlaying the tip of the root(s) and then the root end(s) *per se* (Fig. 20.1). To access the bone, a full-thickness flap must be raised. This means a soft-tissue flap, which consists of gingival and mucosal tissue as well as periosteum. To mobilize the flap various modes of incision can be selected, including horizontal incisions (sulcular and submarginal) and vertical releasing incisions.

It is critical that incisions and flap elevations are carried out in a manner such that soft-tissue healing by primary intention is facilitated. This is secured by:

- Complete and sharp incision of the tissues.
- Avoiding severing of the tissues during flap elevation.
- Preventing drying of the tissue remnants on the root surface during the procedure (see further below).

Flap designs

Triangular flap: a horizontal incision extending one tooth distally and one tooth mesially to the involved area, combined with only one vertical releasing incision (Fig. 20.2), forms the triangular flap. The main advantage of this flap design is easy repositioning and minimal disruption of the vascular supply to the flap. It is indicated for correction of marginally located processes such as perforations, cervical root resorptions or resections of very short roots. If it turns out that the access is too limited, the triangular flap can be converted easily to a rectangular flap by placing an additional releasing inci-

Core concept 20.1 Typical indications for surgical retreatment

- A file fragment that could not be removed blocks the root canal. The top-right radiograph was taken immediately postoperatively and the bottom radiograph after 1 year shows healing. (Radiographs courtesy of Dr T. Kvist.)

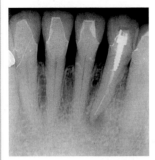
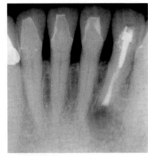
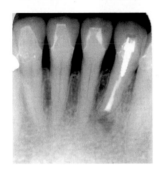

- Grossly overinstrumented and overfilled canal.

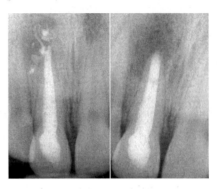

- Failed treatment in spite of adequate root filling results in intracanal treatment. Persistence of a fistula.

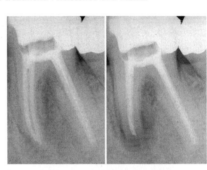

- Apical root canals blocked by ledge.

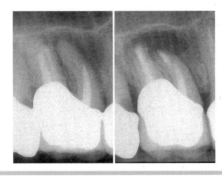

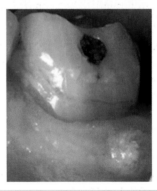

sion at the distal end of the horizontal incision (see below).

Rectangular flap: the rectangular flap is formed by a horizontal incision with two vertical releasing incisions (Fig. 20.3) and is the most frequently used flap in endodontic surgery. The rectangular flap will give excellent surgical access to the apical area in any region. In esthetically critical areas with prosthetic restorations involving submarginally placed crown margins, a postoperative sequel can result in recession, leading to exposure of the crown margins. Using a proper atraumatic

and gentle surgical technique with proper wound management minimizes such esthetic disadvantages.

Submarginal flap according to Ochsenbein–Luebke: the submarginal flap is formed by a scalloped horizontal submarginal incision with two vertical releasing incisions (Fig. 20.4). The submarginal flap is only to be used when there is a broad attached gingiva and when the expected apical lesion or surgical bony access will not involve the incision margins. This flap design has the advantage of preserving the marginal gingiva and does not expose the marginal crestal bone.

Core concept 20.2   Critical steps in surgical retreatment

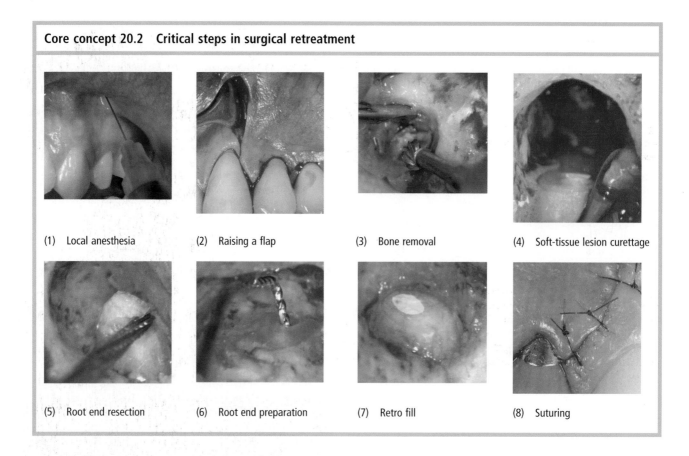

(1)   Local anesthesia   (2)   Raising a flap   (3)   Bone removal   (4)   Soft-tissue lesion curettage

(5)   Root end resection   (6)   Root end preparation   (7)   Retro fill   (8)   Suturing

---

Except for the risk of massive loss of marginal tissue due to a possible insufficient blood supply to the unreflected gingival tissue (see above), the risk of scarring is another disadvantage of this flap design. This is because the flap tends to shrink during surgery, resulting in tension on the flap during and after suturing.

Incisions

Sulcular incision: the scalpel size has to be small enough to allow free movement of the blade within the sulcus and to avoid cutting into the gingiva (Figs 20.5 and 20.6). The scalpel should be kept in constant contact with the tooth. Even so, the incision will sever sulcular epithelium and fibers of the gingival attachment, leaving epithelium and connective tissue at the root surface (Fig. 20.6). These tissue remnants are delicate and easily injured, which can result in impaired healing (17), and should not be allowed to dry out because they facilitate epithelial and gingival reattachment. Interproximally the tissue should be dissected in the middle of the papilla, to preserve its buccal and lingual aspects (Fig. 20.7).

Submarginal incision: the submarginal incision to raise an Ochsenbein–Luebke flap is performed within the attached gingiva and should be at a level where the incision cuts well into the crestal bone (39). The cutting action is a continuous firm stroke with the blade, which separates the tissue all the way to the bone. For easy and precise repositioning of the flap, the incision should not be in a straight line, but scalloped and extending slightly into the interproximal direction. Thus, the contour of the incision should reflect the contour of the marginal gingiva (Fig. 20.8c). The submarginal incision should be at a level that is 2 mm apical to the base of the sulcus (33) in order not to risk subsequent necrosis and recession of the unreflected marginal portion. To size up the width of the attached gingiva, the pocket probing depth has to be determined (Fig. 20.8a). The width of the attached gingiva is then calculated on the basis of the distance from the base of the sulcus to the *linea girlandiformis* (Fig. 20.8b).

In general, healing after this mode of incision is favorable because there is sufficient blood supply from vessels exiting at the crestal bone level and from anastomosing vessels deriving from the papilla.

Where there are deep pockets, this type of incision is contraindicated and a marginal incision should be performed instead. The incision also should not be used when there is danger of having the incision over the bony defect, which increases the risk of postoperative infection. Therefore, the selection of this type of incision

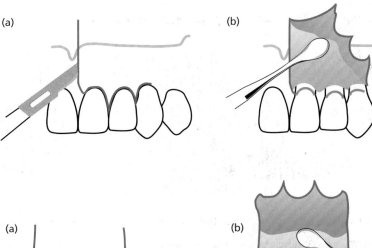

(a)

(b)

Fig. 20.2 (a) Triangular flap requires a sulcular incision, usually with mesial placement of the vertical releasing incision. (b) Flap reflected.

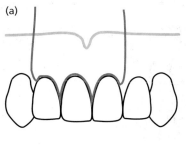
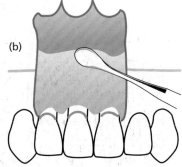

(a)

(b)

Fig. 20.3 (a) Rectangular flap involves two releasing incisions combined with a marginal sulcular incision. The releasing incisions are placed at least one tooth away from the tooth to be operated on, except in the area of the mental foramen, which should not be subjected to vertical incisions. (b) Flap reflected.

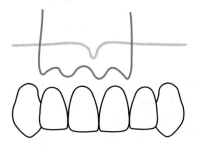

Fig 20.4 An Ochsenbein–Luebke flap is raised by placing a scalloped horizontal incision within the attached gingiva, reflecting the gingival and mucosal tissues (39). For vertical incisions, the same rules apply as for the rectangular flaps.

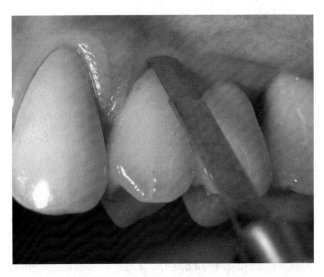

Fig 20.5 Sulcular incision using a microscalpel blade. Note the blade entering into the gingival tissue owing to a small root diameter in the cervical area of the root.

Core concept 20.3 Injection technique

To reduce pain and cardiovascular effects upon injecting an anesthetic solution containing epinephrine:

(1) Aspirate to prevent intravascular administration.
(2) Inject at a slow pace. Speed should not exceed 1–2 ml per minute.
(3) Anesthetize first with half the dose of the solution at a concentration of 1 : 100 000 epinephrine. Wait 3–5 min until initial vasoconstriction and then use 1:50 000 epinephrine.
(4) Use a pulse oxymeter to monitor pulse rate.

---

requires thorough treatment planning. The main advantage is that the original level of the epithelial attachment can be maintained, which is not always the case with the sulcular incision. This is an important esthetic consideration especially with full crowns, where healing after a sulcular incision can result in gingival recession to such an extent that the crown margins become visible.

Vertical incisions: one or two vertical incisions are needed in an endodontic surgical procedure to allow sufficient exposure of the bone. The incision should extend apically enough to prevent tension on the flap during retraction. When cutting in the apical area the blade often does not reach the bone owing to the thickness of the mucosa, therefore a second stroke has to be taken to separate completely the tissue through the periosteum.

The vertical releasing incision is placed usually one tooth laterally to the tooth to be operated on (Fig. 20.3). An exception to this rule is the lower premolar region, where a vertical cut can interfere with the nerve bundles exiting from the mental foramen and cause temporary or permanent paresthesia. In such cases the vertical incision is placed one tooth mesial to the mental foramen. In any case, it is important to determine radiographi-

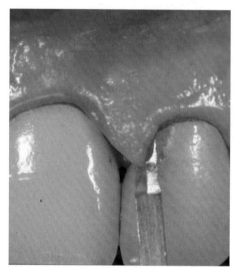

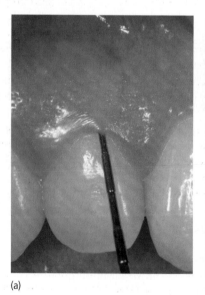

Fig 20.6 Marginal incision leaves small amounts of gingival connective tissue and epithelium on the tooth surface, which should be kept moist and vital for reattachment at the preoperative attachment level.

Fig. 20.7 Dissection of the buccal papilla with a microscalpel. Note complete separation from the lingual portion of the papilla and the preservation of the tissue in all its dimensions.

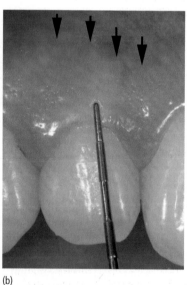
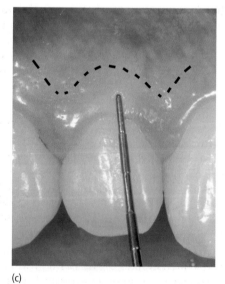

(a)   (b)   (c)

Fig 20.8 (a) Measuring the pocket probing depth is necessary for calculation of the width of the attached gingiva in a submarginal incision procedure. (b) The probe is held on the buccal surface of the gingiva to visualize the base of the probing depth. The attached gingiva represents the distance from the tip of the probe to the linea girlandiformis (arrows). (c) The line represents the location for a submarginal incision.

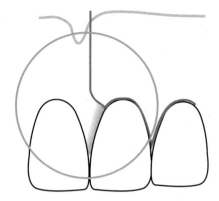

Fig. 20.9   Correct vertical incision preserving the body of the papilla.

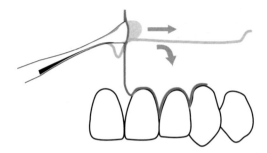

Fig. 20.10   Raising a flap from the releasing incision with a distal–coronal-directed motion, undermining the periosteum.

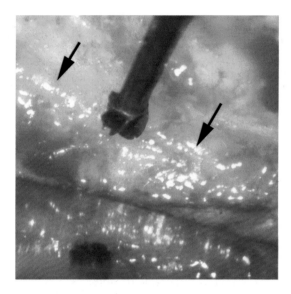

Fig. 20.11   Cut of a small groove in the bone at the base of the flap serves as a rest for the periosteal elevator, giving the assistant a safe position for it so that it will not slip and possibly crush the tissues.

cally the position of the foramen prior to surgery if it is going to be exposed by the flap.

The placement of the vertical incision should be such that the integrity of the papilla is maintained. Figure 20.9 illustrates the correct paramedian releasing incision to be used. Incisions midcrown and incisions that split the papilla should be avoided because they may lead to necrosis of a large portion of the tissue and recessions.

Flap elevation and retraction

After the incision, lifting the tissue from the underlying bone should raise the flap. In the process, the periosteum should not be perforated or torn. To optimize the healing conditions, maintenance of an intact periosteum is essential because it will protect the surgical cavity from being in direct contact with the mucosal tissue, which otherwise can enter the cavity and prevent complete bone fill.

Flap elevation should begin from the releasing incision in an undermining action (Fig. 20.10). The elevating instrument then should be directed toward the marginal ridge. If the periosteum cannot be separated completely from the crestal bone, the flap can be freed by dissecting the unseparated tissue remnants with a scalpel.

Once the flap has been retracted, a small groove should be prepared in the bone with a small round bur. This groove serves as a rest for the retractor, to prevent crushing of the flap during the surgery (Fig. 20.11).

Bone removal

Once the flap has been retracted and held in place, bone usually needs to be removed to uncover the soft-tissue lesion and the apical area of the tooth. A sufficient amount of bone tissue must be eliminated to gain proper access.

It is important that the osseous tissue is managed with caution to prevent postoperative pain and to enhance healing. Heat generation is damaging and should be monitored by using rotating burs under light shaving motions while irrigating with copious amounts of sterile saline (14). Supplementary saline irrigation must be used when cutting deep to uncover, for example, palatal or lingual roots. Excessive pressure during drilling should be avoided at all times. The bone drill, in addition, should be sharp and clean (6). Diamond burs are inefficient and should not be used (38).

Curettage of the soft-tissue lesion

Because the soft-tissue lesion most often represents an inflammatory response to a root canal infection and/or to extruded root filling material, removal of this tissue is not essential *per se* but it needs to be taken out for technical reasons to allow visibility and accessibility to the root tip for the management of the root canal system

---

Advanced concept 20.1 Importance of complete removal of the soft-tissue lesion

Over the years it has been debated extensively whether or not the removal of the soft-tissue lesion is a critical step in the surgical procedure. It has been held that the lesion represents a pathological process and therefore should be removed in its entirety. Given the fact that the soft-tissue lesion actually is a host tissue response to irritants associated with the tooth, most often to a root canal infection, complete curettage should not be necessary. In fact, in a study comparing complete and incomplete removal of periradicular tissues during surgery, no difference in clinical outcome was found in terms of periradicular healing at clinical follow-up (37). It is therefore likely that any inflamed tissue left behind will be incorporated into the new granulation tissue that will form as part of the healing process. Even leaving some epithelial remnants should not jeopardize the healing process. It has been proposed that as long as the irritants of the root canal system are eliminated, the host's defense mechanisms will destroy and eliminate proliferated epithelial cells (56). An exception to this view is the case where bacteria are located within the lesion *per se*, e.g. *Actinomyces* (Chapter 9). These microorganisms appear in nests and can be observed macroscopically as yellow granules. Thus, lesions of this nature may be sustained by the organisms *per se* and should be curetted carefully. Curettage of the soft-tissue lesion diminishes bleeding. Also, from this perspective it is essential to remove as much of the soft-tissue process to enhance the management of the root end for preparation and filling.

(Advanced concept 20.1). Therefore, curettage to remove the soft-tissue lesion has to be performed. This task is greatly facilitated by the use of sharp curettes, because fibrous tissue in the periphery of the lesion often is difficult to detach.

Sometimes the lesion consists of a radicular cyst. By careful dissection the cyst capsule can be released from the adjacent bone and removed in its entirety. If the blood supply of the adjacent tooth (teeth) or other vital structures, such as neurovascular bundles, is endangered, complete removal of the soft-tissue lesion should not be attempted.

Management of bleedings

Hemostasis during endodontic surgery is essential to ensure the successful management of the root end. Hemorrhage control is not only required for visibility and assessment of the root structure but is also necessary to allow insertion and setting of the retrograde root filling material in the absence of moisture.

Several means, described below, can be undertaken to control bleedings.

Proper local anesthesia: hemorrhage reduction is achieved by local anesthesia using a sufficient concentration of the vasoconstrictor (see above). It should be recognized that, even though numbness is achieved soon after the injection, sufficient vasoconstriction takes several minutes to develop.

Proper operation technique: proper handling of the soft tissue minimizes bleeding. Remember that most vessels run parallel to the long axis of the teeth, therefore the releasing incision, for example, should be placed along the long axis of the root to limit the number of blood vessels that may be severed. Furthermore, gentle and atraumatic elevation of the full-thickness flap prevents perforation and tearing of the periosteum. This measure retains the microvasculature within the body of the flap and thus further reduces the risk of bleeding.

Suctioning: suctioning controls localized bleedings. Injured vessels will normally constrict at the first stage of the hemostatic cascade, eventually to be blocked by a fibrin clot. Thus, bleeding ceases spontaneously with time.

Obstruction by mechanical means: slight *hammering* of the bone with a dull object can mechanically obstruct localized hemorrhage from a vessel in the bone. By this measure, the bony space for the vessel is occluded. The procedure is most effective on bleedings from the cortical bone, whereas in loose cancellous bone the effect is less predictable.

Loading the bottom of the bone cavity with a material that mechanically obstructs the openings of the cancellous bone is useful. Two options are available: *bone wax* and *calcium sulfate*. Bone wax has been used for this purpose for many years (54). It has no effect on the clotting and essentially has only a blocking effect. Note that bone wax causes foreign body reaction if left in the cavity after surgery (27), therefore it has to be curetted out completely.

Calcium sulfate in sterile water to a thick mix (48) should be inserted by pressing the material against the cavity walls with a wet cotton pellet. The material sets within minutes. Calcium sulfate is used extensively in general surgery because it is biocompatible (23), resorbs completely and is reported to be osteoinductive (9).

Electrocoagulation: electrocoagulation for hemorrhage control should use bipolar units. The monopolar units frequently used in dental practice for exposing preparation margins before impression are too traumatic owing to the massive heat that these units generate. Bipolar units where the electric current flows only between the two electrodes (usually the branches of the pliers) are much less damaging to the collateral tissues. When monopolar was compared with bipolar electrosurgery, significantly more damage and elevation in lateral tissue temperature was observed (34). For a bipolar coagulation the vessel needs to be grabbed to be effective, otherwise this method is ineffective. Frequently the cut vessels contract and cannot be touched. In such instances, other hemostatic measures should be applied.

Chemicals: small pieces of gauze fitting the bone cavity and saturated with vasoconstrictive agent, e.g. *epinephrine*, effectively control hemorrhage. The systemic effects are usually insignificant owing to the immediate vasoconstriction that is promoted (30). However, the amount of epinephrine given in conjunction with the local anesthetic should be assessed and if the maximum dose is reached then other means of hemorrhage control should be considered.

Ferric sulfate in a concentration of 20%, also known as Monsel's solution, reacts with blood proteins to form a plug that occludes the capillary orifices. The pH is low and the chemical is clearly toxic, which will therefore severely delay healing and in some cases cause abscess formation if left after surgery (36). The dark stain often formed represents agglutinated blood on the bone surface and has to be curetted thoroughly and removed by saline rinses. The bone surface may be freshened with a round drill to remove any remaining coagulated material. Jeansonne *et al.* (28) reported that healing is normal with only a mild foreign-body reaction provided that the surgical wound is thoroughly cleansed prior to wound closure.

Resorbable agents: collagen-based hemostatic materials applied directly to the bleeding area under pressure result in hemostasis within a few minutes. Their potential use in periapical surgery has been demonstrated by Haasch *et al.* (16). If left in the osseous defects there is minimal interference with the wound healing process and the foreign-body reaction is minimal (10).

Surgicel is a substance for hemorrhage control prepared by the oxidation of oxycellulose. Initially it serves as a barrier and then transforms to a sticky mass that will act as an artificial coagulum. The material should be removed from the surgical site after completion of the operation because it can cause foreign-body reaction and impair osseous regeneration (27).

Gelfoam consists of gelatin-based sponges, which promote the disintegration of platelets and cause subsequent release of thromboplastine. This in turn stimulates the formation of thrombin in the sponge spaces (30). If gelfoam is left *in situ*, it will slow down healing initially (4) but after a few months there are no negative effects (47).

Root end resection

Following completion of the surgical access to the root end area, the tip of the root(s) normally has to be cut off at around 2–3 mm (15). This procedure is known under

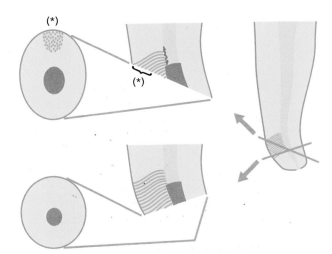

Fig. 20.12 Principle for root end resection. Excessive bevel allows penetration of bacterial elements through dentinal tubules to the resection surface (*). Ideal angulation is square to the long axis of the root (bottom).

different terms, of which apicectomy or apicoectomy are the most common. The rationales for this measure are:

(1) To provide convenient access to the root canal(s) for the apical instrumentation (see below).
(2) To remove any bacterial organisms lodged in accessory and main canals of an apex delta and/or on the surface of the root tip.

The angle of the cut surface should be as square as possible to the long axis of the root to reduce the number of exposed dentinal tubules (Fig. 20.12). Dentinal tubules may serve as pathways for the release of bacterial elements from the infected root canal, especially if the root end filling is short (13). However, occasionally a slight bevel is needed to allow proper access and visual observation of the resected tip (Advanced concept 20.2). Buccally inclined roots do not need a bevel, whereas roots inclined in the opposite direction and roots under a thick bone plate need bevelling. When there is a post in the tooth, the resection should not be performed to the base of it because the seal of the luting cement may be broken.

Following resection, the cut surface should be inspected for the presence of apical ramifications, isthmus formation and possible fracture lines. The inspection needs to be carried out with the use of magnification and if necessary with micromirrors (Fig. 20.13).

Root end preparation

The root canal of the resected root tip needs to be cleaned and shaped to accommodate a retrograde root filling according to the same rationales as for conventional root canal therapy (Clinical procedure 20.1). Thus, the primary objective of this measure is to exclude the root

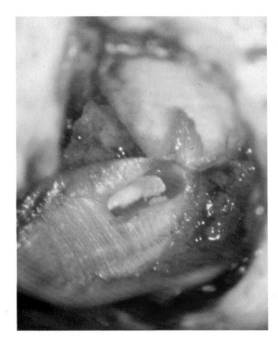

Fig. 20.13   Micromirror view following root end resection and preparation.

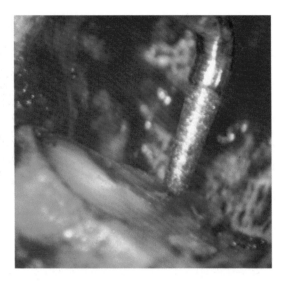

Fig. 20.14   Diamond-coated ultrasonic tip.

Advanced concept 20.2   Beveling of the root end

Gilheany *et al.* (13) have demonstrated that there is no other basis for beveling the root end in endodontic surgery than to achieve convenient access to the root canal system. In fact, an acute bevel in combination with an inadequate root end preparation and filling carries the risk for penetration of bacterial elements along the dentinal tubules or the root end filling, or both, to the resected root surface. *In vitro*, these investigators evaluated, by the hydraulic conductance method, the degree of apical leakage as a function of various depths of retrograde fillings and different cutting angles (0, 30 and 45° to the long axis of the root). Findings were a significant increase of leakage with increased angulation and significantly decreased leakage with increasing depth of the retrograde filling, suggesting that both the permeability of the resected apical dentine and the length of the retrograde filling are significant factors for whether or not the procedure will succeed.

Clinical procedure 20.1   Retrograde hand file preparation

A procedure where the complete root canal is debrided, shaped and filled from the apical end was originally proposed by Nygaard-Östby (46) and later clinically tried and evaluated by Reit and Hirsch (50). Following a small resection of the root tip, the canal is cleaned and enlarged with Hedström files held in a hemostat. The canal is irrigated with 0.5% sodium hypochlorite and sealed with cold laterally condensed or injectable gutta-percha.

Advanced concept 20.3   Isthmuses

The anatomic complexity of the root canal system has been known for years (20), but it was not until recently that the importance of isthmuses in the endodontic surgery of certain teeth was recognized (7). Hsu and Kim (25) studied the resected surfaces of different teeth in the human dentition and observed that in general the chance of isthmus formation is higher when more of the root is resected. With the aid of proper magnification, both anatomical structures, isthmus and ramifications can be detected and effectively treated by the use of ultrasonic instrumentation (see Fig. 20.15).

---

canal as a source of microbial exposure of the organism. The cleaning procedure can be carried out with properly angled ultrasonic root end tips (Fig. 20.14) and with hand-held root canal files or both. Preparation with a small round bur in a micro-handpiece was used for years. Often cavities that are too large and root canals that are insufficiently cleaned resulted from this technique. Also, the cavity frequently became extended to the palatal side of the root and in certain cases even per-

forations occurred. In small and fine roots and very frequently in fused roots, forming an isthmus between them (see Fig. 20.15), this technique is quite unsuitable because the diameter of the smallest bur size may exceed the width of the root (Advanced concept 20.3).

In recent years the use of ultrasonic devices has led to a significant improvement of the apical instrumenta-

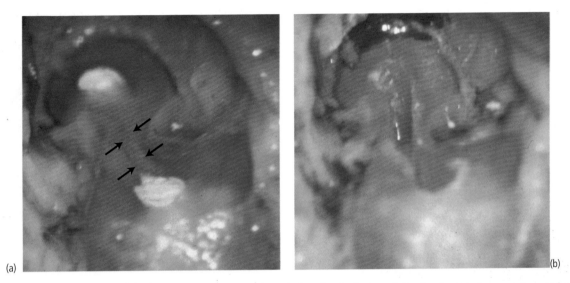

(a)   (b)

Fig. 20.15   (a) The tip of a resected upper premolar displays gutta-percha in the buccal and palatal canals. The fused roots in the connecting area have a fine line (arrowheads) – an isthmus – barely visible in 25× magnification. Failure to diagnose and treat this anatomical structure led to persistence of symptoms after the first surgical treatment. (b) The cleaned retrograde preparation with the isthmus area to be filled.

tion in endodontic surgery. Richman (51) in 1957 used ultrasonically powered chisels to remove bone and to resect teeth. The more recent development of retro-tips in combination with the use of the surgical microscope has not only offset many of the drawbacks from the preparation with rotary instruments but also made it possible to predict the surgical treatments of virtually all teeth.

The ultrasonic energy puts the tip into vibration, which will remove both hard- and soft-tissue elements in the root canal, including root filling material. A light touch has to be applied, because the vibration wave is only effective when the tip is not pressed to the surface during its operation. The methodology offers the following advantages:

(1) An ultrasonic tip is smaller and more delicate than a round bur in a micro-handpiece.
(2) About 3–4 mm of vertical space in the root can be instrumented.
(3) Preparation can be performed at the long axis of the tooth and thus can follow the true path of it, thereby avoiding perforations.

Studies have shown that ultrasonic preparation is superior to conventional preparation with a round bur. The ultrasonic preparation will result in cleaner, more parallel and deeper preparations (62). The drawback of ultrasonics is the reported risk of microcracks and fractures (1, 35). The use of ultrasonically energized file tips has reduced the fracture risk. Powering the files requires much lower energy than for the stiffer root-end tips.

Files furthermore are resilient when tilted during the preparation, which minimizes the wedging forces. An additional advantage of the use of prebend files, commonly used for orthograde instrumentation, is the improved cleaning/shaping and extended preparation further up the canal (61).

Retro fill

The goal of the retrograde filling is to seal the prepared cavity to prevent leakage of tissue fluid to the remainder of the root canal space and the exchange of bacterial elements that may result from such leakage. The significance of the retrograde root filling for a successful outcome has been demonstrated in numerous clinical follow-up studies (12), therefore an important feature of a retrograde root filling is to hermetically seal the root canal space. Furthermore, because the surface of the filling can be quite large, e.g. following cleaning of isthmuses, the material should not vanish by disintegration in tissue fluids over time. Other important requirements are biological compatibility and that the material interferes only minimally with the wound healing process.

Ideally a retrograde root filling should allow new formation of cementum on its surface into which periodontal ligament fibers can insert. Such a tissue response should ensure minimal dissolution of the material over time and thus enhance the long-term prognosis.

Various retrograde filling materials have been employed over the years. Amalgam has enjoyed great acceptance (12) but is currently losing popularity because:

(1) Its sealing ability is questionable (26).
(2) It is difficult to handle during the surgical procedure and amalgam remnants may be left behind in the surgical cavity.
(3) It corrodes, which can lead to disintegration and release of metal ions into the surrounding tissues (42).
(4) Discoloration and tattoos of the gingiva or mucosa may ensue in visible areas, causing non-esthetic disfigurations.
(5) It contains mercury, which is why amalgam is banned for clinical use in several countries.

The most salient problem with amalgam as a retrograde filling material is the poor clinical outcome obtained in several clinical follow-up studies with this material (11, 8).

Alternatives to amalgam are glass ionomer cements, resin composites in combination with dentine bonding (26, 52) and mineral trioxide aggregate (57). Glass ionomers and composites seal the cavity quite well but are technique and moisture sensitive (49).

Excellent experimental (3) and clinical (8) results have been obtained with zinc oxide–eugenol (ZOE)-based cements. The handling of these retrograde filling materials is good but their biological compatibility should be questioned. Release of eugenol causes toxic reactions and will prevent the development of a biological seal at the root end. The toxicity of eugenol depends on the amount of free eugenol in the cement (18). It can be reduced if the cement is mixed to a very dry consistency, leaving little free eugenol in the mix, which also improves its handling. The ZOE-based cements set rapidly when exposed to moisture after condensation. The beveled root surface can be polished in a few minutes, and any excess filling material can be removed from the root end surface.

Another retrograde filling material with clinical potential is an MTA (mineral trioxide aggregate) (57–60). The hydrophilic powder is mixed with water to a creamy consistency, which sets to a hard mass. It seals well, it is reasonably biocompatible and, owing to its hydrophilic properties, is probably the best material to use when moisture control is precarious. However, the material is difficult to handle because of its consistency.

Several authors (55, 13) have pointed out the potential pathway for leakage of bacterial elements at the resected root end along the dentinal tubules. Sealing the entire beveled surface with dentine bonding was therefore proposed and introduced by Rud *et al.* (52). The method includes preparing a slight concavity at the root end and applying a bonding agent, which is followed by the application of a chemically cured composite (Fig. 20.16a,

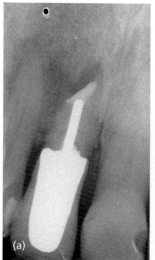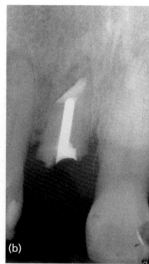

Fig. 20.16   (a) Retrograde filling with resin composite of an upper incisor that had extensive apical root resorption. Healing was uneventful except that the crown later fractured off from the root. (b) Complete bone fill at about 19 months of follow-up. (Courtesy of Dr G. Bergenholtz.)

b). If properly managed, the healing potential is excellent (53).

Flap closure and suturing

Repositioning of the soft tissue to its original position, with the wound edges closely approximated by careful suturing, is normally sufficient for rapid healing. Although the techniques for suturing can be variable, in endodontic surgery usually single sutures are applied to hold the flap in place during the initial healing phase. The sutures are placed in each proximal space and at the vertical releasing incisions.

Atraumatic needles should be used. Select sutures in sizes 6/0 and smaller. Although fine, the needle should still be rigid and have a 3/8 circle with sharp pointed triangular cross-section. The needle length can be a problem in papilla closure, because small suture sizes have rather short needles. The needle length for a comfortable interproximal suture should be at least 12 mm.

The suture material should be non-resorbable because the irritation is considerably less than with a resorbable suture material. They should have a smooth coating or be monofilamentous in sizes 7/0 and smaller. If wound healing is uneventful, sutures can usually be removed within 3 days, at which time an epithelial lining has developed.

The wound healing process after an endodontic surgical procedure consists of:

• Clotting and inflammation.
• Epithelial healing.

- Connective tissue healing.
- Maturation and remodeling of the soft and hard tissues.

These stages are not distinctly separated from each other. They overlap considerably and take place almost simultaneously. Because the original incision disrupted blood vessels, hemostasis has to take place first. Vascular and tissue injury release humoral and cellular mediators that cause a rather complex event of clot formation. The clot connects the wound edges and forms a pathway for the migration of inflammatory and repairing cells. If hemostasis is not complete, blood continues to flow into the wound site and a hematoma may develop. This will delay healing considerably and the coagulum must first be resorbed before connective tissue healing can proceed (21). Applying pressure with soft gauze to the flap for about 5 min after repositioning and suturing can reduce clot and hematoma formation and thereby enhance the healing process.

Under optimal conditions the maturation and remodeling phase of both soft and hard tissue may begin within 5–7 days after surgery. The first step is the formation of an epithelial barrier to protect the underlying connective tissue from irritants of the oral cavity. Sutures can be removed as soon as the epithelial lining has formed, which usually is within 3 days.

Pain control after surgery

The use of an atraumatic operation technique will not only reduce the amount of swelling and enhance the healing process but also lessen postoperative discomfort and pain. In addition to the application of a cold compress to the surgical site to reduce swelling, analgesics with swelling-reducing properties should be prescribed and a dose taken prior to the cessation of the anesthetic effect. Different drugs have various degrees of analgesic and anti-inflammatory effect. Pain perception is elevated in the presence of prostaglandins and an analgesic that slows down the synthesis of prostaglandins will reduce the excitability of the pain receptors to normal levels at the same time as providing pain relief. Inhibition of prostaglandin synthesis will also produce an antiphlogistic effect.

Bone healing

It should be understood that complete bone healing only takes place if the etiology for the inflammatory lesion that led to the surgical procedure is eliminated. If not, an inflammatory lesion will persist that may present itself as a persistent radiolucent bone lesion or recurring swelling or fistulous tract, or both.

In proper healing, the missing structures, bone and cementum will regenerate and within months to a year show up as complete fill of bone in the previous surgical cavity (Fig. 20.17).

In the presence of a defect extending from the buccal to the oral side, bony refill might not take place owing to invasion of cells, derived from mucogingival connective tissue. In such cases protective membranes may be used. Incomplete bony healing results in scar tissue formation (43), which is not considered as a failure (Fig. 20.18).

Prognosis

Information on the outcome of surgical retreatment is abundant. Reported success rates vary between 30% and 90%. Varying inclusion criteria, length of follow-up periods, criteria for evaluation and observer variation render generalized conclusions difficult. However, there seems to be no systematic outcome difference between

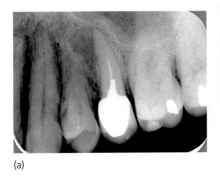

(a)

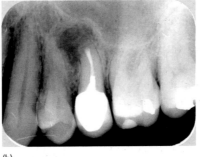

(b)

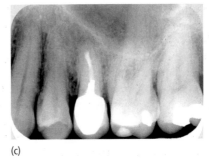

(c)

Fig. 20.17   Successful outcome of an endodontic surgery procedure of an upper second premolar: (a) preoperative radiograph; (b) radiograph immediately postoperatively; (c) 1-year follow-up radiograph with complete bone fill in the previous surgery defect. (Courtesy of Dr Tomas Kvist.)

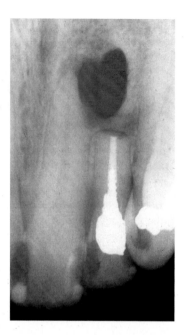

Fig 20.18 Demonstration of a typical image suggesting scar tissue repair after endodontic surgery. Note the bone fill and periodontal ligament space at the tip of the resected lateral incisor. (Courtesy of Dr Johan Warfvinge.)

a surgical and a non-surgical approach to retreatment (2, 19, 32), and as a rough guide three cases out of four might be expected to heal.

> **Core concept 20.4   Scheduling of postsurgical follow-ups**
>
> - *3–5 days:* to check soft-tissue healing and remove sutures.
> - *6 months–1 year:* to check extent of bone fill or clinical signs of persisting infection.

Core concept 20.4 summarizes the scheduling of post-surgical follow-ups.

Among factors that might influence the healing results, the quality of the root filling seal seems to be the most important. Several authors have emphasized that the presence of an initial good quality root filling is essential (22, 40, 44). The choice of root-end-filling material is subjected to controversy and scientific investigations have not singled out one specific material as being superior.

Attention has been called to 'late failures' after apical surgery. Frank *et al.* (11) found that among 104 investigated healed cases 44 were classified 10 years later as failures. Similar relapses of periapical lesions have been reported by Kvist and Reit (32). These findings indicate that healed cases should be included in a recall program.

Case study

Surgery as a primary choice of endodontic treatment

Often endodontic treatment has to be conducted through crowns. When canals are hard to find, substan-

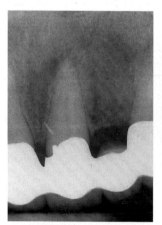
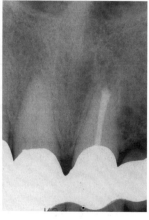

tial amounts of gold and dentine will have to be removed, jeopardizing the retention of the prosthodontic construction. In some situations the risks for such complications may be judged to be too high and a primary surgical approach to endodontic treatment may therefore be carried out.

In this case an acute apical periodontitis was diagnosed in the left central upper incisor. The patient received a full bridge in the upper jaw about 2 years previously. Before the bridge was placed, the incisor was fractured close to the gingival margin but the pulp was found to be vital and had kept its integrity. A cast post was fabricated and retained with parapulpal pins. In the new situation the risk for the post to loosen was judged to be high if the gold mass was penetrated in order to reach the pulp space. Instead, a flap was raised and the root canal cleaned with handfiles in a hemostat in a retrograde direction. The canal was sealed with injectable gutta-percha.

(Images courtesy of Dr C. Reit.)

References

1. Abedi HR, Van Mierlo BL, Wilder-Smith P, Torabinejad M. Effects of ultrasonic root end cavity preparation on the root apex. *J. Endodont.* 1995; 21(Abstr. 41): 225.

2. Allen RK, Newton CW, Brown CE. A statistical analysis of surgical and nonsurgical retreatment cases. *J. Endodont.* 1989; 15: 261–6.

3. Beltes P, Zarvas P, Lambrianidis T, Molyvdas I. In vitro study of the sealing ability of four retrograde filling materials. *Endodont. Dent. Traumatol.* 1988; 4: 82–4.

4. Boyes-Varley JG, Cleaton-Jones PE, Lownie JF. Effect of a topical drug combination on the early healing of extraction sockets in the vervet monkey. *Int. J. Oral Maxillofac. Surg.* 1988; 17: 138–41.

5. Buckley JA, Ciancio SG, McMullen JA. Efficacy of epinephrine concentration in local anesthesia during periodontal surgery. *J. Periodontol.* 1984; 55: 653–7.

6. Calderwood RG, Hera SS, Davis JR, Waite DE. A comparison of the healing rate of bone after the production of defects by various rotary instruments. *J. Dent. Res.* 1964; 43: 207–16.

7. Cambruzzi JV, Marshall FJ. Molar endodontic surgery. *J. Can. Dent. Assoc.* 1983; 49: 61–5.

8. Dorn SO, Gardner AH. Retrograde filling materials: a retrospective success/failure study of amalgam, EBA and IRM. *J. Endodont.* 1990; 16: 391–3.

9. Elkins AD, Jones LP. The effects of plaster of Paris and autogenous cancellous bone on the healing of cortical defects in femurs of dogs. *Vet. Surg.* 1988; 17: 71–6.
Experimental study in dogs showing no difference in the degree of bone healing between autogenous cancellous bone, plaster of Paris and a mixture of plaster of Paris and autogenous cancellous bone. Bone healing was superior to the control with all implants.

10. Finn MD, Schow SR, Schneiderman ED. Osseous regeneration in the presence of four common hemostatic agents. *J. Oral Maxillofac. Surg.* 1992; 50: 608–12.

11. Frank AL, Glick DH, Patterson SS, Weine FS. Long term evaluation of surgically placed amalgam fillings. *J. Endodont.* 1992; 18: 391–8.

12. Friedman S. Retrograde approaches in endodontic therapy. *Endodont. Dent. Traumatol.* 1991; 7: 97–107.

13. Gilheany PA, Figdor D, Tyas M. Apical dentin permeability and microleakage associated with root end resection and retrograde filling. *J. Endodont.* 1994; 20: 22–6.

14. Grunder U, Strub JR. Die Problematik der Temperaturerhöhung beim Bearbeiten des Knochens mit rotierenden Instrumenten – eine Literaturübersicht. *Schweiz. Monatsschr. Zahnmed.* 1986; 96: 965–9.

15. Gutmann JL, Harrison JW. *Surgical Endodontics.* Boston: Blackwell Scientific Publications, 1991; 213–14.

16. Haasch GC, Gerstein H, Austin BP. Effect of two hemostatic agents on osseous healing. *J. Endodont.* 1989; 15: 310–14.

17. Harrison JW, Juroski KA. Wound healing in the tissues of the periodontium following periradicular surgery. I. The incisional wound. *J. Endodont.* 1991; 17: 425–35.
Little difference was found in the temporal and qualitative healing responses to incisional wounds of two flap designs. The submarginal rectangular design showed less predictable results, with a greater intersample variation of wound healing responses in the earlier postsurgical evaluation periods. Vital connective tissue and epithelium, although not visible clinically, remained attached to the root surfaces following reflection of flaps, which included an intrasulcular incision. Preservation of these root-attached tissues seemed to prevent apical epithelial downgrowth along the root surfaces and loss of soft-tissue attachment levels. Preventing dehydration preserved the vitality of root-attached tissues.

18. Hashimoto S, Uchiama K, Maeda M, Ishitsuka K, Furumoto K, Nakamura Y. In vivo and in vitro effects of zinc oxide-eugenol (ZOE) on biosynthesis of cyclo-oxygenase production in rat dental pulp. *J. Dent. Res.* 1988; 67: 1092–6.

19. Hepworth MJ, Friedman S. Treatment outcome of surgical and non-surgical management of endodontic failures. *J. Can. Dent. Assoc.* 1997; 63: 364–71.

20. Hess W. Zur Wurzelkanalanatomie der Wurzelkanäle des menschlichen Gebisses. Zürich: Berichthaus Zürich, 1917; 38–42.

21. Hiat WH, Stallard RE, Butler ED, Badget B. Repair following mucoperiosteal flap surgery with full gingival retention. *J. Periodontol.* 1968; 39: 11–16.

22. Hirsch J, Ahlström U, Henriksson P-Å, Heyden G, Peterson L-E. Periapical surgery. *Int. J. Oral. Surg.* 1979; 8: 173–85.

23. Hogset O, Bredberg G. Plaster of Paris: thermal properties and biocompatibility. A study on an alternative implant material for ear surgery. *Acta Otolaryngol.* 1986; 101: 445–52.

24. Holroyd SV, Requa-Clark B. Local anesthetics. In *Clinical Pharmacology in Dental Practice* (4th edn) (Holroyd SV, Wynn RL, Requa-Clark B, eds). St. Louis: Mosby, 1988; 196–215.

25. Hsu YY, Kim S. The resected root surface. The issue of canal isthmuses. *Dent. Clin. North. Am.* 1997; 41: 529–40.

26. Chong BS, Pitt Ford TR, Watson TF, Wilson RF. Sealing ability of potential retrograde root filling materials. *Endodont. Dent. Traumatol.* 1995; 11: 264–9.
The sealing ability of two potential retrograde root filling materials in extracted teeth – a light-cured glass ionomer cement (Vitrebond) and a reinforced zinc oxide–eugenol cement (Kalzinol) – was compared with that of amalgam. Bacterial leakage occurred in more teeth filled with amalgam compared with both Vitrebond and Kalzinol. Confocal microscopy showed that the size of the marginal gap was the largest with amalgam and smallest with Vitrebond.

27. Ibarrola JL, Bjorgenson JE, Austin BP, Gerstin H. Osseous reaction to three hemostatic agents. *J. Endodont.* 1985; 11: 75–83.

28. Jeansonne BG, Steele PJ, Lemon RR. Ferric sulfate hemostasis. Effect on osseous wound healing: II. With curettage and irrigation. *J. Endodont.* 1993; 19: 174–6.

29. Kim S, Edwall L, Trowbridge H, Chien S. Effects of local anesthetics on pulpal blood flow in dogs. *J. Dent. Res.* 1984; 63: 650–52.

30. Kim S, Rethnam S. Hemostasis in endodontic microsurgery. *Dent. Clin. North Am.* 1997; 41: 499–511.

31. Knöll-Köhler E, Förtsch G. Pulpal anesthesia dependent on epinephrine dose in 2% lidocaine. *Oral Surg.* 1992; 73: 537–40.

32. Kvist T, Reit C. Results of endodontic retreatment: a randomized clinical study comparing surgical and nonsurgical procedures. *J. Endodont.* 1999; 25: 814–17.

33. Lang NP, Löe H. The relationship between the width of keratinized gingiva and gingival health. *J. Periodontol.* 1972; 43: 623–7.

34. Lantis JC II, Durville FM, Connolly R, Schwaitzberg SD. Comparison of coagulation modalities in surgery. *Laparoendosc. Surg. Tech. A* 1998; 8: 381–94.

35. Layton CA, Marshall JG, Morgan LA, Baumgartner JC. Evaluation of cracks associated with ultrasonic root-end preparation. *J. Endodont.* 1996; 22: 157–60.

36. Lemon RR, Steele PJ, Jeansonne BG. Ferric sulfate hemostasis. Effect on osseous wound healing: I. Left in situ for maximum exposure. *J. Endodont.* 1993; 19: 170–73.

37. Lin LM, Gägler P, Langeland K. Periradicular curettage. *Int. Endodont. J.* 1996; 29: 220–27.

38. Lobene RR, Glickman I. The response of alveolar bone to grinding with rotary diamond stones. *J. Periodontol.* 1963; 34: 105–19.

39. Luebke RG. Surgical endodontics. *Dent. Clin. North Am.* 1974; 18, 379–91.

40. Lustmann J, Friedman S, Sharabany V. Relation of pre- and postoperative factors to prognosis of posterior apical surgery. *J. Endodont.* 1991; 17: 239–41.

41. Milam SB, Giovannitti JA. Local anesthetics in dental practice. *Dent. Clin. North Am.* 1984; 28: 493–508.

42. Moberg LE. Electrochemical properties of corroded amalgams. *Scand. J. Dent. Res.* 1987; 95: 441–8.

43. Molven O, Halse A, Grung B. Incomplete healing (scar tissue) after periapical surgery – radiographic findings 8 to 12 years after treatment. *J. Endodont.* 1996; 22: 264–8.

44. Molven O, Halse A, Grung B. Surgical management of endodontic failures: indications and treatment results. *Int. Dent. J.* 1991; 41: 33–42.

45. Nair PNR. New perspectives on radicular cysts: do they heal? *Int. Endodont. J.* 1998; 31: 155–60.

46. Nygaard-Östby B. *Introduction to Endodontics.* Oslo: Universitetsforlaget, 1971; 74.

47. Olson RAJ, Roberts DL, Osbon DB. A comparative study of polylactic acid, Gelfoam and Surgicel in healing extraction sites. *Oral Surg. Oral Med. Oral Pathol.* 1982; 53: 441–9.

48. Pecora G, Baek SH, Rethnam S, Kim S. Barrier membrane techniques in endodontic microsurgery. *Dent. Clin. North Am.* 1997; 41: 585–602.

49. Powers JM, Finger WJ, Xie J. Bonding of composite resin to contaminated human enamel and dentin. *J. Prosthodont.* 1995; 4: 28–32.

50. Reit C, Hirsch J. Surgical endodontic retreatment. *Int. Endodont. J.* 1986; 19: 107–12.

51. Richman MJ. The use of ultrasonics in root canal therapy and root resection. *J. Dent. Med.* 1957; 12: 12–18.

52. Rud J, Munksgaard EC, Andreasen JO, Rud V, Asmussen E. Retrograde root filling with composite and a dentin-bonding agent. *Endodont. Dent. Traumatol.* 1991; 7: 118–25.

53. Rud J, Rud V, Munksgaard EC. Effect of root canal contents on healing of teeth with dentine-bonded resin composite retrograde seal. *J. Endodont.* 1997; 23: 535–41.
Presentation of healing results of 551 periapical surgery cases apically sealed with a dentine-bonded resin composite (Gluma-Retroplast). Success rates varied from 81% to 92%, depending on the root filling quality. Cases with no root filling were the least successful.

54. Selden HS. Bone wax as an effective hemostat in periapical surgery. *Oral Surg.* 1970; 29: 262–4.

55. Tidmarsh BG, Arrowsmith MG. Dentinal tubules at the root ends of apicected teeth: a scanning electron microscopic study. *Int. Endodont. J.* 1989; 22: 184–9.

56. Torabinejad M. The role of immunological reactions in apical cyst formation and the fat of epithelial cells after root canal therapy: a theory. *Int. J. Oral Surg.* 1983; 12: 14–22.

57. Torabinejad M, Watson TF, Pitt Ford TR. The sealing ability of a mineral trioxide aggregate as a retrograde root filling material. *J. Endodont.* 1993; 19: 591–5.

58. Torabinejad M, Higa RK, McKendry DJ, Pitt Ford TR. Effect of blood contamination of dry leakage of root-end filling materials. *J. Endodont.* 1994; 20: 159–63.

59. Torabinejad M, Falah Rastegar A, Kettering JD, Pitt Ford TR. Bacterial leakage of mineral trioxide aggregate as a root end filling material. *J. Endodont.* 1995; 21: 109–12.

60. Torabinejad M, Hong CU, Pitt Ford TR, Kettering JD. Cytotoxicity of four root end filling materials. *J. Endodont.* 1995; 21: 483–92.

61. Velvart P. Das Operationsmikroskop in der Wurzelspitzenresektion. Teil II: Die retrograde Versorgung. *Schweiz. Monatschr. Zahnmed.* 1997; 107: 969–78.

62. Wuchenich G, Meadows D, Torabinejad M. A comparison between two root end preparation techniques in human cadavers. *J. Endodont.* 1994; 20: 279–82.
Twenty anterior teeth in human cadavers were instrumented and obturated with gutta-percha and sealer. After raising a full-thickness flap, the apices of the roots were exposed and beveled at a 45° angle. Half of the apical cavities were prepared with an appropriate-sized Carr alloy tip. The other half were prepared with an inverted cone bur in a slow-speed handpiece. The teeth were extracted, sectioned longitudinally and observed in a scanning electron microscope. The ultrasonic cavities produced more parallel walls and deeper depths for retention. In addition, the ultrasonic tips followed the direction of the canals more closely than those prepared by burs.

Index

Abbreviations: RCT = root canal treatment; ROC = receiver operating characteristic.
Page numbers in **bold** refer to information boxes; page numbers in *italics* refer to figures and tables.

327